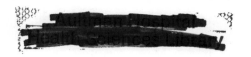

THE CIBA COLLECTION OF MEDICAL ILLUSTRATIONS

VOLUME 5

A Compilation of Paintings on the
Normal and Pathologic Anatomy and Physiology,
Embryology, and Diseases of the

HEART

Prepared by

FRANK H. NETTER, M.D.

Edited by

FREDRICK F. YONKMAN, M.D., Ph.D.

Commissioned and published by

C I B A

OTHER PUBLISHED VOLUMES OF
THE CIBA COLLECTION OF MEDICAL ILLUSTRATIONS
By
FRANK H. NETTER, M.D.

NERVOUS SYSTEM

REPRODUCTIVE SYSTEM

UPPER DIGESTIVE TRACT

LOWER DIGESTIVE TRACT

LIVER, BILIARY TRACT, AND PANCREAS

ENDOCRINE SYSTEM AND
SELECTED METABOLIC DISEASES

KIDNEYS, URETERS, AND URINARY BLADDER

(See page 295 for additional information)

FIRST PRINTING, 1969
SECOND PRINTING, 1971
THIRD PRINTING, 1974
FOURTH PRINTING, 1978

ISBN 0-914168-07-X
LIBRARY OF CONGRESS CATALOG NO.: 53-2151

PRINTED IN U.S.A.

ORIGINAL PRINTING BY COLORPRESS, NEW YORK, N.Y.
COLOR ENGRAVINGS BY EMBASSY PHOTO ENGRAVING CO., INC., NEW YORK, N.Y.
OFFSET CONVERSION BY THE CASE-HOYT CORP., ROCHESTER, N.Y.
FOURTH PRINTING BY THE CASE-HOYT CORP., ROCHESTER, N.Y.

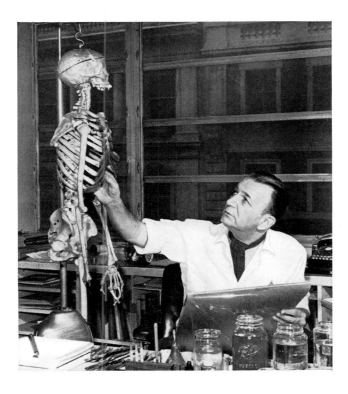

THE ARTIST

Previous books of this COLLECTION *have presented, in various forms, interesting information about Dr. Frank H. Netter. The most recent excellent account, by Mr. Alfred W. Custer, appeared in Volume 4. At this time it seems appropriate to have a unique presentation by one who knows the artist best, his charming wife, Vera. Her original, and quite unaltered, personal comments follow.*

THE EDITOR

What's it like to be married to a genius? I can tell you — it's wonderful! *My* genius doesn't act the way people think a genius is supposed to act. He is a very simple, warm personality who enjoys the ordinary everyday things of life. Indeed, he is so taken up with these matters — with me, with the children, his friends, the stock market, his golf — that I often wonder how he manages to create all the pictures he does. On occasion, when he has completed a large series of pictures, I have asked him, "Frank, how did you manage to do all these?" He has answered me, "You know, darling, the difficult thing about making medical pictures is not the painting at all but rather the study, the thinking, the planning, the creation of a picture so that it says something. Once I have the picture in my mind it is easy to put it on paper." I know that he is thinking about his pictures in the middle of the night when he tosses about restlessly in bed, in the midst of a conversation when he becomes a little detached, or on the golf course when occasionally he makes a poor shot. I know also when he is troubled by a particularly difficult problem; then he sits very quietly and withdrawn, curling a forelock of his hair. But, once the problem is solved he becomes his usual outgoing, friendly self again.

We travel considerably in quest of the knowledge that my husband pictorializes and it is always amazing to me, after having been told of the very great scientist we are to meet, to find the scientist is more impressed in having the opportunity of meeting him. It is this humility and unconsciousness of his own great gift that endears him to so many. At these meetings it is also very interesting to note the great scientist's surprise to find that this artist can converse with him on his own plane regardless of whether the subject be neurophysiology, thoracic surgery, anatomy, biochemistry, orthopedics, or any other phase of medical science. They are always amazed to see how quickly he grasps the essence of the subject and organizes its presentation. The immediate relaxation and response is electric. Most fascinating to me, however, is to see the glow of satisfaction which invariably suffuses the face of the consultant when he sees his lifework graphically depicted and clarified by the pencil and brush of my husband. In most instances these associations have led to long, sincere friendships.

Frank also loves languages and they come to him very naturally but time will never permit him to really study seriously. Once when we were in Switzerland he was somewhat troubled because he learned that the two doctors he had wished to consult that morning at the University spoke no English. That evening I went a little early to meet him at the hospital, expecting to have my ear filled with his frustration at communicating, when, through the door, I was dumbfounded to hear a most familiar voice speaking Italian as though he had never been out of Italy. He says that if he drinks chianti he can talk Italian, if he drinks champagne he can talk French, and if he eats knockwurst he can talk German. (They must have served chianti!)

In English, Frank is very articulate. He is often asked to speak at various medical assemblies because people seem to want to know about his unusual career. Unfortunately, he cannot accept most of these invitations because of time limitations. When he does agree to speak, I become nervous as the day of the address approaches and I see him making no preparation. Just before the meeting he will sit down for fifteen minutes and plan what he will say! He believes that too much preparation makes a speech stilted and dull. Then he gets up on the rostrum and delights his audience with philosophy, narrative, and humor as he speaks extemporaneously.

We live in Manhattan in an apartment overlooking the East River. In the spring I decorate the terrace with colorful plants, but the pride of the terrace is the tomatoes that my husband cultivates and nurtures all spring and summer and then serves with his barbecued steaks. Frank is an early riser but cannot begin the day before the newspaper is delivered so he can see how "Dick Tracy" and his other cartoon friends have fared. His studio is on the lower floor of our duplex and his usual day there begins at eight in the morning and lasts to four in the afternoon, but when he is under pressure he may keep going till six or later. In his early days he would often work until three or four in the morning and sometimes right through the night, but now he abhors such hours and refuses to work at night regardless of the pressure. His work attire surprises even me sometimes. It could consist of a pair of paint-stained slacks and bright plaid shirt and, to my horror, he often neglects to change when he has an outside appointment and ventures forth in this attire with simply the addition of a jacket, even though his closets are full of clothes. On one occasion, when one of the many aspiring students who come to ask his counsel appeared at the house, Frank opened the door in his customary work attire and the young man looked at him and said, "I have an appointment with your father, Dr. Netter." When Frank told him that he was Dr. Netter, his mouth fell open and he said, "But with all those drawings and books I thought you would be an old man." Frank got a real chuckle out of that.

The letters received from all parts of the world in all languages, even from behind the "iron curtain," attest to the great utility of these books and give Frank the strength and desire to go on to the next one, vowing to make each better than the last to the end that those who use them may have the final word in pictorial medicine as it has been given to him.

VERA NETTER

FOREWORD

Heart disease respects no boundaries, no geographic limitations. It occurs in every nation of the world, in both sexes, in all races, and in every stratum of society. Certainly it is the most formidable and challenging of all health problems.

Nonetheless, the past two decades have seen spectacular gains in our knowledge and treatment of most diseases affecting the heart and circulatory system. In some areas, progress has been "literally beyond prophecy." In fact, it is a matter of record that greater overall advances have been made during this short period alone than in all the previous years of recorded human history.

Less than twenty years ago the interior of the heart was an impenetrable anatomic barrier to the surgeon — the last anatomic frontier of the many that surgeons have faced through the ages. Only a few years ago, many physicians and surgeons were pessimistic about any future for open cardiac surgery, predicting that the sick human heart could not tolerate incisions into its walls or intracardiac manipulations of any sort. Therefore, in their estimation, the future of open cardiac surgery was doomed unequivocally to failure.

It is true that before 1952, and total body hypothermia, there had been no successful open-heart surgery; and before 1954, and cross circulation, there had been no regularly successful open-heart surgery by perfusion methods. The key to many of the recent astonishing developments in cardiac therapy has been the development of the technics for extracorporeal circulation and the heart-lung machine.

Today, scores of conditions, hopeless only ten years ago, are being managed successfully in a routine manner by surgery or medical technics developed within this brief span of time.

Another dividend of particular importance has been the creation of a new alliance between the internist and the surgeon, with a resultant significant advance in the mutual knowledge in both fields. The consequence has been the merging of medical cardiology and surgical cardiology into a single vigorous entity.

A startling example of how quickly tomorrow may become yesterday in this field was the dramatic report that the human heart had been successfully transplanted. Because man has long regarded his heart as the primary symbol of life and vitality, the transplantation of this organ has captured the public imagination as has no other therapeutic procedure in this century. However, even this achievement did not come as a complete surprise to certain medical investigators who had clearly foreseen this development as one more step in man's quest to conquer heart disease, and who had worked out in the experimental laboratory the basic technics utilized in this pioneering effort, as illustrated by Dr. Frank H. Netter in the final chapter of this magnificent volume. In fact, it can be said that preparation for the first human-heart transplant really began some fifteen years ago when the technics for successful open-heart surgery were first developed.

Certainly, further knowledge of the involved and challenging immunochemistry of tissue tolerance is the "Gordian knot" of the immediate present which must be "untied" before heart and other organ replacements can become almost routine clinical treatment. But there should not be the slightest doubt that a new "Alexander the Great" will appear to sever this knot and allow the successful homotransplantation

New York City, 1969

and, probably, even heterotransplantation of vital organs.

This entire epic of recent achievements in medical and surgical cardiology has been a brilliant example of the application of fundamental researches in physiology, anatomy, pathology, and biochemistry, leavened with surgeons' skills and the devoted determination of an international consortium of men who maintained and practiced the firm beliefs of John Hunter, the father of scientific medicine and surgery, who stated, "I *think* your solution is just; but why *think?* Why not *try* the experiment?"

Even this brief recounting of some of the milestones of the last two decades serves to emphasize the awe-inspiring magnitude of the task which Dr. Frank Netter assumed when he undertook the creation of this volume. He has illustrated, in a comprehensive manner, much of what is known about the heart — its anatomy and pathology, its embryology, its histology, its physiology, newer aspects of its structure and metabolism, diagnostic aspects of its normal and abnormal functions, and, finally, surgical procedures for all applicable conditions, including cardiac transplantation.

As the artist himself has so aptly stated, "The making of pictures is a stern discipline; one may 'write around' a subject where one is not quite sure of the details, but, with brush in hand before the drawing board, one must be precise and realistic." In regard to the heart, this is a task of such vastness that it heretofore has not been undertaken, and some might well have said that this was indeed an "impossible dream" to achieve. These problems notwithstanding, this volume, larger and more detailed than any in the series to date, has achieved these formidable and all-inclusive objectives in a production of such excellence that it has unprecedented clinical and scientific value. Dr. Netter, to do this, has combined his genius as a great artist with the knowledge, curiosity, and infinite attention to detail typical of an equally great investigator. Moreover, he and his associates of the CIBA Pharmaceutical Company have had the extraordinary perception to select specialists of outstanding knowledge and international recognition to advise in the preparation of both the illustrations and the text discussions that accompany these vivid and dramatic pictorial presentations. The result is a classic volume, with a vast body of up-to-date knowledge, from which even the most experienced investigators, cardiologists, and surgeons will find much that is new and unfamiliar to them. This interchange of the latest knowledge, made so readily assimilable by the unique skill of the artist, cannot help but facilitate the continued astonishing progress that has characterized this dynamic field in the recent past.

And what of the future? Science is an endless frontier. The horizons for future achievements are limited only by the limitations upon one's imagination. No thoughtful seer in this decade is likely to predict that anything is impossible, since his pronouncement may be interrupted by someone else "doing it." In this time of great advances, a continuous and exciting adventure still lies ahead of us. When science fiction is scarcely ahead of scientific achievement, who can see the future? Who can even begin to predict the achievements that will be recounted in a foreword similar to this, written ten years from now? There will, without doubt, be many; let us hope, therefore, that we will continue to have a Dr. Frank Netter to chronicle these events!

C. WALTON LILLEHEI, PH.D., M.D.

CONTRIBUTORS AND CONSULTANTS

The artist, editor, and publishers express their appreciation
to the following authorities for their generous collaboration:

JOHN H. ABEL, JR., Ph.D.

Assistant Professor of Physiology and Anatomy, Colorado State University, Ft. Collins,
Colo.

RALPH D. ALLEY, M.D.

Clinical Associate Professor of Thoracic Surgery, Albany Medical College; Attending
Thoracic Surgeon, Albany Medical Center Hospital, Albany, N.Y.

MARVIN B. BACANER, M.D.

Associate Professor of Physiology, University of Minnesota, Minneapolis, Minn.

MURRAY G. BARON, M.D.

Associate Professor of Radiology, Mount Sinai School of Medicine; Associate Attending
Radiologist, The Mount Sinai Hospital, New York, N.Y.

RUDOLPH C. CAMISHION, M.D.

Professor of Surgery, Jefferson Medical College; Attending Surgeon, Jefferson Medical
College Hospital, Philadelphia, Pa.; Chief, Thoracic and Cardiovascular Surgery and
Attending Surgeon, Cooper Hospital, Camden, N.J.

ALDO R. CASTANEDA, M.D., Ph.D.

Associate Professor of Surgery, University of Minnesota Medical Center, Minneapolis,
Minn.

IGNACIO CHAVEZ RIVERA, M.D.

Head of Teaching, Instituto Nacional de Cardiología de México; Assistant Professor,
School of Medicine, Universidad Nacional Autónoma de México; former Secretary of the
Mexican Society of Cardiology.

ANDRE F. COURNAND, M.D.

Professor Emeritus of Medicine, College of Physicians and Surgeons of Columbia University, New York, N.Y.

J. N. P. DAVIES, M.D., Sc.D., F.C.Path.

Professor of Pathology, Albany Medical College, Albany, N.Y.; formerly Professor of
Pathology, Makerere College Medical School, Kampala, Uganda.

ARTHUR C. DeGRAFF, M.D.

Samuel A. Brown Professor of Therapeutics, New York University School of Medicine;
Visiting Physician, Bellevue Hospital; Attending Physician, University Hospital, New
York University Medical Center, New York, N.Y.; Consultant in Cardiology, Bronx
Veterans Administration Hospital, Bronx, N.Y.

THOMAS A. DOXIADIS, M.D.

Professor of Medicine, Evangelismos Medical Center, Athens, Greece.

JESSE E. EDWARDS, M.D.

Director of Laboratories, Charles T. Miller Hospital, St. Paul, Minn.; Clinical Professor
of Pathology, University of Minnesota, Minneapolis, Minn.

DONALD B. EFFLER, M.D.

Head, Department of Thoracic and Cardiovascular Surgery, Cleveland Clinic Foundation, Cleveland, Ohio.

A. STONE FREEDBERG, M.D.

Associate Professor of Medicine, Harvard Medical School; Director, Cardiology Unit, Beth Israel Hospital, Boston, Mass.

HARRY W. FRITTS, JR., M.D.

Professor of Medicine, College of Physicians and Surgeons of Columbia University, New York, N.Y.

JOHN H. GIBBON, JR., M.D.

Emeritus Professor of Surgery, Jefferson Medical College; Consulting Surgeon, Pennsylvania and Chestnut Hill Hospitals, Philadelphia, Pa.

ALFRED GILMAN, PH.D.

William S. Lasdon Professor of Pharmacology and Chairman of the Department, Albert Einstein College of Medicine, Bronx, N.Y.

LEONARD E. GLYNN, M.D., F.R.C.P., F.C.PATH.

Member of Scientific Staff, Medical Research Council's Rheumatism Research Unit, Taplow, England; Hon. Consultant Pathologist, N.W. Metropolitan Regional Hospital Board.

S. E. GOULD, M.D.

Adjunct Professor of Pathology, University of Miami, Jackson Memorial Hospital, Miami, Flá.; Emeritus Professor of Pathology, Wayne State University School of Medicine, Detroit, Mich.

BRIAN F. HOFFMAN, M.D.

David Hosack Professor of Pharmacology and Chairman, Department of Pharmacology, College of Physicians and Surgeons of Columbia University, New York, N.Y.

CHARLES A. HUFNAGEL, M.D.

Professor of Surgery and Director of Surgical Research Laboratory, Georgetown University Hospital, Washington, D.C.

A. GREGORY JAMESON, M.D.

Director of Cardiology, Department of Medicine, Roosevelt Hospital, New York; Associate Clinical Professor of Medicine, College of Physicians and Surgeons of Columbia University, New York, N.Y.

JAMES R. JUDE, M.D.

Professor of Surgery, University of Miami School of Medicine; Chief of Thoracic and Cardiovascular Surgery, Jackson Memorial Hospital, Miami, Fla.

DAVID KOFFLER, M.D.

Associate Professor, Department of Pathology, Mount Sinai School of Medicine, New York, N.Y.

GEORGE KURLAND, M.D.

Associate Clinical Professor of Medicine, Harvard Medical School; Physician, Chief of Cardiac Clinic and Electrocardiographic Laboratory, Beth Israel Hospital, Boston, Mass.

JOHN S. LaDUE, M.D., Ph.D.

Associate Attending Physician, Memorial Hospital; Assistant Attending Physician, New York Hospital; Associate Professor of Clinical Medicine, Cornell University Medical College, New York, N.Y.

ROBERT S. LITWAK, M.D.

Chief, Division of Cardiothoracic Surgery and Professor of Surgery, Mount Sinai School of Medicine, New York, N.Y.

ALDO A. LUISADA, M.D.

Professor of Medicine and Director of Cardiovascular Research, The Chicago Medical School, University of Health Sciences; Attending Cardiologist, Mount Sinai Hospital, Chicago, Ill.

JAMES R. MALM, M.D.

Professor of Clinical Surgery, College of Physicians and Surgeons of Columbia University, New York, N.Y.

HENRY J. L. MARRIOTT, M.D.

Director of Clinical Research, Rogers Heart Foundation, St. Petersburg, Fla.; Clinical Professor of Medicine (Cardiology), Emory University School of Medicine, Atlanta, Ga.

AUBRE de L. MAYNARD, M.D., F.A.C.S.

Past Director of Surgery (Retired), Harlem Hospital Center; formerly Clinical Professor of Surgery (Retired), College of Physicians and Surgeons of Columbia University; Consulting Surgeon to: Harlem Hospital Center, St. Clare's Hospital, Columbus Hospital, Misericordia Hospital, New York, N.Y., and St. Joseph's Hospital, Barbados, W.I.

LAWRENCE J. McCORMACK, M.D., M.S. (Path.)

Consultant in Pathology, Cleveland Clinic Foundation, Cleveland, Ohio.

HUBERT MEESSEN, Prof. Dr. Dr. h.c.

Director of the Pathologic Institute, University of Düsseldorf, Germany.

G. A. G. MITCHELL, O.B.E., T.D., M.B., Ch.B., M.Sc., D.Sc., Ch.M., F.R.C.S.

Hon. Alumnus, The University, Louvain, Belgium; Chevalier (1st Cl.) Order of the Dannebrog; Professor of Anatomy and Director of the Anatomical Laboratories, The University, Manchester, England.

EMIL A. NACLERIO, M.D., F.A.C.S., F.C.C.P., F.A.C.C.

Chief of the Thoracic Surgical Services, Columbus Hospital, and Attending Thoracic Surgeon, Harlem Hospital Center, Columbia University, New York, N.Y.

IRVINE H. PAGE, M.D.

Director Emeritus, Research Division, Cleveland Clinic Foundation, Cleveland, Ohio.

HANS POPPER, M.D.

Given Professor and Chairman, Department of Pathology, Mount Sinai School of Medicine, New York, N.Y.

JOHANNES A. G. RHODIN, M.D., Ph.D.

Professor and Chairman, Department of Anatomy, New York Medical College, New York, N.Y.

ABEL LAZZARINI ROBERTSON, JR., M.D., Ph.D.

Staff Member, Cleveland Clinic Foundation, Cleveland, Ohio.

NORMAN E. SHUMWAY, M.D., Ph.D.

Professor of Surgery and Head, Division of Cardiovascular Surgery, Stanford University School of Medicine, Palo Alto, Calif.

F. MASON SONES, JR., M.D.

Head, Department of Cardiovascular Disease and Cardiac Laboratory, Cleveland Clinic Foundation, Cleveland, Ohio.

CH. STATHATOS, M.D.

Director, Department of Thoracic Surgery, Evangelismos Medical Center, Athens, Greece.

LODEWYK H. S. VAN MIEROP, M.D.

Professor, Departments of Pediatrics (Cardiology) and Pathology, University of Florida College of Medicine, Gainesville, Fla.; formerly Associate Professor, Departments of Pediatrics (Cardiology) and Anatomy, Albany Medical College, Albany, N.Y.

RICHARD L. VARCO, M.D.

Professor of Surgery, College of Medical Sciences, University of Minnesota, Minneapolis, Minn.

MAURICE B. VISSCHER, M.D., Ph.D.

Regents' Professor and Head of Department of Physiology, University of Minnesota, Minneapolis, Minn.

RICHARD N. WESTCOTT, M.D., F.A.C.C.

Department of Clinical Cardiology and Director, ECG Laboratory, Cleveland Clinic Foundation, Cleveland, Ohio.

PAUL DUDLEY WHITE, M.D.

Clinical Professor of Medicine, Emeritus, Harvard University; Consultant, Massachusetts General Hospital, Boston, Mass.; President, International Cardiology Foundation; Founder, American Heart Association.

TRAVIS WINSOR, M.D., F.A.C.P.

Associate Clinical Professor of Medicine, University of Southern California School of Medicine; Director, Wiley Memorial Heart Research Foundation, Los Angeles, Calif.

BERNARD S. WOLF, M.D.

Professor and Chairman, Department of Radiology, Mount Sinai School of Medicine; Director, Department of Radiology, The Mount Sinai Hospital, New York, N.Y.

INTRODUCTION

With each volume that I have undertaken in THE CIBA COL-LECTION OF MEDICAL ILLUSTRATIONS, I have vowed at the outset to execute it with great expedition and simplicity. But in every case the task has proved to be much more complex and difficult than I had anticipated. As I became involved and absorbed in the subject matter, many facets of the various topics came to light which demanded pictorialization. Just as, when a skin diver plunges beneath the surface of a calm sea, he does not realize what a myriad of hidden phenomena are to come into his view, so have I repeatedly discovered new and marvelous worlds beneath the superficial concepts. But, in the case of this volume on the heart, these factors have been even more pronounced. They were amplified by the fact that the sea of knowledge in which I was swimming kept continuously rising and expanding. New facts were being discovered, new concepts evolved, new methods and technics developed. I had difficulty in keeping abreast of them with my studies as well as with my pencil and brush. But the exploration was always stimulating and inspiring — so much so that I might have gone on indefinitely expanding, revising, and adding, with the result that the book might never have appeared. I therefore had to call a halt, although I am aware that, even as this book goes to press, the pace of progress is accelerating.

The rate of this acceleration becomes evident in the light of a multitude of accomplishments. Somewhat less than three hundred and fifty years ago, William Harvey established the concept of the circulation of the blood, and, since that epochal event, more has been learned about the circulatory system than in the three hundred and fifty thousand years preceding it. In 1902 William Einthoven devised the string galvanometer, and shortly thereafter it was applied, by Sir James Mackenzie and by Sir Thomas Lewis, to the study of the heartbeat, based on the fundamental studies of the cardiac conduction system of Gaskell. Thus, modern cardiology was born some sixty-five years ago. But it continued to grow and mature, nurtured by many, many men and women who are too numerous to mention here. Finally came the advent of cardiac surgery, given tremendous impetus, within the past two decades, by the practical application of extracorporeal circulation. And, just before this book went to press, the first cardiac transplants were performed and we were able to include some-

thing about them herein. Thus, although our knowledge of heart function and heart disease may seem slow in the perspective of a man's lifetime, it has been extremely rapid and, indeed, geometrically accelerating in the light of human history. It is significant also that as each new step forward was made, it necessitated going back and restudying fundamentals. The advent of cardiac surgery necessitated a restudy of heart anatomy; the correction of cardiac anomalies called for a reappraisal of embryology; the discovery of new drugs impelled a deeper analysis of cardiac physiology.

But progress has not ceased. On the contrary, it moves constantly onward at an ever-increasing pace. In the preparation of this volume it has been a great pleasure as well as a great intellectual stimulation to have collaborated with so many men who are catalyzing this progress. And so I herewith express my appreciation to these, my collaborators. Without them, this book would, of course, have been impossible; with them, it was a joy and a great adventure. To have met them, to have come to know them, to have worked with them was a memorable experience. I thank them all for the time they gave me, for the knowledge they imparted to me, for the material with which they supplied me, and above all, for the friendship which they extended to me.

One collaborator in particular, however, I must single out; namely, Dr. L. H. S. Van Mierop, who has become simply "Bob" to me. Here is a man, warm and friendly by nature, forthright and simple in demeanor, yet imbued with an insatiable quest for truth and the comprehension of fundamentals. And his great talents have enabled him to follow this latter bent, so that he is at once clinician, anatomist, embryologist, investigator, student, and teacher. Because of his contributions, I believe that the sections on embryology and on congenital heart disease are both original and classic.

I wish to thank also, Dr. Fredrick F. Yonkman, the Editor, for the care and devotion which he gave to this work. Dr. Yonkman, Mr. A. W. Custer, and other executives of the CIBA Pharmaceutical Company have encouraged and helped me in every way possible. But the concept, and indeed the origination of this series of volumes, must be credited to the foresight and vision of Mr. Paul W. Roder of the CIBA company.

FRANK H. NETTER, M.D.

Remarks by the editor of any new book obviously will vary according to its nature and scope, but one feature emphasized in all previously published books of THE CIBA COLLECTION OF MEDICAL ILLUSTRATIONS warrants repetition, namely, that none of these represents a complete treatise of respective subjects but, hopefully, serves as a valuable ancillary companion to the excellent textbooks available in related medical fields.

In the preparation of this book, Heart (Volume 5), it has been my privilege and pleasure to have worked closely with Dr. Frank Netter. Although I had enjoyed my earlier associations with him in the preliminary development of his work on the autonomic nervous system of Volume 1, and my closer cooperation in revising Part 3 of Volume III, Liver, Biliary Tract and Pancreas, our sustained collaboration during the past few years on this book has led me to a greater appreciation of and admiration for this world-renowned artist as a thorough student, unusual teacher, versatile gentleman, and friend. For me, this has been a very challenging and gratifying chapter in my life as a former teacher, researcher, and administrator in science and medicine.

The preparation of this book has been rewarding also because it not only afforded me renewed contact in collaborating with friends of long standing, but it also resulted in establishing new and firm bonds with other experts in their capacity as consultants. For their complete cooperation in working so conscientiously with Dr. Netter and me, as well as with one another in several instances, I am genuinely appreciative, and I trust that these

collective efforts may result in a ready acceptance of this book as a worthy companion of those comprising THE CIBA COLLECTION OF MEDICAL ILLUSTRATIONS.

Among several special features of this book is the relationship of Section III, Embryology, to Section IV, Congenital Anomalies; in the former, embryologic tissues are *specifically colored* in order that their respective malformed end products or anomalies may be readily recognized during their development. In a sense, this portion of the publication represents a unique monograph within the book itself.

I wish to acknowledge with my sincere thanks the wise counsel and recommendations, given during the early planning of the scope of this book, by Dr. Hans Popper of New York City, Dr. Irvine Page of Cleveland, and Dr. George Wakerlin of Columbia, Missouri. Several discussions with these authorities resulted in attempts to balance the various subjects and consultants included. If any imbalance appears in the minds of some readers, Dr. Netter and I—not these advisers—assume the responsibility for such a consequence.

Besides our collaborating consultants, I wish to thank Dr. Edward A. Boyden, Emeritus Professor of Anatomy at the University of Minnesota, Minneapolis, and Research Professor at the University of Washington, Seattle, for reviewing certain texts for the correct use of anatomic terminology. As noted in the preceding books of this COLLECTION, the Nomina Anatomica, published by Excerpta Medica Foundation, was used as the standard, but in this book, as in certain others, the *Nomina Anatomica* term has not always been chosen. This is true for various reasons; *e.g.*, the author's preference is often predicated on commonly employed clinical terms (usually anglicized) or spelling of the latter in standard medical textbooks and dictionaries. Specific examples include: (1) sinoatrial instead of sinuatrial (*N.A.*); (2) annulus fibrosus for anulus fibrosus (*N.A.*); (3) foregut for anterior intestinal portal; (4) moderator band instead of septo-marginal trabecula, etc. Then, too, when some of these infrequent differences were detected (*e.g.*, venous valve for sinus valve), the plate was already in its final or engraved color-proof form and could not be altered without entailing great expense which could conceivably result in some price increase for the published book. This was undesirable, so we compromised expediently by usually inserting parenthetically in the text the *N.A.* term after the first appearance of the commonly used term.

As a rule, terms appearing in the legend of a plate are in italics in the related text, but frequently, in the latter, other items are also italicized for the sake of emphasis.

Special assistance for which we are grateful was generously given by those investigators footnoted in the text. We also acknowledge gratefully: the assistance of Dr. Anthony Duggan of The Wellcome Museum of Medical Science in London, and Dr. D. S. Ridley of the Department of Medicine, School of Tropical Medicine in London, for background material supplied in connection with the calcification of the heart in endomyocardial fibrosis (page 207); the guidance and advice of Dr. Lawrence Gould and Dr. Peter Hofstra of the U.S. Veterans Administration Hospital, Bronx, New York, regarding surgical procedures as referred to under diseases of the pericardium, on pages 260, 261, and 262; the pathologic material for this same topic made available to us by Dr. Alfred Schwartz of The Jewish Memorial Hospital, New York City; the assistance of Mr. Robert Reed, Medical Artist at the Cleveland Clinic, for making available for study his sketches of operative procedures employed by Dr. Donald B. Effler and his associates (pages 238 to 244). We are also grateful to the authors and their publishers, see SELECTED REFERENCES, for the privilege of including the following:

Page 112   Center and bottom left: after Hertig and Rock.
Page 114   Modified after Davis.
Page 115   Modified in part after Goss.
Page 116   Bottom: redrawn after Davis and Payne.
Page 117   Top: redrawn after Davis and Corner.
            Bottom: after Davis and Heuser.
Page 118   Redrawn after Davis.
Pages 119   Redrawn after Van Mierop, et al.
through 122
Pages 127   Redrawn after Congdon.
and 128
Pages 129   Modified after Grünwald.
and 130
Page 212   From Bargmann, W.: *Histologie und Mikroskopische Anatomie des Menschen*, Thieme, Stuttgart, 6th ed., 1967.

Beyond the call of duty is the gratefully acknowledged, excellent, and diligently meticulous cooperation of Miss Louise Stemmle, Assistant to the Editor, and of her associate, Mrs. Helen Sward. Our joint efforts, combined with the managerial expertise of Mr. Alfred W. Custer of CIBA, were greatly helped by the staffs of Embassy Photo Engraving Co., Inc., Cesareo Studios, and Colorpress. We are appreciative of their keen interest and collaboration as we also are of the exceptional copy editing and valuable suggestions of our literary consultant, Mrs. Anne H. Clark, Destin, Florida. Without their collective and generous consideration, this task would have been still more arduous and less rewarding.

Of special value in this work was the most-appreciated assistance of my wife, Janet;* despite many trying circumstances, her collaboration, editorially and inspirationally, was of great significance throughout. Her quiet forbearance and gentle yet firm assurance and encouragement contributed markedly to the challenging team effort required for the completion of this book.

FREDRICK F. YONKMAN, M.D., PH.D.

*Deceased, November 30, 1968.

CONTENTS

Section I

ANATOMY

by

FRANK H. NETTER, M.D.

in collaboration with

JOHN H. ABEL, JR., Ph.D. and JOHANNES A. G. RHODIN, M.D., Ph.D.
Plates 19 and 20

MURRAY G. BARON, M.D. and BERNARD S. WOLF, M.D.
Plates 21-28

BRIAN F. HOFFMAN, M.D.
Plates 12-14

G. A. G. MITCHELL, O.B.E., T.D., M.B., Ch.B., M.Sc., D.Sc., Ch.M., F.R.C.S.
Plates 17 and 18

F. MASON SONES, JR., M.D.
Plates 29-31

LODEWYK H. S. VAN MIEROP, M.D.
Plates 1-11, 15 and 16

THORACIC CAGE

Before describing the anatomy of the heart, it is desirable to review briefly some of the anatomical features of the thoracic cavity and the organs, in addition to the heart, which it contains.

The thorax proper constitutes the upper part of the body or trunk, and its shape is intermediate between that of a barrel and a truncated cone. This shape is a very favorable one indeed, considering the fact that although much of the time the intrathoracic pressure is subatmospheric, the chest wall still is able to retain its integrity by means of rather thin, light, skeletal elements.

The thoracic cavity occupies only the upper part of the thoracic cage. The abdominal (peritoneal) cavity reaches upward as high as the lower tip of the *sternum* — a circumstance which affords considerable protection to such large and easily injured abdominal organs as the liver, spleen, stomach, and kidneys.

These two cavities are separated by the dome-shaped *diaphragm,* a sheet of tissue consisting of a peripheral muscular part and a central tendinous portion, which closes the thoracic cavity inferiorly. Superiorly, the narrow, upper thoracic aperture, bounded by the upper part of the sternum, the short, stout, first ribs, and the body of the first thoracic vertebra, gives access to the root of the neck and is not closed by any specific structure.

Posteriorly, the thorax is bounded by the bodies of the twelve thoracic vertebrae and the posterior portions of the ribs; anteriorly, by the sternum, the *costal cartilages,* and the anterior portions of the ribs, and, laterally, by the remaining parts of the ribs. The spaces between successive ribs are bridged by the *intercostal muscles.*

The sternum (breastbone) lies anteriorly in the midline and very superficially. The *clavicles* and the first seven pairs of ribs articulate with it. It consists of three parts — the *manubrium* and the corpus sterni (both bony) and the small, cartilaginous *xiphoid process.* The clavicles articulate with the manubrium on its upper border, and the notch between these joints is called the interclavicular or suprasternal notch. Just below the sternoclavicular joints, the cartilages of the first ribs are attached to the sternum. No joint spaces are present here. The manubrium and the body of the sternum are united by fibrocartilage. The

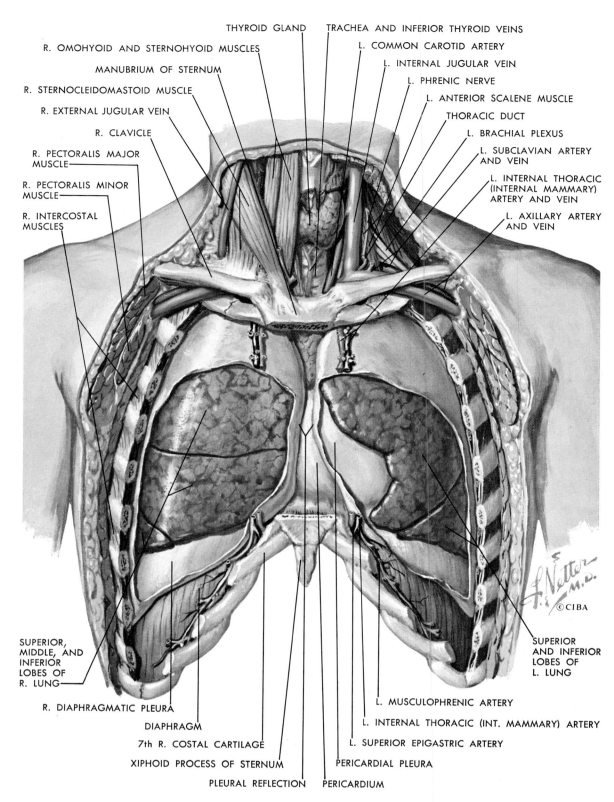

R. OMOHYOID AND STERNOHYOID MUSCLES · THYROID GLAND · TRACHEA AND INFERIOR THYROID VEINS · L. COMMON CAROTID ARTERY · MANUBRIUM OF STERNUM · L. INTERNAL JUGULAR VEIN · R. STERNOCLEIDOMASTOID MUSCLE · L. PHRENIC NERVE · R. EXTERNAL JUGULAR VEIN · L. ANTERIOR SCALENE MUSCLE · THORACIC DUCT · R. CLAVICLE · L. BRACHIAL PLEXUS · R. PECTORALIS MAJOR MUSCLE · L. SUBCLAVIAN ARTERY AND VEIN · R. PECTORALIS MINOR MUSCLE · L. INTERNAL THORACIC (INTERNAL MAMMARY) ARTERY AND VEIN · R. INTERCOSTAL MUSCLES · L. AXILLARY ARTERY AND VEIN · SUPERIOR, MIDDLE, AND INFERIOR LOBES OF R. LUNG · SUPERIOR AND INFERIOR LOBES OF L. LUNG · R. DIAPHRAGMATIC PLEURA · DIAPHRAGM · L. MUSCULOPHRENIC ARTERY · 7th R. COSTAL CARTILAGE · L. INTERNAL THORACIC (INT. MAMMARY) ARTERY · XIPHOID PROCESS OF STERNUM · L. SUPERIOR EPIGASTRIC ARTERY · PLEURAL REFLECTION · PERICARDIAL PLEURA · PERICARDIUM

junction between the manubrium and the body of the sternum usually forms a rather prominent ridge, accentuated by the fact that the two parts of the sternum form a slight angle with each other (sternal angle of Louis). This is a rather important landmark, since the cartilages of the second ribs articulate with the sternum at this point. The third and smallest part of the sternum is the xiphoid cartilage — a thin, spoon-shaped piece attached to the lower end of the sternal body.

Most of the bony thorax is formed by the ribs, of which there are, ordinarily, twelve on each side of the trunk. They consist of a series of thin, curved, rather elastic bones which articulate posteriorly with the thoracic vertebrae and terminate anteriorly in the costal cartilages. The first *seven* pairs attach to the sternum by means of their cartilages, whereas, the eighth, ninth, and tenth pairs articulate with each

other and do not reach the sternum. The eleventh and twelfth pairs are small and poorly developed, ending in free cartilaginous tips. The ribs are thickest posteriorly; they flatten out considerably and become somewhat wider as they curve forward. Along the inferior and inner surface of the posterior part of each rib there is a groove — the sulcus costae — which affords protection to the intercostal vessels and nerve.

The first two and last two ribs differ somewhat from the above description. The *first rib* (see page 3) is very short and relatively heavier. On its superior surface are two grooves, divided by a tubercle — the tuberculum scaleni — which forms the point of insertion of the *anterior scalene muscle.* The groove in front of the muscle is occupied by the *subclavian vein,* whereas the *subclavian artery* follows the groove behind the tubercle. The second rib is longer than the

(*Continued on page 3*)

THORACIC CAGE

(*Continued from page 2*)

first and somewhat resembles the other ribs, except the eleventh and twelfth, which, as stated previously, are small.

The spaces between successive ribs are occupied by intercostal muscles (see page 2). Each external intercostal muscle arises from the lower border of the rib above, runs obliquely downward and medially, and inserts into the upper border of the rib below. Each *internal intercostal muscle* (see page 4) arises from the lower border of the rib above and runs downward and outward to insert on the upper border of the rib below. Between these two muscle layers lie the intercostal vessels, whereas the intercostal nerves lie between the internal and the innermost intercostal muscles.

Many muscles of the upper extremities originate from the chest wall. Among these are the *pectoralis major* and *minor* (see page 2) and the serratus anterior muscles, which originate from the anterior and lateral portions of the chest wall.

From the upper rim of the thoracic cage, several neck muscles originate. The *sternohyoid* (see page 2) and *sternothyroid muscles* are thin, straplike structures which arise from the superior border and posterior surface of the sternum and insert into the hyoid bone and the thyroid cartilage, respectively. The *sternocleidomastoid muscle* (see page 2) arises as a stout sternal head from the upper border of the sternum, adjacent to the sternoclavicular joint, and as a second clavicular head from the medial third of the clavicle. The interval between the two heads is usually visible as a slight depression, behind which the apex of the *lung* rises from the thorax into the root of the neck. Above this interval, the two heads of the sternocleidomastoid muscle unite to form a single muscular belly which passes obliquely upward, backward, and laterally, to insert into the lateral surface of the mastoid process and occipital bone.

Superficial to the sternocleidomastoid muscle, the *external jugular vein* passes perpendicularly downward from its origin at the lower border of the parotid gland, crosses the sternocleidomastoid muscle, and penetrates the deep fascia of the neck to empty into the *subclavian vein*.

Of the deeper neck muscles, the three *scalene* muscles originate from the transverse processes of the cervical vertebrae.

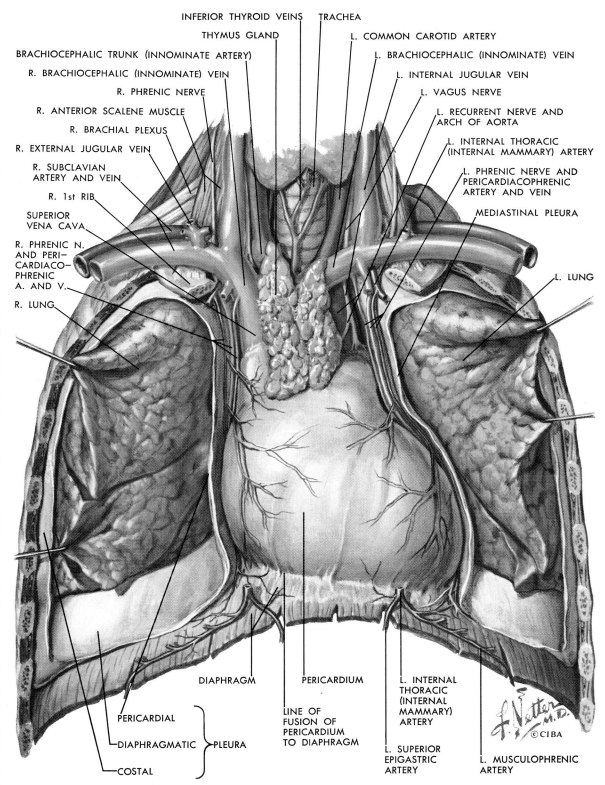

INFERIOR THYROID VEINS — TRACHEA
THYMUS GLAND
BRACHIOCEPHALIC TRUNK (INNOMINATE ARTERY)
R. BRACHIOCEPHALIC (INNOMINATE) VEIN
R. PHRENIC NERVE
R. ANTERIOR SCALENE MUSCLE
R. BRACHIAL PLEXUS
R. EXTERNAL JUGULAR VEIN
R. SUBCLAVIAN ARTERY AND VEIN
R. 1st RIB
SUPERIOR VENA CAVA
R. PHRENIC N. AND PERICARDIACOPHRENIC A. AND V.
R. LUNG

L. COMMON CAROTID ARTERY
L. BRACHIOCEPHALIC (INNOMINATE) VEIN
L. INTERNAL JUGULAR VEIN
L. VAGUS NERVE
L. RECURRENT NERVE AND ARCH OF AORTA
L. INTERNAL THORACIC (INTERNAL MAMMARY) ARTERY
L. PHRENIC NERVE AND PERICARDIACOPHRENIC ARTERY AND VEIN
MEDIASTINAL PLEURA
L. LUNG

DIAPHRAGM
PERICARDIUM
L. INTERNAL THORACIC (INTERNAL MAMMARY) ARTERY
PERICARDIAL
LINE OF FUSION OF PERICARDIUM TO DIAPHRAGM
DIAPHRAGMATIC PLEURA
COSTAL
L. SUPERIOR EPIGASTRIC ARTERY
L. MUSCULOPHRENIC ARTERY

F. Netter M.D. ©CIBA

The *anterior scalene muscle* inserts into the scalene tubercle of the first rib; the medial scalene muscle also attaches to the upper surface of the first rib, but more posteriorly. The posterior scalene muscle inserts on the second rib. The components of the cervical nervous plexus emerge from the groove between the anterior and middle scalene muscles. The anterior scalene muscle is crossed laterally and anteriorly by the *phrenic nerve,* which originates from the cervical plexus and runs downward and behind the subclavian vein to enter the thoracic cavity. The groove between the anterior and middle scalene muscles widens inferiorly to form a triangular opening through which emerge the components of the *brachial plexus* and the *subclavian artery.* The latter, after ascending from the thoracic cavity, crosses the upper surface of the first rib, lying in the groove posterior to the scalene muscle, to enter the axilla. Parallel to the subclavian

artery, but in front of the anterior scalene muscle, runs the *subclavian vein*.

Deep in the lower portion of the neck, under the sternocleidomastoid muscle, is a narrow space bordered anteriorly by the *omohyoid* (see page 2) and strap muscles, posteriorly by the anterior scalene muscle and prevertebral fascia, and medially by the pharynx, esophagus, *trachea*, and *thyroid gland* (see page 2). Enclosed in a common connective-tissue sheath in this space lie the *common carotid artery*, the *internal jugular vein*, and the *vagus nerve*. Of these, the internal jugular vein runs most superficially; the vagus nerve lies beneath, between the common carotid artery and internal jugular veins. On the left side, the *thoracic duct* (see page 2) crosses over the subclavian artery and runs anteriorly to empty into the proximal subclavian vein.

(*Continued on page 4*)

THORACIC CAGE

(Continued from page 3)

Blood for the chest wall is supplied by the *intercostal arteries* and the *internal thoracic (internal mammary) arteries.* After originating from the *aorta*, the posterior intercostal arteries cross the vertebral bodies to enter their corresponding intercostal spaces and pass along the inferior border of the ribs between the internal and external intercostal muscles. Posteriorly, the vessels are well protected by the subcostal groove. The internal thoracic arteries originate from the inferior surface of the subclavian arteries, run downward, lateral to, and (for a short distance) with the *phrenic nerve,* to reach the posterior surface of the anterior chest wall. There they continue their downward course for approximately ¼ inch laterally, to the edges of the sternum, to divide just above the diaphragm into their two terminal branches—the *musculophrenic* and *superior epigastric arteries.* Along their course, the internal thoracic arteries give rise to branches to the *thymus,* mediastinum, and *pericardium* posteriorly, perforating branches to the skin and subcutaneous tissues anteriorly, and, finally, lateral branches which pass along the rib cartilages to anastomose with the posterior intercostal arteries.

The veins of the thoracic wall correspond in their courses with the arteries. The ten lower intercostal veins on the right enter the *azygos vein,* the upper two intercostal veins enter either the azygos or the *brachiocephalic (innominate) vein* (see page 3). The lower intercostal veins on the left side enter the *hemiazygos* or *accessory hemiazygos vein.* The three left superior intercostal veins enter the left brachiocephalic vein by a common stem — the left superior intercostal vein.

The chest wall receives its nerve supply from the intercostal nerves, which accompany the intercostal vessels.

Most of the thoracic cavity is occupied by the two *lungs,* each of which is enclosed by its *pleura.* Each pleura forms a closed sac, invaginated by the lung, so that part of it covers (and is adherent to) the inner surface of the chest wall, the diaphragm, and the mediastinum; these are known, respectively, as the *costal, diaphragmatic,* and *mediastinal pleurae,* and collectively, as the parietal pleura (see page 3). That part of the mediastinal pleura which covers the pericardium is called the *pericardial pleura;* the

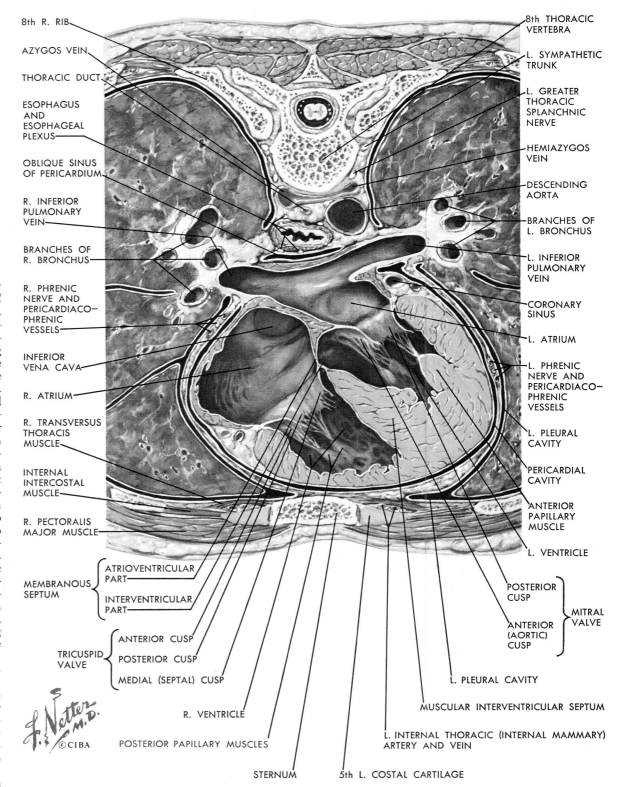

remainder (visceral pleura) covers the lung. The virtual space, between the visceral and parietal pleurae, contains a very small amount of clear fluid. The *pleural reflection* (see page 2), between the costal and diaphragmatic portions of the parietal pleura, lies lower than the corresponding lower edge of the lung. The resulting space, not normally completely filled by the lung even on deep inspiration, is called the recessus costodiaphragmaticus.

The *right lung* consists of three lobes — the *superior, middle,* and *inferior lobes* — and is somewhat larger than the *left lung,* which has two lobes — *superior* and *inferior* (see page 2). The smaller size of the left lung is due to the eccentric position of the heart, which encroaches upon the *left pleural cavity.* Behind the upper *sternum,* the two pleural cavities almost meet; below the fourth-rib cartilage, however, the left costomediastinal reflection deviates

laterally, exposing a small triangular portion of the pericardium which is not covered by pleura. At the same level, the anteroinferior portion of the left superior lobe recedes even more, leaving a portion of the pericardial pleura which is not covered by lung tissue.

The central space between the two pleural cavities is the mediastinum. Arbitrarily, the mediastinum is divided into superior, anterior, middle, and posterior mediastina.

The very shallow anterior mediastinum contains a portion of the *left internal thoracic vessels* and the vestigial *transverse thoracic muscle.*

The superior mediastinum contains the following structures: the thymus gland (see page 3), which, in children after the age of about 12 years, practically disappears, leaving a small pad of fat and areolar tissue; and the brachiocephalic veins, which join each

(Continued on page 5)

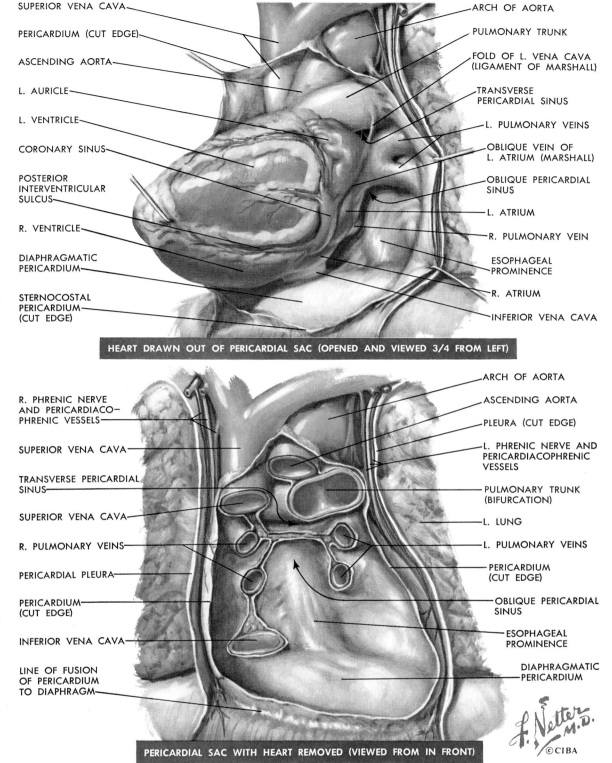

SUPERIOR VENA CAVA
PERICARDIUM (CUT EDGE)
ASCENDING AORTA
L. AURICLE
L. VENTRICLE
CORONARY SINUS
POSTERIOR INTERVENTRICULAR SULCUS
R. VENTRICLE
DIAPHRAGMATIC PERICARDIUM
STERNOCOSTAL PERICARDIUM (CUT EDGE)

ARCH OF AORTA
PULMONARY TRUNK
FOLD OF L. VENA CAVA (LIGAMENT OF MARSHALL)
TRANSVERSE PERICARDIAL SINUS
L. PULMONARY VEINS
OBLIQUE VEIN OF L. ATRIUM (MARSHALL)
OBLIQUE PERICARDIAL SINUS
L. ATRIUM
R. PULMONARY VEIN
ESOPHAGEAL PROMINENCE
R. ATRIUM
INFERIOR VENA CAVA

HEART DRAWN OUT OF PERICARDIAL SAC (OPENED AND VIEWED 3/4 FROM LEFT)

R. PHRENIC NERVE AND PERICARDIACO-PHRENIC VESSELS
SUPERIOR VENA CAVA
TRANSVERSE PERICARDIAL SINUS
SUPERIOR VENA CAVA
R. PULMONARY VEINS
PERICARDIAL PLEURA
PERICARDIUM (CUT EDGE)
INFERIOR VENA CAVA
LINE OF FUSION OF PERICARDIUM TO DIAPHRAGM

ARCH OF AORTA
ASCENDING AORTA
PLEURA (CUT EDGE)
L. PHRENIC NERVE AND PERICARDIACOPHRENIC VESSELS
PULMONARY TRUNK (BIFURCATION)
L. LUNG
L. PULMONARY VEINS
PERICARDIUM (CUT EDGE)
OBLIQUE PERICARDIAL SINUS
ESOPHAGEAL PROMINENCE
DIAPHRAGMATIC PERICARDIUM

PERICARDIAL SAC WITH HEART REMOVED (VIEWED FROM IN FRONT)

THORACIC CAGE

(Continued from page 4)

other on the right to form the *superior vena cava* (see page 3). Posterior to the brachiocephalic veins, the phrenic and vagus nerves descend from the neck. The *phrenic nerves,* accompanied by the *pericardiacophrenic vessels,* run laterally, anterior to the lung roots and along the pericardium, until they reach the diaphragm.

The *aortic arch* ascends from the heart into the superior mediastinum, almost reaches the upper border of the manubrium sterni, courses obliquely backward and to the left over the left main *bronchus,* and continues, as the *descending aorta,* downward, anteriorly and slightly to the left of the vertebral column. Originating from the convexity of the arch, from the proximal to the distal position, are the brachiocephalic, left common carotid, and subclavian arteries.

The *right vagus nerve* (see page 6) passes between the subclavian artery and vein and gives off the right recurrent nerve, which loops around the subclavian artery to ascend along the trachea. The *left vagus nerve* runs between the subclavian vein and the aortic arch, giving rise to the *left recurrent nerve* (see page 3), which similarly loops around the arch to ascend along the trachea.

The trachea descends from the neck, behind the aortic arch, and bifurcates into right and left main bronchi at the level of the sternal angle. Behind the trachea runs the normally collapsed *esophagus* (see page 4), joined by the vagus nerves just beyond the branching off of the recurrent nerves from the vagi. Behind the esophagus, between the azygos vein and the descending aorta, the *thoracic duct* (see page 4) ascends, coursing behind the aortic arch to enter the neck, where it empties into the left subclavian vein.

Against the necks of the ribs, the *sympathetic trunks* descend from the neck, giving off first, at about the level of the sixth rib, the *major splanchnic nerve (greater thoracic splanchnic nerve)* (see page 4) and then the *minor or lesser and lowest thoracic splanchnic nerves.*

The posterior mediastinum is a shallow space containing the lower portions of the esophagus, vagus nerves, descending aorta, azygos and hemiazygos veins, thoracic duct, and sympathetic nerve chains.

The remaining and largest part of the

mediastinum is the middle mediastinum. It contains the *pericardium,* heart, lung roots, and *phrenic nerves.*

The *pericardial cavity* is the third serous cavity contained in the chest, the other two being the pleural cavities. It is roughly conical in shape, with the base of the cone lying posteriorly to the right, and the apex anteriorly to the left. It completely invests the heart and the proximal portions of the great vessels. As with the pleura, one distinguishes a visceral portion of the pericardium overlying the heart and proximal great vessels — usually called the epicardium — as well as a parietal portion.

Of the parietal pericardium, the inferior part is densely adherent to the middle tendinous part of the diaphragm. Most of the lateral and anterior portions are contiguous but not normally adherent to the pleura. A small triangular part of the anterior portion lies directly behind the sternum, separated from it

only by some areolar and fatty tissue, the endothoracic fascia, and the transverse thoracic muscle.

The great vessels enter and leave the pericardial cavity at its base. A curved, transversely running passageway between the arterial and venous poles of the heart is called the *transverse pericardial sinus.* Posteriorly, a blind recess of the pericardial cavity, bordered by the pericardial reflection between the *pulmonary veins* and *inferior vena cava,* is called the *oblique pericardial sinus.* Small recesses exist between the *superior* and *inferior pulmonary veins* on each side and behind the *fold of the left vena cava (ligament of Marshall),* which is a small fold of pericardium running from the left aspect of the *pulmonary trunk* to the *left atrium,* between the neck of the *left auricle* and the *left pulmonary veins.* The fold of the left vena cava contains the vestigial remains of the left common cardinal vein of the embryo.

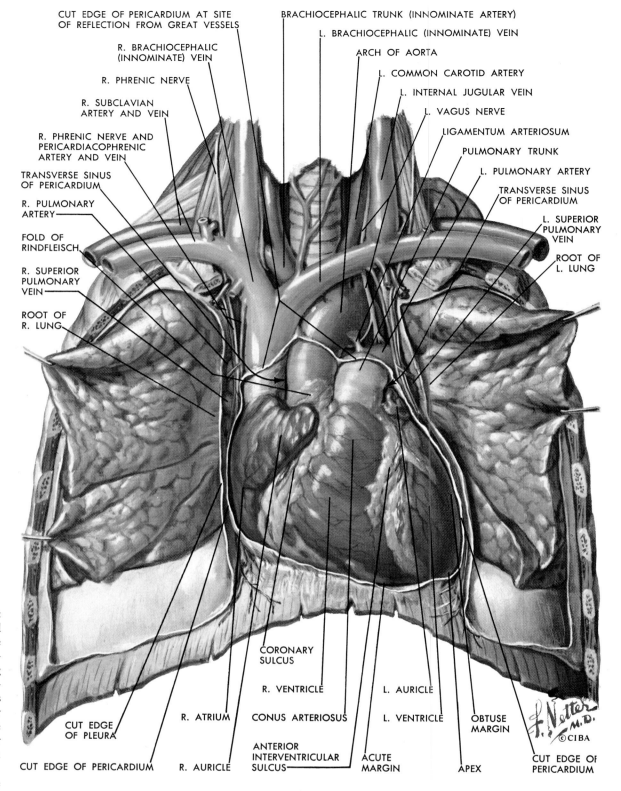

CUT EDGE OF PERICARDIUM AT SITE OF REFLECTION FROM GREAT VESSELS

BRACHIOCEPHALIC TRUNK (INNOMINATE ARTERY)

R. BRACHIOCEPHALIC (INNOMINATE) VEIN

L. BRACHIOCEPHALIC (INNOMINATE) VEIN

ARCH OF AORTA

R. PHRENIC NERVE

L. COMMON CAROTID ARTERY

R. SUBCLAVIAN ARTERY AND VEIN

L. INTERNAL JUGULAR VEIN

L. VAGUS NERVE

R. PHRENIC NERVE AND PERICARDIACOPHRENIC ARTERY AND VEIN

LIGAMENTUM ARTERIOSUM

PULMONARY TRUNK

TRANSVERSE SINUS OF PERICARDIUM

L. PULMONARY ARTERY

R. PULMONARY ARTERY

TRANSVERSE SINUS OF PERICARDIUM

FOLD OF RINDFLEISCH

L. SUPERIOR PULMONARY VEIN

R. SUPERIOR PULMONARY VEIN

ROOT OF L. LUNG

ROOT OF R. LUNG

CORONARY SULCUS

R. VENTRICLE

L. AURICLE

OBTUSE MARGIN

CUT EDGE OF PLEURA

R. ATRIUM

CONUS ARTERIOSUS

L. VENTRICLE

CUT EDGE OF PERICARDIUM

R. AURICLE

ANTERIOR INTERVENTRICULAR SULCUS

ACUTE MARGIN

APEX

CUT EDGE OF PERICARDIUM

Exposure of the Heart

Sternocostal Aspect

Within the *pericardium* lies the heart —a hollow, muscular, four-chambered organ. It is suspended, at its base, by the great vessels. In situ, it occupies an asymmetrical position, with its *apex* pointing anteriorly, inferiorly, and about 60 degrees toward the left. Its four chambers are arranged in two functionally similar pairs, separated from each other by the cardiac *septum* (see page 4). Each pair consists of a thin-walled atrium and a thicker-walled ventricle.

The anatomical nomenclature of the heart has been arrived at by removing it from the body and placing it on its apex, in such a manner that the cardiac septum is in a sagittal plane. This practice has led, in recent years, to some misconceptions and difficulties in orientation among clinicians (cardiologists and surgeons) who deal with the living heart in situ.

On a radiograph of the chest, for example, the left cardiac border is formed by the *left ventricle,* and the right border is formed by the *right atrium,* but not the *right ventricle,* which lies anteriorly. The major and important part of the left atrium lies directly posterior and in the midline in front of the spine and esopha-

gus, allowing the *pulmonary veins* to be as short as possible.

On removing the anterior chest wall and opening the pericardium, most of the presenting part of the heart is formed by the right ventricle, the exposed surface of which is more or less triangular in shape. To its right lies the right atrium.

It is a curious and rather unfortunate circumstance that, in the Anglo-Saxon literature, the term *"auricle"* is often improperly used instead of "atrium." The true auricle is then regrettably called "auricular appendage" instead of "atrial appendage." The latter term is morphologically correct. The incorrect clinical term, "auricular fibrillation," should be replaced by "atrial fibrillation."

The right atrium and ventricle are separated from

each other by the *right atrioventricular (coronary) sulcus* in which runs the right coronary artery, embedded in a variable amount of fat. To the left of the right ventricle, a small segment of the left ventricle is visible, separated from it by the *anterior interventricular sulcus* (groove). The *anterior interventricular (descending) branch* of the *left coronary artery* (see page 17) lies in this groove, again embedded in fat.

Superiorly, the *pulmonary trunk* is seen to originate from the right ventricle and to leave the pericardium just before it bifurcates into its two main branches—the *right* and *left pulmonary arteries.* To its right lies the intrapericardial portion of the ascending *aorta,* the base of which is largely covered by the *right*

(Continued on page 7)

R. PULMONARY ARTERY
L. PULMONARY ARTERY
L. AURICLE
L. SUPERIOR PULMONARY VEIN
L. ATRIUM
L. INFERIOR PULMONARY VEIN
PERICARDIAL REFLECTION
OBLIQUE VEIN OF L. ATRIUM (MARSHALL)
CORONARY SINUS
L. VENTRICLE
APEX

ARCH OF AORTA
R. AURICLE
SUPERIOR VENA CAVA
R. SUPERIOR PULMONARY VEIN
R. ATRIUM
SULCUS TERMINALIS
R. INFERIOR PULMONARY VEIN
CORONARY SULCUS
INFERIOR VENA CAVA
R. VENTRICLE

POSTERIOR ASPECT (BASE) OF HEART

Exposure of the Heart

(Continued from page 6)

L. SUBCLAVIAN ARTERY
L. COMMON CAROTID ARTERY
L. PULMONARY ARTERY
L. SUPERIOR PULMONARY VEIN
L. AURICLE
L. INFERIOR PULMONARY VEIN
OBLIQUE VEIN OF L. ATRIUM (MARSHALL)
L. ATRIUM
PERICARDIAL REFLECTION
CORONARY SINUS
L. VENTRICLE

BRACHIOCEPHALIC (INNOMINATE) ARTERY
SUPERIOR VENA CAVA
ARCH OF AORTA
R. PULMONARY ARTERY
R. SUPERIOR PULMONARY VEIN
R. INFERIOR PULMONARY VEIN
SULCUS TERMINALIS
R. ATRIUM
INFERIOR VENA CAVA
CORONARY SULCUS
POSTERIOR INTERVENTRICULAR SULCUS
R. VENTRICLE

auricle (right atrial appendage). The base of the aorta, including the first part of the right coronary artery, is surrounded by lobules of fatty tissue, the largest and uppermost of which is rather constant and is called the *fold of Rindfleisch*.

Posterior and Diaphragmatic Aspects

After removal of the heart from the *pericardium,* the *posterior* (basilar) and *diaphragmatic aspects* of it can be inspected. The *superior* and *inferior venae cavae* enter the *right atrium,* the long axis of both being inclined slightly forward, and the inferior cava being in a somewhat more medial position. A pronounced groove, the *sulcus terminalis,* separates the right aspect of the superior vena cava from the base of the *right auricle.* As it descends along the posterior aspect of the right atrium, it becomes less distinct.

The *right pulmonary veins* (usually two but, occasionally, three in number), coming from the right lung, cross the right atrium posteriorly, to enter the right side of the *left atrium.* The two *left pulmonary veins* enter the left side of the left atrium, sometimes by a large common stem. The posterior wall of the left

HEART VIEWED FROM BELOW AND BEHIND (DIAPHRAGMATIC ASPECT)

atrium forms the anterior wall of the *oblique pericardial sinus.* Normally, the left atrium is not in contact with the diaphragm.

The bifurcation of the pulmonary trunk lies on the roof of the left atrium, the *left pulmonary artery* coursing immediately toward the left lung, and the *right pulmonary artery* running behind the proximal superior vena cava and above the right pulmonary veins to the right lung.

The *aortic arch* crosses the pulmonary-artery bifurcation after giving off its three main branches — the *brachiocephalic (innominate),* the *left common carotid,* and the *left subclavian* arteries. Variations in this pattern are not uncommon and, usually, are of little significance.

Between the left atrium and the *left ventricle,*

in the posterior (diaphragmatic) portion of the *left atrioventricular groove (coronary sulcus),* lies the *coronary sinus,* into which the cardiac veins enter. It has the appearance of a short, wide vein, but its wall consists of cardiac muscle, and, because of its embryonic origin, it should be considered a true cardiac structure. Its right extremity turns forward and upward to enter the right atrium.

The diaphragmatic surfaces of the *right* and *left ventricles* are separated by the *posterior interventricular* groove or *sulcus.* This sulcus is continuous with the anterior interventricular groove just to the right of the cardiac *apex* which, in a normal heart, is formed by the left ventricle. The posterior interventricular (descending) artery and middle cardiac vein lie in the posterior interventricular sulcus, embedded in fat.

ATRIA AND VENTRICLES

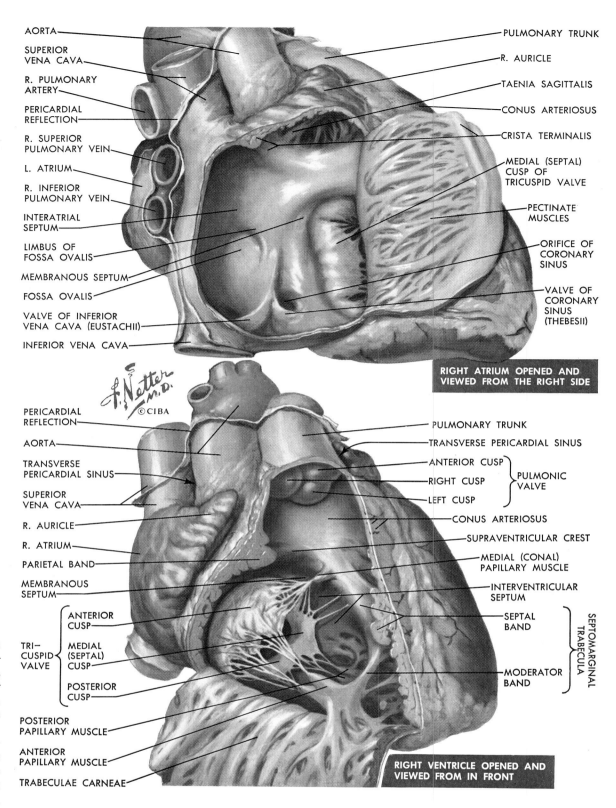

AORTA

SUPERIOR VENA CAVA

R. PULMONARY ARTERY

PERICARDIAL REFLECTION

R. SUPERIOR PULMONARY VEIN

L. ATRIUM

R. INFERIOR PULMONARY VEIN

INTERATRIAL SEPTUM

LIMBUS OF FOSSA OVALIS

MEMBRANOUS SEPTUM

FOSSA OVALIS

VALVE OF INFERIOR VENA CAVA (EUSTACHII)

INFERIOR VENA CAVA

PULMONARY TRUNK

R. AURICLE

TAENIA SAGITTALIS

CONUS ARTERIOSUS

CRISTA TERMINALIS

MEDIAL (SEPTAL) CUSP OF TRICUSPID VALVE

PECTINATE MUSCLES

ORIFICE OF CORONARY SINUS

VALVE OF CORONARY SINUS (THEBESII)

RIGHT ATRIUM OPENED AND VIEWED FROM THE RIGHT SIDE

PERICARDIAL REFLECTION

AORTA

TRANSVERSE PERICARDIAL SINUS

SUPERIOR VENA CAVA

R. AURICLE

R. ATRIUM

PARIETAL BAND

MEMBRANOUS SEPTUM

TRI-CUSPID VALVE { ANTERIOR CUSP / MEDIAL (SEPTAL) CUSP / POSTERIOR CUSP }

POSTERIOR PAPILLARY MUSCLE

ANTERIOR PAPILLARY MUSCLE

TRABECULAE CARNEAE

PULMONARY TRUNK

TRANSVERSE PERICARDIAL SINUS

ANTERIOR CUSP / RIGHT CUSP / LEFT CUSP } PULMONIC VALVE

CONUS ARTERIOSUS

SUPRAVENTRICULAR CREST

MEDIAL (CONAL) PAPILLARY MUSCLE

INTERVENTRICULAR SEPTUM

SEPTAL BAND

MODERATOR BAND

SEPTOMARGINAL TRABECULA

RIGHT VENTRICLE OPENED AND VIEWED FROM IN FRONT

Right Atrium

The *right atrium* consists of two parts: (1) a posterior, smooth-walled part, derived from the embryonic sinus venosus, into which enter the *superior* and *inferior venae cavae,* and (2) a very thin-walled, trabeculated part, which constitutes the original embryonic right atrium.

The two parts of the atrium are separated by a ridge of muscle. This ridge is most prominent superiorly, next to the superior vena caval orifice; it fades out to the right of the inferior vena caval ostium. This ridge is called the *crista terminalis,* and its position corresponds to that of the *sulcus terminalis* (see page 7) externally. It is often stated to be a remnant of the embryonic right venous valve; actually, it lies just to the right of the valve.

From the lateral aspect of the crista terminalis, a large number of *pectinate muscles* run laterally, and more or less parallel to each other, along the free wall of the atrium. In between these pectinate muscles, the atrial wall is paper-thin and translucent.

The somewhat-triangular-shaped superior portion of the right atrium—the *right auricle*—is also filled with pecti-

nate muscles. One of these, originating from the crista terminalis, is usually larger than the others. This one is called the *taenia sagittalis.*

Normally, the right auricle is not well demarcated, externally, from the remainder of the atrium. It forms a ready-made, convenient point of entry for the cardiac surgeon and is used extensively as such.

The anterior border of the inferior vena caval ostium is guarded by a fold of tissue—the *inferior vena caval (eustachian) valve.* It varies greatly in size, and it may even be absent. When very large, it is usually perforated by numerous openings, forming a delicate lace-like structure which is known as the network of Chiari. Just anterior to the medial extremity of the inferior vena caval valve the *coronary sinus* enters the right atrium. Its *orifice,* also, may or may not be guarded by

a valvelike fold, which is termed the *coronary-sinus (thebesian) valve.* Both valves are derived from the very large, embryonic, right venous valve.

The posteromedial wall of the right atrium is formed by the *interatrial septum.* The central, ovoid portion of it is thin and fibrous. It forms a shallow depression—the *fossa ovalis*—in the septum. The remainder of the septum is muscular, and it usually forms a ridge around the fossa ovalis. This is called the *limbus fossae ovalis.* Not infrequently, it is possible to pass a probe under the anterosuperior part of the limbus into the left atrium. In such cases, the foramen (fossa) ovalis is said to be probe-patent. Anteromedially, the tricuspid valve gives access to the *right ventricle.*

(Continued on page 9)

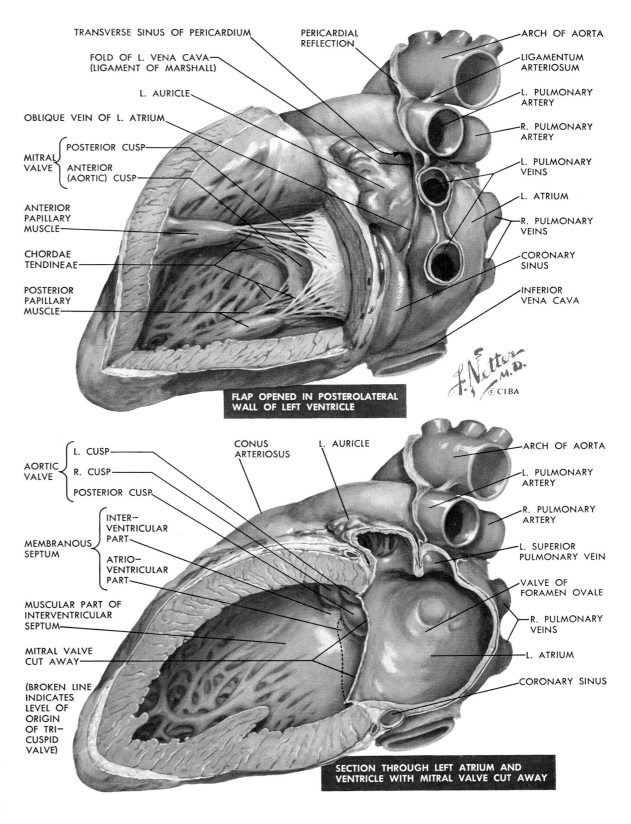

TRANSVERSE SINUS OF PERICARDIUM

PERICARDIAL REFLECTION

ARCH OF AORTA

FOLD OF L. VENA CAVA (LIGAMENT OF MARSHALL)

LIGAMENTUM ARTERIOSUM

L. AURICLE

L. PULMONARY ARTERY

OBLIQUE VEIN OF L. ATRIUM

R. PULMONARY ARTERY

MITRAL VALVE { POSTERIOR CUSP / ANTERIOR (AORTIC) CUSP }

L. PULMONARY VEINS

L. ATRIUM

ANTERIOR PAPILLARY MUSCLE

R. PULMONARY VEINS

CHORDAE TENDINEAE

CORONARY SINUS

POSTERIOR PAPILLARY MUSCLE

INFERIOR VENA CAVA

FLAP OPENED IN POSTEROLATERAL WALL OF LEFT VENTRICLE

AORTIC VALVE { L. CUSP / R. CUSP / POSTERIOR CUSP }

CONUS ARTERIOSUS

L. AURICLE

ARCH OF AORTA

L. PULMONARY ARTERY

R. PULMONARY ARTERY

MEMBRANOUS SEPTUM { INTER-VENTRICULAR PART / ATRIO-VENTRICULAR PART }

L. SUPERIOR PULMONARY VEIN

VALVE OF FORAMEN OVALE

MUSCULAR PART OF INTERVENTRICULAR SEPTUM

R. PULMONARY VEINS

MITRAL VALVE CUT AWAY

L. ATRIUM

(BROKEN LINE INDICATES LEVEL OF ORIGIN OF TRI-CUSPID VALVE)

CORONARY SINUS

SECTION THROUGH LEFT ATRIUM AND VENTRICLE WITH MITRAL VALVE CUT AWAY

ATRIA AND VENTRICLES

(*Continued from page 8*)

Right Ventricle

The *right ventricular cavity* (see page 8) can be divided arbitrarily into a posteroinferior inflow portion, containing the *tricuspid valve,* and an anterosuperior outflow portion, from which the *pulmonary trunk* originates.

The demarcation between these two parts is afforded by a number of prominent muscular bands, as follows: the *parietal band,* the crista supraventricularis (*supraventricular crest*), the *septal band,* and the *moderator band.* Together, these form an almost circular orifice which, in the normal heart, is wide and forms no impediment to flow.

The wall of the inflow portion is heavily trabeculated, particularly in its most apical portion. These *trabeculae carneae* enclose a more or less elongated, ovoid opening. The outflow portion of the right ventricle, often called the *infundibulum,* contains only a few trabeculae. The subpulmonic area is smooth-walled.

A number of *papillary muscles* anchor the *tricuspid-valve cusps* to the right ventricular wall by means of a large number of slender, fibrous strands which are called the *chordae tendineae.* Two of these *papillary muscles*—the *medial* and

the *anterior*—are reasonably constant in position, but they vary in size and shape. The others are extremely variable in every respect.

Approximately where the crista supraventricularis joins the septal band, the small *medial papillary muscle* receives chordae tendineae from the *anterior* and *septal cusps* of the *tricuspid valve.* Often well developed in infants, in adults the medial papillary muscle is, commonly, almost absent or is reduced to a tendinous patch. It is an important surgical landmark, and, because of its interesting embryonic origin, it is of considerable diagnostic value to the cardiac pathologist.

The *anterior papillary muscle* originates from the moderator band. It receives chordae from the *anterior* and *posterior cusps* of the *tricuspid valve.*

In variable numbers, the usually small *posterior* and septal *papillary muscles* receive chordae from the posterior and medial (septal) cusps. Those which originate from the posteroinferior border of the septal band are of some importance in the analysis of certain types of congenital cardiac anomalies.

The *pulmonary trunk* arises superiorly from the right ventricle and passes backward and slightly upward. It bifurcates into *right* and *left pulmonary arteries* (see page 6) just after leaving the pericardial cavity. A short ligament—the *ligamentum arteriosum* (see page 6)—connects the upper aspect of the bifurcation to the inferior surface of the *aortic arch* (see page 6). It is a remnant of the fetal ductus arteriosus (Botallo's duct).

(*Continued on page 10*)

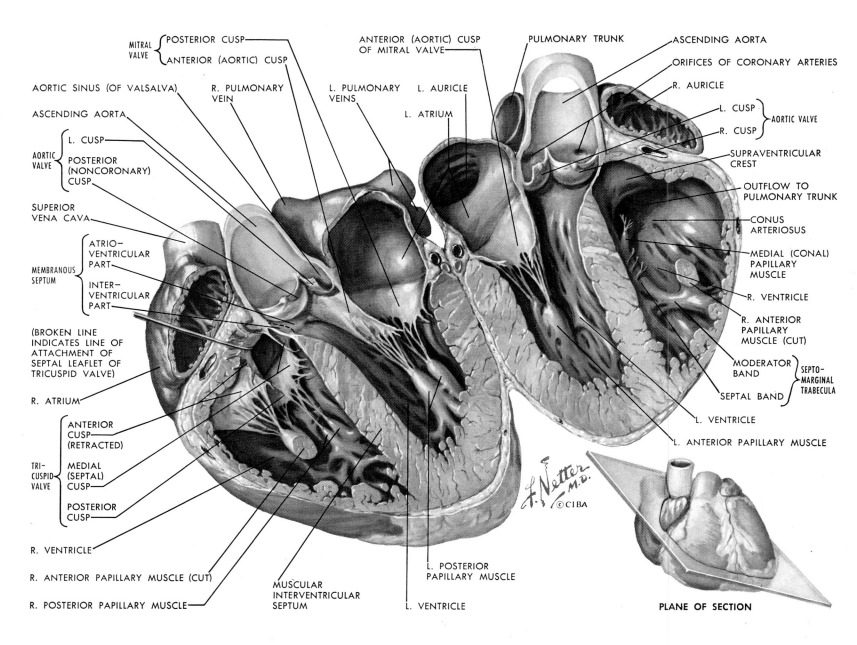

MITRAL VALVE — POSTERIOR CUSP
MITRAL VALVE — ANTERIOR (AORTIC) CUSP
AORTIC SINUS (OF VALSALVA)
R. PULMONARY VEIN
ANTERIOR (AORTIC) CUSP OF MITRAL VALVE
L. PULMONARY VEINS
L. AURICLE
L. ATRIUM
PULMONARY TRUNK
ASCENDING AORTA
ORIFICES OF CORONARY ARTERIES
R. AURICLE
L. CUSP — AORTIC VALVE
R. CUSP — AORTIC VALVE
SUPRAVENTRICULAR CREST
ASCENDING AORTA
AORTIC VALVE — L. CUSP
POSTERIOR (NONCORONARY) CUSP
SUPERIOR VENA CAVA
OUTFLOW TO PULMONARY TRUNK
CONUS ARTERIOSUS
MEMBRANOUS SEPTUM — ATRIO-VENTRICULAR PART
INTER-VENTRICULAR PART
MEDIAL (CONAL) PAPILLARY MUSCLE
R. VENTRICLE
R. ANTERIOR PAPILLARY MUSCLE (CUT)
(BROKEN LINE INDICATES LINE OF ATTACHMENT OF SEPTAL LEAFLET OF TRICUSPID VALVE)
R. ATRIUM
MODERATOR BAND
SEPTO-MARGINAL TRABECULA
SEPTAL BAND
TRICUSPID VALVE — ANTERIOR CUSP (RETRACTED)
MEDIAL (SEPTAL) CUSP
POSTERIOR CUSP
L. VENTRICLE
L. ANTERIOR PAPILLARY MUSCLE
R. VENTRICLE
R. ANTERIOR PAPILLARY MUSCLE (CUT)
R. POSTERIOR PAPILLARY MUSCLE
MUSCULAR INTERVENTRICULAR SEPTUM
L. POSTERIOR PAPILLARY MUSCLE
L. VENTRICLE

PLANE OF SECTION

SECTION I—PLATE 9

ATRIA AND VENTRICLES

(Continued from page 9)

Left Atrium

The *left atrium* consists mainly of a smooth-walled sac, the transverse axis of which is somewhat larger than the vertical and sagittal axes. On the *right,* two or, occasionally, three *pulmonary veins* enter it; on the *left,* there are also two (sometimes one) *pulmonary veins.* The wall of the left atrium is distinctly thicker than that of the right atrium.

The septal surface is usually fairly smooth, with only a somewhat-irregular area indicating the position of the fetal *valve of the foramen ovale.* A narrow slit may allow a probe to be passed from the right atrium to the left atrium.

The *left auricle* is a continuation of the left upper anterior part of the left atrium. Its shape is very variable, for it may be long and also may be kinked in one or more places. Its lumen contains small pectinate muscles, and there usually is a distinct waistlike narrowing, proximally.

Left Ventricle

The *left ventricle* (see also page 9) is shaped like an egg, the blunt end of which has been cut off. Here, both the *mitral* and the *aortic valves* are located adjacent to each other. They are separated by only a fibrous band from which originate most of the *anterior (aortic) cusp of the mitral valve* and the adjacent portions of the *left* and *posterior aortic-valve cusps.* The average thickness of the left ventricular wall is about three times that of the right ventricular wall. Its trabeculae carneae are somewhat less coarse, some being merely tendinous cords. As is the case in the right ventricle, the trabeculae are much more numerous and dense in the apex of the left ventricle. The basilar third of the septum is smooth.

Usually, there are two stout *papillary muscles.* The dual embryonic origin of each of these is often revealed by their bifid apices; each receives *chordae tendineae* from *both* major *mitral-valve cusps.* Occasionally, a third small papillary muscle is present laterally.

Most of the *ventricular septum* is *muscular.* Normally it bulges into the right ventricle — a reflection of the fact that a transverse section of the left ventricle is almost circular. Its muscular portion has approximately the same thickness as the parietal left ventricular wall, and it consists of two layers — a thin layer on the right ventricular side and a thicker layer on the left ventricular side. The major septal arteries tend to run between these two layers.

In the human heart, a variable (but, generally, quite small) area of the septum, immediately below the *right* and *posterior aortic-valve cusps,* is thin and membranous. The demarcation between the muscular and the *membranous* parts of the *ventricular septum* is distinct and is called .the *limbus marginalis.* As seen from the opened right ventricle, the *membranous septum* lies deep to the *supraventricular crest* (see also page 8) and is divided into two parts by the origin of the *medial (septal) cusp* of the *tricuspid valve.* As a result, one portion of the membranous septum lies between the left ventricle and the right ventricle (*interventricular part*); the other, between the left ventricle and the *right atrium* (*atrioventricular part*).

On *sectioning* of the septum in an approximately transverse *plane,* the basilar portion of the ventricular septum, including the membranous septum, is seen to deviate to the right, so that a plane through the major portion of the septum bisects the *aortic valve.* It must be emphasized that the total cardiac septum shows a complex, longitudinal twist and does not lie in any single plane.

VALVES IN OPEN AND CLOSED POSITIONS, DETAILED VALVULAR RELATIONSHIPS

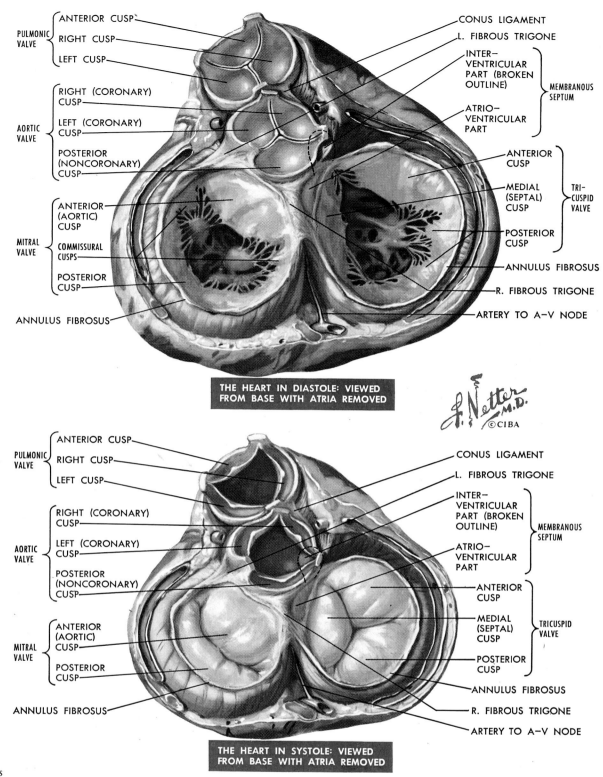

THE HEART IN DIASTOLE: VIEWED FROM BASE WITH ATRIA REMOVED

THE HEART IN SYSTOLE: VIEWED FROM BASE WITH ATRIA REMOVED

Each *atrioventricular-valve apparatus* consists of a number of *cusps, chordae tendineae,* and *papillary muscles.*

The cusps are thin, yellowish-white, glistening membranes, roughly trapezoid-shaped, with fine, irregular edges. They originate from the *annulus fibrosus,* which is a somewhat-ill-defined and rather unimpressive fibrous ring around each atrioventricular orifice. Only at the *right* and *left fibrous trigones* is there more than a token amount of fibrous tissue present.

The atrial surface of the atrioventricular valve is rather smooth (except near the free edge) and not well demarcated from the atrial wall. The ventricular surface is very irregular, owing to the insertion of the chordae tendineae, and is separated from the ventricular wall by a narrow space.

The extreme edges of the cusps are thin and delicate and have a sawtoothlike appearance because of the insertion of equally fine chordae. A little distance away from the edge, the atrial surface of the cusps, particularly in small children, is finely nodular. These nodules are called the noduli Albini. On closure of an atrioventricular valve, the narrow border between the row of nodules and the free edge of each cusp presses against that of the next, resulting in a secure and watertight closure.

The chordae tendineae may be divided into three groups:

The first two groups originate from or near the apices of the papillary muscles. They form a few strong, tendinous cords which subdivide into several thinner strands as they approach the valve edges.

The chordae of the first order insert into the extreme edge of the valve by a large number of very fine strands. Their function seems to be merely to prevent the opposing borders of the cusps from inverting.

The chordae of the second order insert on the ventricular surface of the cusps, approximately at the level of the noduli Albini, or even higher. These are stronger and less numerous. They function as the mainstays of the valves and are comparable to the stays of an umbrella.

The chordae of the third order originate from the ventricular wall much nearer the origin of the cusps. These chordae often form bands or foldlike structures which may contain muscle.

(Continued on page 12)

ASCENDING AORTA

AORTIC SINUSES
(OF VALSALVA)

ORIFICE OF
R. CORONARY ARTERY

MEMBRANOUS
SEPTUM
{ INTER-
VENTRICULAR
PART
ATRIO-
VENTRICULAR
PART }

(BROKEN LINE INDICATES
LEVEL OF ORIGIN OF
TRICUSPID VALVE)

MUSCULAR
INTERVENTRICULAR SEPTUM

ORIFICE OF L. CORONARY ARTERY

NODULUS ARANTII

LUNULA

LEFT
CUSP

POSTERIOR
CUSP

RIGHT
CUSP

AORTIC
VALVE

ANTERIOR (AORTIC)
CUSP OF MITRAL
VALVE

ANTERIOR
PAPILLARY MUSCLE

AORTIC VALVE

VALVES IN OPEN AND CLOSED
POSITIONS, DETAILED VALVULAR
RELATIONSHIPS

(Continued from page 11)

INFERIOR
VENA CAVA

RIGHT
ATRIUM

CHORDAE
TENDINEAE

MEDIAL
(CONAL)
PAPILLARY
MUSCLE

POSTERIOR
PAPILLARY
MUSCLES
(SECTIONED)

SEPTAL
BAND

PARIETAL
BAND

ATRIO-
VENTRICULAR
PART

INTER-
VENTRICULAR
PART
(BEHIND VALVE)

MEMBRANOUS
SEPTUM

POSTERIOR
CUSP

ANTERIOR
CUSP

MEDIAL
CUSP

TRI-
CUSPID
VALVE

POSTERIOR
PAPILLARY
MUSCLE
(SECTIONED)

ANTERIOR PAPILLARY
MUSCLE

TRICUSPID (RIGHT ATRIOVENTRICULAR) VALVE

LEFT
ATRIUM

CHORDAE
TENDINEAE

POSTERIOR
PAPILLARY
MUSCLE

ANTERIOR
PAPILLARY
MUSCLE
(SECTIONED)

ANTERIOR
CUSP

POSTERIOR
CUSP

MITRAL
VALVE

COMMISSURAL
CUSPS

ANTERIOR
PAPILLARY
MUSCLE
(SECTIONED)

MITRAL (LEFT ATRIOVENTRICULAR) VALVE

Occasionally, particularly on the left side, the chordae of the first two orders—even in normal hearts—may be wholly muscular, so that the papillary muscle seems to insert directly into the cusp. This is not surprising, since the *papillary muscles,* the *chordae tendineae,* and most of the *cusps* are derived from the embryonic ventricular trabeculae and, therefore, were all muscular at one time.

The *tricuspid valve* consists of an *anterior,* a *medial (septal),* and one or two *posterior* cusps. The depth of the *commissures* between the cusps is variable, but the commissures never reach the *annulus,* so the cusps are only incompletely separated from each other.

The *mitral (bicuspid) valve* actually is made up of four cusps. These are

two large ones—the *anterior* (aortic) and *posterior* (mural) *cusps*—and two small *commissural cusps.* Here, as in the case of the tricuspid valve, the commissures are never complete, and they should not be so constructed in the surgical treatment of mitral stenosis.

The arterial or semilunar valves differ greatly in structure from the atrioventricular valves. Each consists of three pocketlike cusps of approximately equal size. Although, functionally, the transition between the ventricle and the artery is abrupt and easily determined, this cannot be done anatomically in any simple manner. There is no distinct, circular ring of fibrous tissue at the base of the arteries from which they and the valve cusps arise; rather, the arterial wall expands into three dilated pouches—the sinuses of Valsalva—the walls of which are much thinner

than those of the aorta and of the pulmonary artery. The origin of the valve cusps is, therefore, not straight but scalloped.

The cusps of the arterial semilunar valve are largely smooth and thin. At the center of the free margin of each cusp is a small fibrous nodule which is called the *nodulus Arantii.*

On each side of the nodule of Arantius, along the entire free edge of the cusp, there is a very thin, half-moon-shaped area termed the *lunula.* It has fine striations parallel to the edge, and, near the insertion of the cusps on the aortic wall, the lunulae are commonly perforated. In valve closure, since the entire areas of adjacent lunulae appose each other, such perforations do not cause insufficiency of the valve and are, functionally, of no significance.

ANATOMY OF THE SPECIALIZED CONDUCTION SYSTEM

General Features

The specialized heart tissues include the *sinoatrial (S-A) node, atrioventricular (A-V) node, common atrioventricular (A-V) bundle* or *bundle of His, right* and *left bundle branches,* and peripheral ramifications of these bundle branches which make up the subendocardial and intramyocardial Purkinje network. In addition, there are other fiber groups in the atria which meet some of the criteria — both histological and electrophysiological — for specialization. These constitute *Bachmann's bundle* and the internodal conducting paths of the right atrium.

The body of the sinoatrial node is in the wall of the right atrium, at the junction between the atrium proper and the *superior vena cava.* This junction appears on the epicardial surface as the sulcus terminalis; on the endocardial surface, as the *crista terminalis.* From the main body of the sinus node, extensions run down along the sulcus terminalis toward the A-V node and in a cephalic direction around the dorsal and lateral aspects of the superior vena cava. The atrioventricular node lies in the floor of the right atrium, a variable distance to the left of the coronary-sinus opening. The upper end of the atrioventricular node is in continuity with the atrial myocardium and (see below) fibers of the *internodal tracts.* At the lower end, the nodal fibers change and form the common bundle which passes through the right fibrous trigone along the posterior edge of the *membranous septum* to the apex of the *muscular interventricular septum.* At this point, the common bundle divides into right and left bundle branches which extend subendocardially along both septal surfaces. The left bundle branch rapidly subdivides, forming a broad sheet of fascicles sweeping over the left interventricular septal surface. The right bundle branch extends for some distance without subdivision; one branch usually passes through the *moderator band,* and other parts extend over the endocardial surface of the ventricle. Peripherally, both bundle branches subdivide and form the subendocardial network of *Purkinje fibers* which extend a variable distance into the ventricular walls and are in direct continuity with fibers of the ventricular muscle.

For many years there has been argument about the existence of specialized *atrial* conduction *paths* and about the nature of connections between the *sinoatrial node* and the atrioventricular node. However, until recently, the consensus was that the spread of impulse in the atria did not depend on the existence of specialized conducting paths.

In recent years, evidence obtained from both physiological and anatomical studies has confirmed the existence of specialized atrial fibers localized to form discrete

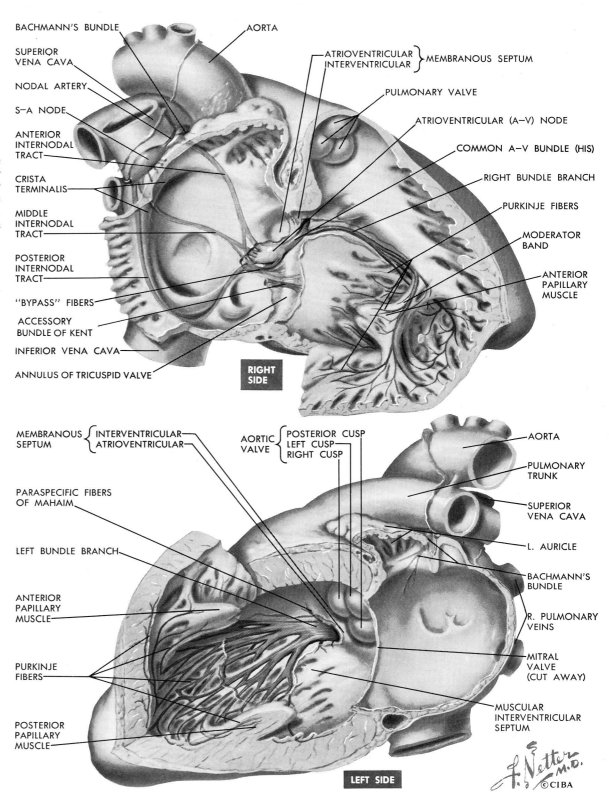

paths. The schematized representation of these paths' distribution is based largely on anatomical studies of the human heart, by James, and on electrophysiological studies of rabbit and puppy atria, by Paes de Carvalho and Wagner. By an intracellular microelectrode to record transmembrane action potentials, Paes de Carvalho demonstrated, in studies of rabbit hearts, the existence of a discrete tract of specialized fibers which coursed around the sinoatrial ring. This tract he called the "sinoatrial-ring bundle." In studies of puppy atria, Wagner showed the existence of physiologically specialized fibers, extending from the head of the sinus node across the interatrial band to the left atrium, following the distribution of Bachmann's bundle. In definitive histological studies of the human atrium, James demonstrated the existence of three discrete internodal paths and the relationship of one of these to Bachmann's bundle. The *anterior*

internodal tract leaves the head of the sinus node and spreads to the left, dividing to form two branches: One extends along the dorsal aspect of the interatrial band to ramify over the left atrium. This subdivision constitutes the specialized fibers of Bachmann's bundle. The other branch curves across the interatrial septum to the region of the atrioventricular node, where it merges with fibers from other nodal tracts. The *middle internodal tract* leaves the posterodorsal margin of the sinus node to cross the interatrial septum and merge at the A-V node with other specialized atrial fibers. This tract corresponds to the bundle described by Wenckebach. The *posterior internodal tract* extends from the tail of the sinus node along the crista terminalis, through the eustachian ridge, to the right superior margin of the atrioventricular node. A description of the interconnections of internodal tracts with the atrium and A-V node follows.

(Continued on page 14)

ANATOMY OF THE SPECIALIZED CONDUCTION SYSTEM

(Continued from page 13)

Physiological evidence suggests that the spread of the sinus impulse to the left atrium and from the sinus node to the A-V node depends normally, and primarily, on activation of the anterior internodal tract and Bachmann's bundle. The physiological significance of these tracts is described in detail below.

The only normal anatomical *communication* between the atria and ventricles of the mammalian heart is the *atrioventricular node* with the common bundle of His. On the atrial side, the atrioventricular node communicates with the atrium through the branched and interweaving fibers of the internodal tracts, and, perhaps, through connections with ordinary atrial musculature. The details of these intercommunications have been described by James. In addition, in studies of the canine A-V node, he has described fiber tracts which appear to bypass the body of the node and connect with distal portions close to the junction of nodal fibers and the common atrioventricular bundle. He also has shown that similar *"bypass" fibers* can be demonstrated in studies of the human atrioventricular node.

In addition to the normal anatomical communications between the atria and ventricles, abnormal ones are found in some hearts. As shown by Truex, these are more frequent in fetal and infantile hearts; occasionally, they persist into adult life. The most common and best-known of such communications was described originally by Kent. The *accessory bundle of Kent* would appear to be a fascicle of ordinary atrial myocardium extending directly from the inferior margin of the right atrium to the upper aspects of the interventricular septum. Although it has not been demonstrated that such connections as the bundle of Kent conduct impulses in the living heart, it has been suggested that they may be the mechanism causing anomalous ventricular excitation in such disorders as the Wolff-Parkinson-White syndrome. Finally, many workers, including Robb and James, have shown that fascicles of atrial myocardium extend through the atrioventricular ring and onto the base of atrioventricular valves. It seems unlikely that these fiber groups are ever responsible for transmission of impulses from the atria to the ventricles.

As shown by Lev, James, and others, there is considerable variation in the bifurcation of the *common bundle* and the distribution of the left bundle branch. Ordinarily, the *left bundle branch* leaves the common bundle as a rather broad fascicle which, frequently, divides into major anterior and posterior divisions. The *right bundle branch* constitutes a smaller prolongation of the common bundle, extending subendocardially along the right side of the interventricular septum. In most hearts, the left bundle branch makes its initial, functional contact with the ventricular myocardium on

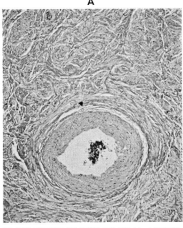

A. SINUS NODE ABOUT CENTRAL ARTERY WITH FIBER TRACTS RADIATING OUT INTO ATRIAL MUSCLE (GOLDNER STAIN, X 10)

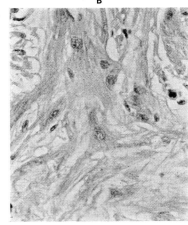

B. NETWORK OF INTERLACING CELLS IN SINUS NODE (GOLDNER STAIN, X 160)

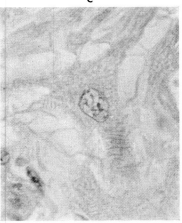

C. DETAIL OF P CELL FROM SINUS NODE (GOLDNER STAIN, X 400)

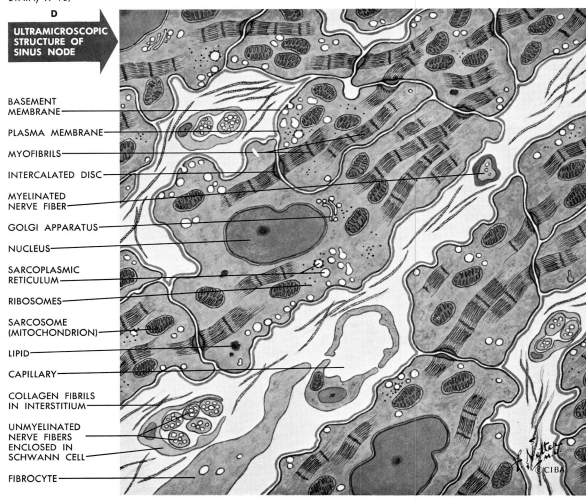

D. ULTRAMICROSCOPIC STRUCTURE OF SINUS NODE

BASEMENT MEMBRANE
PLASMA MEMBRANE
MYOFIBRILS
INTERCALATED DISC
MYELINATED NERVE FIBER
GOLGI APPARATUS
NUCLEUS
SARCOPLASMIC RETICULUM
RIBOSOMES
SARCOSOME (MITOCHONDRION)
LIPID
CAPILLARY
COLLAGEN FIBRILS IN INTERSTITIUM
UNMYELINATED NERVE FIBERS ENCLOSED IN SCHWANN CELL
FIBROCYTE

the left endocardial surface of the interventricular septum some distance beneath the *aortic valve.* The right bundle branch makes its first functional contact with the ventricular myocardium subendocardially near the base of the *anterior papillary muscle.* Sometimes, a small bundle of fibers exits from the left bundle branch and makes contact with the upper dorsal parts of the interventricular septum. This bundle constitutes the *paraspecific fibers of Mahaim.*

Fine Structure of Specialized Cardiac Tissues

The most characteristic anatomical feature of both the human and the canine sinoatrial *(sinus) node* is its relationship to the nodal *(central) artery.* The node completely *surrounds* this artery, which courses through it (usually, as a large, single vessel) and gives numerous branches to the nodal tissue. The collagenous tissue of the artery is continuous with the extensive collagen matrix of the node itself (James). These *collagen fibers* and an extensive *network* of elastic fibers form a mesh through which the nodal tissue is distributed. With increasing age, the relative density of connective tissues is markedly increased (Lev).

In the center of the node, the fibers are distributed in a concentric pattern around the artery (A); in the periphery, their distribution is more *radial,* with some condensation in areas where nodal tissue merges with specialized conduction paths. Nodal fibers are in direct anatomical continuity with fibers of the specialized atrial paths and also with ordinary *atrial muscle* fibers. *Nerve fibers* are numerous within the node, although autonomic ganglion cells appear to be restricted to its periphery (James). Although numerous small veins are found within the node, no consistent pattern of drainage has been demonstrated.

(Continued on page 15)

ANATOMY OF THE SPECIALIZED CONDUCTION SYSTEM

(Continued from page 14)

The *details of cellular* anatomy are shown in parts B and C. Usually the fibers are smaller in diameter than those of the atrial musculature and are gathered in fine bundles which weave through the collagen framework. The majority of fibers are long, thin, and faintly striated, showing a bulging perinuclear clear zone. However, in the central region of the node, James has demonstrated (C) (see page 14) a distinctive cell type (the *P cell*) which is thought to be uniquely related to normal pacemaker activity. These cells are larger than the nodal fibers, have an unusually large, centrally located *nucleus,* and are stellate in shape. They are in continuity with the smaller nodal fibers at many points.

The *ultramicroscopic structure* of the sinoatrial node has been studied by Trautwein, Kawamura, and others (D) (see page 14). Aggregates of irregularly shaped cells are surrounded by a *basement membrane. Myofibrils* are sparse and irregularly arranged, often appearing to be interrupted. Probably because of the irregular packing of myofibrils, *mitochondria* are scattered at random throughout the cytoplasm. The *sarcoplasmic reticulum* also shows less regular distribution than in cardiac muscle fibers; frequently, it appears as invaginations of the outer membrane. No system of T tubules has been described. Cells in apposition are separated only by their respective membranes and a narrow space of approximately 200 angstroms. Where bundles of myofibrils approach the apposed *membranes* on both sides (*intercalated discs*), a thickened, desmosome-like structure is apparent.

The *atrioventricular node* is located beneath a thin flap of atrial muscle just anterior to the ostium of the coronary sinus and just above the insertion of the tricuspid-valve septal cusp. The connections of the A-V node with the atrium above, and with the common bundle below, have been described elsewhere. These relationships, and the general appearance of the node under low magnification, are shown in part A. As in the sinus node, the A-V node is in close anatomical relationship to its nutrient *artery.* This vessel often is eccentrically located and may be divided. In man, the A-V nodal artery arises almost exclusively from the right coronary artery; in dogs, it almost always is a branch of the left circumflex artery (James). The A-V node is rich in venous sinusoids and nerve *fibers;* as in the sinus node, ganglion cells are absent.

Fibers of the A-V node are generally smaller than those of atrial muscle and, as in the sinus node, form a pattern of branching and *interlacing* strands (B and C). The connective-tissue framework is less extensive than in the sinus, but, with age, it still shows a considerable increase in density. Although most cells of the A-V node are small, lightly striated,

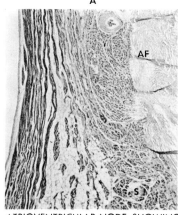

A

ATRIOVENTRICULAR NODE, SHOWING ARTERY, ANNULUS FIBROSUS (AF), INTERVENTRICULAR SEPTUM (S), AND OVERLYING ATRIUM (GOLDNER TRICHROME STAIN, X 10)

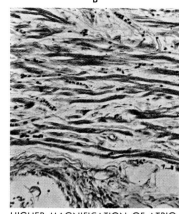

B

HIGHER MAGNIFICATION OF ATRIO-VENTRICULAR NODE: INTERLACING, LOOSELY PACKED FIBERS, AND SEGMENTS OF SMALL ARTERY AND VEIN (HOLMES SILVER STAIN)

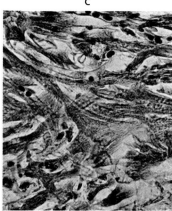

C

HIGH-POWER DETAIL OF ATRIOVENTRICULAR NODAL FIBERS (MASSON TRICHROME STAIN)

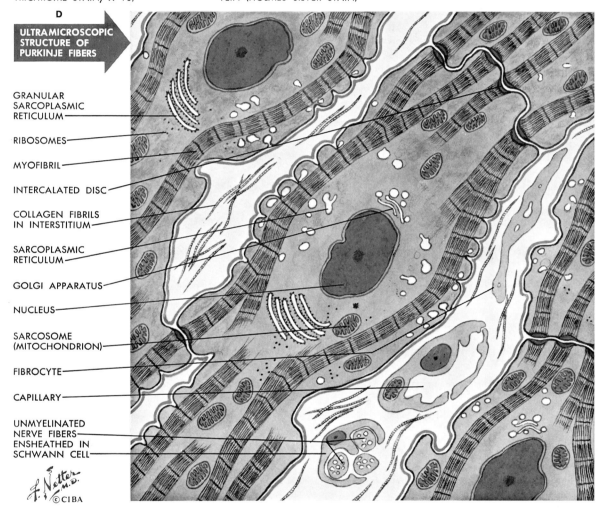

D ULTRAMICROSCOPIC STRUCTURE OF PURKINJE FIBERS

GRANULAR SARCOPLASMIC RETICULUM

RIBOSOMES

MYOFIBRIL

INTERCALATED DISC

COLLAGEN FIBRILS IN INTERSTITIUM

SARCOPLASMIC RETICULUM

GOLGI APPARATUS

NUCLEUS

SARCOSOME (MITOCHONDRION)

FIBROCYTE

CAPILLARY

UNMYELINATED NERVE FIBERS ENSHEATHED IN SCHWANN CELL

and highly branched, some resemble the P cells of the sinoatrial node (Paes de Carvalho, James). As in the sinus, the cellular architecture of the A-V node varies with location; at the region of transition between the node and the common bundle, cells are collected into larger, more regular fascicles, the cells themselves taking on the characteristics of Purkinje fibers. The details of the ultramicroscopic structure of the A-V nodal cells are similar to those of the sinoatrial node.

Typical *Purkinje fibers* are found in the left bundle branch and the periphery of the specialized conducting system of the ventricles; in the common bundle, in the right bundle branch, and at the junction of the Purkinje tissue with ventricular muscle, there is a gradual transition in the fine structure. These fibers are made up of large, fairly regular cells which make contact longitudinally through *intercalated discs* (D). No areas of lateral contact have been described in

detail. The Purkinje cells contain sparse, peripherally located *myofibrils* and a central *nucleus* which usually is surrounded by a clear zone rich in glycogen. *Mitochondria* are frequent and randomly distributed. The *sarcoplasmic reticulum* is clearly evident and usually *granular* in appearance. Present also are T tubules — tubular extensions of the inner layer of the outer membrane which extend across the fiber in the vicinity of the Z line and are thought to be intimately concerned in the process of excitation-contraction coupling. As in other types of cardiac fibers, the intercalated discs show thickenings at the points of attachment of the myofibrils and also show numerous "tight" junctions where the outer layers of the apposed membranes appear to fuse. *Capillaries* and small nerve fibers are distributed in the spaces between the fibers. No specialized nerve endings have been described.

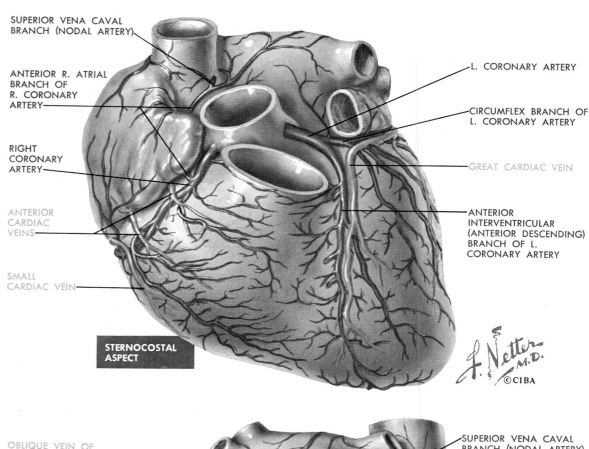

SUPERIOR VENA CAVAL BRANCH (NODAL ARTERY)

ANTERIOR R. ATRIAL BRANCH OF R. CORONARY ARTERY

RIGHT CORONARY ARTERY

ANTERIOR CARDIAC VEINS

SMALL CARDIAC VEIN

L. CORONARY ARTERY

CIRCUMFLEX BRANCH OF L. CORONARY ARTERY

GREAT CARDIAC VEIN

ANTERIOR INTERVENTRICULAR (ANTERIOR DESCENDING) BRANCH OF L. CORONARY ARTERY

STERNOCOSTAL ASPECT

CORONARY ARTERIES AND VEINS

Blood Supply of the Heart

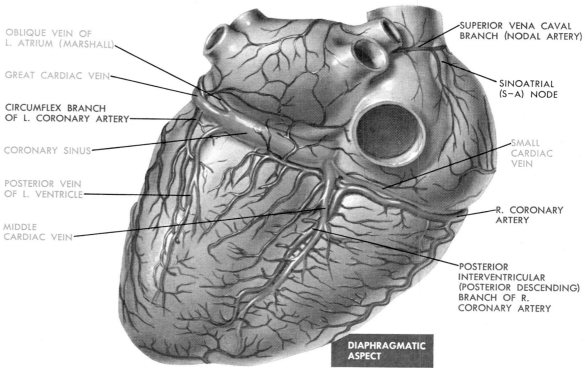

OBLIQUE VEIN OF L. ATRIUM (MARSHALL)

GREAT CARDIAC VEIN

CIRCUMFLEX BRANCH OF L. CORONARY ARTERY

CORONARY SINUS

POSTERIOR VEIN OF L. VENTRICLE

MIDDLE CARDIAC VEIN

SUPERIOR VENA CAVAL BRANCH (NODAL ARTERY)

SINOATRIAL (S–A) NODE

SMALL CARDIAC VEIN

R. CORONARY ARTERY

POSTERIOR INTERVENTRICULAR (POSTERIOR DESCENDING) BRANCH OF R. CORONARY ARTERY

DIAPHRAGMATIC ASPECT

The normal heart and the proximal portions of the great vessels receive their blood supply from two coronary arteries. The *left coronary artery* originates from the left sinus of Valsalva, near its upper border, at about the level of the free edge of the valve cusp. It usually has a short common stem (0.5 to 2 cm) which bifurcates or trifurcates. One branch, the *anterior interventricular (descending) branch*, courses downward in the anterior interventricular groove (largely embedded in fat), rounds the acute margin of the heart just to the right of the apex, and ascends a short distance up the posterior interventricular groove.

The anterior interventricular (descending) branch of the left coronary artery gives off branches to the adjacent anterior right ventricular wall (which commonly anastomose with branches from the right coronary artery) and septal branches (which supply the anterior two thirds and the apical portions of the septum), as well as a number of branches to the anteroapical portions of the left ventricle, including the anterior papillary muscle.

One of the septal branches, originating from the upper third of the anterior interventricular branch, is usually larger than the others and supplies the midseptum, including the bundle of His and bundle branches of the conduction system. Not infrequently, it also supplies the anterior papillary muscle of the right ventricle, by way of the moderator band.

The second (usually smaller) *circum*-

flex branch of the left coronary artery runs in the left atrioventricular sulcus and gives off branches to the upper lateral left ventricular wall and the left atrium. Usually, the circumflex branch terminates at the obtuse margin of the heart, but, in some cases, it reaches the crux (junction of the posterior interventricular sulcus and the posterior atrioventricular groove); in this case, it supplies all of the left ventricle and ventricular septum with blood, with or without the help of the right coronary artery.

In cases where the left coronary artery trifurcates, the third branch, coming off between the anterior interventricular and the circumflex branches, is merely a left ventricular branch which happens to originate from the main artery.

The *right coronary artery* arises from the right

anterior sinus of Valsalva of the aorta and runs along the right atrioventricular sulcus, embedded in fat. It rounds the acute margin to reach the crux, in the majority of cases, and it gives off a variable number of branches to the anterior right ventricular wall. A (usually) well-developed and large branch runs along the acute margin of the heart. Another, the *posterior interventricular (descending) branch*, descends along the posterior interventricular groove, not quite reaching the apex and supplies the posterior third or more of the interventricular septum. The *diaphragmatic* part of the right ventricle is largely supplied by small parallel branches from the marginal and posterior descending arteries, and not from the parent vessel itself. The latter generally crosses

(Continued on page 17)

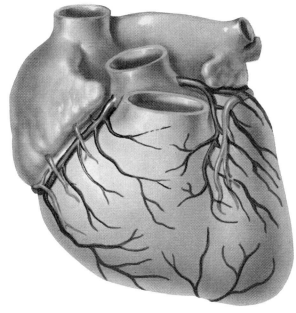

ANTERIOR INTERVENTRICULAR (ANTERIOR DESCENDING)
BRANCH OF L. CORONARY ARTERY VERY SHORT: APICAL
PART OF STERNOCOSTAL SURFACE SUPPLIED BY BRANCHES
FROM POSTERIOR INTERVENTRICULAR (POSTERIOR
DESCENDING) BRANCH OF RIGHT CORONARY ARTERY
CURVING AROUND APEX

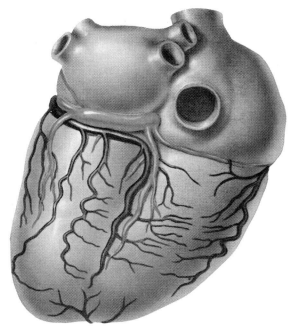

POSTERIOR INTERVENTRICULAR (POSTERIOR DESCENDING)
BRANCH DERIVED FROM CIRCUMFLEX BRANCH
OF LEFT CORONARY INSTEAD OF FROM
RIGHT CORONARY ARTERY

Coronary Arteries and Veins

(Continued from page 16)

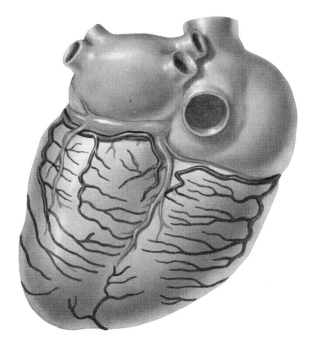

POSTERIOR INTERVENTRICULAR (POSTERIOR DESCENDING)
BRANCH ABSENT: AREA SUPPLIED CHIEFLY BY SMALL
BRANCHES FROM CIRCUMFLEX BRANCH OF LEFT
CORONARY AND FROM RIGHT CORONARY ARTERY

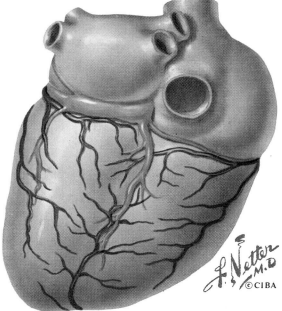

POSTERIOR INTERVENTRICULAR (POSTERIOR DESCENDING)
BRANCH ABSENT: AREA SUPPLIED CHIEFLY BY ELONGATED
ANTERIOR INTERVENTRICULAR (ANTERIOR DESCENDING)
BRANCH CURVING AROUND APEX

the crux, giving off the posterior interventricular branch and a small branch to the atrioventricular node. It terminates in a number of branches to the left ventricular wall.

The posterior papillary muscle of the left ventricle usually has a dual blood supply from both the left and the right coronary arteries.

Of the *right atrial branches of the right coronary artery,* one is of great importance. This branch originates from the right coronary artery, shortly after its takeoff, and ascends along the anteromedial wall of the right atrium. It enters the upper part of the atrial septum, reappears as the *superior vena caval branch (nodal artery)* posterior and to the left of the superior vena caval ostium, rounds this ostium, and runs close to (or through) the *sinoatrial node* (see page 13), giving off branches to the crista terminalis and pectinate muscles.

Variations in the branching pattern are extremely common in the human heart. In about 67 percent of the cases, the right coronary artery is dominant, crosses the crux, and supplies part of the left ventricular wall and the ventricular septum. In 15 percent of the cases, the left coronary artery is dominant (as in dogs and many other mammals), in which case its circumflex branch crosses the crux, giving off the posterior interventricular branch and supplying all of the left ventricle, the ventricular septum, and part of the right ventricular wall.

In about 18 percent of the cases, both coronary arteries reach the crux; this is

the so-called balanced coronary arterial pattern. Not infrequently, there is no real posterior interventricular branch, but the posterior septum is penetrated at the posterior interventricular groove by a large number of branches from either the left coronary artery, the right coronary artery, or both.

The superior vena caval branch, in about 40 percent of the cases, is a continuation of a large *anterior atrial branch* of the left coronary artery rather than of the anterior atrial branch of the right coronary artery.

Finally, it is quite common for the first branch of the right coronary artery to originate independently from the right sinus of Valsalva rather than from the parent artery. Rarely, the second or even the third branch of the right coronary artery arises independently.

Most of the cardiac or coronary veins enter the *coronary sinus.* The three largest are the *great* and *middle cardiac veins* and the *posterior left ventricular vein.* The ostia of these veins may be guarded by unicuspid or bicuspid valves which are fairly well developed. The *oblique vein of the left atrium (Marshall)* enters the sinus near the orifice of the *great cardiac vein.* Its ostium never has a valve. The *small cardiac vein* may enter the right atrium independently, and the *anterior cardiac veins* always do.

Small venous systems exist in the atrial septum — and, probably, also in the ventricular walls and septum — which enter the cardiac chambers directly. These are the thebesian veins. The existence of so-called arterioluminal and arteriosinusoidal vessels is debatable, and the evidence for their presence is inconclusive.

INNERVATION OF HEART I AND II

The heart is supplied by sympathetic and parasympathetic nerves which arise mostly in the cervical region, because, initially, the heart develops in the neck. It later migrates downward into the thorax, carrying its nerves with it.

The *cervical* and upper *thoracic sympathetic*-trunk ganglia contribute cardiac branches, all of which pass through the *cardiac plexus,* usually without forming synapses. They are ultimately distributed to the various layers of the heart wall through the coronary plexuses. Three pairs of sympathetic cardiac nerves are derived from the cervical ganglia of the sympathetic trunks, and others arise from the upper thoracic ganglia.

The *superior cervical sympathetic cardiac nerve* originates by several rootlets from the corresponding *ganglion*. It often unites with the *superior vagal cardiac nerve(s)*, and this *conjoined nerve* then descends behind the carotid sheath, communicating en route through slender rami with the pharyngeal, laryngeal, carotid, and thyroid nerves. On the right side, the conjoined nerve passes posterolateral to the subclavian and brachiocephalic arteries and aortic arch; on the left, it curves downward across the left side of the aortic arch.

The *middle cervical sympathetic cardiac nerve* is often the largest of the cervical cardiac nerves. It is formed by filaments from the *middle* and *vertebral ganglia* of the sympathetic trunk. It usually runs independently to the cardiac plexus but may unite with other cardiac nerves, and it is interconnected with tracheal, esophageal, and thyroid branches of the sympathetic trunks.

The *inferior cervical sympathetic cardiac nerves* consist of filaments arising from the *stellate* (cervicothoracic) *ganglion* and *ansa·subclavia*. They often combine with each other, or with other cardiac nerves, before reaching the cardiac plexus, and inconstant communications exist between them and the *phrenic nerves*.

The *thoracic sympathetic cardiac nerves* are four or five slender branches, on each side, which arise from the corresponding upper thoracic sympathetic-trunk ganglia. They run forward and medially to the cardiac plexus. Some enter it directly; others are united, for variable distances, with filaments destined for the lungs, aorta, trachea, and esophagus.

The vagal (parasympathetic) cardiac branches vary in size, number, and arrangement, but they can be grouped as *superior* and *inferior cervical* and *thoracic vagal cardiac nerves*.

The *superior cervical vagal cardiac*

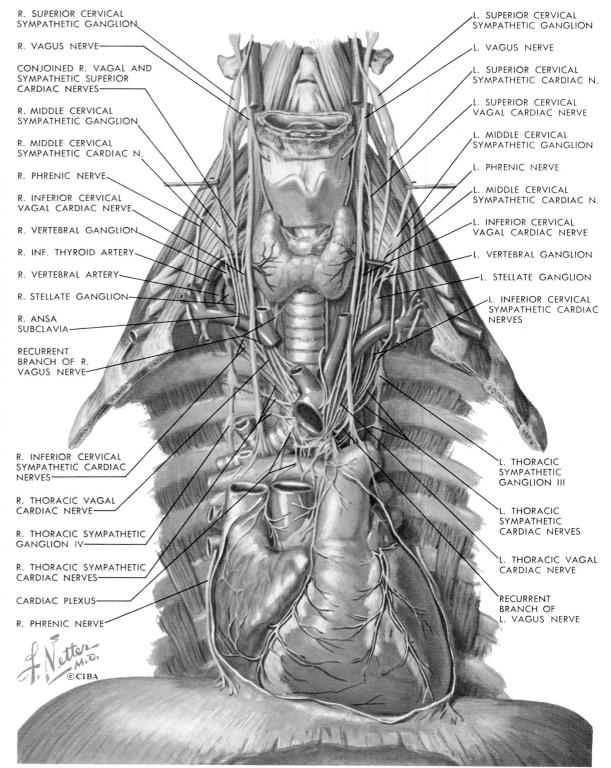

R. SUPERIOR CERVICAL SYMPATHETIC GANGLION
R. VAGUS NERVE
CONJOINED R. VAGAL AND SYMPATHETIC SUPERIOR CARDIAC NERVES
R. MIDDLE CERVICAL SYMPATHETIC GANGLION
R. MIDDLE CERVICAL SYMPATHETIC CARDIAC N.
R. PHRENIC NERVE
R. INFERIOR CERVICAL VAGAL CARDIAC NERVE
R. VERTEBRAL GANGLION
R. INF. THYROID ARTERY
R. VERTEBRAL ARTERY
R. STELLATE GANGLION
R. ANSA SUBCLAVIA
RECURRENT BRANCH OF R. VAGUS NERVE
R. INFERIOR CERVICAL SYMPATHETIC CARDIAC NERVES
R. THORACIC VAGAL CARDIAC NERVE
R. THORACIC SYMPATHETIC GANGLION IV
R. THORACIC SYMPATHETIC CARDIAC NERVES
CARDIAC PLEXUS
R. PHRENIC NERVE

L. SUPERIOR CERVICAL SYMPATHETIC GANGLION
L. VAGUS NERVE
L. SUPERIOR CERVICAL SYMPATHETIC CARDIAC N.
L. SUPERIOR CERVICAL VAGAL CARDIAC NERVE
L. MIDDLE CERVICAL SYMPATHETIC GANGLION
L. PHRENIC NERVE
L. MIDDLE CERVICAL SYMPATHETIC CARDIAC N.
L. INFERIOR CERVICAL VAGAL CARDIAC NERVE
L. VERTEBRAL GANGLION
L. STELLATE GANGLION
L. INFERIOR CERVICAL SYMPATHETIC CARDIAC NERVES
L. THORACIC SYMPATHETIC GANGLION III
L. THORACIC SYMPATHETIC CARDIAC NERVES
L. THORACIC VAGAL CARDIAC NERVE
RECURRENT BRANCH OF L. VAGUS NERVE

F. Netter M.D.
©CIBA

nerve is formed from two or three filaments which leave the *vagus* in the upper part of the neck. It usually unites with the corresponding sympathetic cardiac nerve, and this conjoined nerve then descends to the cardiac plexus (see above).

The *inferior cervical vagal cardiac nerve(s),* one to three in number, arise in the lower third of the neck and often join or communicate with the cardiac branches from the *middle cervical,* vertebral, and/or stellate sympathetic ganglia. If they remain separate, they lie posterolateral to the brachiocephalic artery and aortic arch on the right side, and lateral to the left common carotid artery and aortic arch on the left side.

The *thoracic vagal cardiac nerves* are a series of filaments arising from the vagus nerve of each side, at or below the level of the thoracic inlet, and also from both *recurrent laryngeal nerves,* the left con-

tributing more filaments than the right. They often unite with other cardiac nerves in their passage to the cardiac plexus.

Cardiac Plexus

All the vagal and sympathetic cardiac nerves converge on this plexus, and filaments from its right and left sides surround and accompany the coronary arteries and their branches. The plexus lies between the concavity of the aortic arch and the tracheal bifurcation.

Sometimes, the cardiac plexus is described as consisting of superficial and deep parts, but there is little difference in their depths, and they are intimately interconnected. There is, however, a superficial, tenuous, preaortic plexus over the ascending aorta.

(Continued on page 19)

INNERVATION OF HEART
I AND II

(Continued from page 18)

Several ganglia, in which a proportion of the vagal fibers relay, are present in this plexus. The largest of these — the ganglion of Wrisberg — lies below the aortic arch, between the division of the pulmonary trunk and the tracheal bifurcation. Other smaller collections of parasympathetic cells — the intrinsic cardiac ganglia — are located mainly in the atrial subendocardial tissue, along the atrioventricular sulcus and near the roots of the great vessels; relatively few are found over the ventricles, but enough exist to cast doubt on the view that the ventricular innervation is entirely or predominantly sympathetic.

The cardiac sympathetic and parasympathetic nerves carry both *afferent* and efferent fibers. The afferents transmit impulses, to the central nervous system, from discrete cardiac receptor endings of various types and from terminal networks which are plentiful in such reflexogenous zones as the endocardium around the openings of the caval and pulmonary veins, over the interatrial septum, and in the atrioventricular valves. The efferents carry impulses which are modified reflexly by afferent impulses from the heart and the great vessels. They are under the overall control of the higher centers in the brain, the hypothalamus, and the brain stem.

The pathways illustrated are the more important ones. Afferents from the heart and the great vessels are shown traveling to the cord via the *sympathetic cardiac nerves,* while others are carried upward to *nuclei* in the *medulla oblongata* by the *vagus nerves.* The efferents pursue similar routes, but these travel in a centrifugal direction. The cell bodies of the afferent neurons are situated in the dorsal-root ganglia of the upper four or five *thoracic* spinal *nerves* and in the *inferior vagal* ganglia.

The *preganglionic* parasympathetic fibers are the axons of cells in the *dorsal vagal nuclei,* and they relay in ganglia in the *cardiac plexus* or in intrinsic cardiac ganglia. The *preganglionic sympathetic* fibers are the axons of cells located in the lateral gray columns of the upper four or five thoracic spinal segments. These fibers enter the corresponding spinal nerves and leave them in *white rami communicantes* which pass to adjacent *ganglia* in the *sympathetic* trunks. Some, however, relay in these ganglia, and the postganglionic fibers (the axons of ganglionic cells) are conveyed to the heart in the *thoracic sympathetic cardiac nerves.* Others ascend in the *sympathetic* trunks to form synapses with cells in the *superior, middle,* and *vertebral ganglia,* and the *postganglionic* fibers reach the heart

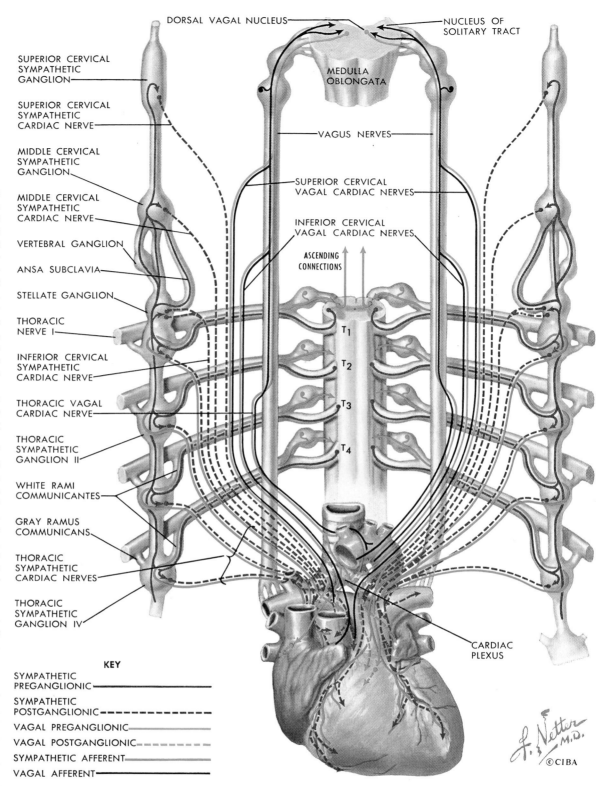

DORSAL VAGAL NUCLEUS
NUCLEUS OF SOLITARY TRACT
MEDULLA OBLONGATA
SUPERIOR CERVICAL SYMPATHETIC GANGLION
SUPERIOR CERVICAL SYMPATHETIC CARDIAC NERVE
MIDDLE CERVICAL SYMPATHETIC GANGLION
MIDDLE CERVICAL SYMPATHETIC CARDIAC NERVE
VERTEBRAL GANGLION
ANSA SUBCLAVIA
STELLATE GANGLION
THORACIC NERVE I
INFERIOR CERVICAL SYMPATHETIC CARDIAC NERVE
THORACIC VAGAL CARDIAC NERVE
THORACIC SYMPATHETIC GANGLION II
WHITE RAMI COMMUNICANTES
GRAY RAMUS COMMUNICANS
THORACIC SYMPATHETIC CARDIAC NERVES
THORACIC SYMPATHETIC GANGLION IV
VAGUS NERVES
SUPERIOR CERVICAL VAGAL CARDIAC NERVES
INFERIOR CERVICAL VAGAL CARDIAC NERVES
ASCENDING CONNECTIONS
T_1 T_2 T_3 T_4
CARDIAC PLEXUS

KEY
SYMPATHETIC PREGANGLIONIC
SYMPATHETIC POSTGANGLIONIC
VAGAL PREGANGLIONIC
VAGAL POSTGANGLIONIC
SYMPATHETIC AFFERENT
VAGAL AFFERENT

F. Netter M.D.
©CIBA

via cardiac branches of these ganglia. Therefore, the parasympathetic relays occur in ganglia near or in the heart, whereas the sympathetic relays are located in ganglia at some distance from the heart. In consequence, the parasympathetic postganglionic fibers are relatively short and circumscribed in their distribution.

Afferent and efferent fibers probably run in all the sympathetic and parasympathetic cardiac nerves, although afferents may not be present in the *superior cervical sympathetic cardiac nerves.* Many afferent vagal fibers from the heart and the great vessels are concerned in reflexes depressing cardiac activity, and, in some animals, they are aggregated in a separate "depressor nerve"; in man, these fibers may run in cardiac branches of the laryngeal nerves.

The thoracic sympathetic cardiac nerves carry many efferent accelerator and *afferent* fibers to and

from the heart and great vessels, and this endows them with an interest disproportionate to their insignificant size. Other cardiac pain afferents run in the middle and *inferior cervical sympathetic cardiac nerves,* but, after entering the corresponding cervical ganglia, they descend within the sympathetic trunks to the thoracic region before passing through rami communicantes into the upper four or five thoracic spinal nerves and so to the cord. According to Arnulf and Hantz, many of the cardiac pain fibers run through the preaortic plexus. For this reason, they advocate excision of this plexus as a simpler and safer alternative to upper-thoracic sympathetic ganglionectomy for the relief of angina pectoris.

Afferent fibers from the pericardium are carried mainly in the phrenic nerves, although those from the visceral serous pericardium are conveyed in the coronary plexuses.

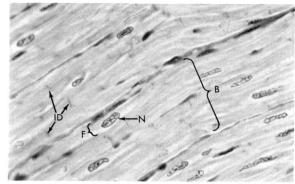

LONGITUDINAL SECTION OF HEART MUSCLE (TRICHROME STAIN, X 400) B=BUNDLE; F=FIBER; ID=INTERCALATED DISCS

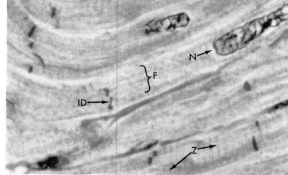

LONGITUDINAL SECTION OF HEART MUSCLE (TRICHROME STAIN, X 1200) N=NUCLEUS; Z=Z LINES

HISTOLOGY OF THE MYOCARDIUM I

The myocardium is composed of specialized striated muscle cells and intervening connective tissue. Each cell (see page 21) possesses a central *nucleus,* a continuous limiting *plasma membrane* (the *sarcolemma*), and numerous contractile *myofibrils* that are separated by varying amounts of *sarcoplasm.* Specialized paired-membrane junctions — the *intercalated discs* — join the cells, end to end, into long *fibers.* The fibers are separated from one another by *intercellular spaces,* of varying widths, containing small amounts of *collagen,* an occasional *fibroblast,* and numerous *capillaries.* Large, lateral, cytoplasmic processes extend from many of the cells to join adjacent fibers and make the myocardium a continuous network of cells. Sheaths of connective tissue separate groups of muscle fibers into long *bundles* which also interconnect. All the muscle fibers within one bundle are parallel; however, adjacent bundles may be parallel, oblique, or even transverse to one another.

The contractile substance of the heart muscle consists of longitudinally arranged myofibrils which extend the full length of each cell and insert into the cytoplasmic surface of the intercalated discs. Each myofibril is divided into a series of repeating units, the *sarcomeres,* which are the fundamental structural and *functional units of contraction.* All the sarcomeres within one cell are in transverse register, giving the cardiac cells a striated appearance. Dark Z *lines* act as a type of transverse septum, dividing the myofibrils into longitudinally arranged sarcomeres. The area between two Z lines is composed of overlapping thick and thin myofilaments. Extending toward the center of the sarcomere from each Z line are thin (50 angstroms) longitudinally oriented actin filaments that produce a light I *band* at both ends of the sarcomeres. Thick (100 angstroms) myosin filaments traverse the central portion of each sarcomere and produce a dense A *band.* The thin filaments are not restricted to the I band, and they interdigitate with the two ends of the thick A-band filaments during diastole. Where there is no intercrescence between *thick* and *thin filaments,* the A band is transected by a lighter H zone. An M *line,*

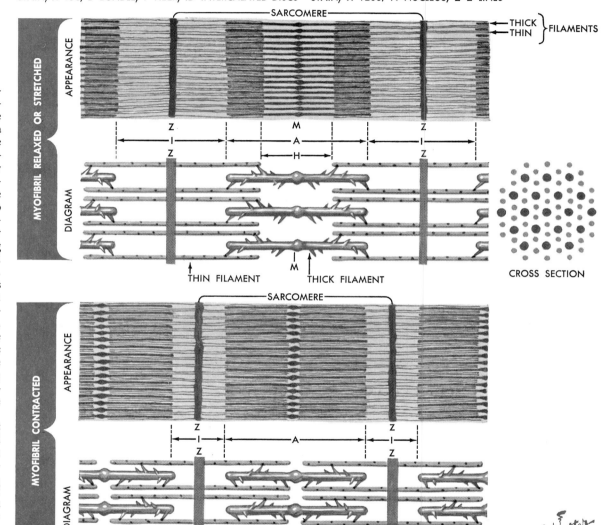

produced by nodular thickenings of the thick myofilaments, bisects the central H disc.

At the level of intercrescence in the A band, six thin filaments are *geometrically arranged* around each thick filament. Each thin filament, in turn, is located at a site equidistant from three thick filaments. The surface of the thin filaments is smooth, whereas that of the thick filaments is studded with minute spines. These spines form an ordered periodic array of interfilamentous bridges between each thick filament and six neighboring thin filaments. Stated differently, each thin filament receives spines from three equidistant thick filaments, at regular intervals along the length of the "overlap region."

During contraction, the length of the A band remains constant, but the I band shortens markedly. In addition, the length of the H band diminishes, and the sarcomere thickens. The thick and thin fila-

ments are believed, by most investigators, to remain constant in length during contraction. One hypothesis explaining these observations is that the thin actin filaments slide past the thick myosin filaments toward the center of the sarcomere. Consequently, the sarcomeres shorten, as evidenced by the decreased distance of any two adjacent Z lines, and the cell as a whole shortens and thickens. During systole the myosin bridges are activated, connect to specific sites on the actin filaments, and produce a force-developing connection between them. Movement is generated by the detachment and reattachment of the spines at active sites farther along the actin filament; this "sweeping" process requires the energy released by ATP (adenosine triphosphate).

During diastole the bridges do not attach firmly to the actin filament, and the muscle fibers, as a whole, lengthen and exhibit plasticity.

HISTOLOGY OF THE MYOCARDIUM II

The heart, as stated previously (see page 20), is composed of a network of branching striated muscle cells with centrally located nuclei. Each cell is bounded by a plasma membrane (sarcolemma) and a mucopolysaccharide-rich *basement membrane*. Minute *pinocytotic vesicles* are present along the cytoplasmic surface of the cells, suggesting that the sarcolemma actively participates in the transport of materials into the cell.

The contractile substance of the heart consists of long parallel myofibrils which exhibit a regular banding pattern and impart a striated appearance to the muscle fiber. Each myofibril is composed of a series of repeating units, the *sarcomeres*, the fundamental units of contraction. The Z lines, which appear as dense structures, act as a kind of continuous transverse septum across each fibril. Two Z lines in longitudinal succession constitute the limits of a sarcomere. Two types of myofilaments extend along the interior of the sarcomeres, overlap at their ends, and, as a consequence, produce the banding effect of the cells. Thick filaments, representing the protein myosin, run along the length of the A band. Thin filaments, presumably actin-containing, extend from each Z line through the I band to the A band, where they overlap with the thick myosin filaments. In diastole, the degree of intercrescence between the thick and thin filaments is relatively small, and a light H band, consisting of thick filaments only, bisects the A band. During contraction, the thin actin filaments slide past the thick myosin filaments, with the consequent disappearance of the I and H bands.

A network of membrane-bounded *intracellular channels* — the *sarcoplasmic reticulum* — is systematically distributed throughout the heart muscle cell. There are two components of this intracellular membranous system, both parts playing important roles in impulse conduction and in muscle contraction and relaxation. One portion consists of a thick-walled tubular network which traverses the myofiber transversely (*T system*) and surrounds the myofibrils at the level of the Z lines. The tubular elements of this network apparently connect with the sarcolemma and may be a result of deep invaginations of it. The second portion of the sarcoplasmic reticulum is the longitudinal component (*L system*) which consists of a series of anastomosing thin-walled tubules that run the length of a sarcomere and form a complex intermittent sleeve around it. The tubules of the longitudinal system anastomose transversely between the sarcomeres, but they are not

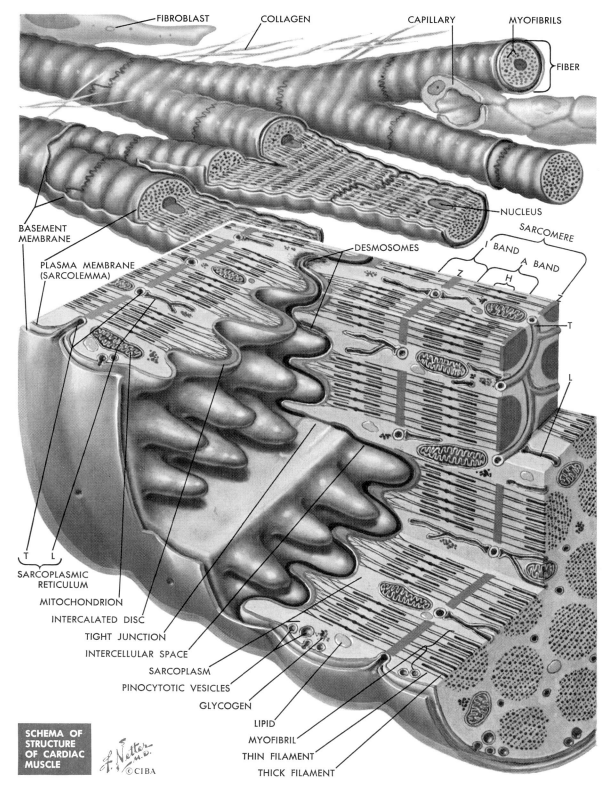

FIBROBLAST — COLLAGEN — CAPILLARY — MYOFIBRILS — FIBER — NUCLEUS — SARCOMERE — I BAND — A BAND — Z — H — Z — T — DESMOSOMES — L — BASEMENT MEMBRANE — PLASMA MEMBRANE (SARCOLEMMA) — T — L — SARCOPLASMIC RETICULUM — MITOCHONDRION — INTERCALATED DISC — TIGHT JUNCTION — INTERCELLULAR SPACE — SARCOPLASM — PINOCYTOTIC VESICLES — GLYCOGEN — LIPID — MYOFIBRIL — THIN FILAMENT — THICK FILAMENT

SCHEMA OF STRUCTURE OF CARDIAC MUSCLE

F. Netter M.D.
© CIBA

continuous longitudinally across the Z lines. No connection between the T system and the longitudinal system has been shown convincingly; however, portions of the T system are prominently dilated, and large vesicles of the longitudinal system, from adjacent sarcomeres, abut directly upon them.

The sarcosomes, or *mitochondria,* of cardiac muscle are large and numerous. They usually are aligned in clumps or columns between the myofibrils. In this position, they can, presumably, satisfy the sarcomeres' unusually high requirement for energy. Large numbers of *glycogen granules* and *lipid droplets* represent localized food stores lying in close conjunction with the mitochondria.

Adjacent cardiac cells are held firmly together by an elaborate, zigzagged, interdigitated region of attachment — the *intercalated discs*. These discs are located at the ends of the cells, at right angles to the

muscle fibers, and at the level of the Z lines. Usually, the cells are not divided across a series of Z lines in register, but the discs occasionally shift the level of one sarcomere to the next Z line, forming steps between the cells. Four types of intercellular relationships are observed along these cell junctions: (1) Dense plaques line the cytoplasmic surface, serving as insertion points for the filaments of the myofibrils. (2) Intermittent *desmosomes,* not associated with the myofibrils, form "intercellular bridges." (3) Along the lateral cell surfaces, at positions where the discs shift one or more sarcomeres, the membranes of the two adjacent cells adhere closely or fuse into *tight junctions*. These junctions are probably involved in the intercellular spread of the excitatory impulse over the muscle. (4) The remaining portion of the two membranes, along the cellular junction, exhibits an intercellular gap of 15 to 20 microns.

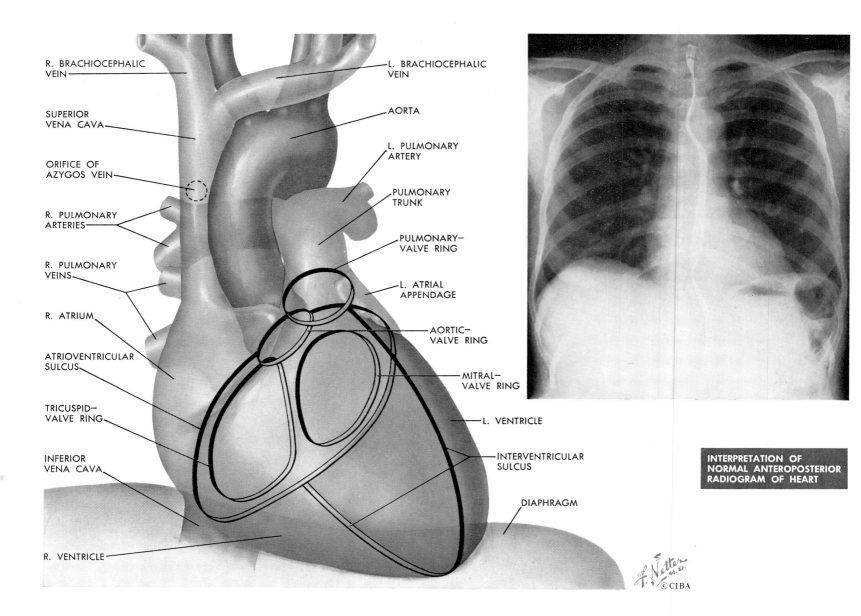

R. BRACHIOCEPHALIC VEIN

SUPERIOR VENA CAVA

ORIFICE OF AZYGOS VEIN

R. PULMONARY ARTERIES

R. PULMONARY VEINS

R. ATRIUM

ATRIOVENTRICULAR SULCUS

TRICUSPID-VALVE RING

INFERIOR VENA CAVA

R. VENTRICLE

L. BRACHIOCEPHALIC VEIN

AORTA

L. PULMONARY ARTERY

PULMONARY TRUNK

PULMONARY-VALVE RING

L. ATRIAL APPENDAGE

AORTIC-VALVE RING

MITRAL-VALVE RING

L. VENTRICLE

INTERVENTRICULAR SULCUS

DIAPHRAGM

INTERPRETATION OF NORMAL ANTEROPOSTERIOR RADIOGRAM OF HEART

RADIOLOGY AND ANGIOCARDIOGRAPHY

Radiology

Radiologic examination forms an integral and essential part of the evaluation of cardiac disease. The size of the heart, the identification of chamber enlargement and of pericardial, cardiac, and coronary calcification, and information regarding the function and hemodynamics of the heart can be determined from a study of chest roentgenograms, from fluoroscopic examination, and from angiocardiographic observations.

The myocardium, valves, and other heart structures have similar radiodensities and therefore cannot be distinguished from one another radiologically unless they are calcified. Similarly, the walls of the cardiac chambers cannot be visually separated from the blood within them unless the opacity of the blood is increased by the injection of a contrast material. The outer borders of the heart can be seen, because the relatively homogeneous cardiac shadow is contrasted against the lucent, air-containing lungs.

The shadow of the heart, as seen on standard roentgenograms or by fluoroscopy, is magnified and somewhat distorted. At the target-to-film or screen distances customarily used, the X-ray beam diverges as it passes through the patient. The structures farther from the film are magnified to a greater extent than are those in close approximation. The distortion can be largely eliminated if the X-ray beam is composed of parallel rather than divergent rays. This is accomplished either by increasing the target-film distance beyond 6 ft (teleroentgenography) or by shuttering down the beam so that only the central 3 to 4 cm are utilized. The latter method (orthodiagraphy) is a fluoroscopic technic in which the border of the heart is traced by the narrow central beam and marked by a pencil on the fluoroscopic screen. The tracing can then be measured and will provide a true index of the heart size in the selected projection. The increased accuracy afforded by these technics is rarely of practical importance, however, and they are little used at present. For most purposes, heart size can be adequately estimated, from the standard 6-ft chest film, by comparing the apparent cardiac size with that of the thorax. Allowances must be made for the degree of inspiration (the higher the diaphragm, the larger the apparent size of the heart) and for the age of the patient. An infant's heart is relatively large in comparison to the chest, whereas an older patient's chest is often small in relation to the heart.

Since the heart is a three-dimensional structure and we see only two borders in any one view, it is necessary to secure films in several projections if the various chambers and great vessels are to be brought into profile. It is also helpful if the esophagus is opacified so that the posterior border of the heart, which abuts on it, can be evaluated. A complete "cardiac series" consists of films made in the frontal, left lateral, 60-degree right anterior-oblique, and 45-degree left anterior-oblique projections. The left anterior-oblique view should be made first, before giving the patient barium, or the esophagus will obscure a portion of the cardiac border. The remainder of the films are exposed with the esophagus filled.

The four films of the cardiac series are usually sufficient for evaluating chamber enlargement. In some instances, however, an overpenetrated or Bucky frontal film of the chest is of help, as it will disclose the shadow of an enlarged left atrium through the cardiac silhouette. At times, the contours of the right atrium and ventricle or the left atrium and ventricle merge with each other, and it is difficult to determine, on the film, the point of transition between the two chambers. This can be accomplished by fluoroscopy, since the phase of pulsation of the atrium is opposite to that of the ventricle.

Plain films of the chest also allow an evaluation of the pulmonary vasculature and the lung changes that may be associated with heart disease. An increase in the size and tortuosity of the pulmonary arteries and veins usually indicates the presence of a left-to-right shunt, whereas a diminution in the prominence of these vessels is associated with a right-to-left shunt. When the

(Continued on page 23)

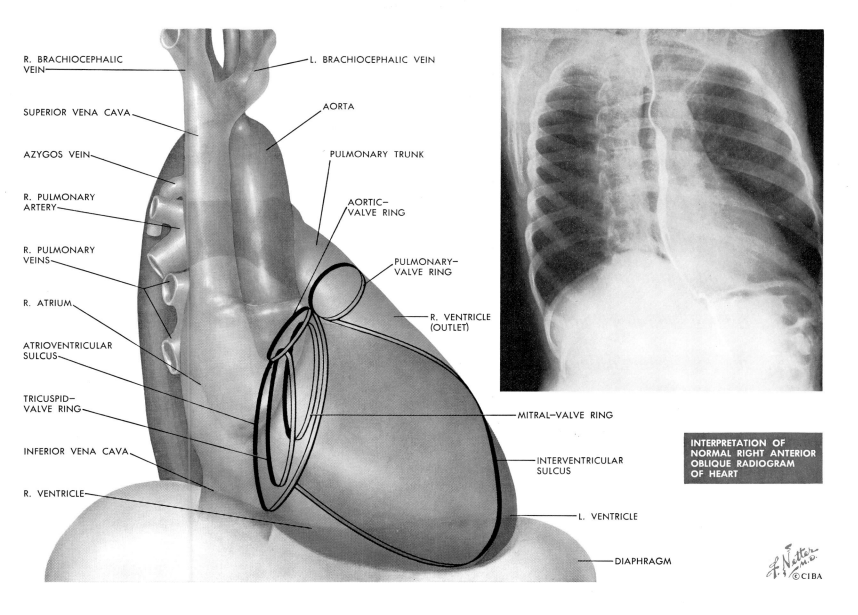

R. BRACHIOCEPHALIC VEIN

L. BRACHIOCEPHALIC VEIN

SUPERIOR VENA CAVA

AORTA

AZYGOS VEIN

PULMONARY TRUNK

R. PULMONARY ARTERY

AORTIC-VALVE RING

R. PULMONARY VEINS

PULMONARY-VALVE RING

R. ATRIUM

R. VENTRICLE (OUTLET)

ATRIOVENTRICULAR SULCUS

TRICUSPID-VALVE RING

MITRAL-VALVE RING

INFERIOR VENA CAVA

INTERVENTRICULAR SULCUS

R. VENTRICLE

INTERPRETATION OF NORMAL RIGHT ANTERIOR OBLIQUE RADIOGRAM OF HEART

L. VENTRICLE

DIAPHRAGM

RADIOLOGY AND ANGIOCARDIOGRAPHY

(Continued from page 22)

pulmonary-artery flow is markedly decreased, as in severe tetralogy of Fallot, the vascular pattern in the lungs often is reticular and nondirectional rather than an orderly radiation of vessels from the lung hilum. This indicates the presence of a significant collateral flow through the bronchial arteries. In congestive failure or in the presence of obstruction on the left side of the heart, as in mitral stenosis, the pulmonary veins become engorged. If this progresses to pulmonary hypertension, the veins, together with the peripheral pulmonary arteries, become quite small while the central pulmonary arteries dilate and become bulbous.

Because the heart is a dynamic structure, considerable information regarding its function can be gained by observing (fluoroscopically) the contraction and expansion of the heart and great vessels. Pulsations can be graphically and permanently recorded by roentgen kymography or electrokymography, but, since the advent of image intensifiers and cine recording, those older methods have been largely superseded.

The pulsations of the two ventricles occur simultaneously and opposite to those of the atria. As the ventricles contract during systole, the atria expand, and vice versa. The aorta and pulmonary artery expand with ventricular systole, as blood is ejected into them. The normal pulsations of the cardiac chambers and the vessels are expansile in nature; i.e., two points on opposite sides of the chamber will move away from each other as the chamber expands, toward each other with contraction. Not uncommonly, following a myocardial infarction, a portion of a ventricle will no longer demonstrate such expansile pulsations. This is because the scarred myocardium cannot contract but simply moves passively with the remainder of the ventricle. If the infarcted area becomes thin, a ventricular aneurysm may result. Fluoroscopically, an aneurysm is seen as a localized bulge, on the ventricular contour, which will pulsate paradoxically. As the ventricle contracts and the intraventricular pressure increases, the aneurysm expands; as the ventricle expands, the aneurysm becomes less prominent, imparting a rocking motion to the cardiac contour.

The dilated, failing heart does not pulsate normally, its borders exhibiting only minimal excursion with systole and diastole. The appearance may be quite similar to the quiet, enlarged cardiac shadow associated with a pericardial effusion. When there is a well-developed layer of epicardial fat, these two conditions can generally be distinguished fluoroscopically. Radiologically, fat appears as less dense and more lucent than heart muscle, blood, or pericardial fluid. Normally, the epicardial fat is not seen, because it lies against the outer border of the heart, near the lucent lungs. Fluid in the pericardial cavity lies outside the epicardial fat, which is then outlined by the denser myocardium on one side and the pericardial fluid on the other. The lucent fat line appears displaced inward and is separated from the outer border of the cardiac silhouette.

Alterations in the character of the pulsations of the great vessels can, at times, provide specific information regarding intracardiac lesions. The two best examples of this are the increased pulsations of the aorta associated with insufficiency of the aortic valve, and the exaggerated pulsations of the pulmonary arteries—the hilus dance—seen in the presence of a large left-to-right shunt.

Fluoroscopy is also the most accurate and sensitive method for detecting and localizing calcification of the various cardiac structures.

Frontal Projection (page 22). Since most chest films are made in the frontal (anteroposterior) projection, this view of the heart usually is seen, and it often provides the first suggestion of the presence of cardiac disease. Enlargement of the left atrium and left ventricle, as well as the right atrium, can be recognized, as a rule, in this projection. The right ventricle, although not border-forming, can produce characteristic changes in the cardiac contour. Because it is the most easily reproducible projection, heart size generally is evaluated in this view.

The upper half of the right contour of the cardiac silhouette is formed by the superior vena

(Continued on page 24)

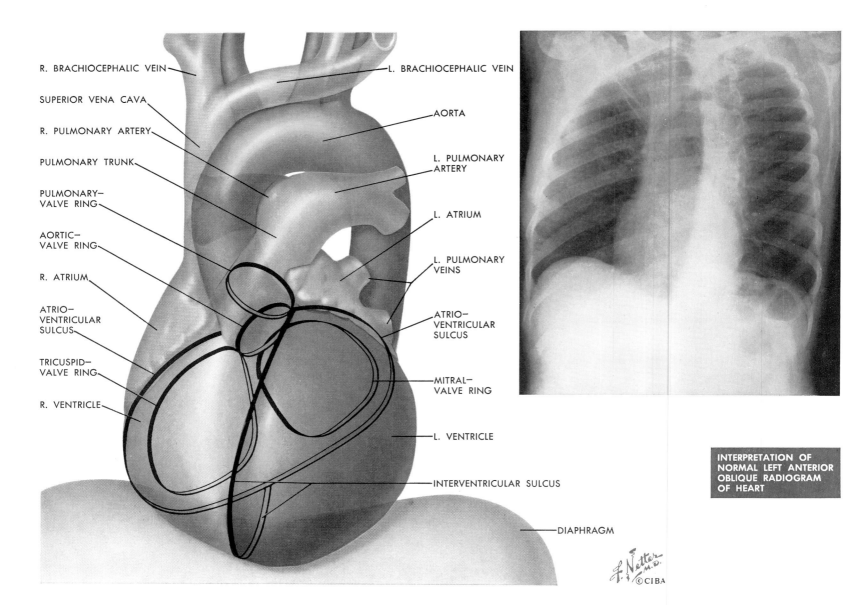

R. BRACHIOCEPHALIC VEIN

SUPERIOR VENA CAVA

R. PULMONARY ARTERY

PULMONARY TRUNK

PULMONARY–
VALVE RING

AORTIC–
VALVE RING

R. ATRIUM

ATRIO–
VENTRICULAR
SULCUS

TRICUSPID–
VALVE RING

R. VENTRICLE

L. BRACHIOCEPHALIC VEIN

AORTA

L. PULMONARY
ARTERY

L. ATRIUM

L. PULMONARY
VEINS

ATRIO–
VENTRICULAR
SULCUS

MITRAL–
VALVE RING

L. VENTRICLE

INTERVENTRICULAR SULCUS

DIAPHRAGM

INTERPRETATION OF
NORMAL LEFT ANTERIOR
OBLIQUE RADIOGRAM
OF HEART

RADIOLOGY AND ANGIOCARDIOGRAPHY

(Continued from page 23)

cava, the lower portion by the lateral wall of the right atrium. The margin of the superior vena cava is straight, but that of the right atrium bulges outward. The angle between these two contours represents the superior aspect of the right atrium. If the patient takes a deep inspiration, an indentation on the right border of the heart can be seen just above the *diaphragm,* identifying the junction of the *inferior vena cava* and the right atrium.

On the left side, the uppermost portion of the cardiovascular silhouette is formed by the distal arch of the *aorta* as it curves posteriorly and inferiorly to become the descending thoracic aorta. This is seen as a localized bulge — the aortic knob — extending from the left side of the mediastinum above the right tracheobronchial angle. This knob usually produces a localized indentation on the left side of the esophagus. In the presence of a right aortic arch, the knob will be on the right side and will displace the esophagus to the left. Immediately below the aortic knob, the main *pulmonary trunk* and *left main pulmonary artery* are border-forming. A small segment of the left cardiac silhouette, below the pulmonary artery, is formed by the *left atrial append-*

age. This segment normally is flat or slightly convex and is continuous with the curve of the left ventricle, which forms the largest portion of the left border of the cardiac contour. It is usually not possible to identify, on films, the point of transition between the normal left atrial appendage and the left ventricle. Fluoroscopically, a reversal in the phase of the pulsations between the two chambers can usually be detected.

The apex of the heart is formed by the left ventricle. In the frontal projection the right ventricle is completely hidden within the cardiac silhouette. Occasionally, if the patient takes a very deep inspiration, a portion of the diaphragmatic surface of the heart, near the cardiac apex, is disclosed. An indentation in this region marks the *interventricular sulcus* between the two ventricles.

Enlargement of the right atrium will cause an outward bowing and an increased curvature of the right heart border. When the right ventricle increases in size, the heart enlarges to the left, the apex is usually lifted, and the groove of the interventricular sulcus appears higher on the apex of the heart than it normally does. As the right ventricle enlarges, it elongates as well as widens, resulting in an elevation of the main pulmonary artery. As the left ventricle enlarges, the cardiac apex is displaced downward and to the left. Often, the entire left cardiac border is displaced to the left, becoming increasingly convex. Left atrial enlargement is detected, in the frontal view, primarily by dilatation of the left atrial

appendage, which produces a localized bulge of the left contour below the pulmonary-artery segment. In addition, the enlarged left atrium often causes an increase in the density of the central portion of the cardiac silhouette and, when sufficiently large, may elevate the left main bronchus. With increasing dilatation, the right border of the left atrium may be seen within the cardiac silhouette to the right of the spine, producing a second curved contour medial to the right atrial margin. With further enlargement, the left atrium may project behind and beyond the right atrium so that the left atrium will form the right border of the cardiac shadow. The border of the right atrium will then be seen within the shadow of the left atrium.

Calcification of the cardiac valves most often occurs secondary to rheumatic valvulitis or bacterial endocarditis and most commonly involves the *mitral* and/or *aortic valves.* In the frontal projection the mitral valve lies to the left of the spine, and, as the heart beats, calcifications on this valve will describe a flat, elliptical trajectory extending downward and to the left. The aortic valve is usually projected over the left side of the spine and moves, in a relatively straight line, upward and slightly to the right. Because of the overlapping shadows of the vertebral bodies, small calcific deposits on the aortic valve may be difficult to detect in the frontal view. The *pulmonic valve* is projected to the left of the spine, at a level higher than the aortic and mitral

(Continued on page 25)

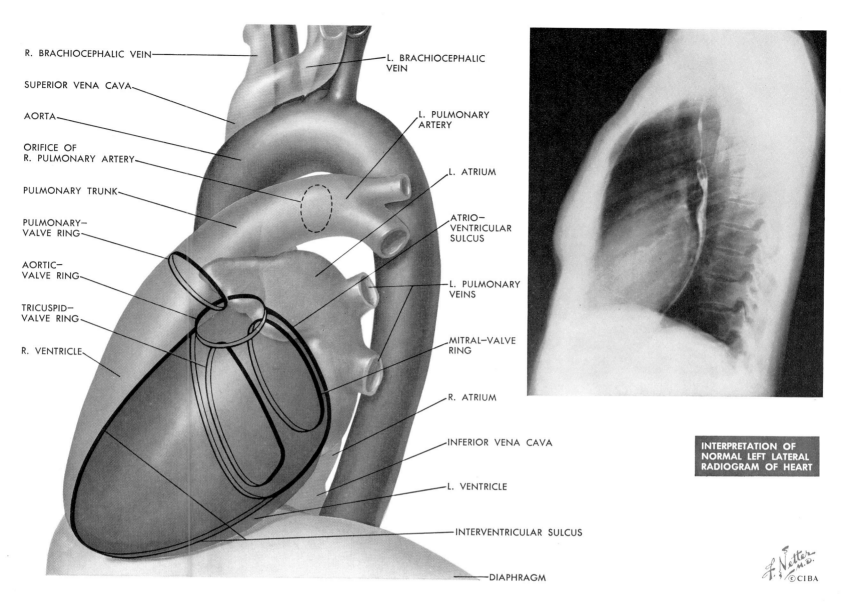

R. BRACHIOCEPHALIC VEIN

SUPERIOR VENA CAVA

AORTA

ORIFICE OF
R. PULMONARY ARTERY

PULMONARY TRUNK

PULMONARY-
VALVE RING

AORTIC-
VALVE RING

TRICUSPID-
VALVE RING

R. VENTRICLE

L. BRACHIOCEPHALIC
VEIN

L. PULMONARY
ARTERY

L. ATRIUM

ATRIO-
VENTRICULAR
SULCUS

L. PULMONARY
VEINS

MITRAL-VALVE
RING

R. ATRIUM

INFERIOR VENA CAVA

L. VENTRICLE

INTERVENTRICULAR SULCUS

DIAPHRAGM

INTERPRETATION OF
NORMAL LEFT LATERAL
RADIOGRAM OF HEART

SECTION I—PLATE 24

RADIOLOGY AND
ANGIOCARDIOGRAPHY

(Continued from page 24)

valves, and moves vertically with the cardiac pulsation. The *tricuspid valve* lies over the spine and moves in a horizontal plane.

Right Anterior-Oblique Projection (page 23). This view is used mainly to evaluate left atrial enlargement and abnormalities of the outflow portion of the right ventricle. It is also the best projection in which to study calcification of the *mitral valve*. During selective left ventricular angiocardiography, it is used to evaluate mitral stenosis or insufficiency, since the mitral valve is seen tangentially, and the left atrium is projected entirely behind the *left ventricle*. This is the only view in which these two chambers do not overlap.

In a properly positioned right anterior-oblique view, the shadow of the spine lies to the right of the cardiac silhouette, and a thin vertical band of air-containing lung separates the two structures. The aortic arch is foreshortened in this view, and the descending aorta partially overlaps the vertebral column.

The right border of the heart is formed by the right posterior aspect of the left atrium, above, and the posterior border of the *right atrium*, below. As the obliquity of the projection is increased, more of the left atrium comes into

profile. The barium-filled esophagus is in contact with this border of the *heart,* and displacement of the esophagus by an enlarged left atrium is best seen in this view.

The uppermost portion of the left border of the cardiovascular silhouette is almost vertical and represents the *ascending aorta.* Just below this segment, the cardiac contour slopes downward and to the left, in a gentle curve, and is formed by the *outflow tract (outlet) of the right ventricle* and the *pulmonary trunk.* The inferior continuation of this curve is formed by the anterior wall of the left ventricle. As in the frontal view, the body of the right ventricle is in contact with the *diaphragm* and cannot be visualized.

The mitral valve is seen almost tangentially and is projected over the midportion of the cardiac silhouette. Because of the lack of confusing, overlapping shadows and because the direction of motion of the mitral valve is perpendicular to the X-ray beam, calcification of this valve is best detected, fluoroscopically, in the right anterior-oblique projection. The elliptical orbit of the valve is directed mainly horizontally. The *aortic valve* is thrown clear of the spine, and, although it is in contact with the upper border of the mitral valve, calcification of the aortic valve can be recognized as it moves mostly in an up-and-down direction. This projection also provides the greatest separation of the aortic and *pulmonic valves.* The latter valve lies at a level higher than the aortic valve, and to its left, touching the left border of the cardiac silhouette. The line of

motion of the pulmonic valve is directed upward and to the right. The *tricuspid valve* is seen almost tangentially and slightly behind the mitral valve. It moves horizontally with the cardiac pulsation and, in the rare instance when the valve is calcified, is easily mistaken for a calcified mitral valve.

Aneurysms of the anterior portion of the left ventricle are best seen in this view.

Left Anterior-Oblique Projection (page 24). This view is very useful in evaluating the size of the *left atrium* and *left ventricle.* The *aortic arch* is seen clearly, because it is oriented roughly parallel to the film and is projected with little foreshortening. A selective left ventricular angiocardiogram, in the left oblique projection, is useful in the detection of a ventricular septal defect, because most of the muscular interventricular septum and a portion of the membranous septum are seen tangentially.

The right border of the cardiac contour is formed by the *right atrium,* above, and the *right ventricle,* below. As the degree of obliquity is increased, more of the right ventricle becomes border-forming. Enlargement of the right atrium will cause an increase in the convexity of the upper right cardiac border; enlargement of the right ventricle usually will produce a more-generalized increase in the curvature of this border.

The left cardiac contour is formed mostly by the left ventricle, except for the upper quarter, which is contributed by the left posterior aspect

(Continued on page 26)

RADIOLOGY AND ANGIOCARDIOGRAPHY

(Continued from page 25)

of the left atrium, directly beneath the left main bronchus. Usually, in a proper 45-degree oblique view, the shadow of a normal left ventricle will not· extend to the left of the shadow of the spine. When this does occur, it indicates an enlargement of the left ventricle. However, this sign must be evaluated cautiously, because, with lesser degrees of obliquity or if the film is not made in full inspiration, a normal left ventricle may not clear the spine. Aneurysms of the posterior left ventricular wall are usually best identified in this view. If the stomach is distended with air, the diaphragmatic surface of the left ventricle can also be evaluated.

The left atrial portion of the cardiac contour is usually straight or minimally convex. An outward bulging in this region denotes left atrial enlargement. This probably is the most sensitive roentgen sign of left atrial enlargement. The esophagus is projected directly over the left atrial segment; therefore, barium must not be given until after this film has been made, because significant degrees of left atrial enlargement could be obscured. With greater degrees of enlargement, the dilated left atrium will push the left main bronchus upward toward the horizontal. The dilated atrium will also encroach on the clear space below the aortic arch.

The greatest length of the aortic arch is seen in this view, and the origins of the great vessels are maximally separated. Thus, this projection is the best for identifying aneurysms of the aortic arch and for opacification studies of the aorta and great vessels.

The *mitral valve* is seen almost directly en face. As a result, calcific deposits on the cusps may be difficult to see, because they move on an axis perpendicular to the fluoroscopic screen, with very little horizontal excursion. In addition, the valve may be hidden partially by the shadow of the spine. Calcification of the *tricuspid valve* can be differentiated from that of the mitral valve because the two valves are completely separated in this projection, the tricuspid valve lying in the right half of the cardiac silhouette. This view is well suited for identifying calcification of the *aortic valve,* which lies in the upper portion of the cardiac silhouette, clear of the spine, and moves along an axis directed upward and to the right. The *pulmonic valve* is situated slightly higher than the aortic valve and moves upward and toward the left.

Lateral Projection (page 25). This view is used primarily for evaluating the presence of right ventricular enlargement, left atrial enlargement, and combined enlargement of the *left atrium* and *left ventricle.* It is also the best view for distinguishing between calcification of the *aortic* and the *mitral valve,* on plain films or on tomograms. A selective right ventricular angiocardiogram, in this projec-

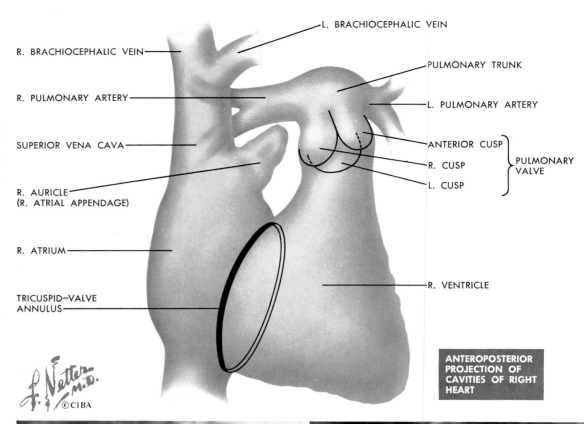

R. BRACHIOCEPHALIC VEIN
R. PULMONARY ARTERY
SUPERIOR VENA CAVA
R. AURICLE (R. ATRIAL APPENDAGE)
R. ATRIUM
TRICUSPID–VALVE ANNULUS
L. BRACHIOCEPHALIC VEIN
PULMONARY TRUNK
L. PULMONARY ARTERY
ANTERIOR CUSP
R. CUSP } PULMONARY VALVE
L. CUSP
R. VENTRICLE

ANTEROPOSTERIOR PROJECTION OF CAVITIES OF RIGHT HEART

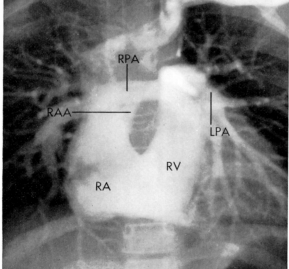

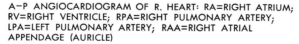

A-P ANGIOCARDIOGRAM OF R. HEART: RA=RIGHT ATRIUM; RV=RIGHT VENTRICLE; RPA=RIGHT PULMONARY ARTERY; LPA=LEFT PULMONARY ARTERY; RAA=RIGHT ATRIAL APPENDAGE (AURICLE)

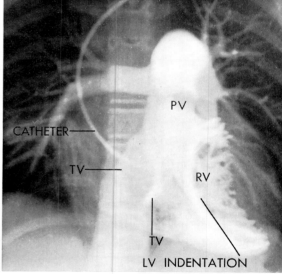

A-P ANGIOCARDIOGRAM: CATHETER IN R. VENTRICLE VISUALIZING VENTRICLE AND R. OUTFLOW TRACT; TV=TRICUSPID VALVE; PV=PULMONARY VALVE

tion, provides the best visualization of the outflow portion of the *right ventricle* and the *pulmonic valve.*

The *heart* is projected clear of the confusing shadows of the sternum and the spine. The anterior margin of the cardiac silhouette is formed by the apex and outflow tract of the right ventricle. Normally, this abuts on the lower quarter or third of the anterior chest wall. The upper two thirds of the anterior cardiac contour are formed by two convex arcs, slanting upward and posteriorly. The lower arc — the more oblique of the two — is formed by the outflow portion of the right ventricle, the upper one by the *ascending aorta.* The radiolucent lung is interposed between these two structures and the sternum. As the right ventricle enlarges, it bulges forward and tends to obliterate more and more of the retrosternal space. Similarly, dilatation and tortuosity, or an aneurysm of the ascending aorta, will encroach on the upper retrosternal space. The upper margin of the aortic

arch, distal to the origin of the great vessels, can usually be identified.

The posterior border of the heart is formed mostly by the posterior wall of the left atrium. Just above the *diaphragm,* small portions of the right atrium and *inferior vena cava* come into profile. When the left ventricle is enlarged, however, it may extend farther, posteriorly, than the *right atrium,* forming the lower portion of the posterior heart border as well. This contour of the heart is evaluated best when the esophagus is filled with barium. The esophagus lies immediately behind the left atrium and left ventricle, and an enlargement of these chambers will indent the anterior wall of the esophagus and displace it posteriorly. If only the left atrium is enlarged, the indentation on the esophagus is localized and occurs at the level of the upper half of the cardiac silhouette, the lower portion of the esophagus being in its normal position.

(Continued on page 27)

RADIOLOGY AND ANGIOCARDIOGRAPHY

(Continued from page 26)

When the left ventricle is enlarged as well, it also pushes the esophagus posteriorly, and the backward curve of the displaced esophagus is then continuous over the entire length of the cardiac silhouette, to the *diaphragm*.

Without the aid of fluoroscopy to identify the axis of motion of valve calcification, localization of a calcific deposit to the mitral or the aortic valve may be difficult. This problem can be resolved in the lateral view. If a line is drawn from the anterior costophrenic sulcus to the point of bifurcation of the trachea, the aortic valve will lie above and in front of this line, while the mitral valve will be below and posterior. The mitral valve moves more or less horizontally in this view, and the aortic valve moves on a vertical axis that is tilted slightly anteriorly and upward. The pulmonic valve is located above the aortic valve and more anteriorly, extending to the anterior border of the cardiac shadow.

Angiocardiography

Roentgen films and fluoroscopy demonstrate only the outer borders of the heart and great vessels. Considerably more information is obtained when the blood is opacified by injecting a contrast medium into the vascular system, so that the inner borders of the cardiac chambers and vessels can be visualized. The structure and motion of the valves can be studied, as can the hemodynamics of the cardiac and pulmonary circulation. The basic requirements for successful angiocardiography are a rapid injection of the contrast material, so that it flows as a radiopaque bolus, and rapid serial roentgenograms of the heart to follow the course of the contrast material. The iodinated contrast medium can be injected into a peripheral vein, whence it is carried to the *heart* via the *superior* or *inferior vena cava,* or it can be injected through a *catheter* directly into a specific cardiac chamber or great vessel. The latter technic, *selective angiocardiography,* provides greater anatomic detail, because the contrast material reaches the chamber as a denser, more-compact bolus and is not diluted in the *right atrium* by nonopaque blood.

A catheter can be placed in the *right atrium, right ventricle,* or *pulmonary trunk* by introducing it into a peripheral vein and then advancing it through the superior or inferior vena cava. In infants less than 4 or 5 days old, the umbilical vein can be used for this purpose. In children, the left atrium can usually be entered by manipulating a catheter in the right atrium, across the foramen ovale. In adults, a similar route is used, the atrial septum being punctured by a transseptal needle and a catheter then being advanced over the needle into the left atrium. The left ventricle is reached by

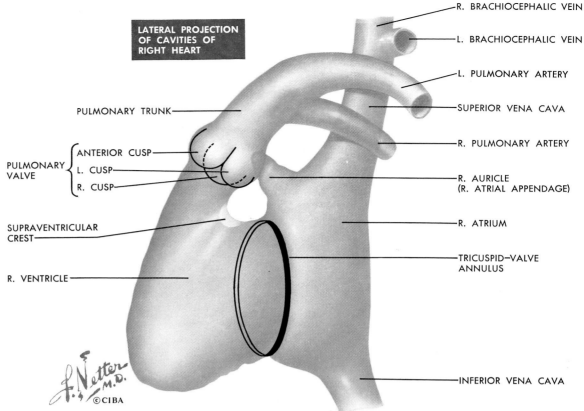

LATERAL PROJECTION OF CAVITIES OF RIGHT HEART

PULMONARY TRUNK

PULMONARY VALVE { ANTERIOR CUSP / L. CUSP / R. CUSP }

SUPRAVENTRICULAR CREST

R. VENTRICLE

R. BRACHIOCEPHALIC VEIN

L. BRACHIOCEPHALIC VEIN

L. PULMONARY ARTERY

SUPERIOR VENA CAVA

R. PULMONARY ARTERY

R. AURICLE (R. ATRIAL APPENDAGE)

R. ATRIUM

TRICUSPID–VALVE ANNULUS

INFERIOR VENA CAVA

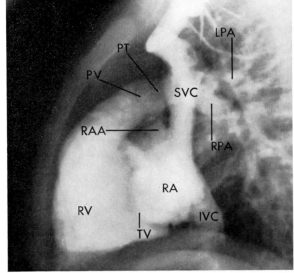

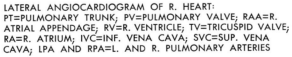

LATERAL ANGIOCARDIOGRAM OF R. HEART: PT=PULMONARY TRUNK; PV=PULMONARY VALVE; RAA=R. ATRIAL APPENDAGE; RV=R. VENTRICLE; TV=TRICUSPID VALVE; RA=R. ATRIUM; IVC=INF. VENA CAVA; SVC=SUP. VENA CAVA; LPA AND RPA=L. AND R. PULMONARY ARTERIES

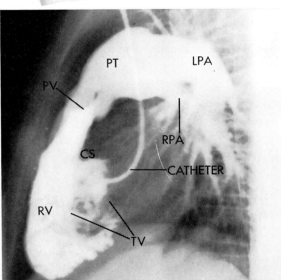

LATERAL ANGIOCARDIOGRAM: CATHETER IN R. VENTRICLE, VISUALIZING VENTRICLE AND OUTFLOW TRACT; CS=SUPRAVENTRICULAR CREST

inserting a catheter into a peripheral artery and passing it retrograde through the aortic valve into the ventricle. If the catheter has the proper curve, it can be manipulated backward through the mitral valve into the left atrium. The left ventricle can also be reached by a transseptal catheter passed from the right atrium into the left atrium and advanced through the mitral valve. The left ventricle can be punctured directly through the anterior chest wall, but angiocardiography by this route has a substantial risk.

Right Heart, Frontal Projection (page 26). The right side of the heart usually can be well visualized by venous angiocardiography as well as by selective injection. In the *frontal (anteroposterior) projection* the superior and inferior venae cavae lie in a straight line to the right of the spine, entering opposite ends of the right atrium. The free wall of the right atrium is thin and is represented by the space between the

right border of the contrast-filled atrium and the right border of the cardiac silhouette. Normally, this measures 2 to 3 mm in diameter. An increase in the width of this space is indicative of a pericardial effusion separating the wall of the right atrium from the pericardium.

The *right atrial appendage (auricle)* extends medially and upward from the upper portion of the right atrium. The *tricuspid valve* lies in an oblique plane relative to the frontal projection, and the line of attachment of its cusps is often seen as an ellipse overlying the spine. The inferior margin of the *tricuspid annulus* lies adjacent to the entrance of the inferior vena cava into the right atrium. The opening of the coronary sinus lies in the same region. This must be kept in mind when catheterizing the right ventricle, since a catheter which has entered the coronary sinus and advanced into the great cardiac vein will

(Continued on page 28)

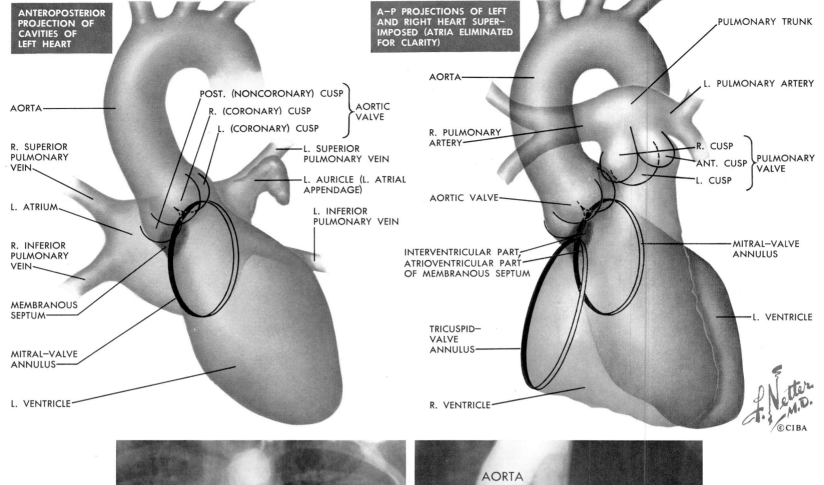

ANTEROPOSTERIOR PROJECTION OF CAVITIES OF LEFT HEART

AORTA

POST. (NONCORONARY) CUSP
R. (CORONARY) CUSP
L. (CORONARY) CUSP
} AORTIC VALVE

R. SUPERIOR PULMONARY VEIN

L. SUPERIOR PULMONARY VEIN

L. AURICLE (L. ATRIAL APPENDAGE)

L. ATRIUM

L. INFERIOR PULMONARY VEIN

R. INFERIOR PULMONARY VEIN

MEMBRANOUS SEPTUM

MITRAL-VALVE ANNULUS

L. VENTRICLE

A–P PROJECTIONS OF LEFT AND RIGHT HEART SUPERIMPOSED (ATRIA ELIMINATED FOR CLARITY)

PULMONARY TRUNK

AORTA

L. PULMONARY ARTERY

R. PULMONARY ARTERY

R. CUSP
ANT. CUSP
L. CUSP
} PULMONARY VALVE

AORTIC VALVE

INTERVENTRICULAR PART,
ATRIOVENTRICULAR PART
OF MEMBRANOUS SEPTUM

MITRAL-VALVE ANNULUS

TRICUSPID-VALVE ANNULUS

L. VENTRICLE

R. VENTRICLE

F. Netter M.D.
©CIBA

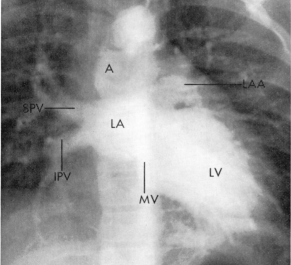

A–P ANGIOCARDIOGRAM OF L. HEART: LA=LEFT ATRIUM;
LV=LEFT VENTRICLE; MV=MITRAL VALVE; A=AORTA;
SPV=SUPERIOR, AND IPV=INFERIOR R. PULMONARY VEINS;
LAA=L. ATRIAL APPENDAGE

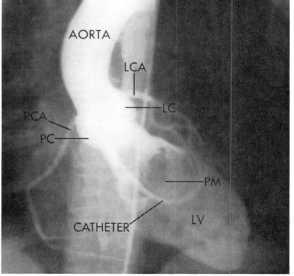

A–P ANGIOCARDIOGRAM: CATHETER IN L. VENTRICLE;
LCA=LEFT CORONARY ARTERY; RCA=RIGHT CORONARY
ARTERY; LC=LEFT CUSP; PC=POSTERIOR CUSP
OF AORTIC VALVE; PM=POST. MITRAL-CUSP ATTACHMENT

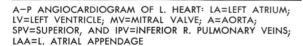

SECTION I—PLATE 27

RADIOLOGY AND ANGIOCARDIOGRAPHY

(Continued from page 27)

follow almost the identical course, in the frontal projection, as one that has crossed the tricuspid valve and lies within the *outflow tract of the right ventricle*. The left border of the ring of the tricuspid valve which forms the left border of the atrium corresponds to the posterior margin of the valve. The right ventricle, in front of the atrium, extends to the right (or anterior) border of the tricuspid valve. Within the elliptical projection of the valve, therefore, the atrium and ventricle overlie each other.

The right ventricle is a roughly triangular-shaped chamber which can be divided into two portions — a large, trabeculated inflow portion and a smooth, narrow outflow tract. In the frontal view these two can be separated by a line drawn from the uppermost margin of the tricuspid valve, downward and to the left, toward the apex of the ventricle. This line will roughly approximate the course of the septal and moderator bands. The inflow tract lies below the line, the outflow tract above the line extending to the *pulmonic valve*. The right border of the inflow portion is formed by the tricuspid valve, the left border by the interventricular septum. The diaphragmatic surface of the right ventricle is a free wall. The right border of the outflow tract is also a free wall and is formed by a sheet of muscle extending from the tricuspid to the pulmonic

valve, lying in front of the root of the aorta. A localized prominence in this muscle, the crista supraventricularis, is projected en face in this view and cannot be identified. The line of attachment of the tricuspid valve can often be seen during diastole, on a selective right ventricular *angiocardiogram*, since contrast material is trapped between the open valve cusps and the walls of the ventricle, while the orifice of the valve is filled by nonopaque blood entering from the atrium.

The pulmonic valve is projected partially en face and is not well visualized in the frontal view. The pulmonary trunk is usually seen well, but its root may be obscured, in part, by the outflow portion of the right ventricle. The *right pulmonary artery* courses almost directly to the right, and its

(Continued on page 29)

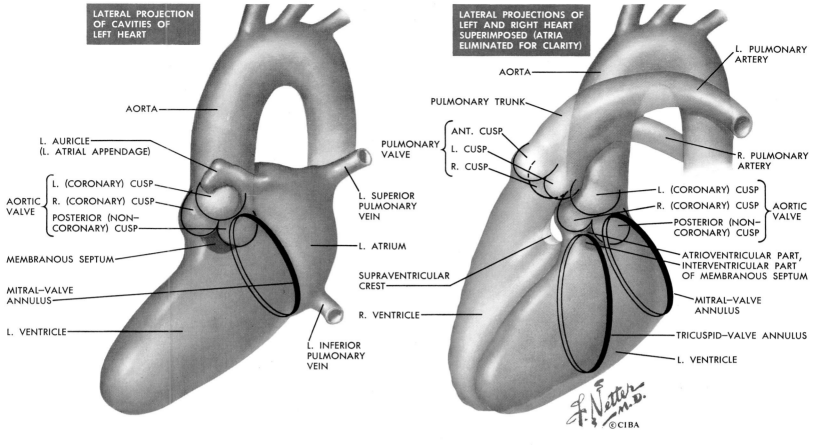

LATERAL PROJECTION OF CAVITIES OF LEFT HEART

AORTA

L. AURICLE (L. ATRIAL APPENDAGE)

AORTIC VALVE { L. (CORONARY) CUSP / R. (CORONARY) CUSP / POSTERIOR (NON-CORONARY) CUSP

MEMBRANOUS SEPTUM

MITRAL–VALVE ANNULUS

L. VENTRICLE

L. SUPERIOR PULMONARY VEIN

L. ATRIUM

R. VENTRICLE

L. INFERIOR PULMONARY VEIN

LATERAL PROJECTIONS OF LEFT AND RIGHT HEART SUPERIMPOSED (ATRIA ELIMINATED FOR CLARITY)

L. PULMONARY ARTERY

AORTA

PULMONARY TRUNK

PULMONARY VALVE { ANT. CUSP / L. CUSP / R. CUSP

R. PULMONARY ARTERY

L. (CORONARY) CUSP

R. (CORONARY) CUSP

POSTERIOR (NON-CORONARY) CUSP

} AORTIC VALVE

ATRIOVENTRICULAR PART, INTERVENTRICULAR PART OF MEMBRANOUS SEPTUM

MITRAL–VALVE ANNULUS

TRICUSPID–VALVE ANNULUS

L. VENTRICLE

SUPRAVENTRICULAR CREST

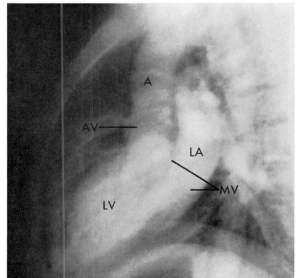

LATERAL ANGIOCARDIOGRAM OF L. HEART: A=AORTA; AV=AORTIC VALVE; LV=L. VENTRICLE; MV=MITRAL VALVE; LA=L. ATRIUM

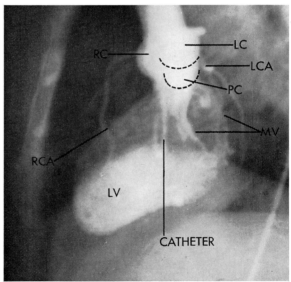

LATERAL ANGIOCARDIOGRAM: CATHETER IN L. VENTRICLE; RC=RIGHT CUSP; LC=LEFT CUSP; PC=POST. CUSP OF AORTIC VALVE; RCA=R. CORONARY ARTERY; LCA=L. CORONARY ARTERY

RADIOLOGY AND ANGIOCARDIOGRAPHY

(Continued from page 28)

greatest length can be seen in this projection, while the *left pulmonary artery* is directed posteriorly and is foreshortened. A steep left anterior-oblique or left lateral view is best for the study of the left pulmonary artery. On a venous angiocardiogram, a portion of the right pulmonary artery is often obscured by contrast material in the superior vena cava or in the right atrium, especially if this chamber is enlarged. Because of this, when performing angiocardiography for a suspected pulmonary-artery thrombus, a selective injection

should be made into the main pulmonary artery rather than into a peripheral vein.

Right Heart, Lateral View (page 27). In the lateral view the *right atrium* is projected almost entirely behind the *right ventricle*. The posterior border of the atrium is a free wall. The interatrial septum lies in an oblique plane and cannot be visualized in either the frontal or the lateral projection. It is seen tangentially only in a steep right posterior-oblique view. The anterior margin of the right atrium is formed by the *tricuspid valve*. The *atrial appendage* arises at a level higher than the valve and extends anteriorly and superiorly. The appendage is roughly triangular in shape, its base being continuous with the atrial cavity. The border of the cavity of the appendage is irregular, because of the pectinate muscles.

The ostium of the coronary sinus lies in the

inferior portion of the atrium just in front of the entrance of the *inferior vena cava*, and the great cardiac vein extends along the posterior aspect of the heart. Therefore, a catheter, passed through the *superior vena cava*, which has entered the great cardiac vein, will curve posteriorly, in the lateral view, rather than anteriorly as it does when it traverses the tricuspid valve to enter the right ventricle.

The right ventricle is best studied by selective angiocardiography because, in the lateral view, the opacified *right atrial appendage*, especially if large, often extends far enough anteriorly to obscure a portion of the *outflow tract or the pulmonic valve*. On a selective study the tricuspid valve can usually be identified as an oblique ring on the posterior aspect of the ventricle. The ante-

(Continued on page 30)

rior border of this ring corresponds to the right margin of the valve. The main body of the right ventricle — the inflow portion — lies directly in front of the tricuspid valve. Just above the upper level of the valve, the ventricle becomes narrowed because of the intrusion of a soft-tissue mass on its posterior aspect. This represents the *crista supraventricularis* and marks the level of the entrance to the infundibulum — the outflow portion of the ventricle. The anterior border of the right ventricular cavity forms a continuous curve to the pulmonic valve.

The pulmonic valve and its cusps are easily identified in the lateral view. This is an ideal projection for the study of pulmonic valvular stenosis, as not only can one see the limitation in the opening of the valve cusps, but the infundibular region of the ventricle can be studied also, and the possibility of associated infundibular stenosis can be evaluated. The *pulmonary trunk* courses upward and backward, continuing the curve of the anterior wall of the right ventricle. The left pulmonary artery is well seen, in the lateral view, as it courses posteriorly, while the right pulmonary artery is foreshortened.

Left Heart, Frontal Projection (page 28). The *left atrium* lies partly above and to the right of the *left ventricle*. The upper border of the atrial cavity in the frontal (*anteroposterior*) view is straight, slanting upward and to the left. The lower margin is bowed downward. The portion of the lower atrial margin that crosses the left ventricular chamber is formed by the inferior margin of the *mitral valve*. The two *superior pulmonary veins* enter the uppermost portion of the atrium, the *inferior pulmonary veins* entering at a slightly lower level. The *left atrial appendage (auricle)*, which often has a hooklike contour in this view, extends to the left border of the heart and overlies the *left superior pulmonary vein*. It may be difficult to distinguish, fluoroscopically, whether a catheter in the *left atrium* has entered the atrial appendage or the left superior pulmonary vein. This can be resolved by viewing the patient in an oblique or lateral projection (since the pulmonary vein extends posteriorly, whereas the appendage lies anteriorly) or by injecting a small quantity of contrast material and outlining the structure.

The left ventricle differs basically from the right in that the inflow (mitral) valve and the outflow (aortic) valve lie adjacent to each other. Indeed, the anterior cusp of the mitral valve arises from a common *annulus* with part of the aortic valve. The body of the left ventricle lies below the two valves rather than being interposed between them, as it is in the *right ventricle*. The left ventricle is roughly oval in shape, with its apex pointing downward and to the left. The trabeculation of the body of the left ventricle is much finer than that of the right ventricle. On a selective left ventricular injection, the inferior portion of the ring of the mitral valve can usually be identified as a curvilinear interface between the contrast material, trapped under the posterior mitral cusp, and the nonopaque blood entering from the left atrium above it. The superior margin of the mitral ring, which is continuous with the aortic ring, usually is not well seen in the frontal view. During ventricular systole, the mitral cusps bulge toward the left atrium, the valve orifice is obscured by the contrast material

in the ventricle, and the line of attachment of the cusps can no longer be observed. Also during ventricular systole, fingerlike indentations, arising from the left and right margins of the ventricle, are often seen intruding into the ventricular lumen, representing the papillary muscles.

The *membranous portion* of the *interventricular septum* cannot be delineated on the *angiocardiogram*. However, its location can be determined in relation to the aortic valve. It lies beneath the anterior portion of the *posterior (noncoronary) cusp* and a small part of the adjacent *right (coronary) cusp* and the commissure between the two. In the frontal projection, the right cusp is seen en face, the *left cusp* forming the left border of the *aortic valve* and the noncoronary cusp the right border. The membranous septum thus forms a segment of the right border of the left ventricle immediately beneath the aortic valve.

The *right coronary artery* arises from the midportion of the aortic valve, in this view, and extends slightly to the right and downward, running in the sulcus between the right atrium and ventricle. The *left coronary artery* originates from the left border of the aortic valve. The anterior descending branch courses downward in the interventricular sulcus overlying the left portion of the left ventricle. The circumflex branch curves to the right, paralleling the inferior attachment of the mitral valve, as it runs in the sulcus between the left atrium and ventricle on the posterior aspect of the heart.

The relationships of the structures on the right and left sides of the heart can be appreciated when the drawings of the two ventricles and their great vessels are *superimposed*. The ventricles are projected on top of one another, for the most part. The outflow tract of the right ventricle is directed upward and toward the left, while blood in the left ventricle reaches the aorta by passing upward and to the right. Thus, the outflow tracts cross each other, the left passing behind the right. Almost the entire right border of the left ventricle is formed by the interventricular septum, the uppermost part being membranous and the remainder muscular. In addition, a segment of the upper left border of the left ventricle also represents the interventricular septum. This is the basal portion of the muscular septum which, on the right side, lies in the lower portion of the infundibulum just above the septal band. The uppermost margin of the tricuspid-valve attachment reaches almost to the aortic valve, and the origin of the septal cusp of the *tricuspid valve* actually crosses the membranous septum. Thus, the membranous septum, on the left side, lies completely within the left ventricle, whereas, on the right side, the anterior portion lies in the right ventricle (interventricular septum), and the posterior portion lies behind the tricuspid valve in the right atrium (atrioventricular septum).

The upper outflow tract of the right ventricle lies above the left ventricle at the level of the aortic sinuses of Valsalva. The pulmonic valve is at a level higher than the aortic valve, the two touching only near the commissures between the right and left cusps.

Left Heart, Lateral Projection (page 29). In the lateral view the *left atrium* is projected almost completely behind the *left ventricle*. The anteroinferior margin of the atrium is formed by the *mitral valve*. The *left atrial appendage (auricle)* arises somewhat above the mitral valve and extends anteriorly, crossing the *aorta* just above the sinuses of Valsalva. If the atrial appendage is sufficiently large, its tip may overlie the *pul-

monic valve*. The posterior border of the atrial cavity is formed by the free wall of the atrium, the pulmonary veins entering its upper and middle portions.

On a selective left ventricular *angiocardiogram*, the line of insertion of the mitral-valve cusps can usually be seen, during diastole, as an opaque ring surrounding the radiolucent blood within the valve orifice. The mitral valve forms the posterior boundary of the ventricle. The upper margin of the mitral valve reaches the *aortic valve* in the region of the commissure between the *left (coronary)* and *posterior (noncoronary) cusps*. The body of the ventricle extends forward and downward from the mitral valve. The posteroinferior border of the body is formed by the free ventricular wall, the entire anterior border being bounded by the *interventricular septum*. The papillary muscles may be seen, in some cases, as radiolucent defects arising from the midportion of the lower border of the ventricle and directed toward the mitral valve.

In this view the *right coronary cusp* of the *aortic valve* is seen tangentially, forming the anterior border of the valve. The left and posterior cusps are projected obliquely and lie posteriorly, with the posterior (noncoronary) cusp always the lower of the two. The *membranous portion* of the interventricular septum, directly below the commissure between the right and noncoronary cusps, is not border-forming. Directly in front of the membranous septum, and comprising the anterior subvalvular border of the ventricle, is the superior portion of the muscular septum.

The *right coronary artery* arises from the upper portion of the right sinus of Valsalva and courses anteriorly, for a short distance, before it curves almost directly downward. The main trunk of the *left coronary artery* is parallel to the X-ray beam and is foreshortened in this view. Its circumflex branch parallels the posterior aspect of the mitral ring. The anterior or descending branch extends anteriorly and downward, overlying the aortic root. It courses over the right sinus of Valsalva, slightly below the origin of the right coronary artery, and then crosses this vessel, so that the lower portion of the anterior descending branch is the most anterior of the major coronary vessels. When the right ventricle is enlarged, the sulcus between the ventricle and the right atrium is displaced anteriorly. The right coronary artery which lies within this sulcus is then seen in the lateral view, completely in front of the left anterior descending branch. In this way, right ventricular enlargement can be recognized on a selective left ventricular angiocardiogram.

When the lateral views of the two ventricles are *superimposed*, it is seen that the *tricuspid valve* lies anterior to the mitral valve. The upper margin of the tricuspid valve demarcates the anterior extent of the *atrioventricular septum*; the mitral valve, the posterior extent. The interventricular portion of the membranous septum lies anterior to the insertion of the tricuspid valve. The *supraventricular crest* is directly in front of the right sinus of Valsalva, so that most of the right ventricular-outflow tract is at a higher level than the left ventricle. Actually, a small portion of the outflow part of the left ventricle, immediately below the commissure between the right and left aortic cusps, does reach the same level as the subpulmonic region of the right ventricle. The outflow tracts are separated in this area by the ventricular septum, and a defect in this region will produce a subpulmonic ventricular septal defect.

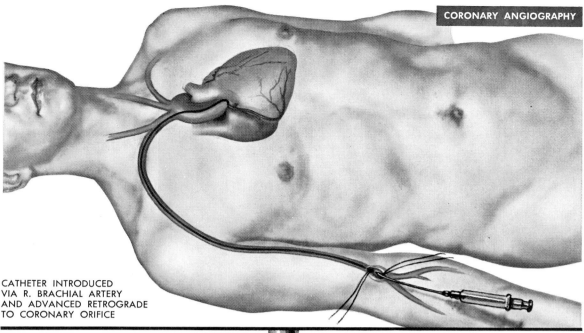

CORONARY ANGIOGRAPHY

SELECTIVE CINE CORONARY ARTERIOGRAPHY

CATHETER INTRODUCED
VIA R. BRACHIAL ARTERY
AND ADVANCED RETROGRADE
TO CORONARY ORIFICE

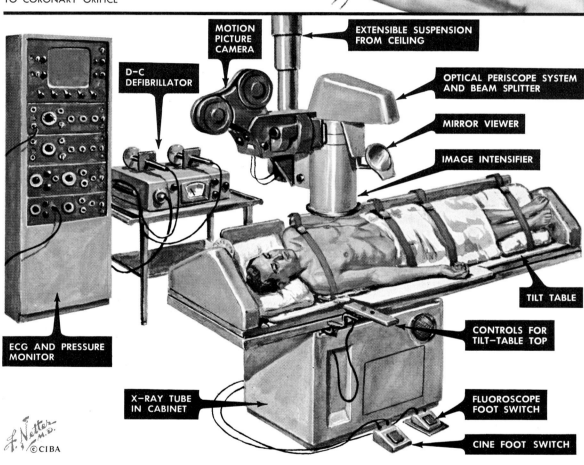

MOTION PICTURE CAMERA

EXTENSIBLE SUSPENSION FROM CEILING

D-C DEFIBRILLATOR

OPTICAL PERISCOPE SYSTEM AND BEAM SPLITTER

MIRROR VIEWER

IMAGE INTENSIFIER

TILT TABLE

CONTROLS FOR TILT-TABLE TOP

ECG AND PRESSURE MONITOR

X-RAY TUBE IN CABINET

FLUOROSCOPE FOOT SWITCH

CINE FOOT SWITCH

The diagnosis of human coronary atherosclerosis depended primarily, until recently, on the ability of the physician to interpret the significance of chest pain described by patients who experience infinitely variable subjective responses to stress. Objective confirmation hinged upon the recognition of transient or persistent electrocardiographic changes which usually indicate the presence of myocardial ischemia, necrosis, or scar-tissue replacement of functioning myocardium. It was thus possible to recognize the presence of coronary atherosclerosis, in the living human, only after the dis-ease process had progressed to a point where arterial obstructions were so severe as to cause transient or permanent secondary changes in the myocardium.

Selective *cine coronary arteriography* provides a clinically useful approach to the precise demonstration of the morphologic characteristics of the human coronary-artery tree (see pages 16 and 17). In the study of more than 10,500 patients representing all phases of the natural history of coronary atherosclerosis, only 9 deaths have been attributable to this arteriographic procedure.

Technic

Under local anesthesia the *right brachial artery* is mobilized routinely in the right antecubital fossa immediately above its bifurcation. An 8-French woven *catheter*, 80 cm long, with a special tip which tapers to a 5-French diameter in its distal 2 in., is passed *retrograde* from the right brachial artery directly into the ascending aorta. The catheter tip is *introduced* directly, first into one and then into the other *coronary orifice*, under direct vision, utilizing a 6-in. *image* amplifier (*intensifier*) equipped with either an *optical system* or a closed-circuit television unit to provide direct visualization during the procedure.

Pressure measurements from the catheter tip are *recorded* constantly with a Statham P-23 D-b strain gauge, to permit immediate recognition of arterial

(*Continued on page 32*)

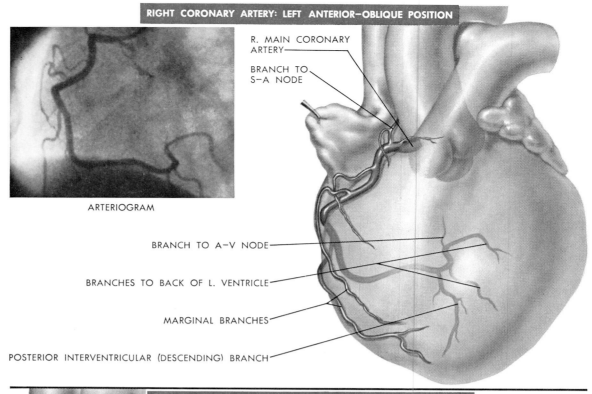

RIGHT CORONARY ARTERY: LEFT ANTERIOR–OBLIQUE POSITION

R. MAIN CORONARY ARTERY

BRANCH TO S–A NODE

ARTERIOGRAM

BRANCH TO A–V NODE

BRANCHES TO BACK OF L. VENTRICLE

MARGINAL BRANCHES

POSTERIOR INTERVENTRICULAR (DESCENDING) BRANCH

SELECTIVE CINE CORONARY ARTERIOGRAPHY

(Continued from page 31)

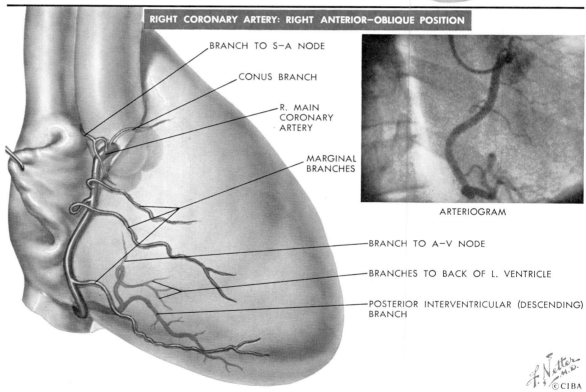

RIGHT CORONARY ARTERY: RIGHT ANTERIOR–OBLIQUE POSITION

BRANCH TO S–A NODE

CONUS BRANCH

R. MAIN CORONARY ARTERY

MARGINAL BRANCHES

ARTERIOGRAM

BRANCH TO A–V NODE

BRANCHES TO BACK OF L. VENTRICLE

POSTERIOR INTERVENTRICULAR (DESCENDING) BRANCH

occlusion by the catheter tip. The *electrocardiogram* also is *monitored constantly*.

Multiple small doses of contrast medium are injected directly into the orifice of each *coronary artery,* with the patient positioned in varying *right and left anterior-oblique projections* (see pages 23 and 24). Individual projections for each patient are selected on the basis of direct fluoroscopic visualization, in an effort to photograph all segments of each vessel in a plane perpendicular to that of the X-ray beam. Usually, four to six *arteriograms* of each artery are made, in *varying* right and left anterior-oblique projections. An

average of 4 to 6 ml of 70 percent Hypaque®, injected manually with a 10-ml syringe, is required for adequate *opacification* of individual coronary vessels. Positioning the patient in multiple right and left anterior-oblique projections is facilitated greatly by the use of a rotating X-ray *tilt table,* which permits the patient to be rotated quickly as much as 60 degrees, in either direction, from the supine position.

The passage of the contrast medium through *all branches of the coronary tree* is recorded with a 35-mm *motion-picture camera* at a rate of 60 frames per second, using Eastman Double X negative film. Individual exposures are limited to a range from 3 to 5 milliseconds with a square-wave X-ray pulsing system.

After each coronary artery has been *opacified* effec-

tively in the appropriate projections, the catheter tip is passed across the aortic valve into the left ventricle. Pressure measurements are recorded in the left ventricle. Its cavity then is opacified selectively, with 40 ml of 90 percent Hypaque®. Left ventriculography is performed routinely in the right anterior-oblique projection. This provides a clear-cut demonstration of localized left ventricular aneurysms or areas of the ventricular myocardium which show impaired contractility due to interstitial scar-tissue replacement or grossly impaired myocardial perfusion. Left ventriculography also permits the ready identification of associated mitral- or aortic-valve lesions or severely impaired left ventricular function due to gen-

(Continued on page 33)

SELECTIVE CINE CORONARY ARTERIOGRAPHY

(*Continued from page 32*)

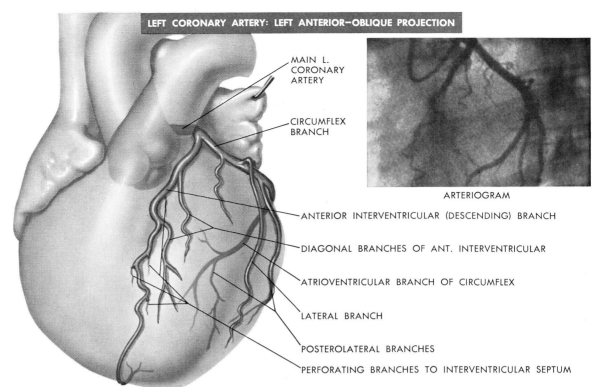

LEFT CORONARY ARTERY: LEFT ANTERIOR-OBLIQUE PROJECTION

MAIN L. CORONARY ARTERY

CIRCUMFLEX BRANCH

ARTERIOGRAM

ANTERIOR INTERVENTRICULAR (DESCENDING) BRANCH

DIAGONAL BRANCHES OF ANT. INTERVENTRICULAR

ATRIOVENTRICULAR BRANCH OF CIRCUMFLEX

LATERAL BRANCH

POSTEROLATERAL BRANCHES

PERFORATING BRANCHES TO INTERVENTRICULAR SEPTUM

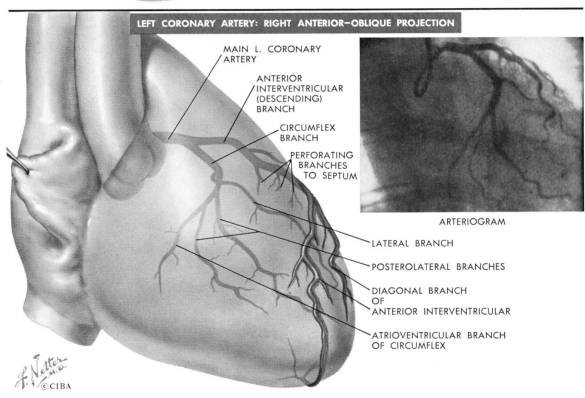

LEFT CORONARY ARTERY: RIGHT ANTERIOR-OBLIQUE PROJECTION

MAIN L. CORONARY ARTERY

ANTERIOR INTERVENTRICULAR (DESCENDING) BRANCH

CIRCUMFLEX BRANCH

PERFORATING BRANCHES TO SEPTUM

ARTERIOGRAM

LATERAL BRANCH

POSTEROLATERAL BRANCHES

DIAGONAL BRANCH OF ANTERIOR INTERVENTRICULAR

ATRIOVENTRICULAR BRANCH OF CIRCUMFLEX

eralized preexisting myocardial injury.

Upon completion of the procedure, the catheter is withdrawn, and the brachial arteriotomy is carefully closed by direct suture.

Clinical Applications

Using the technic described above, *distal radicles* of the human coronary-artery tree, as small as 100 to 200 microns in lumen diameter, may be demonstrated routinely. Segmental lumen-diameter variations of the major branches due to atherosclerosis, which result in no more than a 10 percent reduction in lumen diameter, are demonstrable. More-advanced obstructive lesions, which are capable of limiting myocardial perfusion, are visualized easily. When the vessels are opacified selectively, the presence, the sites of origin, and the distribution of effective intercoronary collateral channels, which compensate for severe obstructive lesions, may be defined precisely. In patients demonstrating angiographically normal vessels, the presence of coronary atherosclerosis may be ruled out.

Coronary arteriography has proved to be essential for the selection of patients with coronary atherosclerosis who may benefit by the application of surgical technics designed to improve myocardial perfusion, and for objectively assessing the results of such procedures. Severe localized obstructions in major proximal arteries may now be overcome by direct surgical attack. In other instances, the demonstration of more-diffuse obstructive lesions provides an objective basis for planning specific sites for internal-mammary-artery implantation, to compensate for perfusion deficits in one or more areas of the left ventricular myocardium. If the involved heart muscle has been replaced by scar tissue, demonstrable by left ventriculography, surgical revascularization is contraindicated.

Postoperatively, repeated coronary *arteriograms* and selective internal-mammary arteriograms permit long-term assessment of the effectiveness of such surgical technics, as well as the evolving state of the basic disease process in individual patients.

Section II

PHYSIOLOGY AND PATHOPHYSIOLOGY

by

FRANK H. NETTER, M.D.

in collaboration with

MARVIN B. BACANER, M.D. and MAURICE B. VISSCHER, Ph.D., M.D.
Plates 1-4

IGNACIO CHAVEZ RIVERA, M.D.
Plate 55

ANDRE COURNAND, M.D., A. GREGORY JAMESON, M.D., and HARRY W. FRITTS, JR., M.D.
Plates 5-9

JOHN H. GIBBON, JR., M.D. and RUDOLPH C. CAMISHION, M.D.
Plates 59-61

ALFRED GILMAN, Ph.D.
Plates 62-66

BRIAN F. HOFFMAN, M.D.
Plates 10-11

JAMES R. JUDE, M.D.
Plates 56-58

JOHN S. LaDUE, M.D., Ph.D.
Plates 53-54

ROBERT S. LITWAK, M.D.
Plates 33-34

ALDO A. LUISADA, M.D.
Plates 35-52

HENRY J. L. MARRIOTT, M.D.
Plate 32

TRAVIS WINSOR, M.D., F.A.C.P.
Plates 12-31

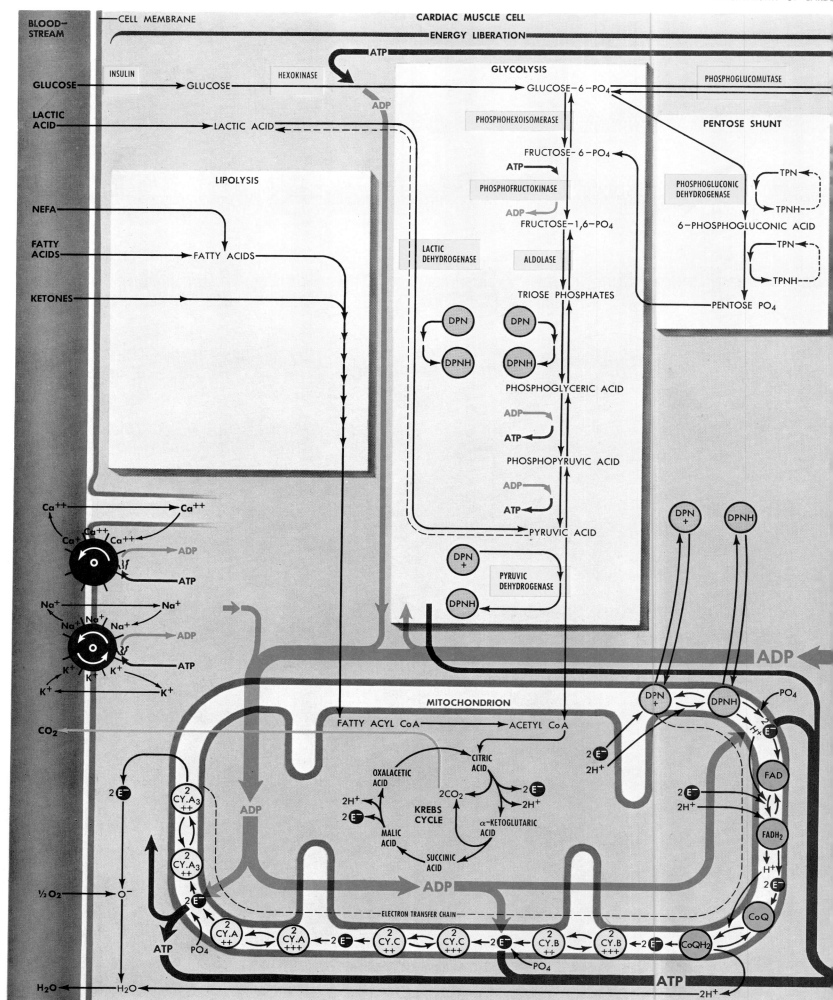

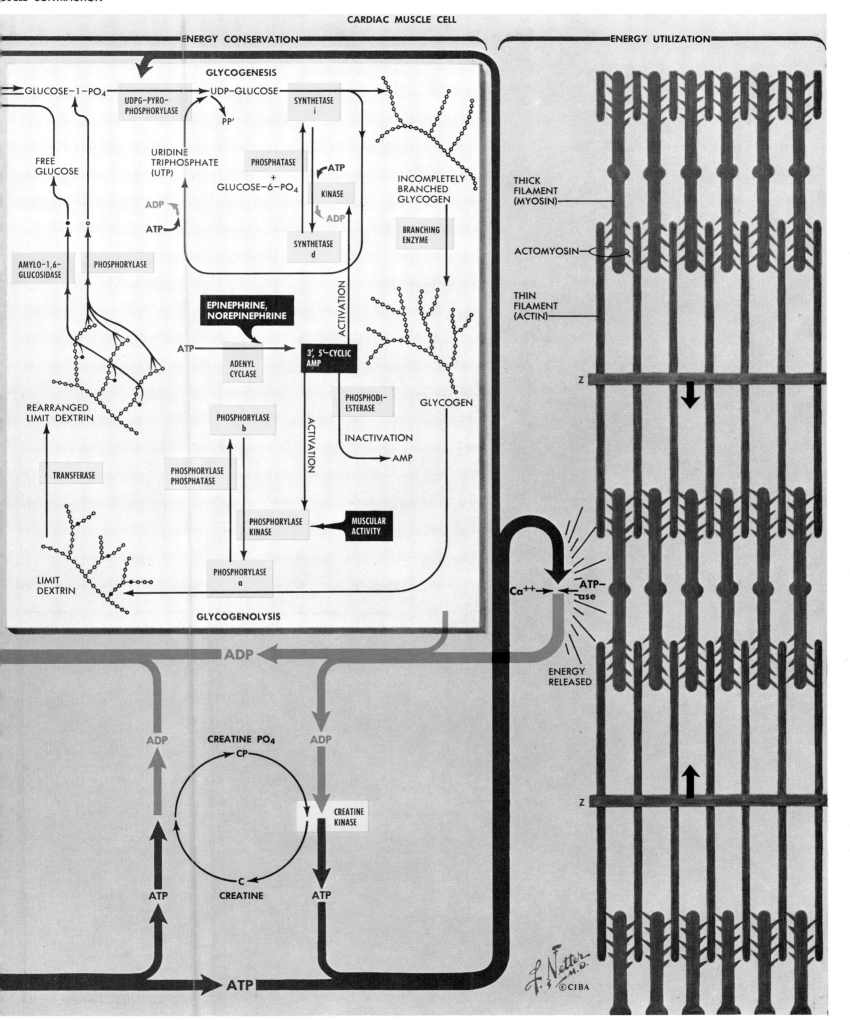

CARDIAC MUSCLE CELL

ENERGY CONSERVATION

ENERGY UTILIZATION

GLYCOGENESIS

GLUCOSE–1–PO₄

UDPG-PYRO-
PHOSPHORYLASE

UDP-GLUCOSE

SYNTHETASE
i

PP'

FREE
GLUCOSE

URIDINE
TRIPHOSPHATE
(UTP)

PHOSPHATASE
+
GLUCOSE–6–PO₄

ATP

KINASE

ADP

ATP

ADP

INCOMPLETELY
BRANCHED
GLYCOGEN

THICK
FILAMENT
(MYOSIN)

AMYLO-1,6-
GLUCOSIDASE

PHOSPHORYLASE

SYNTHETASE
d

BRANCHING
ENZYME

ACTOMYOSIN

THIN
FILAMENT
(ACTIN)

EPINEPHRINE,
NOREPINEPHRINE

ACTIVATION

ATP

ADENYL
CYCLASE

3', 5'-CYCLIC
AMP

REARRANGED
LIMIT DEXTRIN

PHOSPHODI-
ESTERASE

GLYCOGEN

Z

PHOSPHORYLASE
b

ACTIVATION

INACTIVATION

AMP

TRANSFERASE

PHOSPHORYLASE
PHOSPHATASE

PHOSPHORYLASE
KINASE

MUSCULAR
ACTIVITY

Ca⁺⁺

ATP–
ase

ENERGY
RELEASED

LIMIT
DEXTRIN

PHOSPHORYLASE
a

GLYCOGENOLYSIS

ADP

ADP

ADP

ADP

CREATINE PO₄

CP

CREATINE
KINASE

C

CREATINE

ATP

ATP

Z

ATP

BIOCHEMISTRY OF CARDIAC MUSCLE

The heart may be viewed as a chemodynamic machine which liberates *energy* stored in carbon-carbon and carbon-hydrogen bonds of substrate fuels, such as fats and carbohydrates, and then utilizes this energy to perform mechanical work. In the case of the heart, the machine is a positive-displacement pump which accelerates a mass of blood through the circulatory system.

The metabolic process in heart muscle may be divided into three phases (as promulgated by Olson): (1) *energy liberation*, (2) *energy conservation*, and (3) *energy utilization*. A schematic representation of these processes and their interrelationships is depicted.

The process of energy liberation includes the chemical reactions that break down *fatty acids, glucose, pyruvate,* and *lactate,* which are the principal substrates utilized by the heart, into 2-carbon fragments that may enter the common-terminal oxidative pathway of the *Krebs tricarboxylic acid cycle.* By this process, the free energy released from the substrate bonds is *transferred* by *hydrogen electrons* along the electron transport chain of enzymes (located in the *mitochondrion*) to *oxygen,* which is the ultimate electron acceptor.

The phase of energy conservation includes, principally, the process of *oxidative phosphorylation.* According to current views, the free energy liberated from the oxidizable substrate is not used directly in the contractile process but is used, instead, to form high-energy ester bonds between phosphoric acid residues and certain organic compounds. In the mammalian heart the free energy of the hydrogen electrons is transferred to the terminal phosphate bond of adenosine diphosphate *(ADP)* and creatine to form the high-energy compounds adenosine triphosphate *(ATP)* and *creatine phosphate (CP),* where the energy is stored for later use. The formation of glycogen in the *myocardial cell* also results in the storage of some energy and may be included in the phase of energy conservation.

Energy utilization includes the processes by which energy, stored in the terminal phosphate of ATP and CP, is channeled into the contractile process whereby mechanical work is performed. Also, ATP is used to perform chemical work in driving a variety of chemical reactions, in the metabolic pathway, that require energy.

The stepwise *chain* of chemical-mechanical events in heart contraction may be illustrated by following a molecule of glucose, which is a prime 6-carbon sugar substrate, through the metabolic cycle. Glucose is brought via capillary *blood* and, with the help of *insulin,* crosses the capillary and myocardial *cell*

membrane into the sarcoplasm, where it enters the biochemical factory by phosphorylation to *glucose-6-phosphate,* under the enzymatic influence of *hexokinase.* This reaction requires energy, which is supplied by ATP. The glucose-6-phosphate thus formed may follow one of three paths: (1) be incorporated into *glycogen,* (2) undergo direct oxidation through the reactions of the *pentose shunt,* or (3) continue in the mainstream of carbohydrate metabolism, that of *glycolysis* via the Embden-Meyerhof series of reactions.

The steps in glycolysis lead to the formation of 2 identical molecules of the 3-carbon compound, *pyruvic acid.* The heart is, essentially, an aerobic organ which is rich in the respiratory enzymes necessary to carry out the oxidative reactions of the Krebs cycle. These are located within the numerous mitochondria of the cardiac cell, in close proximity to the contractile fibers. Pyruvic acid, derived from glycolysis or from the capillary blood, is quickly converted to acetyl coenzyme A *(acetyl CoA),* under the influence of the enzyme *pyruvic dehydrogenase* and 5 cofactors present within the mitochondrion. The 2-carbon "acetyl" fragment of the acetyl CoA complex then is attached to the 4-carbon *oxalacetate* by means of a condensing enzyme, and the resulting product—*citric acid*—continues around the "wheel" of the Krebs tricarboxylic acid cycle. This continuous cyclic process results in the breakdown of the "acetyl" by decarboxylation, with the release of CO_2 and the regeneration of oxalacetate, which is then available to combine with another molecule of acetyl CoA and make another trip around the cycle. The net result of this process is the complete oxidation of 1 molecule of the 3-carbon pyruvate to 3 molecules of CO_2 and the associated release of the energy previously trapped between the bonds. The bond energy, released from the 2-carbon acetyl fragment in the form of hydrogen electrons, is transferred to produce 1 molecule of ATP-, *DPNH-* (reduced diphosphopyridine nucleotide), and *FADH₂-* (flavin adenine nucleotide) bound electrons which are then transported around the electron transport chain. The DPNH- and FADH₂-bound hydrogens or their electrons $(H \rightarrow H^+ + e)$ are fed into the electron transport chain, and the energy of this electronic current is tapped off in the electron transport system in three places, resulting in the phosphorylation of ADP to ATP. In the cytochrome system the electron is finally combined with molecular oxygen $(\frac{1}{2}O_2)$ to form *water.*

In the process of breaking down glucose to pyruvate via the Embden-Meyerhof scheme, there is a yield of 4 moles of ATP. However, 2 moles of ATP are required in the two kinase reactions (hexokinase and phosphofructokinase), and therefore there is a net gain of only 2 ATPs in anaerobic glycolysis. In the presence of oxygen there is further oxidation of the 2 pyruvate molecules in the Krebs cycle, which yields at least another 30 ATPs.

When not enough oxygen is present for pyruvate to be oxidized in the Krebs cycle, anaerobic glycolysis may be sustained by the oxidation of DPNH (formed during the breakdown of the *triose phosphate* to *phosphoglyceric acid*) by pyruvate which is converted to lactic acid. This reaction is catalyzed by the enzyme *lactic acid dehydrogenase.*

Glycolysis is of limited value in energy production, representing a release of only 9 percent of the energy content of glucose. Under normal conditions where oxygen is plentiful, lactic acid, coming from other tissues such as *exercising muscle,* is used as a substrate, by conversion to pyruvate, which then enters the Krebs cycle.

A second path that glucose-6-phosphate may follow is conversion to glycogen. Under the enzymatic influence of *phosphoglucomutase,* glucose-6-phosphate is converted to *glucose-1-phosphate* which then reacts enzymatically with *uridine triphosphate* (UTP) to form *UDP-glucose-1-phosphate* or uridine-diphosphoglucose (UDPG). Under the influence of the enzyme glycogen *synthetase,* the UDPG is transferred to *incompletely branched glycogen* composed of 1:4 glucose linkages. Another enzyme rearranges the branch points to form 1:6 linkages.

The breakdown of glycogen follows a path that is completely different from that of its synthesis.

Under the influence of *phosphorylase* and a debranching enzyme, glycogen is broken down through a series of steps leading to the release of glucose-1-phosphate which is readily converted back into glucose-6-phosphate.

The cardiac concentration of glycogen is very constant at about 0.5 percent; however, it is not an inert storage substrate but is an actively exchanging metabolic pool. When radioactive C^{14}-labeled glucose is infused for 4 hours into the circulation of the actively contracting heart, about 30 percent of the cardiac glycogen is found to be C^{14}-labeled. This means a turnover rate of about 8 percent per hour, with the infused C^{14}-labeled glucose appearing as C^{14}-labeled glycogen, and old glycogen breaking down to free glucose-1-phosphate to participate in active metabolism while the total concentration of cardiac glycogen remains almost constant.

Two enzymes that are important in the regulation of glycogen concentration are glycogen synthetase, which catalyzes glycogen synthesis, and phosphorylase, which catalyzes breakdown. Each of these enzymes exists in both active and inactive forms, and their interconversion requires additional enzymes and cofactors. *Norepinephrine* and *epinephrine* exert an important influence on the activation of phosphorylase b to the active form, phosphorylase a, for glycogen breakdown. Glycogen may be considered as a high-energy fuel, readily available for rapid entry into the glycolytic cycle. In hypoxia, glycolysis, as well as the breakdown of glycogen itself, becomes greatly accelerated.

The third pathway for glucose-6-phosphate metabolism is via the pentose shunt. The energy released from glucose-6-phosphate in this path is transferred to the *TPNH* formed. There is no direct generation of ATP, and it is not known if the TPNH formed in the cytoplasm can be oxidized in the mitochondria to generate ATP. However, TPNH can be used in various synthetic reactions, such as the synthesis of fatty acids and sterols.

Nonesterified fatty acids (NEFA) enter the cell and combine with albumin. They are an important fuel for the heart. The NEFA are broken down by the process of β-oxidation, which splits off 2-carbon fragments that ultimately end up as acetyl CoA moieties which are oxidized via the Krebs cycle. Although glucose, when available, is the preferred substrate, fatty acids may provide up to 80 percent of the energy requirements of the heart, in the absence of glucose.

The ATP formed during substrate oxidation is the metabolic "currency" of the cell; i.e., all the chemical and mechanical work performed by the cell is paid for by the breakdown of ATP into ADP. Creatine phosphate is a reserve energy source, which can be used to phosphorylate ADP to ATP if the metabolic generation of ATP is interrupted.

Although ATP appears to be the immediate source of energy for muscle contraction, the mechanism by which its chemical energy is coupled to contraction of the cardiac fibers is not known. The current hypothesis of muscle contraction visualizes the muscle-fiber proteins as interdigitating *myosin* (thick) and *actin* (thin) *filaments.* Between these filaments are crossbridges composed of the protein meromyosin. *Calcium (Ca)* is known to be a critical coupling factor in contraction, because, in its absence, excitation-contraction coupling is lost.

The current concept of muscle contraction that is most widely accepted, but not proved, is the sliding-filament model (see page 20). In this view the thin filaments are drawn toward each other by *the* changing reactivity of the crossbridges. The crossbridge, which is fixed to the thick filament, is postulated to be linked by a calcium bond to the thin filament. Electrical depolarization shifts the calcium portion, breaking the link and shifting the position of the thin filament to align with a different crossbridge. In the process, ATP is broken down by the change in proximity of the tip of the crossbridge moving toward the myosin (thick filament), which is a structural protein, and calcium-dependent ATPase (the enzyme that breaks down ATP to ADP). However, it should be emphasized that, as yet, no model fits all the facts or adequately accounts for the contractile process.

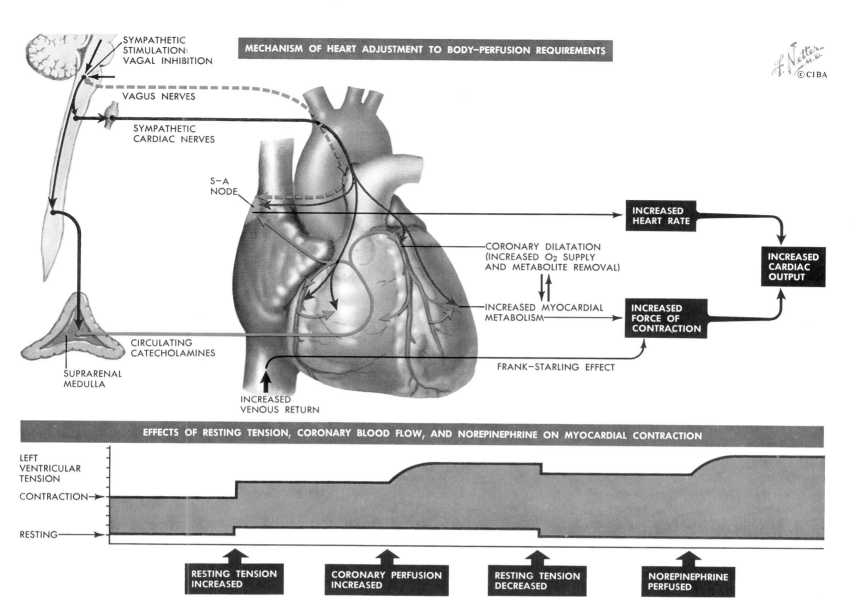

SECTION II—PLATE 2

MECHANISM OF CARDIAC ADJUSTMENT TO BODY-PERFUSION REQUIREMENTS

The *heart* must adapt its performance to widely varying needs of the body, in order that each organ will receive enough blood to support its metabolic requirements. The limits of adaptation range from the minimum work needs during sleep to the maximum demands while performing heavy exercise.

The normal heart adjusts its work output to its load by utilizing any or all of a number of available mechanisms which enable it to augment or diminish its performance level. The heart can *increase its work output* by *increasing the rate* at which it contracts and by *increasing the force of contraction,* thereby ejecting more blood with each stroke. The force of contraction can be augmented by humoral and neural mechanisms which alter the *metabolic state of the myocardium* or by stretching the myocardium to *increase its resting length or tension.*

The heart, like all striated muscle, responds to stretch, under increased tension at rest, by a more vigorous contraction. This response is intrinsic and "instantaneous"; *i.e.,* it occurs in the next contraction after a stretch, and is maintained during the period of stretch. The metabolic state of the myocardium is influenced by the rate of coronary blood flow, which determines the rate of delivery of *oxygen* and metabolic substrates as well as the "washout" of CO_2 and *metabolites.* Under a given

resting load or initial tension, the heart produces more contractile tension when its oxygen supply is increased by increasing its coronary blood flow; by the same mechanism, tension development declines when blood flow and oxygen delivery fall. This concept is of great importance in understanding the mechanism of diminished cardiac working capacity in states where blood flow to the myocardium is impaired, as in coronary arteriosclerosis, or when coronary-perfusion pressure falls, as in all shock states. Changing the rate of oxygen delivery by altering *coronary perfusion* causes a slow and progressive change in contractile tension, in sharp contrast to the instantaneous effect observed when resting tension and length are altered. It should be noted that after coronary perfusion has been *increased to augment myocardial metabolism* and contractile tension, *decreasing the resting tension* to its initial level leaves the contractile tension proportionally greater than initially. Thus, the magnitude of contractile tension, for a given amount of stretch, is also influenced by the metabolic state of the myocardium which had been previously altered by changing coronary-perfusion pressure.

Dilatation of the coronary vessels occurs by the release of metabolites during contraction and recovery, and by the direct action of *catecholamines* released from *sympathetic-nerve endings* in the myocardium. Catecholamines, released from the *suprarenal medulla,* enter the myocardium via the coronary arteries and have a similar effect on coronary-artery caliber.

Still another mechanism, that of catecholamines, for changing energy output and, therefore, work capacity of the heart, is shown in the upper and lower panels of the diagram. *Epinephrine* and *norepinephrine* greatly increase the tension production

and work capacity of the heart under otherwise constant conditions. This is a most important adaptive mechanism that influences myocardial metabolism and contraction directly at the cellular level, as well as by an indirect effect on coronary flow through coronary dilatation. It should be observed that the direct tension-augmenting effect of catecholamines is slow and progressive; it is very similar to the tension-augmenting effect seen when oxygen delivery is changed by increasing coronary perfusion.

Increasing the heart rate effectively augments cardiac output as long as the stroke output is not diminished disproportionately. As the heart rate increases greatly, the diastolic period, during which the venous return fills the heart, becomes progressively shortened, and stroke output declines. Faster heart rates cannot account for all the increase in cardiac output per minute. Possible increase in heart rate is limited to two or three times the resting level; since heavy exercise may require up to ten times the resting cardiac output, stroke output must also increase. Normally, the heart ejects only 50 to 60 percent of its volume with each stroke; hence, a more forceful contraction increases stroke volume by ejecting a greater portion of this residual volume.

Any simplistic view of regulatory mechanisms in the heart is unwarranted. The work capacity of the myocardium is influenced by a variety of factors, and although those illustrated and referred to above appear to be the important ones, it must be recognized that others are sometimes of critical significance. For example, suprarenal-cortical-hormone deficiency, thyroid-hormone deficiency, calcium, potassium, and defects in acid-base concentration can be crucial to the work capacity and, hence, the ability of the heart to adjust to changes in the imposed load.

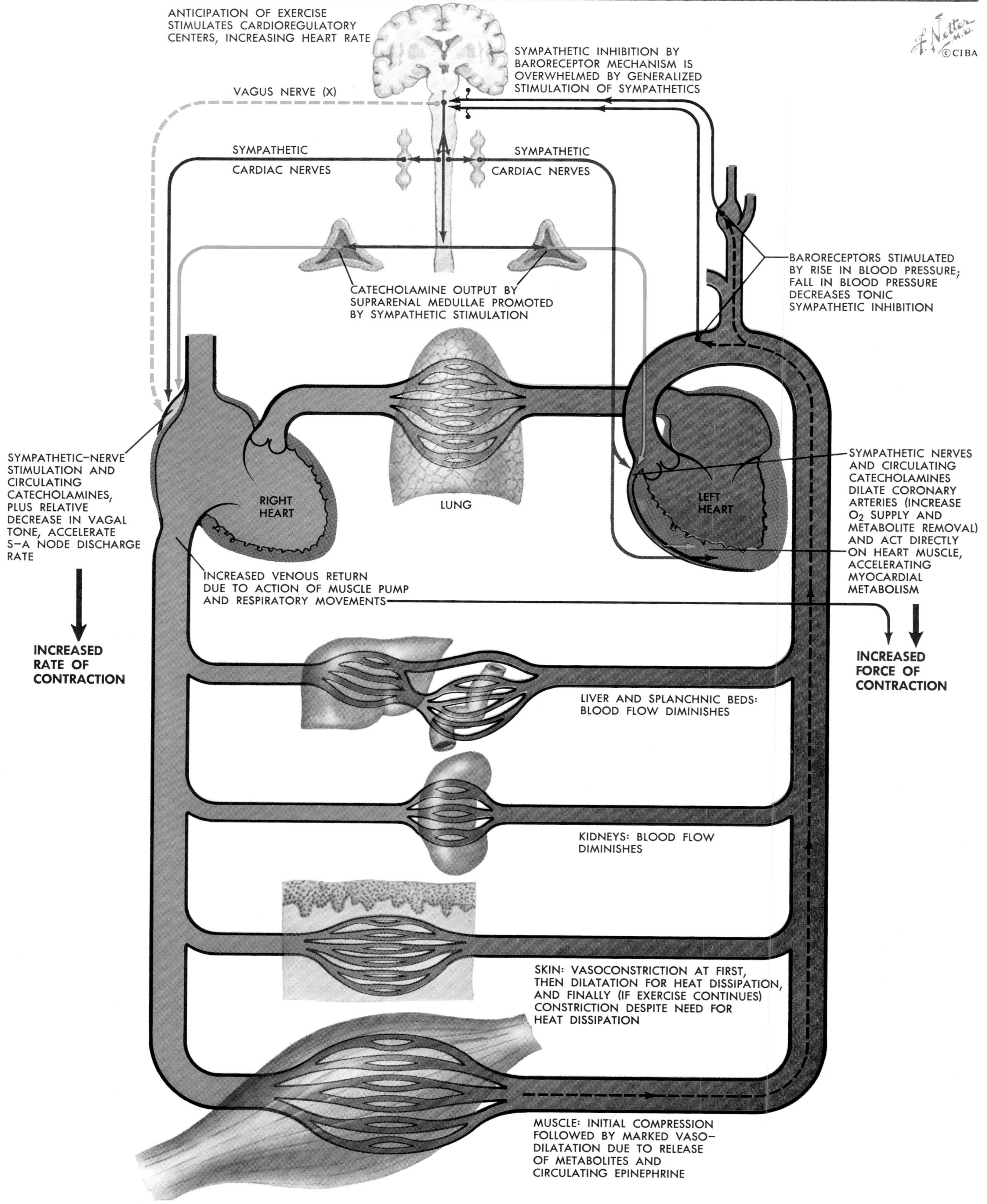

ANTICIPATION OF EXERCISE
STIMULATES CARDIOREGULATORY
CENTERS, INCREASING HEART RATE

SYMPATHETIC INHIBITION BY
BARORECEPTOR MECHANISM IS
OVERWHELMED BY GENERALIZED
STIMULATION OF SYMPATHETICS

VAGUS NERVE (X)

SYMPATHETIC
CARDIAC NERVES

SYMPATHETIC
CARDIAC NERVES

BARORECEPTORS STIMULATED
BY RISE IN BLOOD PRESSURE;
FALL IN BLOOD PRESSURE
DECREASES TONIC
SYMPATHETIC INHIBITION

CATECHOLAMINE OUTPUT BY
SUPRARENAL MEDULLAE PROMOTED
BY SYMPATHETIC STIMULATION

SYMPATHETIC–NERVE
STIMULATION AND
CIRCULATING
CATECHOLAMINES,
PLUS RELATIVE
DECREASE IN VAGAL
TONE, ACCELERATE
S–A NODE DISCHARGE
RATE

RIGHT
HEART

LUNG

LEFT
HEART

SYMPATHETIC NERVES
AND CIRCULATING
CATECHOLAMINES
DILATE CORONARY
ARTERIES (INCREASE
O$_2$ SUPPLY AND
METABOLITE REMOVAL)
AND ACT DIRECTLY
ON HEART MUSCLE,
ACCELERATING
MYOCARDIAL
METABOLISM

INCREASED VENOUS RETURN
DUE TO ACTION OF MUSCLE PUMP
AND RESPIRATORY MOVEMENTS

INCREASED
RATE OF
CONTRACTION

INCREASED
FORCE OF
CONTRACTION

LIVER AND SPLANCHNIC BEDS:
BLOOD FLOW DIMINISHES

KIDNEYS: BLOOD FLOW
DIMINISHES

SKIN: VASOCONSTRICTION AT FIRST,
THEN DILATATION FOR HEAT DISSIPATION,
AND FINALLY (IF EXERCISE CONTINUES)
CONSTRICTION DESPITE NEED FOR
HEAT DISSIPATION

MUSCLE: INITIAL COMPRESSION
FOLLOWED BY MARKED VASO-
DILATATION DUE TO RELEASE
OF METABOLITES AND
CIRCULATING EPINEPHRINE

CIRCULATORY RESPONSE TO EXERCISE

The healthy man adjusts his cardiac output to his oxygen needs, during *exercise,* up to a maximum which depends on his state of conditioning. In disease, too, there is regulation, and the maximum output attainable is contingent on the degree and type of the disorder.

Cardiac output increases proportionately to the increase in heart rate, if the stroke output remains the same. As the heart rate accelerates, the duration of systole is shortened only slightly, but the diastolic period is, proportionately, shortened much more, thus decreasing the time available for filling during diastole. Limitation of the stroke output occurs when the heart rate exceeds 180 to 200 beats per minute, because the filling is inadequate.

In the normal person who is not athletically trained, the cardiac output is increased, at best, two and one half to three times by increasing heart rate. One reason for the expanded exercise capacity of trained athletes is that their resting heart rates are low and their resting stroke volumes are high. The fully conditioned athlete may have resting heart rates as low as 40 beats per minute, and the heart can, therefore, have nearly a fivefold increase before reaching rates at which filling times are so low as to limit the stroke output.

Filling rates depend on the adequacy of the pressure gradient in the venous system, which, in turn, is governed by reflexes that control the capacity of the venous bed. The phasic contraction of the *skeletal muscles,* during exercise, acts as a *pump* by squeezing *venous blood* toward the heart.

The heart rate at rest is normally maintained at a low value by tonic vagal inhibition of the *sinoatrial* pacemaker. Increased pacemaker activity augments the heart rate (1) by *decreasing* the *vagal* impulse rate, (2) by augmentation in the *sympathetic-nerve* discharge rate, and (3) by increases in the concentration of *circulating catecholamines* from the *suprarenal medullae* and from sympathetic-nerve endings elsewhere in the body. During heavy exercise there may be an increase in cardiac output up to tenfold, and, since a maximum increase in the heart rate can, at best, triple the cardiac output, obviously the additional volume must result from an increase in the stroke output.

There are several mechanisms which *increase the strength of myocardial contraction* and its capacity to perform stroke work. Catecholamines increase the cardiac work capacity, even at constant heart rates, by their direct effects on the metabolic processes and the contractile apparatus. They also increase the work capacity by *increasing the oxygen* delivery to the myocardium, through a direct *vasodilator effect* upon the *coronary vasculature.* In anticipation of muscular activity and as a result of proprioceptive impulses from the muscle reaching the brain, the sympathetic system is activated. This results in an elevated systemic blood pressure, which is usually sustained during exercise, and which directly increases the coronary perfusion by an elevation of the driving head of pressure. Oxygen delivery to the myocardium is increased, and this accelerates the rate of *myocardial oxidative metabolism.*

Readjustment and redistribution of the peripheral circulation occurs, during exercise, by sympathetic, humoral, and metabolic regulation of the vascular caliber, which *decreases the blood flow* to the *abdominal viscera* and other *noncritical vascular beds,* while the blood flow to working *muscles* is *increased.* The elevation of blood pressure that occurs during exercise would be expected to excite the *baroreceptor* mechanism and lower the heart rate. However, by some unexplained mechanism (possibly catecholamine effects), the baroreceptor control is overcome, and the heart rate remains high, despite a significant *increase in blood pressure. Blood flow to the skin* increases, in order to *dissipate* the excessive *heat* produced by the increase in metabolic rate.

For many years, a change in stroke output was considered to be mediated primarily by the effect of an increased stretch of the heart, resulting from augmented venous return. However, it has been clearly demonstrated that the diastolic size of the heart, during exercise, either remains unchanged or actually gets smaller. Such evidence directly contradicts the concept that adaptation of heart performance, in exercise, is mediated by the stretch mechanism.

Actually, the adjustment to changes in load, during exercise, is accomplished by a combination of factors: A change in heart rate is effected by sympathetic discharge, which causes the release of catecholamines locally at the *sinoatrial node,* and by circulating catecholamines which enter the heart via the coronary circulation. An increased force of contraction is effected by the augmented oxygen delivery through the improved coronary flow and catecholamine activity. The enhanced coronary blood flow is mediated by an increase in the coronary-perfusion pressure, which, in turn, is mediated by the catecholamine effects on the coronary and peripheral vascular caliber, as well as by the increased release of local metabolites, which causes coronary dilatation. These adjustments enable the heart to maintain a metabolic equilibrium by increasing its rate of oxidative recovery to support the increase in work output required of it.

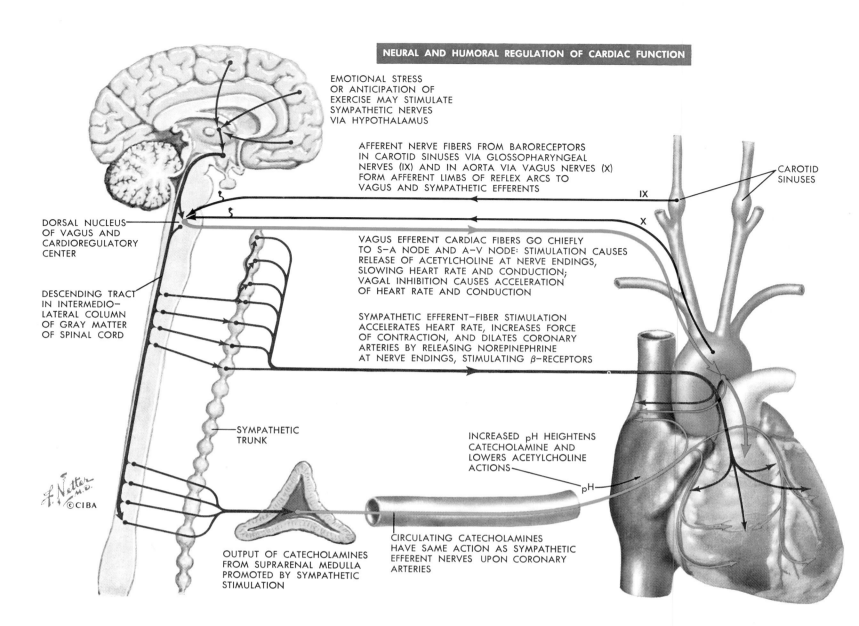

EMOTIONAL STRESS
OR ANTICIPATION OF
EXERCISE MAY STIMULATE
SYMPATHETIC NERVES
VIA HYPOTHALAMUS

AFFERENT NERVE FIBERS FROM BARORECEPTORS
IN CAROTID SINUSES VIA GLOSSOPHARYNGEAL
NERVES (IX) AND IN AORTA VIA VAGUS NERVES (X)
FORM AFFERENT LIMBS OF REFLEX ARCS TO
VAGUS AND SYMPATHETIC EFFERENTS

IX

X

CAROTID
SINUSES

DORSAL NUCLEUS
OF VAGUS AND
CARDIOREGULATORY
CENTER

VAGUS EFFERENT CARDIAC FIBERS GO CHIEFLY
TO S-A NODE AND A-V NODE: STIMULATION CAUSES
RELEASE OF ACETYLCHOLINE AT NERVE ENDINGS,
SLOWING HEART RATE AND CONDUCTION;
VAGAL INHIBITION CAUSES ACCELERATION
OF HEART RATE AND CONDUCTION

DESCENDING TRACT
IN INTERMEDIO-
LATERAL COLUMN
OF GRAY MATTER
OF SPINAL CORD

SYMPATHETIC EFFERENT-FIBER STIMULATION
ACCELERATES HEART RATE, INCREASES FORCE
OF CONTRACTION, AND DILATES CORONARY
ARTERIES BY RELEASING NOREPINEPHRINE
AT NERVE ENDINGS, STIMULATING β-RECEPTORS

SYMPATHETIC
TRUNK

INCREASED pH HEIGHTENS
CATECHOLAMINE AND
LOWERS ACETYLCHOLINE
ACTIONS

pH

OUTPUT OF CATECHOLAMINES
FROM SUPRARENAL MEDULLA
PROMOTED BY SYMPATHETIC
STIMULATION

CIRCULATING CATECHOLAMINES
HAVE SAME ACTION AS SYMPATHETIC
EFFERENT NERVES UPON CORONARY
ARTERIES

SECTION II—PLATE 4

Neural and Humoral Regulation of Cardiac Function

The efferent innervation of the heart is controlled by both the sympathetic and the parasympathetic systems (see pages 18 and 19). *Afferent fibers* accompany the *efferents* of both systems. The *sympathetic fibers* have positive chronotropic (rate-increasing) and positive inotropic (force-increasing effects). The *parasympathetics* have a negative chronotropic effect and may be somewhat negatively inotropic, but the latter effect is, at most, small and is masked, in the intact circulatory system, by the increased filling which occurs when the diastolic filling time is increased.

The heart is normally under the restraint of *vagal inhibition,* and, consequently, bilateral

vagotomy increases the heart rate. *Vagal stimulation* not only *slows the heart* but also *slows conduction* across the *atrioventricular (A-V) node.* Sectioning of the cardiac sympathetics does not lower heart rate, under normal circumstances.

The totally denervated heart loses some (but surprisingly little) of its capacity to respond to changes in its load. The denervated heart still responds to *humoral* influences, more slowly and less fully, but it is remarkable how well the secondary mechanisms, such as the *suprarenal medullary output of catecholamine,* can substitute for the primary mechanism that controls heart rate in exercise.

The *nervous mechanisms* controlling heart

rate are several. The *baroreceptor reflexes,* with afferent arms from the *carotid sinus,* the *arch of the aorta,* and *other pressoreceptor zones,* operate as negative-feedback mechanisms to regulate pressure in the arteries. They affect not only heart activity but also the bore of the resistance vessels in the vascular system.

The heart is also affected reflexly by afferent impulses via the autonomic nervous system. The response, in such instances, may be either tachycardia or bradycardia, depending on whether the sympathetic or the parasympathetic system is activated more strongly in particular individuals. Tachycardia is the common response in excitement.

CARDIAC CATHETERIZATION

Right-Heart Catheterization

Cardiac catheterization, first attempted by Forsmann on himself in 1928, has proved practicable and has been developed by Cournand, Richards, and their co-workers. It is now a common technic in both clinical and research laboratories.

Technic. The primary goal of *right-heart catheterization* is to reach and study, by the use of a *catheter*, the conditions existing in the chambers and great vessels of the right side of the heart. In these procedures a radiopaque flexible *catheter* (there are various designs) is *introduced into a vein*, usually the *basilic*, which has been isolated by a cutdown, using local anesthesia. After introduction into the vein, the catheter is manipulated under fluoroscopic control, and with constant ECG control, downstream through the venous system to the *right atrium*, and eventually into the *right ventricle* and *pulmonary artery*. Frequently, the catheter is *wedged*, being cautiously advanced into the most-peripheral *branch* of the pulmonary artery that will accept the catheter tip. A pressure recorded from the wedge position has essentially the same mean pressure as the *left atrium* and the same, but delayed, phasic features.

Occasionally in adults, frequently in children, and particularly *in infants*, instead of using a basilic vein, the catheter is preferably introduced into a *saphenous vein* and is advanced to the femoral and iliac veins and then up the *inferior vena cava* to reach the right atrium.

Manipulation of the catheter to reach any part of the right heart is usually not difficult except in those cases in which normal anatomic configurations or relations are disturbed, as congenital heart disease.

Diagnostic Procedures. The position of the catheter in the fluoroscopic image may indicate some departure from the intracardiac course normally taken by a catheter. Examples include passage into a persistent left *superior vena cava* through the coronary sinus from the right atrium, passage through a patent ductus arteriosus, and traversal of an interatrial or *interventricular septal defect*.

Blood can be sampled for oxygen or other analysis, and pressures can be measured through the catheter from any point reached. Oxygen samples can be used to determine the site of entry into the right heart and the size of a left-to-right intracardiac shunt in congenital heart disease, and oxygen values from the pulmonary artery can be used, with other data, to calculate the pulmonary blood flow by application of the Fick principle (see page 44). Blood samples drawn through the catheter and then through a densitometer permit identification of left-to-right shunts, following injection through the catheter of suitable dyes into selected locations. Measurement of pressures through the catheter,

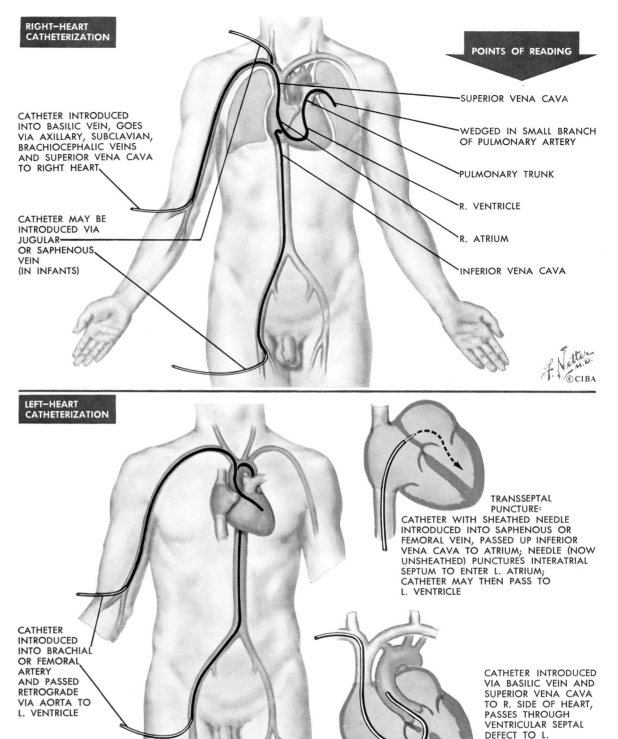

RIGHT–HEART CATHETERIZATION

CATHETER INTRODUCED INTO BASILIC VEIN, GOES VIA AXILLARY, SUBCLAVIAN, BRACHIOCEPHALIC VEINS AND SUPERIOR VENA CAVA TO RIGHT HEART

CATHETER MAY BE INTRODUCED VIA JUGULAR OR SAPHENOUS VEIN (IN INFANTS)

POINTS OF READING

SUPERIOR VENA CAVA

WEDGED IN SMALL BRANCH OF PULMONARY ARTERY

PULMONARY TRUNK

R. VENTRICLE

R. ATRIUM

INFERIOR VENA CAVA

LEFT–HEART CATHETERIZATION

CATHETER INTRODUCED INTO BRACHIAL OR FEMORAL ARTERY AND PASSED RETROGRADE VIA AORTA TO L. VENTRICLE

TRANSSEPTAL PUNCTURE: CATHETER WITH SHEATHED NEEDLE INTRODUCED INTO SAPHENOUS OR FEMORAL VEIN, PASSED UP INFERIOR VENA CAVA TO ATRIUM; NEEDLE (NOW UNSHEATHED) PUNCTURES INTERATRIAL SEPTUM TO ENTER L. ATRIUM; CATHETER MAY THEN PASS TO L. VENTRICLE

CATHETER INTRODUCED VIA BASILIC VEIN AND SUPERIOR VENA CAVA TO R. SIDE OF HEART, PASSES THROUGH VENTRICULAR SEPTAL DEFECT TO L. VENTRICLE, THENCE TO AORTA (MAY ALSO PASS THROUGH ATRIAL SEPTAL DEFECT)

using external pressure transducers, permits the measurement of the level of pressure and a determination of the phasic form of the pressure in any location. Pressures recorded as a catheter traverses a valve permit an evaluation of the site and degree of valvular stenosis.

Special sensors at the tip of a catheter have been designed for the detection and recording of intracardiac ECGs, pressures, and phonocardiograms.

Complications. Brief arrhythmias, vasovagal episodes, and minor degrees of phlebitis may be observed. More serious complications are rare.

Left-Heart Catheterization

Technic. The aim of *left-heart catheterization* is the study of conditions in the chambers and vessels of the left heart. In congenital heart disease the catheter

may reach the left side of the heart from a right-heart chamber, passing through a septal defect or a patent ductus arteriosus.

More commonly, the left heart is approached by *retrograde passage* of the catheter from its point of insertion into a peripheral *artery*, by arteriotomy, or, less commonly, by percutaneous technic. The catheter is manipulated under fluoroscopic control, in a retrograde direction, through the artery to the *aorta* and, frequently, across the aortic valve into the *left ventricle*. Entry into the *left atrium*, retrograde through the mitral valve, is often possible. Approach to the left atrium can also be accomplished by passage of the catheter from a right-groin vein up to the right atrium, introduction of a long special needle into the catheter, and *puncture of the interatrial septum* by the *unsheathed needle*. The catheter can then be

(Continued on page 44)

43

CARDIAC CATHETERIZATION

(Continued from page 43)

advanced into the left ventricle, using the needle as a guide. Direct percutaneous needle puncture of the apex of the left ventricle (not illustrated) may be employed to reach the left ventricle.

Diagnostic Procedures. Sampling and pressure measurements do not differ from right-heart procedures. Estimations of valvular abnormalities are possible by simultaneous pressure measurements on both sides of the valve. Dye curves are useful in cardiac-output determinations and in estimating valvular insufficiency.

Complications. Arrhythmias comprise the most common complication. They frequently respond to simple catheter withdrawal, however, and rarely require electroconversion. Other complications include arterial spasm and, exceptionally, occlusion of the artery. Perforations of the walls of an artery of the aorta, or of a heart chamber, have been reported. Fluid should never be forced through a catheter from which blood cannot be withdrawn.

The Fick Principle

In broadest outline, the *Fick principle* states that if the amount of a tracer material added to a flowing fluid is known, as well as the concentration of the trace material in the fluid proximal and distal to the point where mixing occurs, then the volume of fluid flowing past the mixing point per unit of time can be calculated.

Because of the conditions that must be fulfilled, a rigorous application of this principle to the cardiopulmonary system is impossible. Application only to instantaneous flow, the immediate mixing of the tracer material with the fluid, and the absence of any fluctuation in the addition rate of the tracer material or of the rate of fluid flow are among the limiting conditions. Nevertheless, the laboratory application of the principle for measuring pulmonary blood flow yields satisfactory results, using *oxygen* for the tracer material.

Method. For the clinical measurement of pulmonary blood flow, the fasting unsedated patient lies supine on the catheterization table, while a *catheter* and an *indwelling arterial needle* are positioned in the *pulmonary* and a *peripheral artery,* respectively. The patient's expired air is collected in a *spirometer* for a period of 2 minutes, and *samples of mixed venous blood* from the pulmonary artery and *arterial blood* from the peripheral artery are withdrawn through the catheter and needle, respectively, for 1 minute in the middle of the gas-collection period. The total volume of expired air, along with the oxygen concentrations of the expired and inspired air, are used to calculate the *oxygen consumption.* This figure is used, with the values of arterial and mixed venous O_2 *content,* to calculate the pulmonary blood flow, or *cardiac output,* by substitution in the equation shown.

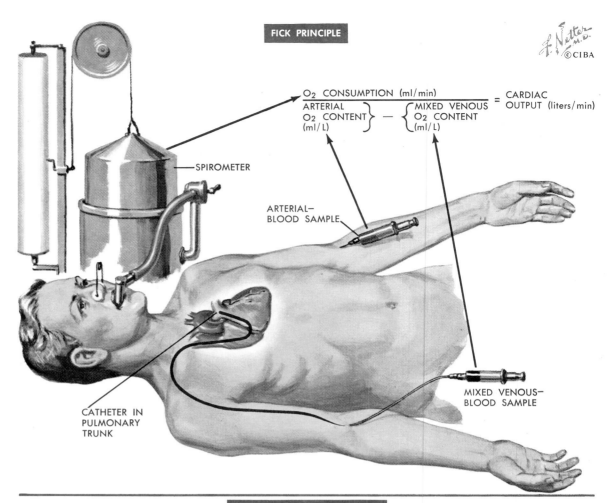

FICK PRINCIPLE

$$\frac{O_2 \text{ CONSUMPTION (ml/min)}}{\left.\begin{matrix} \text{ARTERIAL} \\ O_2 \text{ CONTENT} \\ \text{(ml/L)} \end{matrix}\right\} - \left\{\begin{matrix} \text{MIXED VENOUS} \\ O_2 \text{ CONTENT} \\ \text{(ml/L)} \end{matrix}\right.} = \begin{matrix} \text{CARDIAC} \\ \text{OUTPUT (liters/min)} \end{matrix}$$

SPIROMETER

ARTERIAL–BLOOD SAMPLE

MIXED VENOUS–BLOOD SAMPLE

CATHETER IN PULMONARY TRUNK

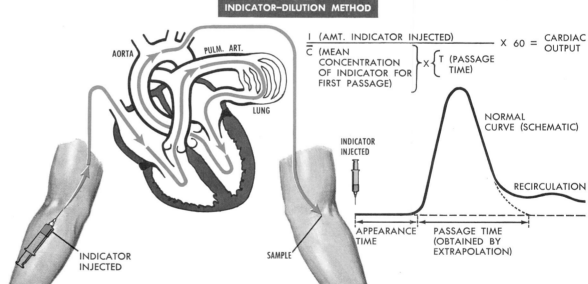

INDICATOR–DILUTION METHOD

AORTA — PULM. ART. — LUNG

$$\frac{I \text{ (AMT. INDICATOR INJECTED)}}{\bar{C} \left.\begin{matrix}\text{(MEAN} \\ \text{CONCENTRATION} \\ \text{OF INDICATOR FOR} \\ \text{FIRST PASSAGE)}\end{matrix}\right\}} \times \left\{ T \begin{matrix}\text{(PASSAGE} \\ \text{TIME)}\end{matrix}\right. \times 60 = \begin{matrix}\text{CARDIAC} \\ \text{OUTPUT}\end{matrix}$$

INDICATOR INJECTED

NORMAL CURVE (SCHEMATIC)

RECIRCULATION

INDICATOR INJECTED

SAMPLE

APPEARANCE TIME

PASSAGE TIME (OBTAINED BY EXTRAPOLATION)

Analyses. Chemical methods are in general use for the gas analyses, and chemical, oximetric, or spectrophotometric methods are used in the blood gas analyses.

Reproducibility. Performed, as outlined, with due care to avoid possible errors in sampling and analyses in a patient in a "steady state" of metabolic activity, the measurement of the pulmonary blood flow yields a mean value for the measurement period with a reproducibility of about 5 percent.

Indicator-Dilution Method

The *indicator-dilution method* for determining the *cardiac output* is based on the same general principle as that of the Fick method just described.

In the indicator-dilution method a given amount of a tracer *dye,* usually indocyanine green, is *injected*

almost instantaneously into the peripheral vein or, alternatively, into the *pulmonary artery,* and continuous *sampling* through a densitometer is carried out downstream, usually from a peripheral artery. The *time* required for the dye to *appear* at the sampling site is called the *appearance time.* The dye *concentration* first rises rapidly to a peak and then returns toward the base line until its downward course is interrupted by the appearance of recirculated dye that has made a complete circuit of the shortest paths the blood follows through the systemic circulation. Because the midportion of the downward limb of the curve, up to recirculation, is exponential in character, it is possible to *extrapolate* it, essentially to zero concentration, on a semilogarithmic plot, and thus to eliminate the concentration of recirculated dye. Then replotting the curve on the original coordinates and

(Continued on page 45)

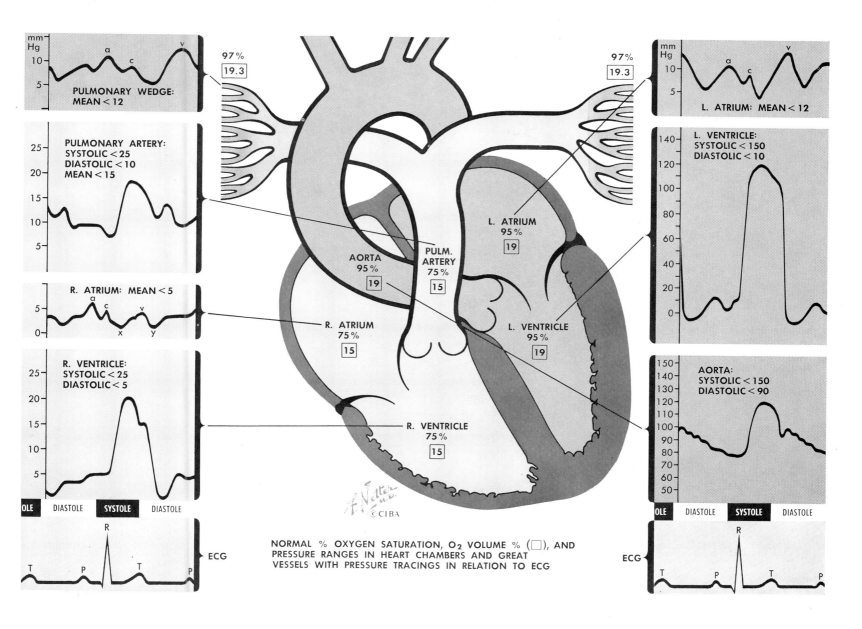

NORMAL % OXYGEN SATURATION, O₂ VOLUME % (▢), AND PRESSURE RANGES IN HEART CHAMBERS AND GREAT VESSELS WITH PRESSURE TRACINGS IN RELATION TO ECG

CARDIAC CATHETERIZATION

(Continued from page 44)

standardization of the curve permit calculation of the *mean concentration* ($\bar{c}$) of dye for the time of its passage, as well as the *passage time* (T) itself. Substitution of these values, along with the figure for the amount of dye injected, in the equation shown yields a value for the cardiac output.

Standardization is usually accomplished by mixing known amounts of blood and dye and measuring the optical density of the mixtures in the densitometer.

Possible Errors. The most common errors result from faulty standardization technics, inaccurate measurement of the amount of dye injected, or improper extrapolation of the dye curve to eliminate the effect of the recirculated dye.

Reproducibility. The method measures the *mean* flow for the measurement period. Properly performed, the dye-dilution method has a reproducibility of 5 percent and yields values in close correspondence with those of the Fick method.

Normal Oxygen and Pressure

Normal Oxygen Saturations in the Heart and Great Vessel. In the venae cavae, *right atrium, right ventricle,* and *pulmonary arteries,* the *oxygen saturation* is *normally* close to *75 percent* (content *15 volume percent*). There are small phasic variations in the saturation of blood sampled from the right-heart chambers. The variation is maximal in the right atrium, where contributions of blood from the renal veins (with a relatively high saturation), from the hepatic veins (with a relatively low saturation), from the coronary sinus (with a very low saturation), and from the lower inferior vena cava and superior vena cava (with intermediate saturations), meet and start mixing. The mixing is probably complete by the time the blood reaches the pulmonary artery. In the *pulmonary-wedge* position, nearly saturated blood (97 to 99 percent) can be withdrawn through the wedged catheter, approximating the values of pulmonary venous blood.

Blood leaving the capillary bed is at least *97 percent saturated* (oxygen content, *19.3 volume percent* for an O₂ capacity of 20 volume percent). Blood entering the *left atrium* is slightly less saturated, owing to its admixture with blood passing through pulmonary arteriovenous and other small shunts.

Normal Intracardiac Pressures

Atrial and Wedge Pressures. The phasic *pressures* in the right atrium, left atrium, and pulmonary-artery wedge position (the latter, essentially, a slightly delayed left atrial pressure) have the same overall characteristics. Small differences in the amplitude and timing of the phasic features are seen. In normal sinus rhythm the pressure pulse in these chambers is characterized by an *a* wave produced by the atrial contraction which begins with completion of the atrial P wave in the *ECG.* In the ECG the P wave is followed, after a brief delay, by the QRS signaling the depolarization of the ventricular myocardium. Immediately following depolarization, ventricular contraction begins. The atrioventricular valves close, and the *c* waves in the atrial pressure curves are produced by changes in the dimensions of the atria and by bulging of the valves into the atria, secondary to ventricular contraction. Following the *c* wave, there is a drop in pressure to a low value (the *x* descent) in response to further atrial volume changes during continued ventricular contraction. During the remainder of *systole,* continuous venous inflow produces a rise in pressure (the *v* wave). The peaks of the *v* waves coincide with the opening of the mitral and tricuspid valves. A pressure drop in the atria (the *y* descent) accompanies the transfer of blood from the atria into the ventricles.

Ventricular Pressures. Except for the level of the peak systolic pressures in the left ventricle, which is approximately five times that in the right, the phasic pressures in the right and left ventricles are similar in contour. The ventricles begin to

(Continued on page 46)

CARDIAC CATHETERIZATION

(Continued from page 45)

contract approximately 60 milliseconds following the QRS in the ECG, the right preceding the left, and this action is associated with closure of the atrioventricular valves, resulting in elevated ventricular pressures. During the subsequent period of sequential myocardial contraction, lasting 10 milliseconds and 40 milliseconds, respectively, for the right and left ventricles, there are no volume changes (the period of isovolumic contraction). When the ventricular pressures exceed the end-*diastolic* pressures in the pulmonary artery and aorta, the semilunar valves open, and ejection begins. During the ejection period, the right ventricle and pulmonary artery, and the *left ventricle* and *aorta*, have the same phasic pressures until, systole being completed, the semilunar valves close, and the pressures begin to drop in the ventricles. This is followed by the brief period of isovolumic relaxation. As soon as the ventricular pressures fall below the pressures in the atria, the atrioventricular valves open; diastole starts and proceeds with venous filling of the common ventricular and atrial chambers, leading to superposable pressures in the atria and ventricles.

Aortic and Pulmonary-Artery Pressures. As noted above, during ejection the ventricular pressures and the pressures in the *aorta* or pulmonary artery are identical and are characterized by a smooth rise to a peak, and then a steady fall to the dicrotic notch, signaling the closure of the aortic and pulmonary valves. This is followed by a steady decrease in pressure as a "runoff" of blood from the arterial system into the venous system occurs through the capillary beds. This is abruptly terminated by the next ejection.

Abnormal Oxygen and Pressure Findings

Ventricular Septal Defect. In cases of *ventricular septal defect,* a shunt of saturated (95 percent) blood is ejected during systole by the *left ventricle* through the defect into the *right ventricle,* under the influence of the normally occurring pressure difference between the two ventricles. There the *shunted* blood contaminates the less-saturated mixed venous blood. Thus, an increased volume of blood with a greater-than-normal O_2 saturation (i.e., 85 percent) flows into the *pulmonary artery*. In the majority of cases, the volume of blood shunted depends on the systolic pressure difference between the two ventricles and on the size of the defect. The increase in O_2 saturation of the blood in the pulmonary artery is in direct proportion to the volume of the shunt.

The *pressures* in the pulmonary artery and right ventricle are usually elevated somewhat, owing to the increased pulmonary vascular resistance which is secondary to the failure of neonatal involution to take place in the normal prenatal

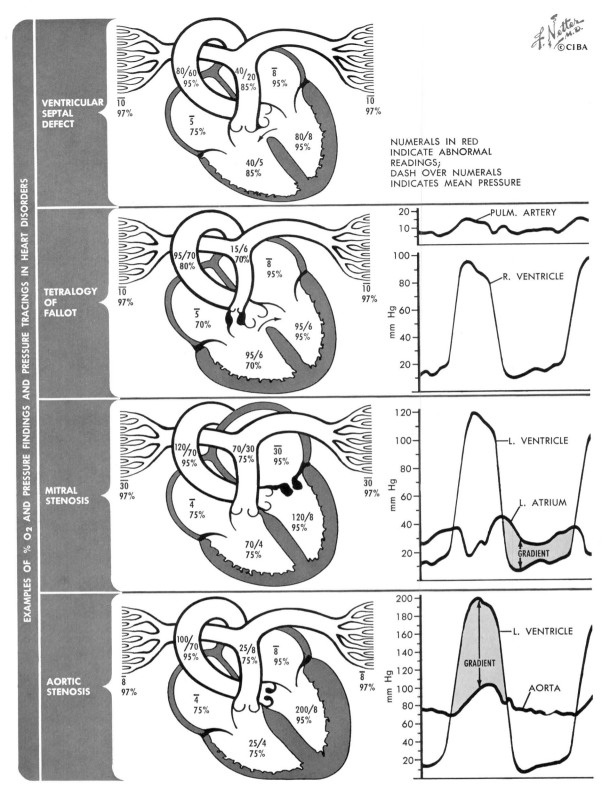

NUMERALS IN RED INDICATE ABNORMAL READINGS; DASH OVER NUMERALS INDICATES MEAN PRESSURE

EXAMPLES OF % O₂ AND PRESSURE FINDINGS AND PRESSURE TRACINGS IN HEART DISORDERS

VENTRICULAR SEPTAL DEFECT

TETRALOGY OF FALLOT

MITRAL STENOSIS

AORTIC STENOSIS

medial hypertrophy of the small arteries. The pressures may be greatly elevated by subsequent intimal and other pathologic changes. Eventually, following the development of very high right-ventricle pressures, the shunt may be reversed, and desaturated blood may flow from the right to the left ventricle and the systemic arteries.

Tetralogy of Fallot. The basic abnormalities in the *tetralogy of Fallot* are pulmonary stenosis, valvular or infundibular interventricular septal defect, disproportion in the diameter between (and, usually, some degree of displacement of) the aorta and pulmonary artery, with secondary right ventricular hypertrophy. Because of the pulmonary stenosis which significantly increases normal outflow resistance, the right ventricular hypertension may reach systemic levels; this results in a *shunt* of unsaturated blood through the defect, with a mild reduction of O_2 saturation in

the left ventricle and a greater reduction in the *aorta* and systemic arteries. The latter causes the cyanosis characteristic of these patients. The greatly reduced pulmonary blood flow reaches full saturation in the lungs.

Systolic pressure in the right ventricle reaches the level of the aortic pressure; however, distal to the pulmonary stenosis the pressures are lower than normal, and the pressure contour is often distorted.

Mitral Stenosis. The obstacle to diastolic flow from the left atrium to the left ventricle, following narrowing of the mitral valve, causes an elevation of the left atrial pressures and, eventually, a reduction in left ventricular flow. A pressure *gradient* across the mitral valve, throughout diastole, can be demonstrated by simultaneous pressure measurements in the left atrium and the left ventricle. Roughly, this gradient

(Continued on page 47)

Cardiac Catheterization

(*Continued from page 46*)

is inversely proportional to the square of the cross-sectional area of the valve orifice and is directly proportional to the square of the volume flow. The gradient is greater with increases in the degree of *stenosis* and during exercise. The left atrial hypertension is accompanied by pulmonary venous hypertension which results in right ventricular hypertension, increased right ventricular work, and hypertrophy. At first, diastolic pressures in the pulmonary artery and left atrium are identical, until the pulmonary vascular resistance is increased because of pathologic changes in the vascular bed, resulting in a gradient between the two pressures. Acute bouts of left atrial hypertension lead to pulmonary edema, whereas chronic pulmonary-artery hypertension may eventually cause right ventricular failure.

Aortic Stenosis. In *aortic stenosis*, obstruction to the ejection of blood from the ventricle into the aorta, owing to infundibular, valvular, or supravalvular stenosis, results in an abnormally high pressure in the left ventricle and an abnormally low pressure in the aorta and, hence, a systolic pressure gradient across the valve.

Progressive obstruction to left ventricular outflow magnifies these effects and leads to left ventricular hypertrophy and, eventually, to acute or chronic left ventricular failure.

Abnormal Indicator-Dilution Curves

The use of the *indicator-dilution* method, as described previously (see page 44), results in dye curves of different characteristic contours, depending on various pathologic situations, some of which are outlined below.

Left-to-Right Shunt. In an uncomplicated *ventricular* septal defect *there is a left-to-right shunt* circuit in which blood circulates through the defect to the right ventricle, then to the *lungs,* back to the left heart, and through the defect again. Some blood may make several such circuits before entering the systemic circulation. Therefore, dye *injected* into a peripheral vein will mix with the blood passing through the right heart and will be divided between the systemic flow and the flow through the shunt circuit. Thus, the recorded *dye curve* has a *slower* rate of rise and reaches a *peak* that is *lower than normal*. Furthermore, the downslope (*disappearance slope*) of the curve is characterized by a *hump* (distinct from and earlier than the normal recirculation hump) and is *prolonged*.

Right-to-Left Shunt. In a relatively unusual form of *atrial* septal defect, where there is increased pulmonary vascular resistance, a *right-to-left shunt* carries unsaturated blood from the right to the left atrium. Part of the dye injected into a peripheral vein reaches the left heart directly, and the remainder follows the

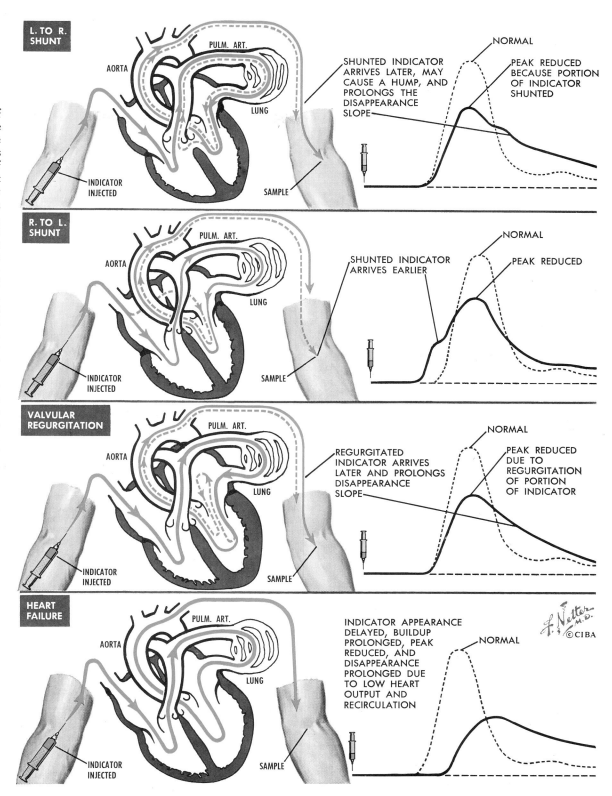

normal circuit through the lungs. This causes an *early hump* on the ascending limb of the *dye curve* and a *peak* dye concentration *lower than normal* by an amount proportional to that appearing earlier.

Valvular Regurgitation. In mitral *regurgitation* during ventricular systole, blood returns through the mitral valve into the enlarged left atrium, where it mixes with blood entering the atrium from the pulmonary veins.

Dye injected into a peripheral vein reaches the left ventricle where, during systole, it is both ejected into the aorta and forced back into the left atrium. With each successive heart cycle, dye passes back and forth between the two chambers, becoming progressively more dilute.

The *dye curve* recorded is characterized by a *reduced peak* concentration and a *delayed downslope*.

Heart Failure. In *heart failure* there are dilatation of one or more chambers of the heart, increased diastolic

blood volume in those chambers, increased venous blood volume, slowed circulation time, and reduced systolic stroke output. This results in a greater dilution of the dye injected into a peripheral vein, as well as a slower rate of ejection. Because of these abnormalities, a *dye curve* recorded from a peripheral artery is characterized by a *delayed appearance*, a *late* and *reduced peak* concentration, and a *prolonged disappearance time*, the latter being the result of significant *recirculation* before all the injected dye has passed the *sampling* site in its sluggish first passage.

The prolonged disappearance time and the accompanying diminished or absent recirculation hump, singly or in combination, tend to produce curves lacking a truly exponential portion of the downslope, so that elimination of recirculation is impossible. Therefore, such curves are invalid for the calculation of cardiac output.

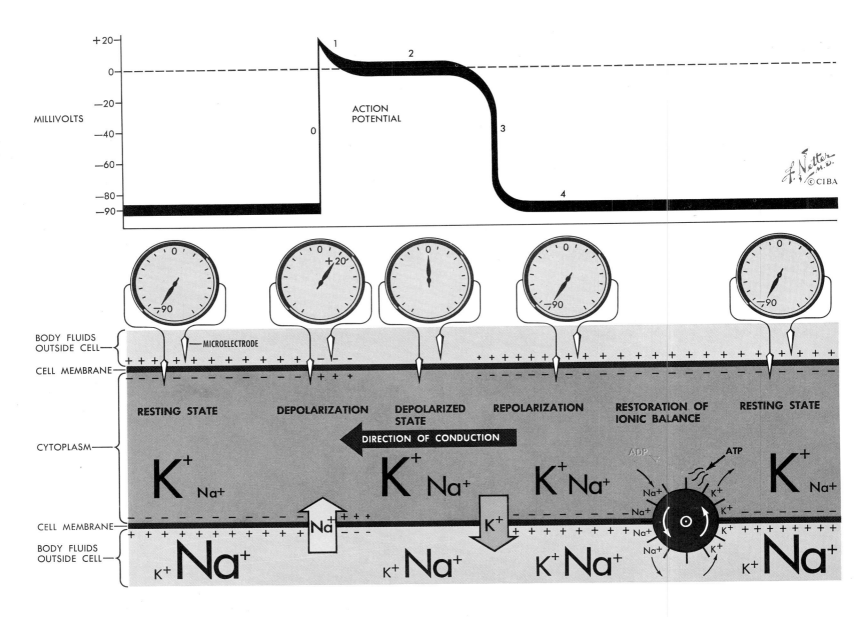

ACTION POTENTIAL

MILLIVOLTS: +20, 0, −20, −40, −60, −80, −90

BODY FLUIDS OUTSIDE CELL — MICROELECTRODE

CELL MEMBRANE

RESTING STATE   DEPOLARIZATION   DEPOLARIZED STATE   REPOLARIZATION   RESTORATION OF IONIC BALANCE   RESTING STATE

CYTOPLASM

DIRECTION OF CONDUCTION

CELL MEMBRANE

BODY FLUIDS OUTSIDE CELL

PHYSIOLOGY OF THE SPECIALIZED CONDUCTION SYSTEM

General Considerations

Under normal conditions, heart activation results from an impulse originating in a cell or cell group, which constitutes the pacemaker, and from the propagation of this impulse to all fibers of the atria and ventricles. Arrival of the electrical signal at the contractile fibers of the heart initiates contraction. Regular rhythmic activity requires the presence of specialized automatic fibers. Coordinated contraction of the atria and ventricles requires a system which distributes the electrical impulse to the muscle fibers of these chambers in the proper sequence and at the proper time. Both of these functions are performed by *specialized* groups of cardiac fibers. The automaticity which underlies pacemaker activity is a unique property not only of the fibers in the sinoatrial node but also of other groups of specialized atrial fibers and the cells of the His-Purkinje system. The conduction system is composed of the fibers of the internodal tracts, Bachmann's bundle, the atrioventricular node, the bundle of His, the bundle branches, and the peripheral Purkinje fibers. The cells of the conduction system, in addition to having a characteristic histological appearance, possess unique electrical properties. These properties, and the basis for electrical activity of all cardiac fibers, can best be understood by recording the transmembrane potentials through intracellular *microelectrodes.*

Basis for Transmembrane Potentials

Cardiac *cells,* like other excitable mammalian tissues, have an intracellular ionic composition which differs from that found in the extracellular fluids. For our consideration, the most important ions are sodium (Na^+) and potassium (K^+). The relative magnitudes of the concentrations of these ions are indicated by the sizes of the symbols in the illustration. Intracellular K concentration is approximately thirty times greater than the extracellular concentration, whereas intracellular Na concentration is approximately thirty times less. Because of this difference, and because the resting membrane is more permeable to K than to Na, the *membrane* of the *resting* fiber is polarized. The magnitude of this polarization (the transmembrane resting potential) can be measured by inserting a microelectrode inside the cell and measuring the potential difference across the membrane. This is shown schematically both as the recorded voltage (−90 mv) and as an oscilloscopic tracing.

With the onset of excitation, there is a change in the permeability of the membrane which permits Na ions, carrying a positive charge, to move rapidly down their electrochemical gradient, across the membrane, and inside the fiber. This sudden influx of positive charge, carried by Na^+, actually *reverses* the transmembrane potential so that the inside becomes 20 to 30 mv more positive than the *outside.* The inward Na^+ current is represented here by the large arrow; the resulting change in transmembrane potential is shown as the upstroke (*phase 0*) of the oscilloscopic tracing. After excitation there is a period of variable duration (*phases 1 and 2*) when the membrane potential remains close to zero. This period, often described as the plateau of the trans-

membrane *action potential,* results from a decrease in Na and K permeability. Subsequently, *repolarization,* or restoration of the normal resting potential, takes place because of an increase in K permeability and an efflux of K^+ from the cells. The phase of rapid repolarization (phase 3) is followed by a period of stable resting potential (*phase 4*) until the arrival of the next wave of excitation.

In order to maintain the normal concentration gradients for these ions, an active transport system, often referred to as a "pump," must extrude the sodium which has entered and pump in an equivalent amount of potassium. The pump is represented by the wheel with gates.

The accompanying figure is a representation of a longitudinal section of a single fiber during propagation of the impulse. The activity (*conduction*) is spreading from right to left. At the extreme left of the tracing, the resting potential has not yet been changed by the coming wave of excitation; at the right, repolarization is complete, and the resting potential has been restored. In the middle of the figure, the current flow associated with excitation is shown under the upstroke (phase 0) of the action potential; the currents associated with repolarization appear under phase 3. The relative magnitude and polarity of the transmembrane potential are suggested by the plus and minus signs inside and outside the membrane. Propagation, or the spread of the impulse, occurs because a change in transmembrane potential at one point, during phase 0, causes a local longitudinal potential difference. This produces a flow of current across the membrane in advance of the action-potential upstroke, resulting in excitation of the next adjacent segment of the fiber. Since, during propagation, these processes are

(Continued on page 49)

48

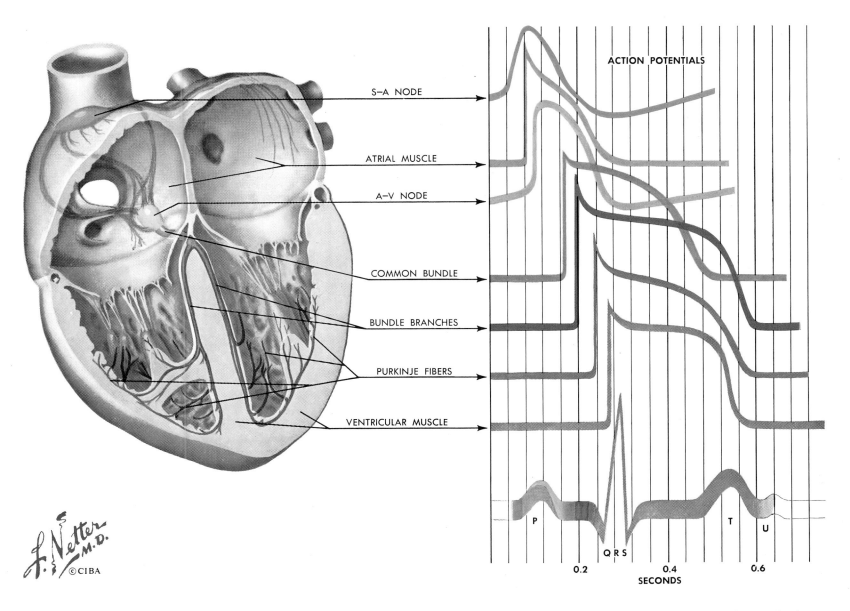

ACTION POTENTIALS

S-A NODE

ATRIAL MUSCLE

A-V NODE

COMMON BUNDLE

BUNDLE BRANCHES

PURKINJE FIBERS

VENTRICULAR MUSCLE

P   QRS   T   U

0.2   0.4   0.6
SECONDS

PHYSIOLOGY OF THE SPECIALIZED CONDUCTION SYSTEM

(Continued from page 48)

continuous, activity spreads from its point of origin throughout all excitable fibers.

Transmembrane Potentials of Specialized Fibers

The description just given applies, in general, to all cardiac fibers. However, records of transmembrane *action potentials* recorded from cells in different parts of the heart show special characteristics which are important in understanding the initiation and spread of the normal cardiac impulse.

Sinoatrial Node and Atrium. This trace *(S-A node)* is recorded from a single automatic fiber in the sinoatrial node. The record shows two points of importance: (1) There is no steady resting potential; instead, after repolarization, the transmembrane potential decreases spontaneously. It is this slow, spontaneous *depolarization* (see page 48) during phase 4 which causes the automatic activity of sinus fibers. A similar cause of automaticity has been recorded from all the specialized cardiac fibers capable of normal pacemaker activity. (2) The rate of rise of the upstroke of the action potential is low. This causes slow conduction of the impulse within the node. The action potential recorded from an ordinary *atrial muscle* fiber is shown below that recorded from the sinoatrial node. Here, the upstroke is rapid and the resting potential steady.

Atrioventricular Node. Action potentials recorded from fibers of the *A-V node* resemble those shown for sinus fibers. The extremely slow spread of the impulse through the A-V node results largely from the low rate of rise of the action potential. The phase-4 depolarization shown probably causes automatic activity only in fibers of the lower node in close proximity to the common bundle.

His-Purkinje System. The action potentials recorded from the fibers of this part of the specialized conduction system *(Purkinje fibers)* have three important characteristics: (1) The rate of rise of the action potential is high, and thus conduction is rapid. (2) The duration of the action potential is great, and thus the refractory period is long. (3) Under appropriate conditions, each of these fiber groups (not shown) may develop spontaneous phase-4 depolarization and become an automatic pacemaker.

The bottom trace *(ventricular muscle)*, recorded from an ordinary muscle fiber of the ventricle, is included to contrast the time of excitation and action-potential duration with the other records.

Sequence of Excitation and the Electrocardiogram

The seven tracings of transmembrane action potentials indicate the normal sequence of heart activation in relation to the schematic electrocardiogram shown below them. The coloring of the ECG trace suggests the temporal relationship of each type of action potential to the normal electrocardiogram, and also the contribution of electrical activity in each type of cell to the ECG recorded from the body surface.

Activity of pacemaker fibers in the sinoatrial node precedes the first indication of activity in the electrocardiogram (the *P wave*) and cannot be demonstrated in the body-surface leads. Depolarization of atrial muscle fibers, in a sequence largely determined by the specialized atrial paths shown, causes the P wave. Repolarization of atrial fibers ordinarily is not seen in the ECG. Activity reaches the upper part of the A-V node early during the P wave. Propagation through the node is slow, and excitation of fibers in the His bundle does not occur until the middle of the *P-R interval*. The spread of activity through the *common bundle*, the *bundle branches,* and parts of the Purkinje system precedes the earliest excitation of ventricular muscle. There is no indication in the ECG of excitation of the fibers of the His-Purkinje system. The *QRS complex* results from activation of the muscle fibers of the ventricles. The isoelectric *S-T segment* corresponds to the plateau of the ventricular action potential, and the *T wave* results from repolarization of ventricular fibers. The *U wave* corresponds in time with repolarization of the specialized fibers of the bundle branches and Purkinje system, and it may reflect this event as recorded at the body surface.

From these traces it is clear that, although the normal sequence of heart activation results from the anatomical distribution and unique electrical properties of specialized cardiac cells, there is no signal recorded in the electrocardiogram which corresponds to these events. Thus, the sequence of excitation of the specialized tissues can be determined only by implication when noting the temporal characteristics of the P and QRS complexes and their interrelationships. Finally, since excitation and the resulting depolarization cause contraction of the myocardial fibers, the coordinated mechanical activity of the heart depends on the anatomical distribution and the electrical properties of the specialized cardiac fibers.

THE ELECTROCARDIOGRAM

Introduction

An electrocardiogram is a graph of voltage variations plotted against time. The variations result from the depolarization and repolarization of the cardiac muscle, which produces electric fields that reach the surface of the body where electrodes are located. An electrocardiographic machine is a galvanometer which records voltage variations, usually on paper tape. The first such machine was developed by Wilhelm Einthoven in 1906. It consisted of a silver-plated quartz string situated in a fixed magnetic field. Voltage variations from the body passed through the string, and the interaction of the electric fields between the magnet and the string resulted in the string's movement, which was photographed. Currently, vacuum tubes and transistorized instruments are employed instead of the string galvanometer.

Since the development of a practical method of recording the electrocardiogram, much has been learned about the electrophysiology of the heart. The major contribution was by Einthoven, winner of a Nobel prize, who described the vector concept and pointed out that the action current of the heart, often called the "accession" or "regression" wave, can be represented by a *vector* which has magnitude, direction, and sense. The magnitude of the voltage of the accession wave is the length of the *arrow shaft,* the direction is determined with respect to a *line of reference,* and the sense is indicated by the presence of an *arrowhead* on the shaft. In its simplest concept, the vector represents the magnitude of a single *dipole, i.e.,* a paired electric charge, minus and plus. Likewise, the electric effect of a group of dipoles can be represented by a vector.

The Normal Electrocardiogram

The electrocardiogram is a record of voltage variations plotted against time. The paper on which the electrocardiogram is recorded is ruled in *1-mm*-spaced lines, horizontally and vertically. When the tracing is properly standardized (a *1-mv* change produces a *10-mm* stylus deflection), each vertical space represents a voltage change of *0.1 mv,* and each

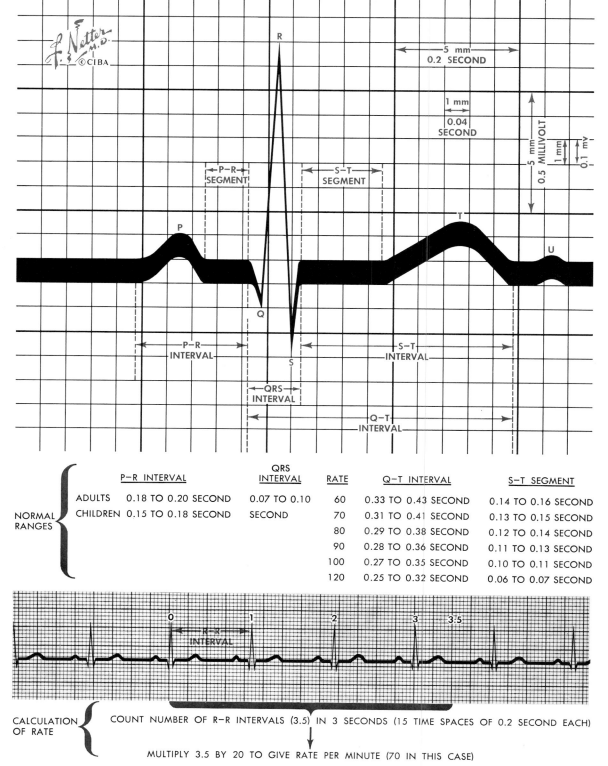

			QRS INTERVAL	RATE	Q-T INTERVAL	S-T SEGMENT
NORMAL RANGES		P-R INTERVAL				
	ADULTS	0.18 TO 0.20 SECOND	0.07 TO 0.10	60	0.33 TO 0.43 SECOND	0.14 TO 0.16 SECOND
	CHILDREN	0.15 TO 0.18 SECOND	SECOND	70	0.31 TO 0.41 SECOND	0.13 TO 0.15 SECOND
				80	0.29 TO 0.38 SECOND	0.12 TO 0.14 SECOND
				90	0.28 TO 0.36 SECOND	0.11 TO 0.13 SECOND
				100	0.27 TO 0.35 SECOND	0.10 TO 0.11 SECOND
				120	0.25 TO 0.32 SECOND	0.06 TO 0.07 SECOND

CALCULATION OF RATE { COUNT NUMBER OF R-R INTERVALS (3.5) IN 3 SECONDS (15 TIME SPACES OF 0.2 SECOND EACH)

MULTIPLY 3.5 BY 20 TO GIVE RATE PER MINUTE (70 IN THIS CASE)

horizontal space a time interval of *0.04 second*. Each fifth line, horizontal and vertical, is heavy. The time interval between the heavy lines is *0.2 second*. The voltage change between two heavy lines is *0.5 mv.*

A *P* wave is the result of atrial depolarization. This wave should not exceed 2.5 mm (0.25 mv) in height in *lead II* (see page 51), nor should the duration be greater in this lead than 0.11 second. The *P-R interval,* which includes the P wave plus the *P-R segment,* is a measure of the time interval from the beginning of atrial depolarization to the beginning of ventricular depolarization. This interval should not be greater than *0.2 second* for rates over *60 beats per minute.* The *Q* wave is the first downward deflection of the *QRS complex,* and it represents septal depolarization (see pages 52 and 53). The *R* wave is the *first positive* or *upward deflection* of the QRS complex, and, normally, this is due to apical left ventricular depolar-

ization. The S wave is the *first negative deflection* following the R wave, and it is due to depolarization of the posterior basal region of the left ventricle. The voltage of the R wave in the precordial leads (see page 51) should not exceed 27 mm. The *Q-T interval* is measured from the beginning of the QRS complex to the end of the T wave, and this includes the QRS complex, *S-T segment,* and T-wave intervals. (The latter two constitute the *S-T interval.*) The Q-T interval varies with the cardiac rate and should not be greater than *0.43 second* for rates above 60. The total QRS interval should not exceed *0.1 second.*

The *cardiac rate* may be determined by *counting the number of R-R intervals within 16 vertical heavy time lines (15 time spaces) and multiplying by 20.* The first interval counted is coincident with the zero time line.

ELECTROCARDIOGRAPHIC LEADS AND REFERENCE LINES

Leads

The conventional electric connections used for recording the electrocardiogram are the *limb leads, augmented limb leads,* and *precordial leads.*

Limb Leads. These are bipolar, for they detect electric variations at two points and display the difference. *Lead I* is a connection between electrodes on the left arm and the right arm. The galvanometer is between these points of contact. When the left arm is in a positive field of force with respect to the right arm, an upward (positive) deflection is written in lead I. *Lead II* is the connection between the left-leg and right-arm electrodes. When the left leg is in a positive field of force with respect to the right arm, an upward deflection is written in this lead. *Lead III* is a connection between the left leg and the left arm. When the left leg is in a positive field of force with respect to the left arm, a positive deflection is written in lead III.

Augmented Limb Leads. These are unipolar, for they register the electric variations in potential at one point (right arm, left arm, or left leg) with respect to a point which does not vary significantly in electric activity during cardiac contraction. The lead is augmented by virtue of the type of electric connection, which results in a trace of increased amplitude, as compared to the older Wilson unipolar lead connections. *Lead aV_R* inscribes the electric potentials of the right arm with respect to a null point, which is made by uniting the wires from the left arm and the left leg. *Lead aV_L* records the potentials at the left arm in relation to a connection made by the union of wires from the right arm and the left foot. *Lead aV_F* reveals the potentials at the left foot in reference to a junction made by the union of wires from the left and right arms.

Precordial Leads. These are unipolar and are recorded in chest positions 1 through 6. The *V* designation indicates that the movable electrode registers the electric potential under the electrode with respect to a V or central terminal connection, which is made by connecting wires from the right arm, left arm, and left leg. The electric potential of the central terminal connection does not vary significantly throughout the cardiac cycle; therefore, the recordings made with the V connection show the electric variations that are taking place under the movable precordial electrode. Position V_1 is at the fourth intercostal space to the right of the ster-

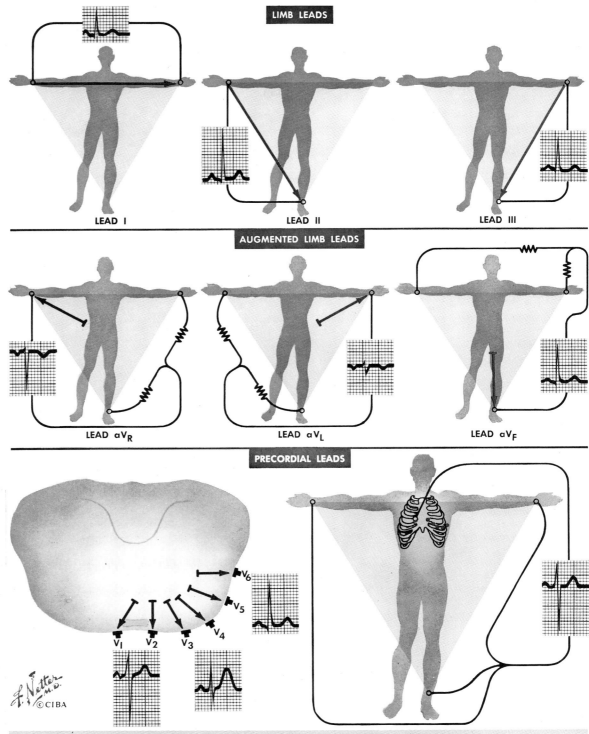

LIMB LEADS

LEAD I   LEAD II   LEAD III

AUGMENTED LIMB LEADS

LEAD aV_R LEAD aV_L LEAD aV_F

PRECORDIAL LEADS

V_6 V_5 V_4 V_1 V_2 V_3

WHEN CURRENT FLOWS TOWARD RED ARROWHEADS, UPWARD DEFLECTION OCCURS IN ECG
WHEN CURRENT FLOWS AWAY FROM RED ARROWHEADS, DOWNWARD DEFLECTION OCCURS IN ECG
WHEN CURRENT FLOWS PERPENDICULAR TO RED ARROWS, NO DEFLECTION OR BIPHASIC DEFLECTION OCCURS

num; V_2 is at the fourth intercostal space to the left of the sternum; V_4 is at the left midclavicular line in the fifth intercostal space; V_3 is halfway between V_2 and V_4; V_5 is at the fifth intercostal space in the anterior axillary line; and V_6 is at the fifth intercostal space in the left midaxillary line.

At times, other precordial-lead placements are helpful; *e.g.,* those elevated 2 in. above the usual positions (EV_1, EV_2, etc.), which may help to detect infarcts of the myocardium; those placed 2 in. below the usual positions (LV_1, LV_2, etc.) when the heart is unusually low in the thorax, as in patients with pulmonary emphysema; or those to the right of V_1 (designated V_3R, V_4R, etc.), which are used to differentiate right bundle-branch block and right ventricular hypertrophy from the normal condition. Leads farther to the left are designated V_7, V_8, etc. These are used to explore the left ventricle when it is directed posteriorly.

Reference Lines

For the various leads, the reference lines of Einthoven are shown in the plate as *red arrows.* For example, the line of reference for lead I is a line which connects the left- and right-arm electrodes. An accession wave (often expressed as a vector), directed toward the arrowhead of any of the red arrows, results in an upward (positive) deflection in the electrocardiogram. If the electric activity, or accession wave, is directed toward the tail of the reference arrow, a downward (negative) deflection is written, but if this wave is perpendicular to the line (90 degrees), no deflection — or a small biphasic one — will be written. The height of the electrocardiographic wave is proportional to the magnitude of the projection of the accession-wave vector on a reference line (see pages 52 and 53).

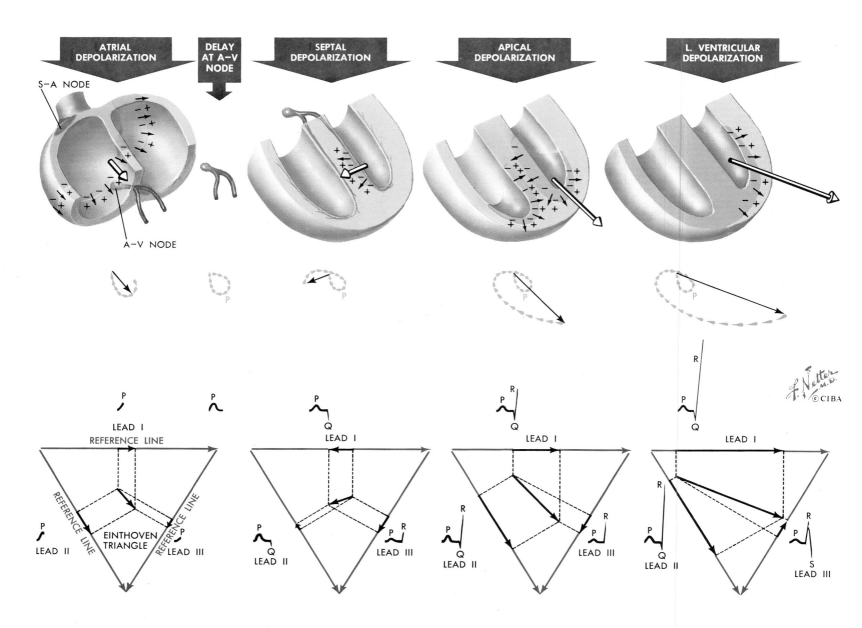

CARDIAC DEPOLARIZATION AND REPOLARIZATION AND MEAN INSTANTANEOUS VECTORS

Depolarization

Atrial Depolarization and Mean Vectors. The cardiac impulse originates in the sinus node and starts the process of *atrial depolarization* by lowering the resistance of the cell membrane, allowing neutralization or reversal of certain dipoles (see page 48). This leaves an electric-wave front, an accession wave, which is preceded by positive forces and followed by negative ones. Normally, this wave is initiated at the *sinoauricular (S-A) node,* but, early (*i.e.,* during atrial depolariza-

tion), the wave spreads toward the foot and *A-V node.* Toward the end of atrial depolarization, the accession wave is directed toward the left atrium and left arm. The early atrial-depolarization wave may be represented as a vector, the length of which indicates the magnitude (strength) of the voltage generated by the accession wave. The late atrial-depolarization voltage is represented by a second vector, the length of which is a measure of the voltage generated at this point in time. If one connects the heads of these vectors with their points of origin, a loop is formed; this is the *P loop* of the vectorcardiogram (VCG). The P loop, as seen in the frontal plane, is shown herewith. A mean P vector can be determined from the instantaneous vectors 1 and 2 by using the parallelogram law. To derive the mean vector from two instantaneous vectors, a parallelogram is completed. The instantaneous vectors are drawn as originating from a common point of origin *E.*

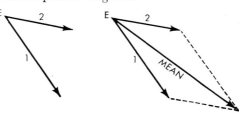

The parallelogram is completed by drawing a line

from each arrowhead, parallel to the opposite vector. The *mean vector* is an *arrow connecting E* with the *opposite angle of the parallelogram.* The mean vector indicates the average direction taken by the atrial accession wave, and its magnitude as the wave travels over the atria.

One can analyze the mean atrial-depolarization vector against the *Einthoven-triangle* reference frame to predict the type of *P waves* that will appear in *leads I, II, and III.* If one projects the mean vector against the *reference line* of lead I, there will be a projected vector, the length of which is proportional to the amplitude of the P wave in that lead. The direction of the wave (up or down) is determined by the direction of the projected atrial vector with respect to the polarity of the reference line. The direction of the P wave will be upward when the projected vector points in the same direction as the reference arrow for that lead, and negative when the opposite relationship exists.

Just before atrial depolarization is complete, depolarization of the A-V node begins; however, the nodal-depolarization process is of such low magnitude that the electrocardiographic instrument is unable to detect these changes, and it is not until the interventricular septum is invaded that a QRS complex begins. Normally, there is a time interval from the end of the P wave to

(Continued on page 53)

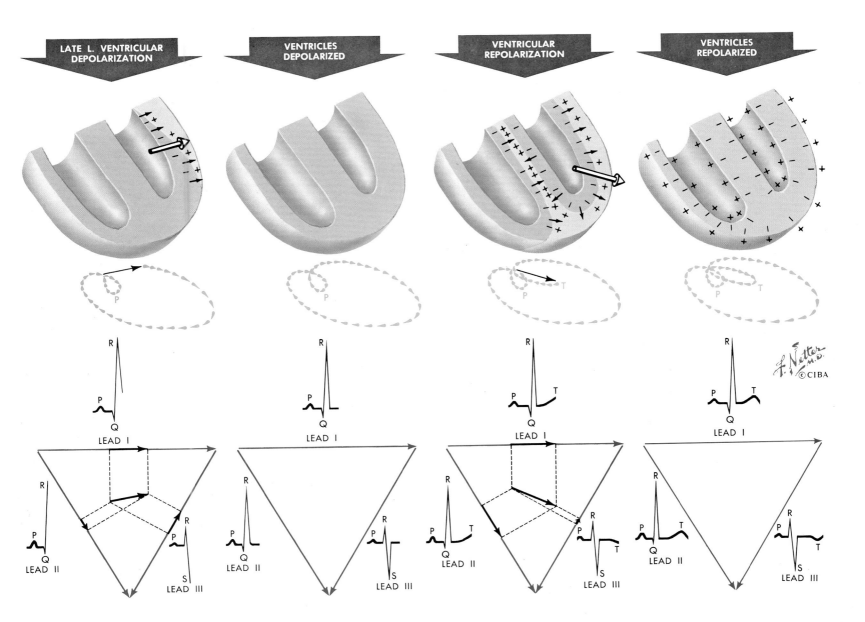

CARDIAC DEPOLARIZATION AND REPOLARIZATION AND MEAN INSTANTANEOUS VECTORS

(Continued from page 52)

the beginning of the QRS complex (known as the P-R segment), which is usually opposite in direction to the P wave and is a result of atrial repolarization.

Septal Depolarization. The *first* important electric movement in *septal depolarization* normally begins at the left side of the septum, moves to the right, and results from the fact that branches of the bundle of His enter the septum at a higher level on the left than on the right. The septal left-to-right movement is of importance, since it writes the normal septal Q *wave* in leads I, aV$_L$, and V$_6$. If the first electric movement is analyzed (using the Einthoven reference frame), it is evident that a Q wave will initiate the QRS complex, in leads I and II, and an R *wave* in lead III.

Apical Depolarization. A *second* electric movement of significance is *apical depolarization*, which follows the early depolarization of the right ventricle. Projection of the second instantaneous vector onto the Einthoven triangle indicates that leads I, II, and III will develop R waves at this time.

Left Ventricular Depolarization. Depolarization of the right ventricle occurs quickly and is completed early because of the thinness of this structure compared to that of the left ventricle. A *third* significant electric movement is toward the lateral wall of the left ventricle. At this time, the amplitude of the R waves is increased in leads I and II, and S waves appear in lead III. The forces, at this point in time, are strong, since there are no counterforces from the right ventricle, and the left ventricular muscle mass is thick.

Left Late Ventricular Depolarization. A *fourth,* or late, instantaneous vector exists toward the base of the left ventricle and occurs just before the end of the *ventricular-depolarization* process. This force results in a deepening of the S *waves* in lead III and an accentuation of the amplitude of the R waves in leads I and II.

Ventricles Depolarized. When the dipoles are removed or reversed, and consequently there are no potential differences on the body as a result of electric changes affecting the heart, the heart is in the *depolarized state.* The myocardium is in a refractory condition during this period, and a myocardial stimulus will fail to elicit a contraction. Since there are no voltage differences, the electrocardiographic trace returns to the base line in all leads; it is during this time that the S-T segment is written.

Repolarization

Repolarization of the ventricles is a very complex process which might be looked upon as a vector appearing opposite to the wave of depolarization. As a result, the development of positive (upward) T waves is shown in the standard leads I and II. The normal direction of T waves in lead III is variable.

Ventricles Repolarized. Finally, each cell of the myocardium becomes repolarized, with a preponderance of negative charges inside the cell and positive charges outside. The heart is now ready for its next stimulation and contraction. The heart muscle is thus in a *receptive state,* and a stimulus will elicit a contraction. Now the trace is *isoelectric,* since there are no net potential differences on the body surface.

THE SPATIAL VECTORCARDIOGRAPHIC LOOP

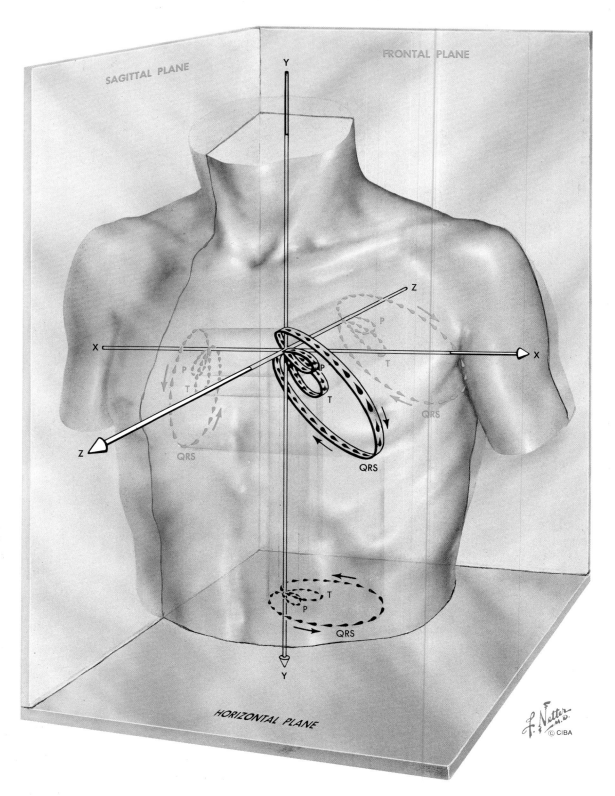

The vectorcardiographic system is a method for displaying the action current of the heart. A three-dimensional or spatial voltage loop is produced by this action current. This can be projected on the *frontal, horizontal,* and *sagittal reference planes.* The spatial-vector loop is made up of numerous instantaneous spatial vectors.

Several reference-frame systems are in use, but only the Frank orthogonal (X, Y, Z) system is shown in the plate. Three major loops — the *P, QRS,* and *T* — occur with each cardiac contraction. These are made by plotting electrically the action current of the heart from any two orthogonal leads (at an angle of 90 degrees to each other). The loop usually consists of a series of dots placed 2 milliseconds apart. Each dot is shaped like a teardrop, with the blunt end leading, so that the direction of the loop movement can be determined.

Frontal-Plane Projection

The frontal-plane projection is a plot of the X axis (from left to right) against the Y axis (foot to head). Electrodes placed on the left and right arms or sides of the body record electric variations between these two electrodes. At the same time, electrodes on the head and foot record electric variations occurring between them. By putting the side-to-side leads on the horizontal beam of a cathode-ray scope, and the foot-to-head leads on the vertical beam of the scope, and recording the two simultaneously, a loop or frontal-plane vectorcardiogram (VCG) is recorded.

Sagittal-Plane Projection

The sagittal-plane projection consists of a plot of the Y axis against the Z axis (front to back).

Horizontal-Plane Projection

The horizontal-plane projection is made by a plot of Z against X (left to right).

From these three projections — frontal, horizontal, and sagittal — one may visualize the spatial loop (three dimensions) as shown in the plate.

Spatial Magnitude and Distortions

In conventional vectorcardiography, one records on the scope, and then on photographic film, three loop projections of the spatial vector, including the frontal, the horizontal, and, usually, the left sagittal projections. From these is visualized the three-dimensional or spatial loop, which must have given rise to the three projections. With the aid of modern computers, it is now possible actually to record the magnitude of the spatial vector as well as its projections.

The vectorcardiogram is of extreme importance in showing the balance of electric forces which are present at any point in time. In cardiac disease these components are unbalanced, as is clearly shown in the vectorcardiogram. For example, with hypertrophy of a chamber there is an overbalance of forces toward the hypertrophied muscle, distorting the vectorcardiographic loop in this direction. Also, when normal forces are destroyed, as with myocardial infarcts, the forces are directed away from the infarcted area, and the loop again is distorted.

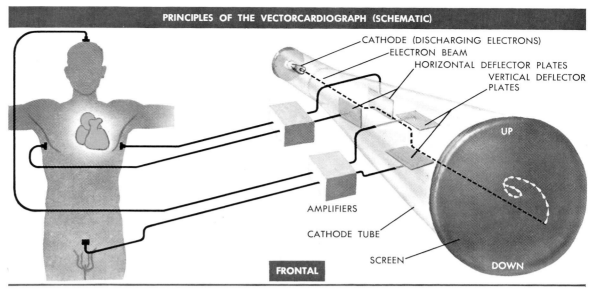

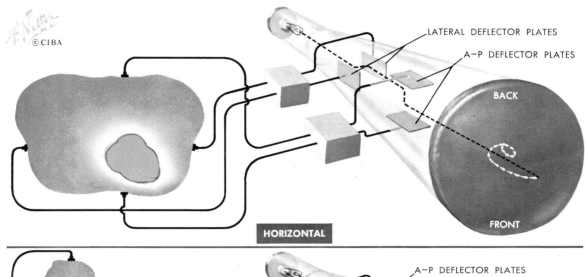

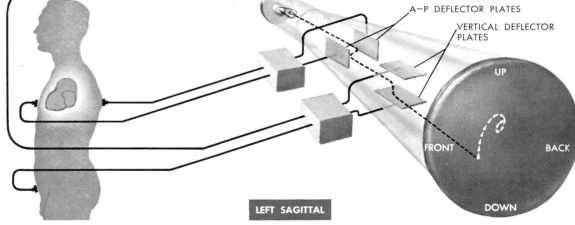

PRINCIPLES OF THE VECTORCARDIOGRAPH

The vectorcardiographic instrument is merely an X-Y plotter — *i.e.,* a device which plots forces in two directions at one time. In its simplest concept, the *vectorcardiograph* plots voltage variations occurring in one direction against those occurring in a different direction. The instrument is electronic, with *electrodes* placed on the surface of the body. These electrodes pick up the heart current and lead it, through *amplifiers,* to a *cathode-ray tube.* The tube *discharges an electron beam,* which passes through a pair of *horizontal* and *vertical plates* to a phosphor *screen.* On striking the screen the beam produces luminous spots. A beam interrupter is employed to interrupt the trace every 2 milliseconds to make timing possible. Each point is shaped electronically, so that a teardrop outline is formed. The blunt end of the teardrop is the leading edge, and the pointed end is the trailing edge. By observing the form of these time dots, it is possible to visualize the direction in which the beam is moving.

The vectorcardiographic machine has been so built that the body potentials will be displayed in a standard way, the types of electric connections being referred to as *frontal, horizontal,* and *left sagittal.* A schematic concept follows.

Frontal Projection

Lead X, left to right: A positive potential under the left arm, as compared to the right, results in a movement of the cathode-ray beam to the right of the screen, as viewed from the front. Here, the left side of the body is positive, the right relatively negative. The cathode beam, when displaced to the right side of the screen, indicates this relationship.

Lead Y, foot to head: A positive potential at the foot, with respect to the head, moves the beam *downward* on the cathode-ray screen. Thus, a point on the screen below the center of the heart indicates this relationship.

Horizontal Projection

Lead X, left to right: A positive potential on the left of the body, compared to the right, results in a movement of the cathode-ray beam to the right of the screen, as viewed from the front.

Lead Z, *front to back:* A positive force in the front of the body, as compared to the back, produces a downward deflection of the beam on the screen.

Left Sagittal Projection

Lead Z, front to back: A positive force in the front of the body, compared to the back, produces a deflection to the left of the screen.

Lead Y, foot to head: A positive potential at the foot, with respect to the head, results in moving the beam to the bottom of the cathode-ray screen.

Other Lead Systems

About nineteen different types of electric connections have been devised, but only a few of these record the voltage variations from the body, in the X, Y, and Z axes, with equal accuracy. Some of the lead systems are complex and require the application of many electrodes to the body; others are highly inaccurate and produce distortions in one plane or another, *e.g.,* amplifying the heart voltages from front to back while failing to amplify adequately the forces from head to foot. The Frank leads appear to be a good compromise between simplicity and accuracy, and they are employed by many physicians who are using vectorcardiography in a practical way.

The system described above was oversimplified.

NORMAL VECTOR-CARDIOGRAPHIC LOOP AND DERIVATION OF THE ELECTRO-CARDIOGRAM IN VARIOUS LEADS

FRONTAL PLANE

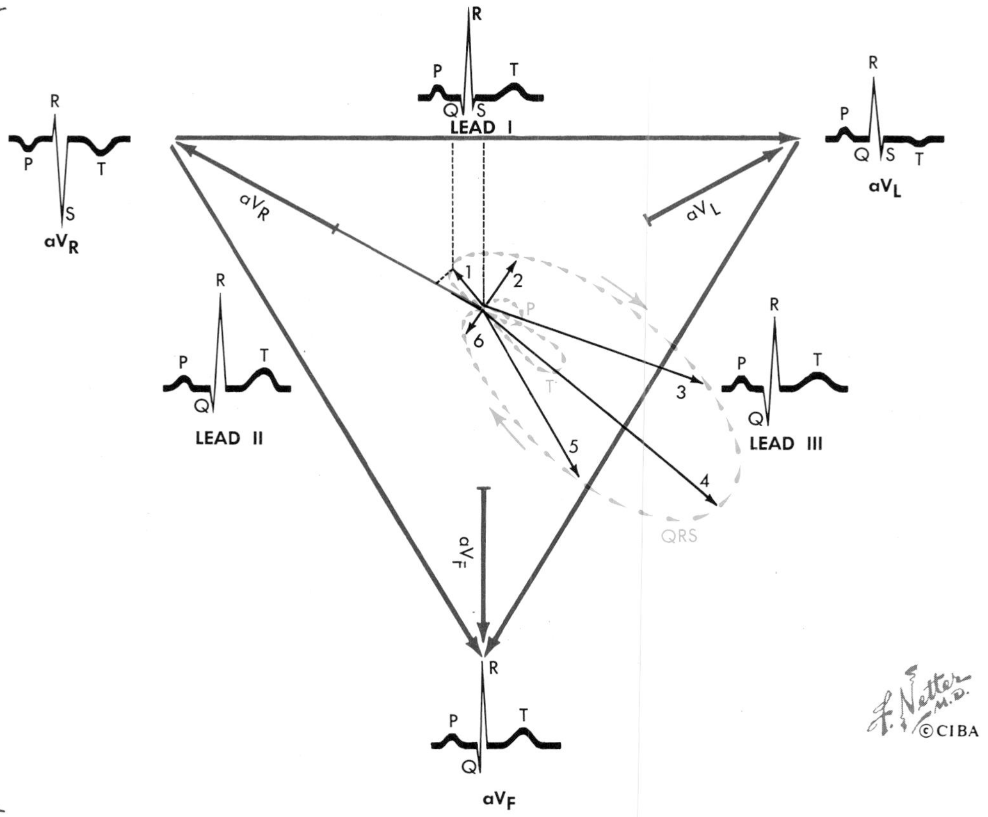

HORIZONTAL PLANE

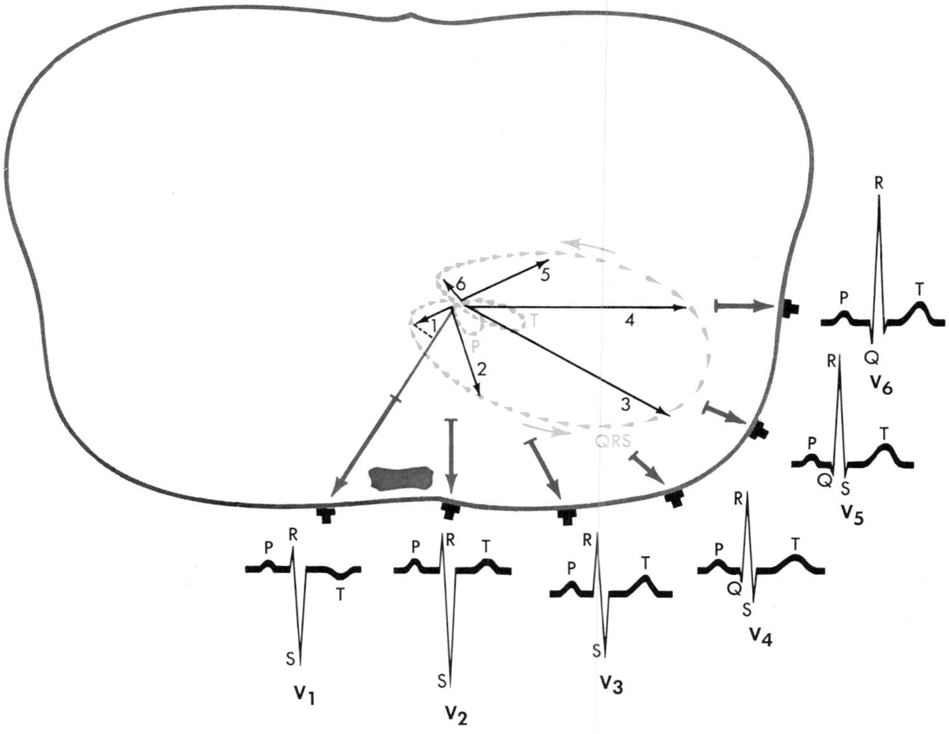

Normal Vectorcardiographic Loop and Derivation of the Electrocardiogram

There is a definite relationship between the frontal and horizontal *vectorcardiographic loops* and the conventional twelve-lead *electrocardiogram.* The diagram shows the bipolar *leads I, II,* and *III,* which ordinarily are analyzed on the Einthoven triangle; in addition, the augmented unipolar *leads* aV_R, aV_L, and aV_F, which are analyzed on the triangle reference system drawn inside Einthoven's triangle, are displayed. The inside augmented or triaxial frame consists of three reference arrows pointing toward the right arm, the left arm, and the left leg. In principle, a heart vector pointing toward the head of an arrow of *any* reference line will write an *upward deflection* in that lead. If directed perpendicular to any reference line, no deflection — or a small one — will be written in that lead; if pointing away from the head of the reference arrow, a negative deflection will be written in that lead. The magnitude of any deflection in the electrocardiogram is proportional to the magnitude of the vector projected on a line of reference.

For example, let us take the first instantaneous vector (1) in the *frontal plane,* which points from the region of the A-V node toward the right shoulder. As the projected vector points toward the right-arm electrode, an *R wave* is written in lead aV_R. As the vector points away from the lead-I reference arrow, the trace writes a *Q wave* in that lead. If the vector points slightly away from the augmented unipolar left-arm-lead reference arrow, a very small Q wave is written in that lead. As the projected vector points away from the head of the aV_F reference arrow, there is a Q wave in that lead. The vector points away from the head of the lead-II reference arrow, and Q waves are written in that lead.

In the *horizontal plane* the projection of the first vector points toward the reference arrow which runs from the A-V node to the V_1 position, and an *R wave* is written in that lead. The projected vector points also toward a line running from the A-V node to the V_2 position, and the R wave is still being written. A Q wave is written in leads V_5 and V_6 because the projection, on reference lines 5 and 6 of the first vector, points away from the head of the reference line.

Each instantaneous vector of the loop can be analyzed in this way. The first vector (1) produces little or no deflection in V_4. This vector points away from the V_4 reference line which connects the A-V node with the V_4 chest position and, therefore, writes a Q wave in this lead. This is true also for V_5 and V_6.

It is necessary to emphasize that each wave of the electrocardiogram is the result of an infinite number of successive vectors which act in the same or in the opposite direction, and it is the net effect of these vectors, at any point in time, which determines the size and shape of the tracing. The time sequence of the occurrence of these vectors is important; *e.g.,* in lead V_1 the R wave is early and is produced by the early vector (number 1 in the drawing), but the S wave, a late deflection, is produced by the late vectors (numbers 4, 5, and 6 in the drawing).

RIGHT AXIS DEVIATION (IN NORMAL)

LEFT AXIS DEVIATION (IN NORMAL)

AXIS DEVIATION IN A NORMAL SUBJECT

The *mean* electric axis of the *P, QRS,* and *T* waves, in the normal individual, often reflects the anatomic position of the heart in the chest; however, an abnormal axis can be caused by disease of the heart. This plate deals with normal variations in the vectorcardiographic loop. The QRS and T loops, in the frontal plane, vary between −30 *and* +110 *degrees* and, in the horizontal plane, between +30 *and* −30 *degrees,* measured from the left arm.

In right axis deviation, in the frontal plane, the P and QRS loops are directed toward the right, often to +90 *degrees*. Electrocardiographically, there are tall R waves in *leads II, III, aV_F, V_2,* and *V_3*.

Left axis deviation is characterized by a QRS loop which points toward the left shoulder blade (left, up, and back). The mean electric axis is often close to −30 in the frontal plane, and, in the horizontal plane (toward the back), approaches the −30 position. The S waves are deep in leads V_1 and V_2, and the R waves are tall in *leads I, aV_L, V_5,* and *V_6*.

It is important to understand the relationship between the position of the heart in the chest and the electrocardiogram, for the heart's position has a profound influence on the tracing. The concept is complex, because the heart can rotate around an anteroposterior axis, a transverse axis, and an anatomical axis which runs from the base to the apex of the heart. Actually, the heart can rotate from front to back, side to side, and around the anatomic axis, all simultaneously. The rotation around the anatomic axis is the most difficult to visualize. Rotation here consists of turning around an axis which runs from the valvular base of the heart

through the septum, finally emerging from the apex. An observer at the left of a subject would see the emerging axis at the apex of the heart. If the observer could then visualize a clock at the base of the heart, he could also visualize any rotational change around the axis and could designate the direction of rotation as clockwise or counterclockwise.

In a patient with an intermediately placed heart, the right ventricle is in front, to the right, and superior to the left ventricle, and the left ventricle is in back, below, and to the left of the right ventricle. Now, if one were to put an electrode directly on the right ventricle, a "right ventricular complex" (small r, large S, and inverted T) would be recorded. If an electrode were placed directly on the left ventricle, a "left ventricular complex" (small q, large R, and upward T) would be recorded. An electrode on the body or on a limb, facing one ventricle or the other,

will record in the lead the type of complex which is typical of that ventricle. In the intermediate heart position, neither the right nor the left ventricle directly faces the aV_L or aV_F electrode; thus, these leads have small complexes which do not look exactly like the right or left ventricular complexes. With inspiration and the descent of the diaphragm, or in a subject with an asthenic body build, the heart rotates clockwise, causing the left ventricle to face the foot and the right ventricle to face the left arm. Thus, typical complexes of a left ventricular type will be recorded from lead aV_F, whereas aV_L will record complexes of a right ventricular type. In an obese or pregnant subject, or during expiration with a high diaphragm, the heart rotates counterclockwise, and left ventricular (predominantly positive) complexes are recorded in lead aV_L, right ventricular (predominantly negative) complexes in lead aV_F.

RIGHT ATRIAL ENLARGEMENT

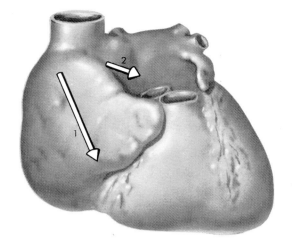

LEFT ATRIAL ENLARGEMENT

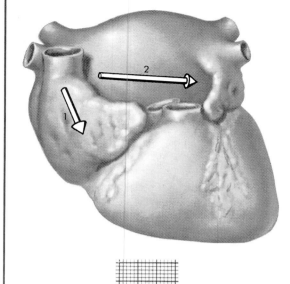

ATRIAL ENLARGEMENT

Enlargement of the right atrium, as compared to the left, occurs in patients with cor pulmonale, pulmonary hypertension, or tricuspid or pulmonary stenosis. As a result, the first atrial electric movement predominates, and the electrical axis of the P wave generally is toward the foot and to the front. As a consequence, the P waves in *lead I* are small, but they are tall in *leads II, III,* and *aV_F,* often exceeding the upper limit of normal (2.5 mm) for lead II. The vector loop is *down, forward,* and large. Moderately tall P waves are present in leads V_1 and V_2.

Right Atrial Enlargement

Right atrial enlargement is found when there is a pressure or flow overload in the right atrium, as compared to the left. The pressure is increased characteristically in the right atrium in patients with tricuspid stenosis, and the "P pulmonale" picture of right atrial enlargement occurs. Here, the P waves are tall, peaked, narrow, and unnotched (easily seen in leads II, III, and aV_F), with a tendency toward right axis deviation.

Left Atrial Enlargement

By contrast, *left atrial enlargement* causes the electrocardiographic picture of "P mitrale." This usually is due to mitral stenosis or regurgitation incident to rheumatic heart disease. Here, the P waves are notched and wide in lead II, with a tendency to left axis deviation,

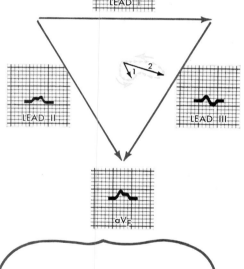

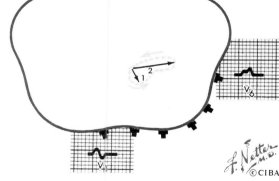

but, typically, they are normal in height. There is enlargement of the left atrium, as compared with the right; therefore, the electric forces are directed toward the left axilla. Characteristically, the P waves in lead II are wide, being 0.12 second or more. The loop of the P wave is unusually large and shows a left axis deviation. Wide, notched P waves also are seen in lead V_6. With left atrial enlargement, the late P vectors are large as compared to the early ones.

Enlargement of Both Atria

When both right and left atria are enlarged, the P waves are tall — more than 2.5 mm in lead II — and wide, being 0.12 second or longer in this lead. Notching is present. This condition occurs when

mitral-valve disease prevails in the presence of an interatrial septal defect or when multiple valvular defects are present. The atrial T waves or the repolarization waves of the atria are normally small, often being undetectable or lost in the QRS complexes. Normally, the T wave is discordant with the P wave, in that a positive P wave is usually followed by a very small, negative T wave. Generally, the area under the atrial T wave is a little smaller than that under the P wave.

With enlargement of the P waves, in either "P mitrale" or "P pulmonale," the atrial T waves enlarge in proportion to the increased size of the P waves, with resultant depression of the P-R segments. Large atrial T waves often call attention to atrial abnormalities and are helpful *diagnostically*.

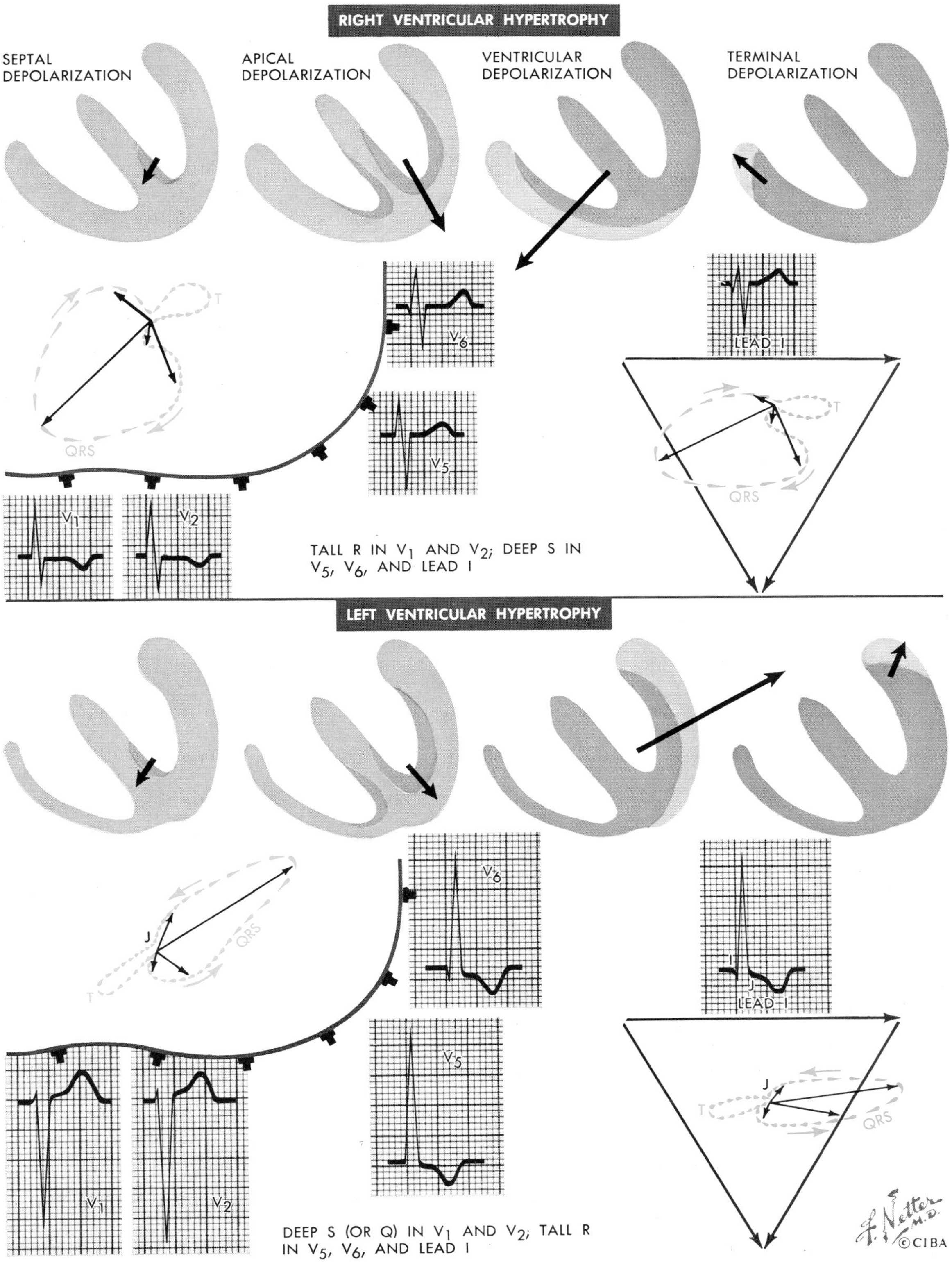

VENTRICULAR HYPERTROPHY

Various terms have been used to describe the electrocardiographic picture of ventricular hypertrophy; these include ventricular preponderance, strain, systolic or diastolic overload, enlargement, and hypertrophy. Some of these describe a functional state of overwork of one ventricle as compared to the other, or they refer to an anatomic condition with increased muscle of one ventricle compared to the other. Ventricular preponderance is an all-inclusive term which, in its broad sense, includes most conditions, and the word "enlargement" covers both hypertrophy and dilatation.

Right Ventricular Hypertrophy

The *QRS* forces are directed to the right because of the thick right ventricle, which distorts the horizontal loop to the right and forward and is associated with *tall R waves,* relative to the normal, in *leads V_1 and V_2,* and *deep S waves* in *leads V_4 and V_5.* The R/S amplitude ratio in lead V_1 is abnormal, indicating a tall R wave with respect to the depth of the S wave. Normally, this ratio should be less than 1. Characteristically, the S-T segments and T waves are opposite in direction to that portion of the QRS complex of greatest area (usually the R wave), and also the *T loop* is opposite to the QRS loop. Thus, the R wave is up and the T wave is down in leads V_1 and V_2, but in leads V_5 and V_6 the S wave is always down and the T wave is up.

Right ventricular hypertrophy may be caused by congenital or acquired heart disease, and the hypertrophy may result from a pressure or volume overload. As a consequence, the right ventricular muscle thickens with respect to the left, and a right ventricular preponderance develops. Since it is the net electric change of the whole heart which writes the electrocardiogram and vectorcardiogram, the QRS electric forces are directed, in general, from the left to the right of the heart and of the body. Usually, the direction of the electric forces will be from the smaller muscle mass toward the larger one; *i.e.,* from the normal toward the hypertrophied ventricle.

Left Ventricular Enlargement

The large muscle mass of the *left hypertrophied ventricle,* compared to the right, distorts the QRS loop toward the left scapula. This results in small R waves and deep S waves in leads V_1 and V_2, with high R waves and small or no S waves in leads V_5 and V_6. Again, the S-T segments and T waves are opposite in direction to the major deflection of the QRS complex, which means that, in lead V_1, the deep S wave is associated

RIGHT VENTRICULAR HYPERTROPHY

SEPTAL DEPOLARIZATION   APICAL DEPOLARIZATION   VENTRICULAR DEPOLARIZATION   TERMINAL DEPOLARIZATION

TALL R IN V_1 AND V_2; DEEP S IN V_5, V_6, AND LEAD I

LEFT VENTRICULAR HYPERTROPHY

DEEP S (OR Q) IN V_1 AND V_2; TALL R IN V_5, V_6, AND LEAD I

with a *positive* S-T segment and T wave, whereas, in lead V_6, the tall R wave is associated with a *negative* S-T segment and T wave. In the horizontal loop, the early forces in the patient are from left to right and to the front, later toward the left scapula, finally returning to the zero point. When the shifts of the S-T segments are characteristic of left ventricular enlargement, there is an open QRS-T loop in the vectorcardiogram; *i.e.,* the beginning and the end of a QRS complex are at different levels, and, usually, a T wave follows which is 180 degrees discordant with the major portion of the QRS loop. The frontal loop is displaced toward the left shoulder, with discordant QRS and T-wave relationships. An open loop may be seen here also. The *J point* is the junction between the end of the QRS complex and the beginning of the T wave in the electrocardiogram. A point just in front of the J point, which is the end of the P-R interval and the beginning of the QRS complex, is called the *I point.* The open loop in the vectorcardiogram is found when the I and J points in the electrocardiogram are at different horizontal levels. Usually, in a normal subject, the I and J points are on the same level, often on the isoelectric line. With severe left ventricular hypertrophy the J point shifts below the I point in lead V_5, and in severe right ventricular hypertrophy J is below I in lead V_1. The I-J relationships are also changed by digitalis, hypokalemia, myocardial infarction, myocardial ischemia, pericarditis, and bundle-branch block.

Right and Left Ventricular Hypertrophy

When both of these conditions exist, the muscle with the greater degree of hypertrophy will dominate the electrical picture.

COMPLETE RIGHT BUNDLE-BRANCH BLOCK

A–V NODE

BLOCK   BLOCK   BLOCK

QRS

P   T

V₆

V₅

LEAD I

R

r

S   V₁   V₂

QRS

P   T

QRS DURATION GREATER THAN 0.12 SECOND:
MAJOR QRS DEFLECTION (DURATION) DOWNWARD
IN LEAD I AND L. CHEST LEADS, UPWARD IN R. CHEST
LEADS; P AND P–R INTERVAL NORMAL

COMPLETE LEFT BUNDLE-BRANCH BLOCK

BLOCK

A–V NODE   BLOCK   BLOCK

P   QRS

T

R

V₆

V₅

R

R   ATYPICAL

TYPICAL

LEAD I

T   P   QRS

V₁   V₂

S   S

QRS DURATION GREATER THAN 0.12 SECOND:
MAJOR QRS DEFLECTION (DURATION) UPWARD IN
LEAD I AND L. CHEST LEADS, DOWNWARD IN R. CHEST
LEADS; P AND P–R INTERVAL NORMAL

F. Netter ©CIBA

BUNDLE-BRANCH BLOCK

Bundle-branch *block* is a term indicating disease in, or an altered transmission through, certain branches of the conduction system of the heart. Blocks may occur in either the left or the right ventricle or, possibly, both.

In this condition a characteristic change is a widening of the QRS complex greater than 0.1 second. When the *duration* of this *complex* ranges from 0.1 to 0.12 second, the block is *incomplete*; if it is *greater than 0.12 second*, a *complete bundle-branch block* exists. With a *complete right bundle-branch block*, the first 0.04 second of the QRS complex is normal in configuration but the last portion is abnormal. With a *left bundle-branch block,* the total duration of the wave is written by an abnormal depolarization wave, and the tracing is very abnormal.

Blocks may be *typical* or *atypical*. A typical block has a lesion only in the bundle of His or one of its branches, and there is no associated lesion. An atypical block has, in addition to the bundle-branch block, some other lesion, such as a myocardial infarct. A typical block has T waves which are opposite in direction to the wave of greatest duration in the QRS complex, *i.e.,* T is opposite to S in a right bundle-branch block in V_6, but T is opposite to r in lead V_1. An atypical block does not necessarily follow this rule.

Right Bundle-Branch Block

Only a small defect in the right bundle of His is necessary to block the right bundle. The first electric movement is a normal one from the left side of the septum to the right; this writes the usual septal Q wave in leads V_5 and V_6. The next movement is through the left ventricle from the endocardium to the epicardium, and this writes a normal R wave in leads V_5 and V_6. Finally, there is a slow progression of the activation wave through the septum and the Purkinje system on the right and through the right ventricle, which requires more time. As a result, there is a wide S wave in leads V_5 and V_6, and the duration of the S wave is usually greater than that of the R wave in the QRS complex. This order of depolarization — right, then left, then right — registers, in lead V_1, an r, an S, and an R′ wave, and here the duration of the R′ wave is greater than that of the R wave. In the vectorcardiogram one sees the electromotive forces going first to the right, then to the left, and then back to the right again. There is a slowing down

of the writing of the VCG (dots are closer together) during late ventricular depolarization, because the activation of the right ventricle is slow. The horizontal-plane vectorcardiogram is to the right, then to the left, and then to the right front, whereas the frontal-plane vectorcardiogram is right, then left, then right, and often up. It is to be recalled that in a right bundle-branch block the first part of the QRS loop is normal, but the last part is abnormal.

Right bundle-branch block often is caused by arteriosclerosis or prolonged strain on the right ventricle, as in pulmonary hypertension or pulmonary stenosis.

Left Bundle-Branch Block

A block in the left bundle of His alters the entire ventricular-depolarization pathway. Ventricular depolarization starts from the right side of the septum

and progresses toward the left front, writing small r waves in leads V_1 and V_2. The voltage next swings toward the left near the cardiac apex, then toward the left base, writing tall R waves in leads I, V_5, and V_6, and S waves in leads V_1 and V_2. The electric movement is generally toward the left scapula, and, characteristically, the S-T segments and T waves are *opposite* in direction to the *major deflection of the QRS* complex. When this QRS complex and T-wave relationship occurs, the tracing is characteristic of *typical* left bundle-branch block. When the QRS complex and the T wave are *not opposite* or are concordant, the tracing is referred to as *atypical*, and it is probable that some other lesion, such as a myocardial infarction, is present as well as the block.

Left bundle-branch block is caused by arteriosclerosis, myocardial infarction, cardiac failure, or severe strain on the left ventricle, as in hypertension.

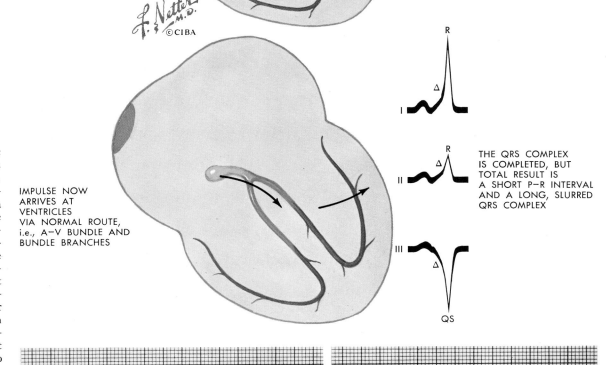

IMPULSE ORIGINATES AT S—A NODE, PASSES THRU ATRIUM, IS DELAYED AT A—V NODE BUT PASSES RAPIDLY THRU ACCESSORY BUNDLE OF KENT

P WAVE IS NORMAL, BUT ALMOST IMMEDIATELY THEREAFTER △ WAVE APPEARS DUE TO ARRIVAL OF IMPULSES AT VENTRICLES VIA ABNORMAL ROUTE, RESULTING IN SHORT OR ABSENT P—R SEGMENT

IMPULSE NOW ARRIVES AT VENTRICLES VIA NORMAL ROUTE, i.e., A—V BUNDLE AND BUNDLE BRANCHES

THE QRS COMPLEX IS COMPLETED, BUT TOTAL RESULT IS A SHORT P—R INTERVAL AND A LONG, SLURRED QRS COMPLEX

PAROXYSMAL TACHYCARDIA → NORMAL, AFTER QUINIDINE

WOLFF-PARKINSON-WHITE SYNDROME

The *Wolff-Parkinson-White complex* is often referred to as *false bundle-branch block* or the *bundle of Kent syndrome*. It is important to distinguish true bundle-branch block from false bundle-branch block, the former having a high incidence of organic heart disease. About 20 per cent of the patients with false bundle-branch block have organic heart disease and 80 percent have the functional disorder only. It has been postulated that there is an *accessory muscle bundle,* connecting the atria to the ventricles, over which depolarization occurs rapidly from atria to ventricles, resulting in ventricular preexcitation. The syndrome is most commonly seen in young subjects who have frequent attacks of supraventricular or even ventricular tachycardia. Between attacks of rapid heartbeating, the *QRS complexes* ordinarily are typical of the picture seen in false bundle-branch block. This consists of a *short P-R interval* (usually less than 0.11 second), a QRS complex which is widened by a △ *wave,* and, usually, a QRS complex whose duration is from 0.11 second to 0.14 second. Actually, the P-R interval is decreased by the amount the QRS complex is increased, so that the P-J interval remains quite normal.

The upstroke of the R *wave in lead I,* in a patient with a right-side bundle of Kent, is usually *slurred* because of the △ wave which exists at the beginning of the QRS complex. If, however, the bundle of Kent connects the left atrium to the left ventricle, depolarization will be from left to right, and this will produce, in lead I, QRS complexes which are primarily negative. Most commonly, however, the bundle of Kent is on the right, with the accession wave going from right to left and a △ wave appearing at the beginning of the QRS complex in lead I. Of course, the bundle of Kent

could be posterior or anterior, in which case different configurations of the trace would result.

The short P-R interval can be explained by an *abnormal* muscle communication, the bundle of Kent, or a connecting band of tissue between the *atrium* and the *ventricle.* The *impulses from the sinus node* travel more rapidly through the bundle of Kent than through the *A-V node* and bundle of His. The widening of the QRS complex and the slurring of the upstroke of the R wave in lead I are explained by the depolarization wave entering the right ventricle early and without delay, through the abnormal connection between the atria and the ventricles. Since the depolarization process through the ventricles is longer than normal, because of its abnormal direction, the QRS complex is exceptionally wide. After the early depolarization of the ventricle from the bundle of Kent has begun, the normal atrial impulses, which

were *delayed at the A-V node,* enter the ventricle by the normal pathway, and the depolarization of the ventricles is completed in a normal fashion. Thus, the terminal portions of the QRS complexes are normal.

The bundle of Kent predisposes to attacks of *paroxysmal tachycardia* by facilitating retrograde conduction into the atria with the initiation of circus movements or antegrade conduction in the Kent pathway with retrograde conduction in the His-Purkinje system. Therefore, all young individuals complaining of attacks of tachycardia should have an electrocardiogram during a period of normal heart rate to determine if a false bundle-branch block exists.

Quinidine is often used successfully to block the accession wave as it passes through the bundle of Kent. Digitalis is usually ineffective and given alone may be dangerous because of 1:1 conduction to the ventricle in certain atrial arrhythmias.

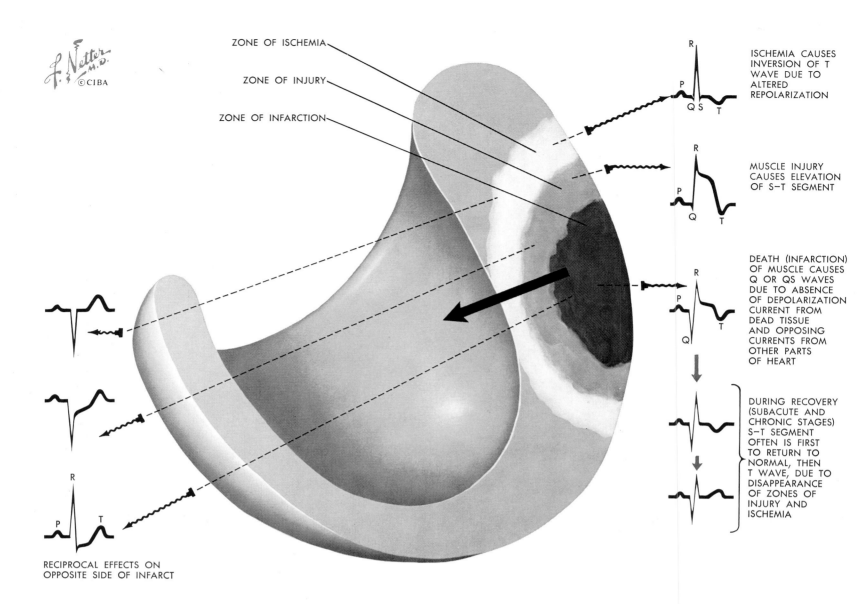

ZONE OF ISCHEMIA
ZONE OF INJURY
ZONE OF INFARCTION

ISCHEMIA CAUSES INVERSION OF T WAVE DUE TO ALTERED REPOLARIZATION

MUSCLE INJURY CAUSES ELEVATION OF S-T SEGMENT

DEATH (INFARCTION) OF MUSCLE CAUSES Q OR QS WAVES DUE TO ABSENCE OF DEPOLARIZATION CURRENT FROM DEAD TISSUE AND OPPOSING CURRENTS FROM OTHER PARTS OF HEART

DURING RECOVERY (SUBACUTE AND CHRONIC STAGES) S-T SEGMENT OFTEN IS FIRST TO RETURN TO NORMAL, THEN T WAVE, DUE TO DISAPPEARANCE OF ZONES OF INJURY AND ISCHEMIA

RECIPROCAL EFFECTS ON OPPOSITE SIDE OF INFARCT

MYOCARDIAL ISCHEMIA, INJURY, AND INFARCTION

Infarcted myocardium is *dead heart muscle* resulting, usually, from an occluded artery. Electrically, one might divide the *infarcted muscle* into three zones: the *zone of infarction* or tissue death, the *zone of injury,* and the *zone of ischemia.* Dead heart muscle is that which has been destroyed so that *polarization* of the cell is not possible. Injured cardiac muscle has cell membranes which are never fully polarized, and this usually results from a deficient arterial blood supply. Ischemic muscle is myocardial tissue in which *repolarization* is impaired. This often is due to a lack of blood supply or other causes.

Minor degrees of cardiac disturbances can produce the so-called ischemic changes.

Infarction produces *Q or QS waves* in the electrocardiogram; injury, *S-T segment shifts;* and ischemia, *T-wave changes.* An electrode placed directly over an acute myocardial infarct "looks through" the dead area and records impulses from the opposite side of the heart, writing Q waves in the electrocardiogram. An electrode immediately adjacent to the dead infarcted area writes, primarily, shifts of the S-T segments because the electrode is over the zone of injury. Still more distal to the dead area is the ischemic zone, and an electrode over this site produces only T-wave changes. *After recovery* from myocardial infarction, the dead zone remains unchanged, and Q or QS waves tend to persist, whereas the S-T segments and T waves usually *return to normal.* An electrode placed across the heart *opposite the infarct* records changes which are *reciprocal* with those gained from electrodes placed over the infarct.

The electrocardiogram is often interpreted with respect to the duration and timing of a myocardial infarct, as follows:

An *acute* infarct is characterized by large shifts of the S-T segments in some of the leads. These changes last only a few days.

In *subacute* infarction the S-T segments usually return, after a few days, to the isoelectric line, and abnormal coved T waves develop.

These waves, as a rule, last for a few weeks.

Finally, in a *chronic* infarct, the S-T segments and T waves become nearly normal, and only persistent abnormal Q or QS waves remain to reveal the presence of the infarct. The chronic stage is reached 2 to 3 months after the inception of the infarct, but this timing is variable.

With an acute attack of angina pectoris, ischemia and injury of the heart occur, but there is no infarct. As a consequence, changes in the S-T segments and T waves develop during the attack, but, characteristically, they disappear with the cessation of pain.

It is not unusual to find a patient, with or without anginal symptoms and showing a normal electrocardiogram at rest, who develops an abnormal tracing with exercise. Normally, even severe exercise, such as marathon running, does not produce an abnormal electrocardiogram such as that seen in coronary arteriosclerosis. In abnormal cases with coronary stenosis, exercise results in negative shifts of the S-T segments in lead V_4 and other leads, revealing the existence, at that time, of subendocardial ischemia. With rest, the tracing returns to normal within a few minutes.

A *diagnosis* of myocardial infarction is sometimes impossible because of the location of the infarct. For example, an intramural infarct which does not involve the epicardium or endocardium cannot be detected by electrocardiography or vectorcardiography.

LOCALIZATION OF ANTERIOR INFARCTS

Infarcts of the myocardium may occur in various locations on the anterior wall of the left ventricle.

Anterolateral Infarct

These infarcts are *anterolateral* in position and are due to *occlusion of the anterior interventricular branch of the left coronary artery,* in which case there is a loss of the initial R waves in the precordial leads (V_3 through V_5) which overlie the infarct. A Q wave is commonly present in *lead I* as well. There is a discordant relationship between the S-T segments and the T waves in *leads I and III.* The shifts of the S-T segments are upward in lead I and downward in lead III, and the T waves face toward each other, *i.e.,* down in lead I and up in lead III. The plate shows a rather typical subacute anterolateral myocardial infarct.

Anterior (Anteroseptal) Infarct

A small, strictly *anterior* or *anteroseptal myocardial infarct* disrupts only a small number of anteriorly positioned forces. As a consequence, there is a loss of the initial R waves in leads V_2 and V_3 but, often, not in leads V_4, V_5, and V_6. Since the forces moving in the frontal plane of the body are not disturbed by this infarct, the limb leads remain normal, and in the plate we see *leads I, II, and III* giving no indication of this infarct.

This kind of infarct usually is due to *occlusion of a right division of the ante-*

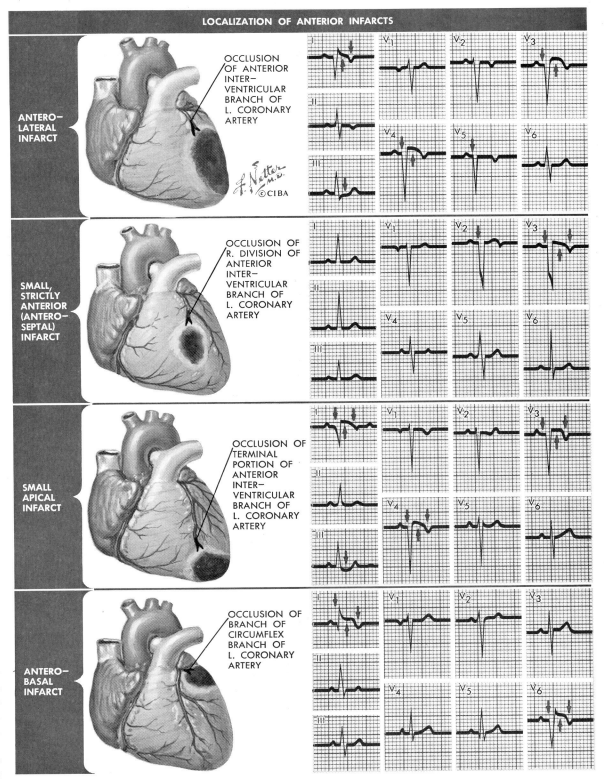

LOCALIZATION OF ANTERIOR INFARCTS

ANTERO-LATERAL INFARCT — OCCLUSION OF ANTERIOR INTER-VENTRICULAR BRANCH OF L. CORONARY ARTERY

SMALL, STRICTLY ANTERIOR (ANTERO-SEPTAL) INFARCT — OCCLUSION OF R. DIVISION OF ANTERIOR INTER-VENTRICULAR BRANCH OF L. CORONARY ARTERY

SMALL APICAL INFARCT — OCCLUSION OF TERMINAL PORTION OF ANTERIOR INTER-VENTRICULAR BRANCH OF L. CORONARY ARTERY

ANTERO-BASAL INFARCT — OCCLUSION OF BRANCH OF CIRCUMFLEX BRANCH OF L. CORONARY ARTERY

rior intraventricular branch of the left coronary artery.

Apical Infarct

A *small apical infarct* disturbs the electric forces moving in the frontal plane of the body, resulting in a loss of the normal R waves (Q waves) in lead I. Because of the slight anterior position of the infarct, there is a loss of R waves in leads V_3 and V_4 as well. The plate shows a subacute infarct with discordant shifts of the S-T segments in leads I and III (up in I and down in III), the T waves being opposite to the segment shifts.

An apical infarct is usually due to *occlusion of the terminal portion of the anterior interventricular branch of the left coronary artery.*

Anterobasal Infarct

An *anterobasal myocardial infarct* destroys the electromotive forces on the lateral aspect of the left ventricle. It therefore disrupts the forces that are moving in the frontal plane of the body but does not significantly distort the anteroposterior forces. There is, however, a loss of initial R waves (Q waves) in lead V_6. The loss of forces here influences lead I also, with Q waves in this lead. If the infarct is acute, there will be positive shifts of the S-T segments in leads I and V_6, followed by inverted T waves.

This type of infarct results from *occlusion of a branch of the circumflex branch of the left coronary artery.*

LOCALIZATION OF POSTERIOR INFARCTS

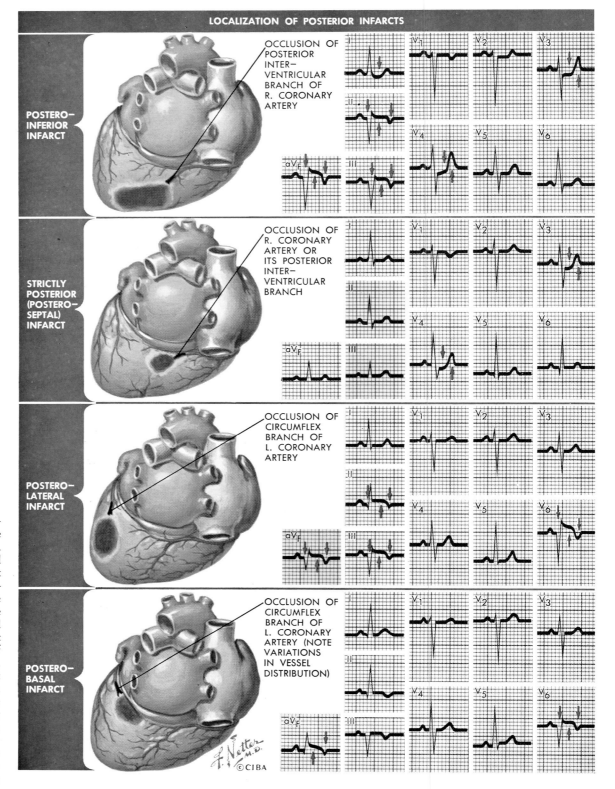

LOCALIZATION OF POSTERIOR INFARCTS

POSTERO-INFERIOR INFARCT — OCCLUSION OF POSTERIOR INTER-VENTRICULAR BRANCH OF R. CORONARY ARTERY

STRICTLY POSTERIOR (POSTERO-SEPTAL) INFARCT — OCCLUSION OF R. CORONARY ARTERY OR ITS POSTERIOR INTER-VENTRICULAR BRANCH

POSTERO-LATERAL INFARCT — OCCLUSION OF CIRCUMFLEX BRANCH OF L. CORONARY ARTERY

POSTERO-BASAL INFARCT — OCCLUSION OF CIRCUMFLEX BRANCH OF L. CORONARY ARTERY (NOTE VARIATIONS IN VESSEL DISTRIBUTION)

LOCALIZATION OF POSTERIOR INFARCTS

Posteroinferior Infarct

These infarcts are usually readily apparent on the electrocardiogram, because they show large Q waves in *leads II, III,* and *aV_F.* The infarct may be referred to as diaphragmatic in position, since it occurs in that portion of the heart adjacent to the diaphragm. In the subacute stage the shifts of the S-T segments are negative in *leads I, V_3,* and *V_4,* elevated in lead III. Lead aV_F is probably the most revealing lead because of the presence of large Q waves, elevated S-T segments, and inverted T waves. A posterior infarct is often diagnosed when the Q wave in lead aV_F is at least 25 percent of the amplitude of the R wave, particularly when this exists with the breath held in deep inspiration.

A *posteroinferior infarct* is usually produced by *occlusion of the posterior interventricular branch of the right coronary artery.*

Posterior (Posteroseptal) Infarct

A *strictly posterior infarct* is often situated over the interventricular septum and is referred to as a *posteroseptal infarct.* Because of the location of this infarct, the R waves in V_1 and V_2 tend to be tall; and in V_5 and V_6 they tend to be small. One may detect negative S-T segment shifts in leads V_3 and V_4 which are persistent for at least a few days. As far as the twelve standard leads are concerned, this infarct is in a blind spot. The loss of muscle mass is small, and the voltage changes are slight. The precordial leads are far from the infarct, making detec-

tion difficult or impossible. The infarct can be discovered by an esophageal lead, but this procedure is uncomfortable for the patient. In such a case, blood-transaminase tests (page 92) are important.

Usually, this infarct is due to *occlusion of the right coronary artery or its posterior interventricular branch.*

Posterolateral Infarct

This infarction is often due to *occlusion of the circumflex branch of the left coronary artery.* Here, the lateral and posterior walls of the left ventricle are involved.

The precordial lead which faces the infarct most directly is lead V_6 and, consequently, there are Q waves in this lead. If the infarct is subacute, there will be elevated S-T segments and inverted T waves. Since lead aV_F also faces the infarct, this lead will

resemble lead V_6. The area of injury often spreads considerably wider than the area of muscle death; for this reason, one sees elevated S-T segments and inverted T waves in leads II, III, and aV_F.

Posterobasal Myocardial Infarction

This condition is generally due to *occlusion of the circumflex branch of the left coronary artery.* Here, the infarct is high at the base of the heart.

Since the infarct is small and high at the base, there will be some reflection of its presence in lead V_6, with Q waves, elevated S-T segments, and inverted T waves. As in the posterolateral infarct, the area of injury and ischemia may spread in a wide zone around the infarction, so that even lead aV_F may show abnormally elevated S-T segments and inverted T waves.

SINUS AND ATRIAL ARRHYTHMIAS

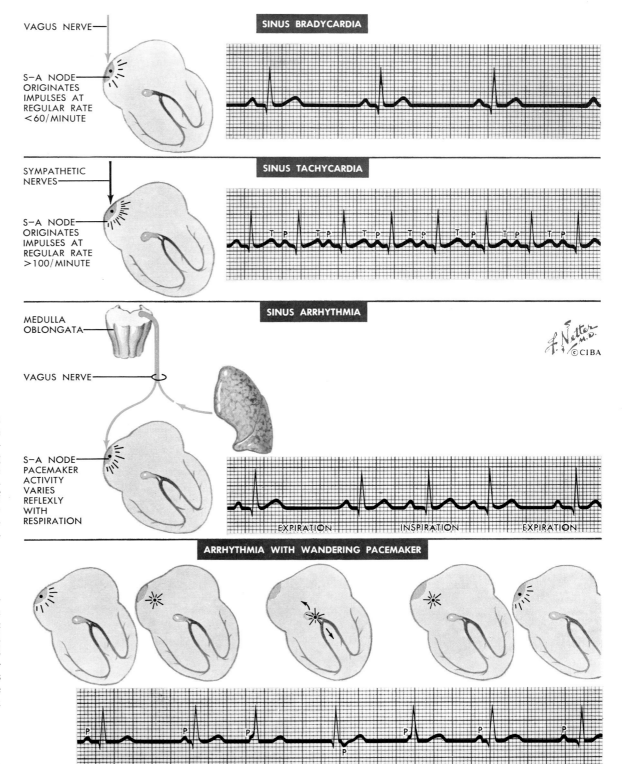

VAGUS NERVE

S-A NODE ORIGINATES IMPULSES AT REGULAR RATE <60/MINUTE

SINUS BRADYCARDIA

SYMPATHETIC NERVES

S-A NODE ORIGINATES IMPULSES AT REGULAR RATE >100/MINUTE

SINUS TACHYCARDIA

MEDULLA OBLONGATA

VAGUS NERVE

S-A NODE PACEMAKER ACTIVITY VARIES REFLEXLY WITH RESPIRATION

SINUS ARRHYTHMIA

EXPIRATION   INSPIRATION   EXPIRATION

ARRHYTHMIA WITH WANDERING PACEMAKER

Certain *arrhythmias* are caused by a disturbance at the sinus node. These include *sinus bradycardia, sinus tachycardia, sinus arrhythmia,* and *wandering pacemaker.* The sinus node is under the control of the *parasympathetic* and *sympathetic nerves,* and altered function of these nerves may influence cardiac activity. The *S-A node* is depressed by parasympathetic *(vagus)* functions or stimulated by sympathetic activity.

Sinus Bradycardia

In this condition the *sinus node originates impulses at a slow rate — less than 60 beats per minute. Sinus bradycardia* is common in patients with high vagal tone, hypothyroidism, and increased intracranial tension, during athletic training, and during treatment with digitalis and/or reserpine. Usually, the slow rate is due, in part at least, to vagal inhibition of the sinus node.

Sinus Tachycardia

Sympathetic-nerve stimulation or the blocking of vagus nerves can produce this condition. The *sinus node originates impulses at a rate greater than 100 beats per minute,* and close inspection of these curves shows that there is some variation in the R-R interval. It is important to observe this variation in order to differentiate *sinus tachycardia* from atrial tachycardia, in which there is no significant variation between the R-R intervals. Sinus tachycardia is found in patients after exercise or smoking, in hyperthyroidism, anxiety, toxic states, fever, anemia, and diseases involving the heart or lungs, and from other causes. Sinus tachycardia is characterized by a slowing of the pulse rate during carotid-sinus pressure, and by the gradual return of the rate to its previous basic level upon release of such pressure. This is in con-

trast to the reaction to carotid pressure in atrial tachycardia, which may cause the rhythm to change abruptly to a sinus rhythm.

Sinus Arrhythmia

Sinus arrhythmia is a variation in cardiac rate during breathing or, sometimes, with other organ function, such as contraction of the spleen. The arrhythmia is commonly found in children or in patients with Cheyne-Stokes respiration. Usually, afferent impulses from the lungs travel to the cardiac center, with efferent impulses traveling over the vagus nerve to the sinus node. The *pacemaker activity at the node varies reflexly with respiration.* Generally, there are about five cardiac beats to each respiratory cycle. With *expiration* the cardiac rate is slow; with *inspiration* it is more rapid.

Wandering Pacemaker

A *wandering pacemaker* is present when, with each beat, the pacemaker changes its position in the atrium, often traveling down to and into the A-V node and back to the sinus node again. This occurs when there is a variation in the vagal tone at the sinus node or there are changes in sympathetic stimulation. In the electrocardiogram, the P-R interval becomes progressively shorter, and the *P waves* often disappear within the QRS complexes or may even appear *after* the QRS complexes. In lead II, at times, the P waves may be *inverted* because the atria are depolarized from the A-V node to the sinus node, instead of in the usual direction. A wandering pacemaker is not a serious irregularity; it is often transient and may, at times, be stopped by anticholinergic agents such as propantheline bromide (Pro-Banthine®).

PREMATURE CONTRACTIONS

Three common terms are employed to describe certain abnormal cardiac contractions. These are *premature contractions* (beats occurring early in time), ectopic beats (beats with sites of origin outside the sinus node), and extrasystoles (added beats). Only extrasystoles are truly added or additional beats, and, often, these are interpolated or are added between two normal beats without interfering with the basic rhythm (not illustrated).

Atrial Premature Contractions

These are due to an irritability of the atria, with early contractions emanating from an impulse in the atria outside of the S-A node. One may differentiate atrial from ventricular premature contractions by measurement of the compensatory pause. With atrial premature contractions the compensatory pause is incomplete, whereas with ventricular premature contractions it is complete.

The measurement of the compensatory pause for atrial premature beats is made as follows: Select the atrial premature beat (P wave) which appears different from the *P waves* of the basic mechanism and is premature in time. This is the atrial premature contraction. Measure the time interval from the premature P wave to the P wave immediately in front, and add this interval to the time interval between the premature P wave and the P wave immediately following ($<2X$). This total time duration is shorter than the time between two normal P-P intervals which do not include a premature contraction ($2X$).

Nodal Premature Contractions

These contractions occur as a result of stimulation of the A-V node. Usually, there is retrograde conduction starting at the A-V node, with an accession wave moving over the atria from the A-V node to the S-A node, and P waves of an abnormal form are written. At times, there is no retrograde conduction, and P waves and atrial contraction do not occur. Often, the stimulus at the A-V node is vagal or is due to disease.

High A-V Nodal Rhythm. This condition prevails when the *head* of the A-V node becomes the pacemaker, and atrial depolarization occurs in a retrograde fashion from the A-V node to the S-A node. With nodal premature contractions, *inverted* P waves are written in *leads II, III, and aV_F* because of retrograde auricular depolarization. The P-R interval is short, P waves precede the QRS complexes, and the QRS and T waves are of normal configuration.

Middle Nodal Rhythm. When the junctional tissue is stimulated below the A-V node near its *center,* atrial and ventricular

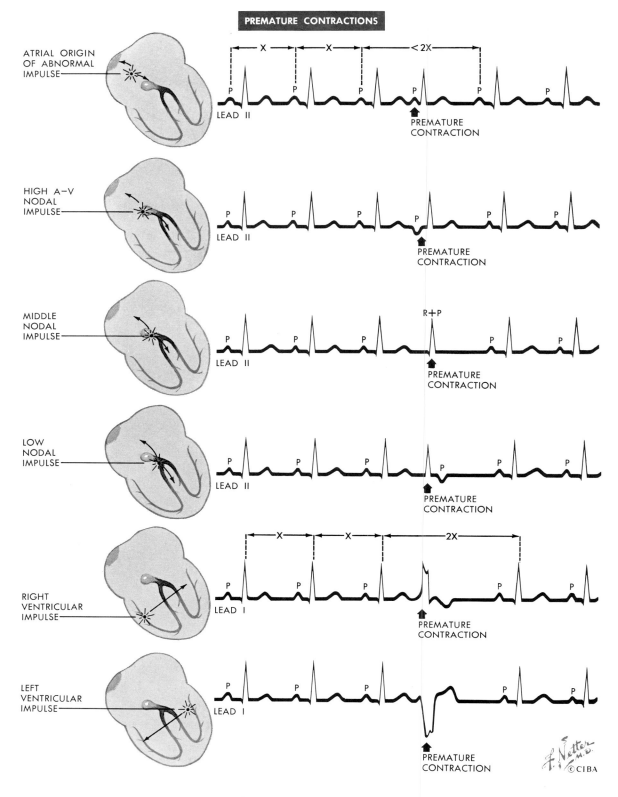

PREMATURE CONTRACTIONS

ATRIAL ORIGIN OF ABNORMAL IMPULSE

LEAD II — PREMATURE CONTRACTION

HIGH A-V NODAL IMPULSE

LEAD II — PREMATURE CONTRACTION

MIDDLE NODAL IMPULSE

LEAD II — R+P — PREMATURE CONTRACTION

LOW NODAL IMPULSE

LEAD II — PREMATURE CONTRACTION

RIGHT VENTRICULAR IMPULSE

LEAD I — PREMATURE CONTRACTION

LEFT VENTRICULAR IMPULSE

LEAD I — PREMATURE CONTRACTION

depolarizations occur simultaneously. Here, the P waves fall within the QRS complexes, and the summation complexes ($QRS+P$) are slightly different in appearance from the normal QRS complexes of the basic mechanism.

Low Nodal Impulse. If the pacemaker is *low* in the junctional tissues, the ventricles are depolarized before the atria, the QRS complexes are written first, and *inverted* P waves in leads II, III, and aV_F are written later.

Right Ventricular Impulse

The P-wave rhythm is not disturbed. The ventricles contract early from a stimulus in the region of the right ventricle. The accession wave travels from right to left and, moving in this direction, produces *upright* QRS deflections in *lead I.* The duration of

this complex is long, because the pathway is abnormally long. It measures greater than 0.10 second, and it is followed by S-T segments and T waves which are opposite in direction to the major deflections of the QRS complexes. The compensatory pause is complete; *i.e.,* the time interval between two normal QRS complexes which do not contain an ectopic beat is the same as the time from a QRS complex before the ectopic QRS beat to the QRS complex which follows this beat.

Left Ventricular Impulse

A pacemaker in the wall of the left ventricle produces an accession wave which travels from left to right, resulting, in *lead I,* in negative (*inverted*) wide QRS complexes with positive (*upward*) S-T segments and T waves, and complete compensatory pauses.

SINUS ARREST, BLOCK, AND A-V BLOCK

Sinus Arrest

Sinus arrest is usually a functional condition in which the sinus node fails to send impulses to the atria, resulting in a period of cardiac asystole. Eventually, recovery occurs. The first beat after the asystole may be a normal sinus beat (known as a *sinus escape* beat), or the *A-V node may take over* for the first beat, originating from a pacemaker in the A-V node (called a *nodal escape* beat). Here, the P wave may be detectable when there is *retrograde atrial conduction*. In this case, *inverted* P waves either precede or follow the *QRS complexes in leads II, III, and* aV_F, or there may be no retrograde conduction and hence no P waves. A ventricular escape beat has all the characteristics of a ventricular ectopic beat. Escape beats of these various types may precede sinus rhythm, sinus bradycardia, sinus tachycardia, nodal rhythm, ventricular tachycardia, or other cardiac rhythms or arrhythmias.

Sinoauricular Block

In this condition the *sinus node is blocked* organically or chemically. The block may occur *intermittently,* in which case every other beat may fail to appear. The sinus node recovers slowly after depolarization, and the refractory period is such that only every other beat is written. Periodically, in some cases, more than one beat is skipped. In other cases the *S-A node is more severely diseased,* and repolarization of the P wave occurs very slowly. Then an *A-V nodal rhythm develops* and takes over the role of pacemaker, and the P waves are *inverted* in leads II, III, and aV_F.

Atrioventricular Block

Atrioventricular block often is classified as a first-, second-, or third-degree A-V block. A *first-degree* A-V block has a *prolonged P-R interval.* A *second-degree* A-V block is characterized by the *occasional dropping of a QRS complex.* A *third-degree* A-V block shows a *complete dissociation* between atrial and ventricular contractions. With a first-degree A-V block, the P-R interval is long, exceeding 0.2 second for rates above 60. With a second-degree A-V block, an occasional P wave is not followed by a QRS complex. Normally, there is, of course, one P wave for every QRS complex, but, with a second-degree block, there may be seven P waves for every six QRS complexes (or some other ratio of P to QRS). This degree of block would be designated 7:6. A complete A-V block may be of two types: (1) The pacemaker may be in the junctional tissue, with QRS complexes essentially normal in appearance and not wide, or (2) the pacemaker may be in a ventricle, and the QRS complexes will be wide and abnormal in shape. In either case, there will be a complete dissociation between the beating of the atria and the ventricles. There also will be two different frequencies — one around 76 beats per minute, which represents the atrial-depolarization rate, and the other around 30 beats per minute, which is the ventricular-depolarization rate.

Clinically, these arrhythmias are important, because a very slow rate, due to any cause, markedly decreases cerebral, coronary, and other organ circulation, which results

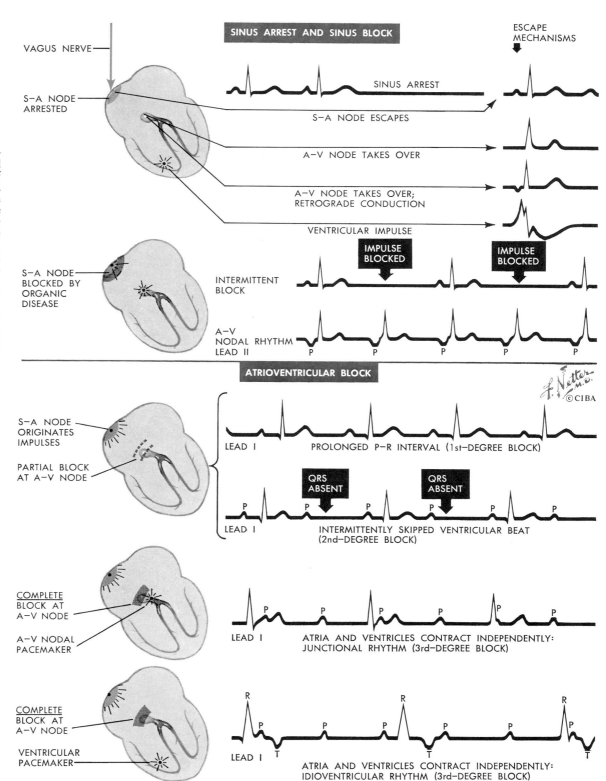

in tissue damage and, often, death. Every effort should be made, by medical or surgical means, to maintain a normal rate. Drugs, such as isoproterenol, and pacemakers may be of great benefit.

Morgagni-Adams-Stokes Syndrome (Adams-Stokes; Stokes-Adams). The Stokes-Adams syndrome refers to attacks of syncope due to severe bradycardia (often less than 20 beats per minute) or prolonged asystole (frequently 10 seconds or more). The collapse results from cerebral ischemia during cessation of effective ventricular output. The syncope occurs more readily when the patient is standing than in the supine position. The attacks usually occur when there is a failure of ventricular contraction in patients with complete heart blocks, due to either ventricular flutter fibrillation, ventricular asystole, or a combination of both. The attacks usually are limited to cases of organic complete heart block in which syncope, with or without convulsions, occurs in the absence of an effective idioventricular pacemaker, and this should be distinguished from other forms of syncope, *e.g.,* that which may occur in the *normal* heart as a result of *vagal reflexes* from a sensitive or compressed carotid sinus.

Because of the widespread use of cardiac pacemakers, knowledge of the life history of heart block and of the Stokes-Adams syndrome becomes important. The *prognosis,* in patients with complete heart block and Stokes-Adams syndrome, is grave. In one series, 30 percent of the patients died within 6 months of the onset of syncope, whereas only 20 percent survived for 4 years or longer.

Treatment is important. Digitalis should be stopped if the block is due to this agent. Potassium should not be administered, because of its myocardial depressant action. Isoproterenol can increase the cardiac irritability and accelerate the rate. Electrical defibrillation may be necessary if ventricular fibrillation is present. Mouth-to-mouth breathing and cardiac compression are temporary helpful measures. Most important is the use of temporary — and then permanent — *cardiac pacemakers,* which have been lifesaving in a large number of patients (see pages 71 and 72).

TACHYCARDIA, FIBRILLA- TION, AND ATRIAL FLUTTER

Paroxysmal Tachycardia

There are four forms of *paroxysmal tachycardia* — *atrial, atrial with block, nodal,* and *ventricular.*

Paroxysmal Atrial Tachycardia. This condition is due to a *pacemaker in the atria* which gives rise to rapid regular impulses at a rate above 100 beats per minute, often as much as 180. Usually, one can identify *P waves,* although sometimes the P and T waves fall on each other. The R-R intervals are regular. The condition is characterized by an abrupt beginning and ending. The *onset* and end often occur within the course of a single beat. Carotid-sinus pressure may cause a sudden reversion to sinus rhythm, which is diagnostic of this condition.

Paroxysmal Atrial Tachycardia with Block. It is important to recognize *paroxysmal atrial tachycardia with block,* since it is due, usually, to *digitalis intoxication.* It has all the characteristics of paroxysmal atrial tachycardia, but, occasionally, a *QRS complex* fails to appear; *i.e.,* there is a block at the *A-V node.* Otherwise, the condition is the same as paroxysmal atrial tachycardia. When digitalis is the cause, it should be withdrawn and the patient treated with potassium, insulin, glucose, anticholinergic drugs, etc.

Paroxysmal Nodal Tachycardia. This disturbance is characterized by *inverted P waves* in *leads II, III,* and *aV_F,* owing to retrograde atrial conduction. The P waves fall before, within, or after the QRS complexes. Retrograde conduction may occur. Paroxysmal nodal tachycardia often is caused by disease of the A-V node.

Ventricular Tachycardia. This condition is due to rapid impulse formation in a ventricle. The arrhythmia is serious and often associated with the toxic effects of digitalis, quinidine, or procainamide, or it may be due to serious organic cardiac disease. The ventricular rate is more rapid than the atrial rate, and close inspection of the tracing allows one to identify occasional P waves occurring at the basic atrial rate, usually 76 per minute. The ventricular contractions are generally more than 100 beats per minute and may be 140 or 160. The QRS complexes are wide, with T waves which are discordant with the QRS complexes, and the P-R intervals are not precisely identical.

Atrial Fibrillation

This condition is due to the presence of *multiple* islands of abnormal myocardium in various states of *refraction,* so that the *atrial-depolarization wave* must wind its way in and out of these islands of tissue, resulting in electric potentials of low voltage with variable directions. Only some of these impulses are transmitted through the A-V node; hence all the R-R intervals are different, owing to the irregularity of conduction. Rheumatic heart disease, hyperthyroidism, and

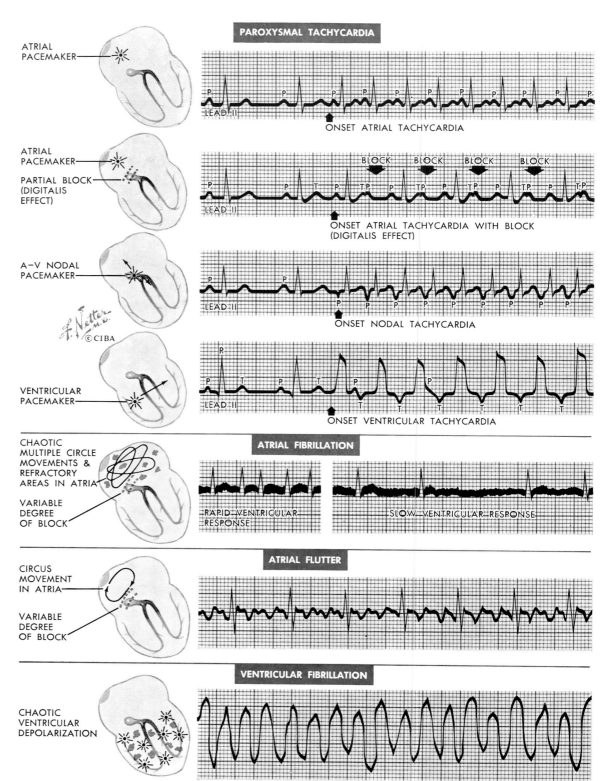

arteriosclerotic heart disease are common causes of this condition. With atrial fibrillation there are no consistently identifiable P waves in the tracing. The *ventricular* rate may be *rapid or slow,* depending on the degree of conduction through the A-V node and on the presence of heart failure, digitalis, and other factors. If the rate is rapid and heart failure is present, the rate can be slowed greatly by digitalis, and sinus rhythm often can be accomplished by cardioversion.

Atrial Flutter

This disturbance is due either to a *circus movement* or to a low atrial pacemaker which fires regularly at a rapid rate, usually about 220 beats per minute. Often, there is a *variable block* at the A-V node, so that only every other beat, or every third or fourth beat, is transmitted to the ventricles. In *leads II, III,* and *aV_F,* there usually are *inverted P waves* followed by *atrial T waves,* or a continuous atrial activity from the circus movement is present. These waves have a sawtooth appearance. Arteriosclerotic heart disease, hyperthyroidism, and rheumatic heart disease are common causes of this condition.

Ventricular Fibrillation

Multiple periodic ventricular pacemakers result in erratic depolarization of the ventricles, producing a tracing which resembles distorted sine waves that are irregular in amplitude and duration. The waves may be of high or low voltage. With this condition, there is no effective pumping of the heart. Severe organic cardiac disease or the toxic effects of digitalis or quinidine sometimes produce a similar condition. Ventricular fibrillation often is associated with sudden death, and the *treatment* of choice is the immediate application of electrical defibrillation, which may be lifesaving.

EFFECT OF DRUGS AND ELECTROLYTES ON ELECTROCARDIOGRAMS

Commonly employed drugs affecting the *electrocardiogram* are *digitalis* and *quinidine,* or allied agents. The effect on the tracing depends on the dose of the drug, the rate of excretion, the responsiveness of the patient, and the previous abnormalities of the electrocardiogram. Typical effects of these drugs on an essentially normal electrocardiogram (ECG) are indicated.

Small doses of digitalis and allied drugs, such as ouabain and squill, produce a *mild digitalis effect (A)* with sagging *depression of the S-T segments,* negative J shifts, and lowering of the T waves. The Q-T intervals may be shortened slightly because of increases in the rate of ventricular repolarization. Digitalis usually slows the cardiac rate and atrioventricular conduction because of vagal depression of the S-A and A-V nodes. With large doses *(B)* a further *depression of J* occurs, with sagging of the S-T segments and a distinct *decrease in the Q-T intervals,* which fall outside of normal limits. With *toxic* doses there is a depression of the A-V conduction tissue, with prolonged P-R intervals, and a state of ventricular irritability, with *ventricular ectopic beats* which may be single or multiple and, not uncommonly, multifocal *(C)*. *Coupling* is common, and atrial fibrillation or flutter, with paroxysmal atrial tachycardia, and block or variable degrees of *A-V block* may occur.

Quinidine and related drugs, such as procainamide (Pronestyl®) and lidocaine hydrochloride (Xylocaine®), tend to depress the electric activity of the atria and ventricles. Characteristically, the P waves increase in duration, with a slight increase in amplitude. If fine *atrial fibrillation* is present *(D)*, quinidine, in moderate doses, causes coarse atrial fibrillation, with increased amplitudes and durations *(E)* of the atrial-depolarization waves. With larger doses of quinidine in atrial fibrillation, *sinus rhythm* may be established, and, characteristically, notching of the T waves occurs *(F)*. After toxic doses of quinidine, there are *widening of the QRS complexes* and secondary *T-wave changes (G)*, so that the T waves point in a direction opposite to the major deflection of the QRS complexes. The Q-T intervals are increased in duration, because of depression of the depolarization and repolarization processes. Finally, cardiac irregularities, such as ventricular tachycardia or fibrillation, develop with toxic doses of quinidine.

As far as the ECG is concerned, *potassium* and *calcium,* as well as their relative concentrations, are the most important *electrolytes*. Acidosis also has an effect. Other electrolytes, such as sodium and magnesium, which are known to affect the ECG in experimental animals, do not produce changes in man, because they

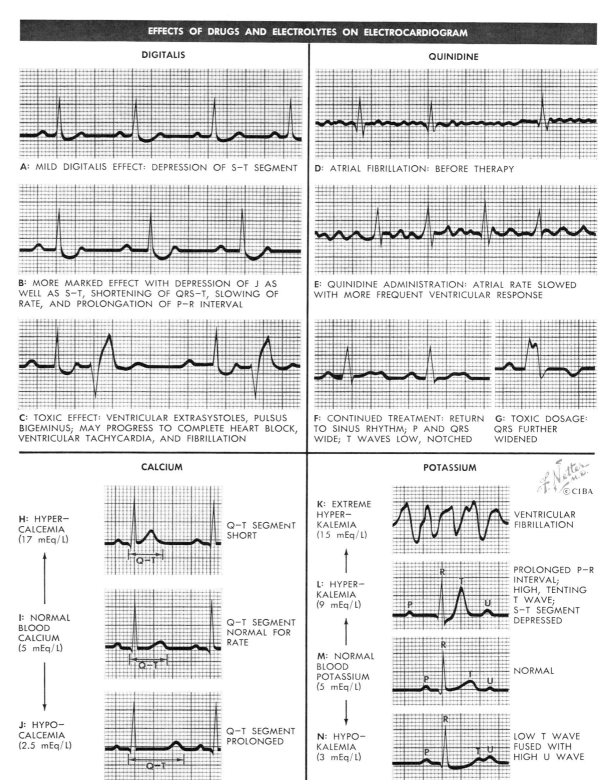

EFFECTS OF DRUGS AND ELECTROLYTES ON ELECTROCARDIOGRAM

DIGITALIS

A: MILD DIGITALIS EFFECT: DEPRESSION OF S-T SEGMENT

B: MORE MARKED EFFECT WITH DEPRESSION OF J AS WELL AS S-T, SHORTENING OF QRS-T, SLOWING OF RATE, AND PROLONGATION OF P-R INTERVAL

C: TOXIC EFFECT: VENTRICULAR EXTRASYSTOLES, PULSUS BIGEMINUS; MAY PROGRESS TO COMPLETE HEART BLOCK, VENTRICULAR TACHYCARDIA, AND FIBRILLATION

QUINIDINE

D: ATRIAL FIBRILLATION: BEFORE THERAPY

E: QUINIDINE ADMINISTRATION: ATRIAL RATE SLOWED WITH MORE FREQUENT VENTRICULAR RESPONSE

F: CONTINUED TREATMENT: RETURN TO SINUS RHYTHM; P AND QRS WIDE; T WAVES LOW, NOTCHED

G: TOXIC DOSAGE: QRS FURTHER WIDENED

CALCIUM

H: HYPER-CALCEMIA (17 mEq/L) — Q-T SEGMENT SHORT

I: NORMAL BLOOD CALCIUM (5 mEq/L) — Q-T SEGMENT NORMAL FOR RATE

J: HYPO-CALCEMIA (2.5 mEq/L) — Q-T SEGMENT PROLONGED

POTASSIUM

K: EXTREME HYPER-KALEMIA (15 mEq/L) — VENTRICULAR FIBRILLATION

L: HYPER-KALEMIA (9 mEq/L) — PROLONGED P-R INTERVAL; HIGH, TENTING T WAVE; S-T SEGMENT DEPRESSED

M: NORMAL BLOOD POTASSIUM (5 mEq/L) — NORMAL

N: HYPO-KALEMIA (3 mEq/L) — LOW T WAVE FUSED WITH HIGH U WAVE

© CIBA

do not fall to the low levels of concentration found in experimental situations.

Hypercalcemia may be encountered in patients with hyperparathyroidism. The electrocardiogram is characterized by *shortening of the Q-T intervals,* often with increased amplitudes of the T waves *(H)*. The T waves begin immediately after the ending of the QRS complexes, so the QRS complexes and T waves appear compressed.

Hypocalcemia increases the duration of the S-T and Q-T intervals (J). The QRS complexes and T waves merely appear to be widely separated from each other by long S-T segments which often are isoelectric.

Hyperkalemia depresses the atria, the A-V node, and the ventricles but has less effect on the sinus node. As a consequence, increases in concentrations of potassium produce *prolonged P-R intervals (L)*, *high T waves,* sinoauricular block with small or absent mechanical contractions of the atria, tenting of the T waves (tall and narrow at the base), intraventricular block with widening of the QRS complexes, *abnormal shifts of the S-T segment,* and, finally, ventricular standstill or *ventricular fibrillation (K)*.

Hypokalemia, which frequently results from the administration of diuretics or cortisone, or from vomiting, diarrhea, surgical suction, or a low intake of potassium, causes an *amplitude loss in the T waves (N)* and a prominence of the U waves, with easily measured Q-U intervals. In some leads the T and U waves are clearly separated, but in others they may *fuse,* causing a T-U complex. Deviations of the S-T segment (either depressions or elevations) may occur. Hypokalemia associated with other abnormal states (such as myocardial ischemia and infarction) or with cardiac drugs (such as digitalis and quinidine) is difficult to recognize.

MISLEADING ELECTROCARDIOGRAPHIC FINDINGS

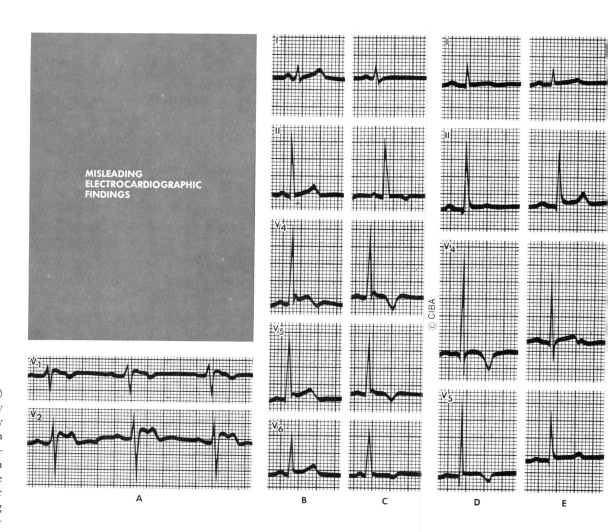

MISLEADING ELECTROCARDIOGRAPHIC FINDINGS

© CIBA

A   B   C   D   E

Having an electrocardiogram (ECG) taken is generally regarded as an entirely safe procedure, and, indeed, it usually is. However, anything that can result in unmerited hospitalization, lack of insurability, serious financial reverses, and even suicide should never be regarded as quite harmless. Yet all these, as well as other calamities, have befallen some unwitting victims of electrocardiography, as the following clinical vignettes illustrate.

A healthy young dentist of 32 developed pain in the front of his chest. After consulting an eminent cardiologist, he found himself encased in an oxygen tent because of some *saddle-shaped S-T elevation,* in his right chest leads (A), which was not recognized as a normal variant. He lost several thousands of dollars through hospitalization and absence from his practice. Labeled as a "suspected coronary" case (although the diagnosis was quite unconfirmed), he was then unable to obtain life insurance without a heavy rating and, of course, developed a disabling cardiac neurosis until, after 3 years, the still-unchanged ECG was recognized for what it was.

A hale and hearty football player, 19 years of age, developed prenuptial chest pain. No one could blame the physician for taking an ECG — "just to be sure" — in place of an adequate history, but he was culpable indeed. Impressed by the *ST-T* changes (B) he saw, he referred the athlete to a cardiologist who, likewise impressed, incarcerated him in the hospital. This disturbing turn of events inverted his labile T waves (C) and "confirmed" the cardiac diagnosis. After 5 weeks of imprisoned normalcy, football was eliminated, a cardiac neurosis was generated, and the nuptials were postponed for 6 months before tentative consummation thereof. Finally, at an (apparently) more-enlightened center, these changes were recognized for what they

were, and, still with his fluctuating ST-T pattern, he was acquitted, with a clean bill of health and an admonition to love happily ever after.

A bus driver was stricken with a chest pain and submitted to an ECG. This was not "normal," and he was put to bed for several weeks, with a diagnosis of "angina." No bus company wanted a driver with angina, so, when he was released from unwarranted captivity, he could find no work. Disconsolate, he finally threw himself into a river, leaving behind a sick wife and four children. Dragged from the river, his body yielded a normal myocardium with unobstructed coronaries.

A schoolboy of 18, chasing a friend down the street, reached out to grab him and collapsed, with chest pain, on the sidewalk. Transported to a nearby emergency room, he was subjected to the inevitable ECG, which disclosed an unconventional *ST-T* pattern (D). After a month's detention in the hospital, he was forbidden to take part in sports and was advised to leave school and acquire a home tutor, which he did. A year later, another center suspected the true insignificance of the electrocardiographic pattern, "righted" the ST-T deviations with ingested potassium (E), and, by cineangiography, demonstrated a normal coronary tree.

We cannot explain why some normal persons have such offbeat tracings, any more than we can explain the variation in distribution of the normal coronary tree. Inverted T waves frequently are attributed to "juvenility" and the high ST takeoff to "early repolarization," but this adds little of value and gives satisfaction only to those who like to disguise ignorance with polysyllables.

The moral of all this is that we who undertake to interpret electrocardiograms at least should be well

aware of the kinds of suspicious-looking patterns that may be merely normal variants, as well as the many physiologic stimuli that can upset a normal electrocardiogram and simulate disease. But this is not enough, since suspicion alone cannot prove the point; many suspect patterns are indistinguishable from the mimicked pattern of disease, and we must know how to gather more clues. There are some helpfully discriminating tests with which we should be familiar and know when to apply them. Innocently inverted T waves may "right" themselves when a tracing is obtained with the patient fasting, yet how many of us make a point of securing a tracing with the patient unfed before condemning him for an abnormal electrocardiogram? Exercise, which often exaggerates the electrocardiographic changes of organic disease, "improves" the ST-T pattern of the disease mimic. In a patient whose suspicious changes result from anxiety, the simple expedient of putting him to sleep with a hypnotic may restore the tracing to "normal." If hyperventilation is the cause of such changes, simple holding of the breath or a dose of propantheline bromide (Pro-Banthine®) may eliminate them. In other circumstances, performing the Valsalva maneuver may absolve the "abnormalities." A large dose of potassium salts (which, of course, must never be given in the absence of guaranteed good renal function) often "rights" the innocently inverted T wave but seldom restores the negative waves seen in disease.

One cannot overemphasize our obligation to be familiar with such variables and their proper interpretation, for we hardly can depart further from the Hippocratic ideal—"to help, or at least to do no harm" —than when we, through professional ignorance, turn a healthy man into a cardiac cripple.

PACEMAKER IMPLANTATION IN TREATMENT OF COMPLETE HEART BLOCK

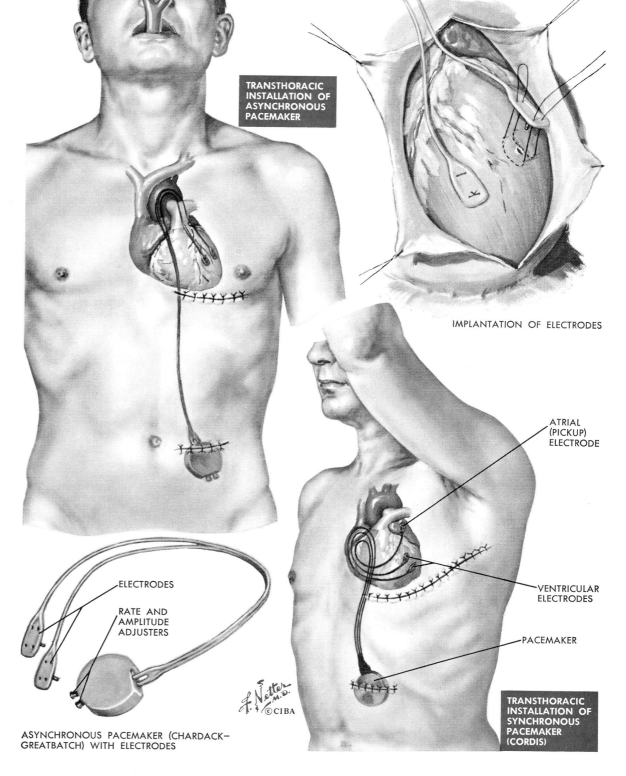

TRANSTHORACIC INSTALLATION OF ASYNCHRONOUS PACEMAKER

IMPLANTATION OF ELECTRODES

ELECTRODES

RATE AND AMPLITUDE ADJUSTERS

ASYNCHRONOUS PACEMAKER (CHARDACK–GREATBATCH) WITH ELECTRODES

ATRIAL (PICKUP) ELECTRODE

VENTRICULAR ELECTRODES

PACEMAKER

TRANSTHORACIC INSTALLATION OF SYNCHRONOUS PACEMAKER (CORDIS)

The sudden onset of complete heart block portends a highly unfavorable prognosis unless effective therapy is instituted. Prior to the introduction of electrical methods of cardiac pacing, by Callaghan, Bigelow, and Zoll, therapeutic measures were primarily pharmacologic and were designed to improve atrioventricular conduction and stimulate idioventricular pacemaker foci. Research, notably by Chardack, Zoll, Kantrowitz, and Nathan, led to the development of totally implantable pacemakers. These presently represent the treatment of choice in patients with chronic heart block who have (1) episodes of syncope or convulsions owing to ventricular bradycardia, (2) cardiac failure secondary to the bradycardia, and (3) unstable ventricular rhythms associated with the heart block.

Technics of Permanent Pacemaker Implantation, with Thoracotomy

Asynchronous Pacemaker. A temporary electrode catheter is positioned in the right ventricular-outflow tract, prior to thoracotomy, to ensure predictable pacing during anesthetic induction and the exposure of the heart through the left fifth intercostal space. Two *Chardack* helical-coil *electrodes,* each partially encased in a Silastic® sleeve, are *implanted* in the left ventricular myocardium. The distal ends of the electrodes are tunnel-communicated to a subcutaneous abdominal pocket and connected to a pulse generator.

The rate and amplitude of the pulse can be altered percutaneously, at any time after implantation, by the insertion of a needle with a triangular cross section into the readily palpated adjustment nipples. Stimulating thresholds generally approximate 1.5 to 2 milliamperes, and the pulse generator is adjusted to provide at least twice the threshold requirements at a rate of 64 to 72 beats per minute.

Synchronous Pacemaker. Nathan and his co-workers have devised an implantable synchronous pacemaker which senses each P wave by means of a third electrode sutured to the left atrium. The pulse generator amplifies the signal, introduces a time delay which is approximately equal to a normal P-R interval, and finally initiates ventricular depolarization through two electrodes implanted in the left ventricular myocardium, employing the technic described above. Thus, essentially normal electromechanical relationships between the atria and ventricles are maintained. Physiologically induced alterations in the atrial rate cause the ventricles to follow in a synchronous fashion. A blocking device prevents excessive ventricular rates, should atrial tachycardia or flutter occur. If atrial fibrillation is present and the fibrillary (F) waves are detected, an irregular but rate-controlled ventricular response is observed. When the F waves are small and undetected, the pacer's automatic idioventricular circuit drives the ventricles asynchronously at 52 beats per minute. Similarly, if the intrinsic *atrial* rate is

(Continued on page 72)

PACEMAKER IMPLANTATION IN TREATMENT OF COMPLETE HEART BLOCK

(Continued from page 71)

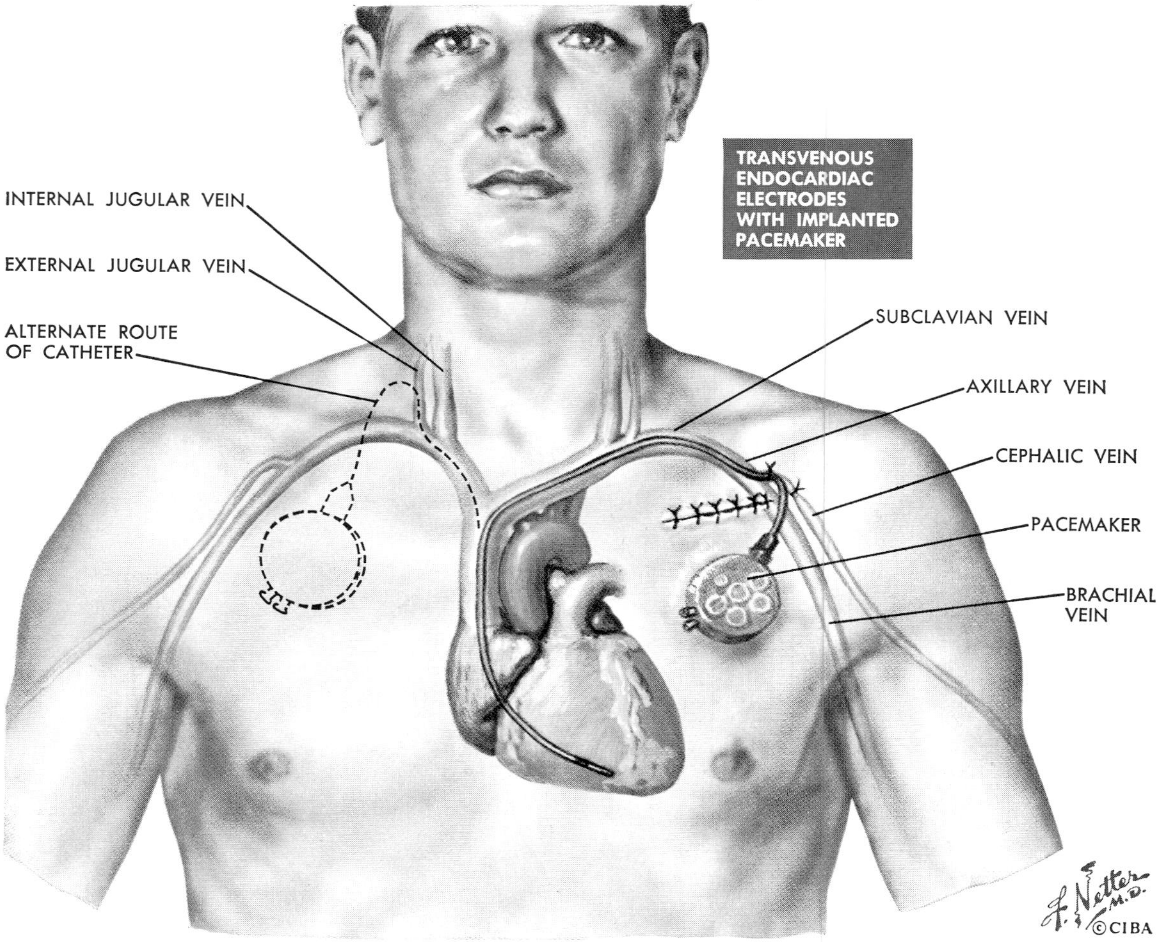

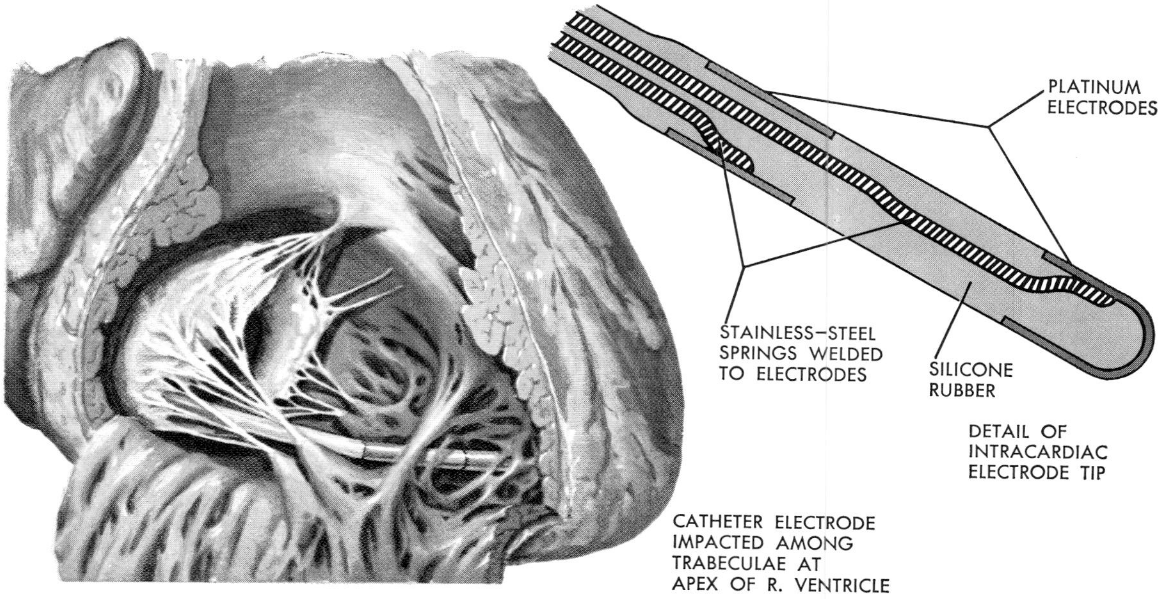

INTERNAL JUGULAR VEIN

EXTERNAL JUGULAR VEIN

ALTERNATE ROUTE OF CATHETER

TRANSVENOUS ENDOCARDIAC ELECTRODES WITH IMPLANTED PACEMAKER

SUBCLAVIAN VEIN

AXILLARY VEIN

CEPHALIC VEIN

PACEMAKER

BRACHIAL VEIN

PLATINUM ELECTRODES

STAINLESS–STEEL SPRINGS WELDED TO ELECTRODES

SILICONE RUBBER

DETAIL OF INTRACARDIAC ELECTRODE TIP

CATHETER ELECTRODE IMPACTED AMONG TRABECULAE AT APEX OF R. VENTRICLE

below 52 per minute, or if the P-wave potential is below the sensing *amplitude* of the *pacemaker* ($\pm$1 millivolt), the ventricles will again be driven by the idioventricular circuit.

Transvenous Electrode Pacemaker

The ability to maintain lengthy periods of ventricular pacing through a *catheter electrode* with an external generator, as suggested by Furman, led to the development of totally implantable catheter-electrode–generator systems. Their major advantage lies in the avoidance of thoracotomy; the entire implantation is performed under local anesthesia. Chardack's catheter consists of a *Silastic®* tube which contains two separate helical coils of *stainless steel* welded to *platinum-electrode contact terminals*. Two stainless-steel stylets, placed in the lumina of the coils, provide additional stiffness during manipulation of the catheters.

Implantation is performed under fluoroscopic guidance with an image intensifier. An incision is made below the clavicle, the *cephalic vein* is identified in the deltopectoral groove, and the catheter is inserted in this vein, close to its junction with the *axillary vein*. The catheter is passed into the *apex of the right ventricle*, where it is *impacted* in the multiple *trabeculae* seen in this area, so that the electrode tips make firm contact with the ventricular myocardium. Once the

electrode has been satisfactorily positioned, the stylets are withdrawn, the pulse generator is connected to the electrode catheter, and the unit is placed in a subcutaneous pocket.

An *alternative method of catheter insertion* utilizes the *external jugular vein*. This requires a second incision over the vein, and the catheter must be tunneled over or under the clavicle to the infraclavicular pouch.

"Demand" Pacemaker. Approximately 10 percent of the patients who have undergone pacemaker implantation have a temporary return of sinus rhythm, so that a potential hazard, that of electrically induced ventricular arrhythmias initiated in the vulnerable period following ventricular depolarization, is introduced. This has led to the recent development of a

"demand" pacemaker in which the stimulus cannot be fired during the vulnerable period, because the pulse-generator output is inhibited for a definite time period by a signal derived from the previous ventricular depolarization. Thus, if the pacemaker is set at a rate of 60, the pulse generator would not fire until a 1-second asystolic period had been exceeded. Any conducted or ectopic ventricular depolarization would inhibit the unit for an additional second.

Implanted cardiac pacemakers have substantially improved the *prognosis* of patients suffering from complete heart block. These individuals can often return to active daily life and, generally, require no supplementary medication. Elective pulse-generator replacement is presently advised after a 30-month period of use.

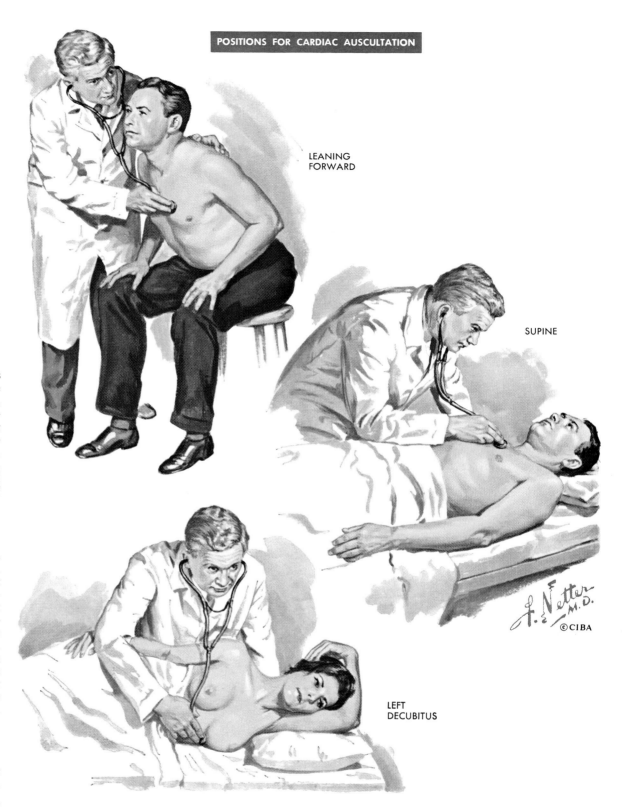

POSITIONS FOR CARDIAC AUSCULTATION

LEANING FORWARD

SUPINE

LEFT DECUBITUS

AUSCULTATORY POSITIONS AND AREAS; EVENTS IN CARDIAC CYCLE

The basic instrument of *auscultation* is the human ear. Although the stethoscope has technical advantages, it often distorts, decreases, or selectively emphasizes certain vibrations. Frequently, the naked ear is superior to the stethoscope in the detection of *low-pitched* vibrations (*sound III, sound IV,* see page 75, gallops), first, because it is a larger collector of sound and, second, on account of the fusion of auditory with palpatory perception.

The Position of the Patient

In auscultation, various *positions* can be used. The patient may be sitting, *supine,* lying on the *left* side, or bent *forward.* The first, third, and fourth positions increase the contact of the apex with the chest wall, and these are preferred for mitral or left ventricular sounds and *murmurs.* The left-side position causes tachycardia and accentuates the *rumbling* murmur of *mitral stenosis.* The bent-forward posture is preferred for *aortic diastolic murmurs,* whereas the supine is best for pulmonic and tricuspid murmurs.

Areas of Auscultation

The conventional designations of mitral, tricuspid, aortic, and pulmonary areas of auscultation have been used in the past. Revision of the areas named and different interpretations of their meanings have been suggested, by Luisada, Shah, and Slodki, according to the chamber or vessel in which a given sound or murmur is best recognized by intracardiac phonocardiography; *i.e.,* it has been proposed to divide the thorax into seven areas: *left ventricular, right ventricular,* left atrial, right atrial, *aortic, pulmonary,* and descending thoracic aortic.

Left Ventricular Area. The apical area (so-called "mitral" area) is the best location for detecting not only the *murmur of mitral stenosis* or *insufficiency* but also the *left ventricular* or atrial gallops and the *aortic component of the second sound* (A component of II, see page 75). The *murmurs of aortic stenosis and insuffi-*ciency (especially the latter) also are often heard well at this location. However, these vibrations are picked up over a larger area formed by the entire left ventricle, centering around the apex beat and extending to the fourth and fifth left interspaces medially and to the anterior axillary line laterally. In cases with *ventricular enlargement,* the sound shifts to either the left or the right.

Right Ventricular Area. The so-called "tricuspid" area should be renamed "right ventricular." In this location, not only the *murmurs of tricuspid* stenosis and insufficiency but also the right ventricular and atrial gallops and the *murmurs of pulmonary insufficiency* and *ventricular septal defect* can be well heard.

The right ventricular area includes the lower part of the sternum and the fourth and fifth interspaces, 2 to 4 cm to the left and 2 cm to the right of the sternum. This area may extend also to the point of maximal impulse, in the presence of severe *right ventricular enlargement,* the "apex," in such patients, being formed by the right ventricle.

Aortic Area. The aortic component of the second *heart sound* and the murmurs of aortic-valve defects are often heard well at the *third left interspace* (Erb's point) (see page 77), which in the past, was called the "auxiliary aortic" area. This point is frequently more revealing than is the second right interspace, except in cases with dilatation of the ascending aorta, where the manubrium or the second right interspace may be more informative. The term "aortic" area should designate both the aortic root and part of the ascending aorta. The vibrations heard best in this area include the murmurs caused by *aortic stenosis, aortic insufficiency,* augmented flow across the aorta or dilatation of the ascending aorta, and abnormalities

(Continued on page 74)

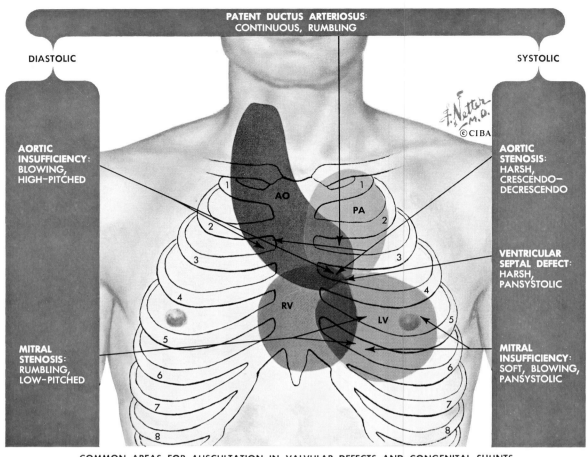

PATENT DUCTUS ARTERIOSUS:
CONTINUOUS, RUMBLING

DIASTOLIC

SYSTOLIC

AORTIC
INSUFFICIENCY:
BLOWING,
HIGH-PITCHED

AORTIC
STENOSIS:
HARSH,
CRESCENDO-
DECRESCENDO

VENTRICULAR
SEPTAL DEFECT:
HARSH,
PANSYSTOLIC

MITRAL
STENOSIS:
RUMBLING,
LOW-PITCHED

MITRAL
INSUFFICIENCY:
SOFT, BLOWING,
PANSYSTOLIC

AUSCULTATORY POSITIONS AND AREAS; EVENTS IN CARDIAC CYCLE

(Continued from page 73)

of the arteries of the neck, as well as the aortic *ejection click* and the aortic component of the second heart sound.

Pulmonary Area. The term "pulmonary" area should refer to the *pulmonary artery* rather than the pulmonary valve. The murmurs of *pulmonary stenosis* and *insufficiency,* the murmur caused by increased flow or dilatation of the pulmonary artery, the pulmonary ejection click, the *pulmonary component (P component of II) of the second sound* (see page 75), and the *murmur of patent ductus arteriosus* are heard best in this location.

The pulmonary area is formed by the second left interspace near the sternal edge; it extends upward to the clavicle and downward to the third left interspace near the sternal margin, but it may extend also posteriorly at the level of the fourth and fifth dorsal vertebrae.

Most Significant Auscultatory Findings

Sounds. The *first sound (I)* is often louder over the left ventricular area (apex and midprecordium); the *second sound (II)* is frequently louder over the aortic and pulmonary areas (base). The first sound is a long noise of *lower* tonality; the second sound is shorter and sharper. In normal adolescents or young people, the first sound may be split. The best area for hearing this split sound is at the third left interspace. This splitting is not influenced by respiration.

The loudness of the first sound is decreased in myocarditis, myocardial infarct, myocardial fibrosis, hypothyroidism, mitral insufficiency *(soft),* aortic insufficiency, and pericarditis with effusion. It is increased in mitral stenosis, systemic hypertension, and hyperthyroidism.

The *second sound* is frequently *split,* during inspiration, in normal children and young people. The best area for hearing this splitting is the third left interspace, close to the sternum (Erb's point). The second sound has an increased loudness of the aortic component in systemic hypertension, coarctation of the aorta, and aortitis. A decreased loudness of this

COMMON AREAS FOR AUSCULTATION IN VALVULAR DEFECTS AND CONGENITAL SHUNTS

AO=AORTIC AREA (MURMURS OF AORTIC STENOSIS AND AORTIC INSUFFICIENCY)

PA = PULMONARY-ARTERY AREA (MURMURS OF PULMONARY STENOSIS AND INSUFFICIENCY)

RV = RIGHT VENTRICULAR AREA (MURMURS OF TRICUSPID-VALVE DISEASE)

LV=LEFT VENTRICULAR AREA (MURMURS OF MITRAL STENOSIS AND MITRAL INSUFFICIENCY)

3rd L. INTERSPACE (MOST MURMURS OF PULMONARY, AORTIC, AND TRICUSPID ORIGIN, AND OF VENTRICULAR SEPTAL DEFECT; SPLITTING OF 2nd SOUND)

ARROWS POINT TO BEST AREAS FOR AUSCULTATION

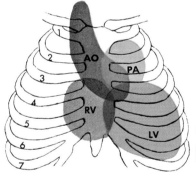

PROJECTION OF AUSCULTATORY
AREAS IN ISOLATED
LEFT VENTRICULAR ENLARGEMENT

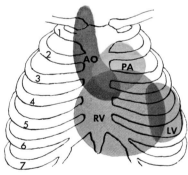

PROJECTION OF AUSCULTATORY
AREAS IN ISOLATED
RIGHT VENTRICULAR ENLARGEMENT

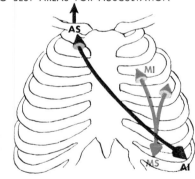

USUAL TRANSMISSION OF "INFLOW"-
AND "OUTFLOW"-TRACT MURMURS OF
LEFT HEART: AS=AORTIC STENOSIS; AI=
AORTIC INSUFFICIENCY; MS=MITRAL
STENOSIS; MI=MITRAL INSUFFICIENCY

component characterizes aortic stenosis. (The aortic component may be so delayed as to follow the pulmonary component—a paradoxical splitting.) The second sound has an increased loudness of the pulmonary component in pulmonary hypertension. There is decreased loudness in pulmonary stenosis. (The pulmonary component not only is smaller but also is delayed, causing a wider splitting.)

The second sound has a wider, fixed splitting in conditions presenting a diastolic overload of the right heart and in right bundle-branch block, owing to delay of the pulmonary component. Cases with left bundle-branch block may present such a delay of the aortic component as to cause paradoxical splitting.

The *third sound (III)* is usually normal in children and adolescents. It may be audible over either the left or the right ventricular area in ventricular overload, myocarditis, tachycardia, or heart failure.

The *atrial sound (IV)* is never heard in normal hearts. It is audible over either the left ventricular area (more commonly) or the right ventricular area (less commonly) in ventricular overload, myocarditis, tachycardia, atrial flutter, and complete or incomplete A-V block or obstruction. It is then called atrial gallop.

A left atrial gallop is frequently heard in aortic stenosis or systemic hypertension. A right atrial gallop is often heard in pulmonary stenosis or pulmonary hypertension. A slightly different type is the "summation" gallop, which is due to the summation of sounds III and IV (see page 79). This is most commonly encountered in cases with tachycardia and grade-1 A-V block.

A *systolic click* (see page 78) can be heard over either the pulmonary (pulmonary *ejection sound*) or the aortic area (aortic ejection sound). These clicks

(Continued on page 75)

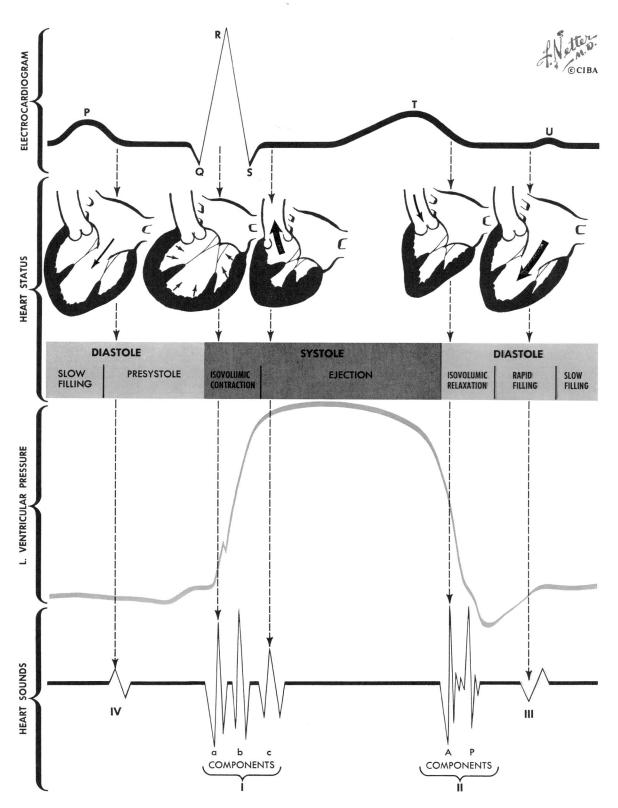

AUSCULTATORY POSITIONS AND AREAS; EVENTS IN CARDIAC CYCLE

(Continued from page 74)

are caused by either an increased loudness of the third component of sound I, in the case of the aorta, or a *new* sound, of equivalent significance but not usually present, as in the case of the pulmonary artery. They occur whenever there is either a dilatation of the aorta or pulmonary artery or a narrowing of the aortic or pulmonary valve (usually with post-stenotic dilatation).

A diastolic snap or click can be heard in the fourth left interspace, close to the sternum, over the entire left ventricular area or even over the entire precordium. This is the mitral opening snap that is most often heard in mitral stenosis. Occasionally, it can be heard also in diastolic overload of the left heart (mitral insufficiency, patent ductus). A tricuspid opening snap is audible over the right ventricular area in cases of tricuspid stenosis. It can be heard, occasionally, in diastolic overload of the right ventricle (tricuspid insufficiency, atrial septal defect, ventricular septal defect).

Murmurs. Murmurs are significant findings of auscultation.

The regurgitant murmur of A-V-valve insufficiency is *blowing*, prolonged, and *soft*, in either *decrescendo* or *pansystolic* and, occasionally, in *crescendo*. Whereas the murmur of mitral insufficiency is maximal over the left ventricular area and easily audible at the left axilla, that of tricuspid insufficiency is maximal over the right ventricular area and is well heard over the right precordium. Inspiration or inspiratory apnea increases the loudness of the tricuspid murmur but decreases that of the mitral murmur.

The murmur of A-V-valve stenosis is a typical, *low-pitched rumble* (see page 74) which acquires higher pitch and greater loudness in presystole if there is sinus rhythm. It is heard best, in mitral stenosis, in the fourth left intercostal space, halfway between the apex and the sternal border; in tricuspid stenosis, over the right ventricular area. This murmur becomes louder in inspiration or inspiratory apnea.

The regurgitant murmur of semilunar-valve insufficiency is a soft, high-pitched, blowing, occasionally musical, murmur in decrescendo. In aortic insufficiency the murmur is loudest in the third left interspace, and it can be followed along the left sternal border and toward the apex; if the ascending aorta is dilated, the murmur is louder in the second right interspace and can be followed downward along the right sternal border. In pulmonary insufficiency the murmur is loudest over the second left interspace and can be followed downward from the upper left to the lower right part of the sternum.

The stenotic murmur of the semilunar valves is the loudest of all murmurs. It is *harsh,* starts a bit after sound I, and is often preceded by an ejection click. It often has a crescendo-decrescendo quality and ends before sound II. In aortic stenosis it is maximal in the third left or second right interspace. It is readily heard over the suprasternal notch and the carotid arteries, and it can be heard at the apex.

In subaortic stenosis, especially of the muscular type, it is maximal over the left ventricular area. In pulmonary stenosis the murmur is best heard over the pulmonary area. It radiates moderately downward and often can be heard in the back (pulmonic areas).

The murmur caused by a ventricular septal defect is long, harsh, and pansystolic. It is heard best over the right ventricular area.

The murmur caused by patency of the ductus arteriosus is a continuous one, with accentuation in late *systole* and early *diastole*. It is best heard over the first and second intercostal spaces. In complicated "ductus," especially in children, the murmur may be only *systolic*.

Friction Rubs. These sounds can be heard over various areas. They resemble the noise made by rubbing new leather, and they usually are heard in both systole and diastole, *i.e.,* "to-and-fro" rubs.

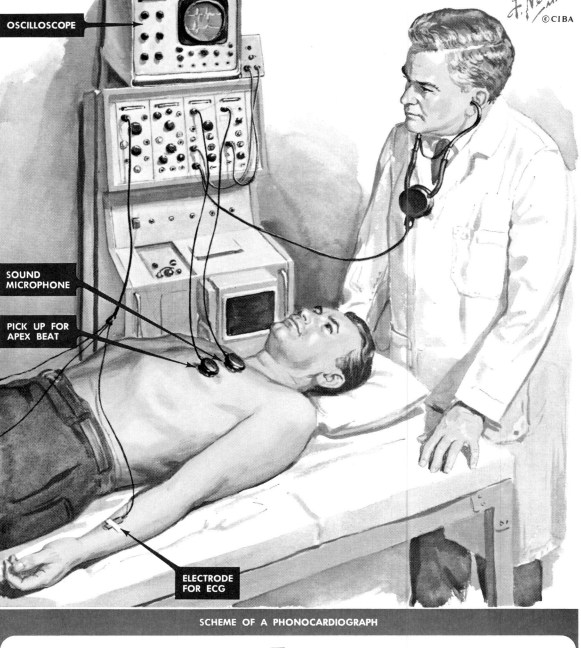

OSCILLOSCOPE

SOUND
MICROPHONE

PICK UP FOR
APEX BEAT

ELECTRODE
FOR ECG

PHONOCARDIOGRAPHY

The Vibratory Phenomenon of the Precordium

The total displacement of the wall of the precordial area constitutes a complex wave caused by the dynamic action of the heart. The spectrum of vibration, generated by the heart and transmitted to the body surface, ranges from about 1 to 1500 cps (cycles per second) in certain patients with heart disease. It overlaps only partly the auditory band.

The Phonocardiograph

Phonocardiography is the graphic registration of the various bands of the vibratory spectrum. No system of phonocardiography can simultaneously register, with equal clarity and detail, the adjoining bands. Therefore, in order to record the high-frequency, low-energy components, it is necessary to attenuate the low-frequency components. The frequency spectrum is subdivided into adjoining bands through the use of band-pass or high-pass filters. The frequency band passing through the *filter* is then amplified to the desired level for recording. The essential elements of a *phonocardiograph* include the transducer, *filters, amplifier,* recording system, and *transcribing system.*

Normal Cardiac Cycle in the Phonocardiogram

Presystole. The *phonocardiogram,* in the medium-frequency range (30 to 60 cps), seldom reveals a diphasic or triphasic slow wave (sound IV, see page 77). Higher bands show no waves in this phase.

Ventricular Systole. The phonocardiogram, in the medium-low range (50 to 150 cps), indicates a small initial vibra-

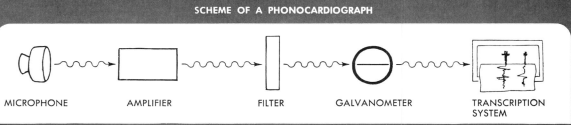

SCHEME OF A PHONOCARDIOGRAPH

MICROPHONE   AMPLIFIER   FILTER   GALVANOMETER   TRANSCRIPTION SYSTEM

tion, of low frequency and magnitude, during the mechanoacoustic interval. It then shows a central phase of large vibrations which can often be subdivided into various groups.

Medium-High and High-Frequency Vibrations (150 to 1000 cps). In these bands the first heart sound (*sound I*) often becomes split into two phases, according to two possible occurrences: (1) The first possibility, more commonly found in young individuals, consists of two groups of vibrations, separated by 30 to 40 milliseconds, which originate in the left ventricle (close splitting). (2) The second possibility, more common in mature individuals, consists of two groups of vibrations, separated by 60 to 70 milliseconds, which originate, respectively, in the left ventricle and the aorta, but, occasionally, in the pulmonary artery (wide splitting). The second of these two vibrations (third component of the first sound) could be called the

ejection sound (see page 78), in analogy with the clinical term, ejection click. It is due to vibrations arising in one of the major arteries (usually the aorta) at the beginning of ventricular ejection.

Occasionally, three groups of vibrations occur, *i.e.,* the first two normal groups plus a small ejection sound.

Isovolumic Relaxation Period. The medium-low-frequency tracing (50 to 150 cps) usually records from two to four large vibrations which comprise the second heart sound (sound II). Frequently, two larger components can be recognized within the central part of this sound — the aortic (A) and pulmonic (P) components respectively (see page 75).

The medium-high-frequency and high-frequency (150 to 1000 cps) tracing reveals two large vibrations (aortic and pulmonary components) which usually emerge (except in older individuals) and

(Continued on page 77)

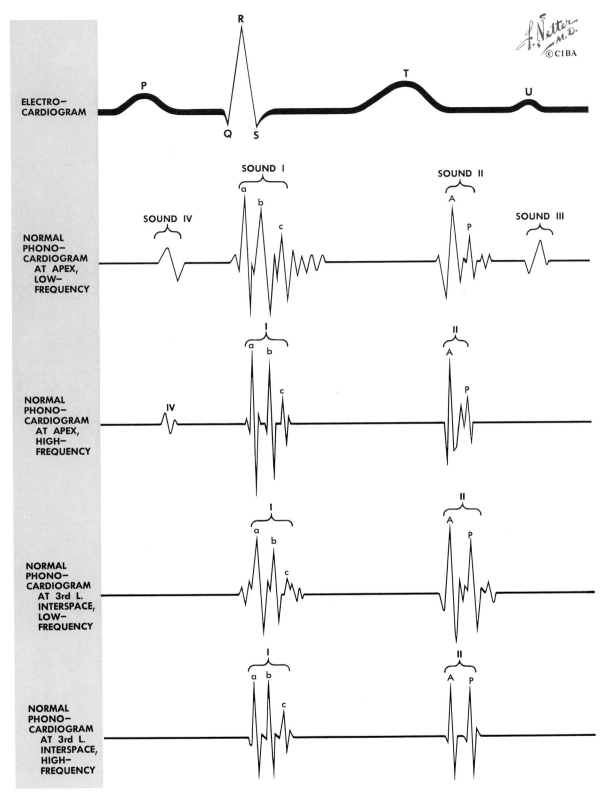

ELECTRO-CARDIOGRAM

SOUND I

SOUND II

SOUND IV

NORMAL PHONO-CARDIOGRAM AT APEX, LOW-FREQUENCY

SOUND III

NORMAL PHONO-CARDIOGRAM AT APEX, HIGH-FREQUENCY

NORMAL PHONO-CARDIOGRAM AT 3rd L. INTERSPACE, LOW-FREQUENCY

NORMAL PHONO-CARDIOGRAM AT 3rd L. INTERSPACE, HIGH-FREQUENCY

PHONOCARDIOGRAPHY

(Continued from page 76)

are widely separated during inspiration.

Protodiastole. In this phase, usually, the phonocardiogram of normal individuals shows no vibrations. In rare exceptions a small vibration corresponds to the opening of the mitral valve, and this should be called the mitral-opening sound.

Diastole. This phase (see page 75) can be divided into *rapid filling* (early diastole) and *slow filling* (middiastole). Phonocardiograms of normal individuals usually reveal no vibrations. However, in normal children and adolescents, a small, low-pitched vibration is often recorded in early diastole (sound III).

Time Relationship of Phonocardiographic and Electrocardiographic Waves

Since an *electrocardiogram* (ECG) is usually recorded with the phonocardiogram, the following time relationships between the two tracings should be known: (1) Sound IV, whenever present, falls at the end of the *P* wave and always precedes the *Q* wave of the ECG. (2) The first group of vibrations of sound I coincides with either the *R* wave or the *RS* slope of the ECG. (3) The *Q-I* interval is less than 0.07 second in normal subjects. (4) The aortic component of sound II falls at the end of the *T* wave of the ECG. Abnormal vibrations (opening snap, sound III, see page 79) have no coincidence with the electrocardiogram.

Abnormal First and Second Sounds

First Sound. Increased intensity of the first sound (*sound I*) occurs in tachycardia as associated with hyperthyroidism, anemia, emotional upset, fever, and exercise. A loud first sound with a normal rate

suggests either a short conduction time or *mitral stenosis* (see page 79).

LEFT VENTRICULAR OR SYSTEMIC HYPERTENSION. A wide splitting (see page 79) of the first sound is often present in *aortic stenosis* or systemic hypertension, owing to increased loudness of the third component (*c*) of the first sound (so-called *ejection sound*).

RIGHT VENTRICULAR OR PULMONARY HYPERTENSION. Whenever pressure rises considerably in the right ventricle, right ventricular components are probably recorded and may contribute to the character of the first sound. With dilatation of the pulmonary artery or moderate pulmonary stenosis, one often finds a wide splitting of the first sound. This is due to auscultation of the first component (*a*) of the first sound plus a loud third-component ejection sound which is most likely the result of an abnormal jet of blood in the pulmonary artery, causing a sudden distention of the wall.

MITRAL STENOSIS. Since mitral-valve closure occurs only when the *left ventricular pressure* (see page 75) has risen above that of the left atrium, closure of the mitral valve is delayed, occurring during the rapid rise of pressure. Subsequent to mitral closure, this rise is extremely fast, a fact which causes the loudness of the sound and its "snapping" quality.

BUNDLE-BRANCH BLOCK. Often, a small, prolonged first sound is heard, especially in left bundle-branch block. Audible splitting of the first sound may be due to: (1) simulation of splitting owing to a *presystolic gallop;* (2) normal close splitting, owing to audibility of the first (*a*) and second (*b*) components; and (3) abnormal wide splitting, because the first (*a*) and third (*c*) components are audible.

MYOCARDITIS. The first sound is often faint and muffled. Since the magnitude of the first component

(Continued on page 78)

PHONOCARDIOGRAPHY

(Continued from page 77)

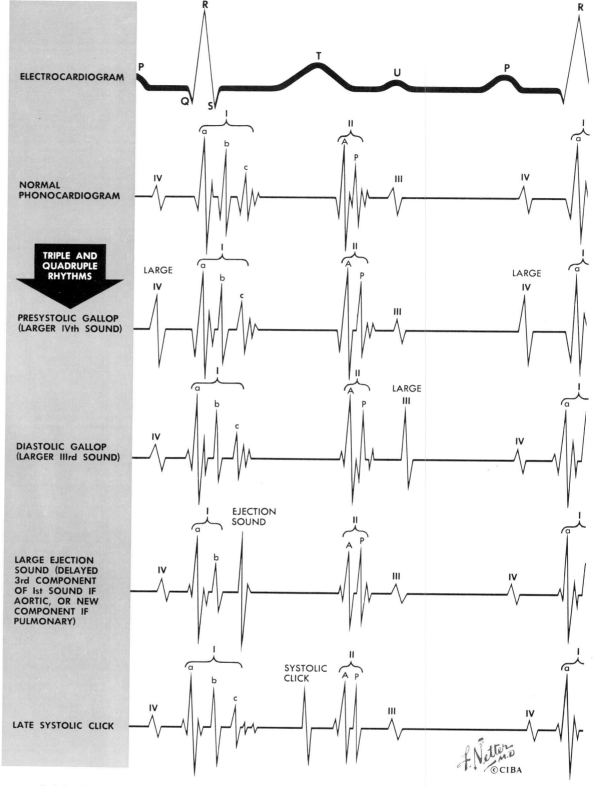

of the first sound is closely related to the rapidity of contraction (first derivative of left ventricular pressure), weakening of the sound (slower rise of pressure) is logical.

MYOCARDIAL INFARCTION. In myocardial infarction the first sound is often weak and is formed by vibrations of *low frequency*. Part of the energy developed by the normal sections of the left ventricle is absorbed by the elastic distention of the infarcted area; therefore, the pressure rise will occur more slowly. Since the magnitude of the first component of the first sound is closely related to the rapidity of rise, this will cause a decrease of the first sound.

AORTIC INSUFFICIENCY. Certain patients with *aortic insufficiency* (see page 79) exhibit a remarkable decrease of the first sound, owing to incomplete closure of the left ventricular chamber by the aortic valve. Thus, a slower rise of pressure will occur during the tension period.

MITRAL INSUFFICIENCY. Patients with *mitral insufficiency* often have a small first sound. A mechanism similar to that of aortic insufficiency has actually been demonstrated; *i.e.*, the escape of blood through the damaged mitral valve causes a slower rise of pressure in the left ventricle and an attenuation of the first large component of the first sound.

THYROID DISEASES. The first sound is loud and booming in thyrotoxicosis, whereas it is weak and poorly heard in hypothyroidism. This is explained by opposite changes in the speed of contraction, as a result of the endocrine disorder.

Second Sound. DIASTOLIC OVERLOAD. *Diastolic* overload of one ventricle prolongs ejection, with a normal or shorter duration of the isometric tension phase. This is typically observed in diastolic overload of the right ventricle (atrial

septal defect) and may play some role in diastolic overload of the left (mitral insufficiency, patent ductus arteriosus). Therefore, in all these cases there will be an abnormal second sound (sound II), with wider splitting of a normal type *(A-P)* in right ventricular overload, and a single second sound or paradoxical splitting (P-A) in left ventricular overload.

SYSTOLIC OVERLOAD. In systemic hypertension the left ventricular systole is definitely prolonged. However, because the left ventricle dominates cardiac dynamics, the right ventricular systole is also prolonged; therefore, no typical change of the A-P interval occurs. Left ventricular failure would tend to *delay* the *aortic component,* thus causing paradoxical splitting (P-A) of the second sound. Pulmonary hypertension does not seem to cause changes in the splitting of the second sound, whereas right ventricular failure causes an appreciable splitting through

prolongation of the right ventricular systole (the *pulmonary component* being large and *delayed* [A-P]). In aortic stenosis, several factors are involved. These are: (1) left ventricular overload and hypertension (minor change); (2) possible left ventricular failure (delay of the aortic component); and (3) a lower level of aortic pressure (delay of valve closure). On account of (2) and (3), paradoxical splitting (P-A), with a small aortic component, is often observed in severe aortic stenosis. In pulmonary stenosis one finds similar factors: right ventricular overload and hypertension, possible right ventricular failure, and a lower level of pulmonary-artery pressure. Therefore, a regular but wider type of splitting (A-P), with a small pulmonary component, is often observed in severe cases.

BUNDLE-BRANCH BLOCK. In right bundle-branch

(Continued on page 79)

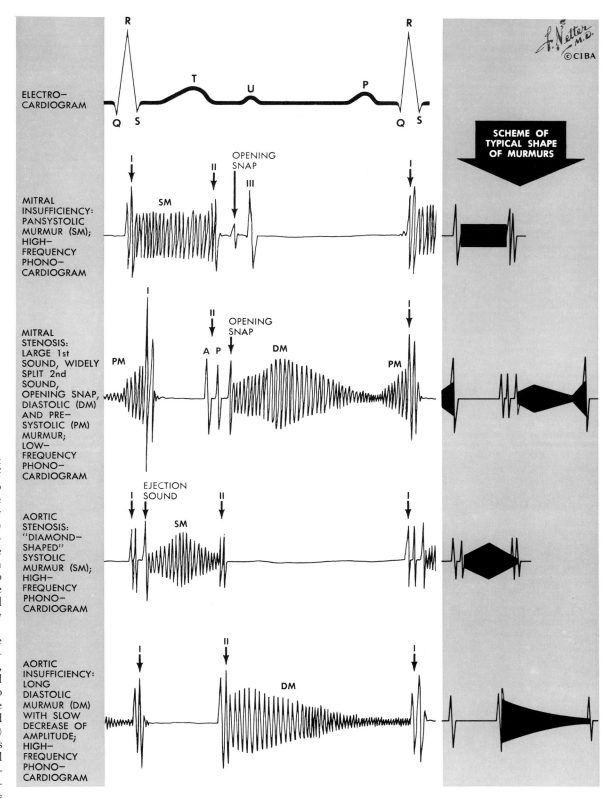

ELECTRO-CARDIOGRAM

SCHEME OF TYPICAL SHAPE OF MURMURS

MITRAL INSUFFICIENCY: PANSYSTOLIC MURMUR (SM); HIGH-FREQUENCY PHONO-CARDIOGRAM

MITRAL STENOSIS: LARGE 1st SOUND, WIDELY SPLIT 2nd SOUND, OPENING SNAP, DIASTOLIC (DM) AND PRE-SYSTOLIC (PM) MURMUR; LOW-FREQUENCY PHONO-CARDIOGRAM

AORTIC STENOSIS: "DIAMOND-SHAPED" SYSTOLIC MURMUR (SM); HIGH-FREQUENCY PHONO-CARDIOGRAM

AORTIC INSUFFICIENCY: LONG DIASTOLIC MURMUR (DM) WITH SLOW DECREASE OF AMPLITUDE; HIGH-FREQUENCY PHONO-CARDIOGRAM

PHONOCARDIOGRAPHY

(Continued from page 78)

block, delayed activation of the right ventricle causes delayed contraction of this chamber and delayed ejection into the pulmonary artery. As a result, there is delayed closure of the pulmonary valve, causing a wide splitting (A-P) of the second sound. In left bundle-branch block, delayed activation of the left ventricle causes delayed contraction of this chamber and delayed ejection into the aorta, resulting in delayed closure of the aortic valve. The second sound will be either single or paradoxically split (P-A).

In complex malformations with a large communication between the two ventricles and with pulmonary hypertension, there is no splitting, and a single second sound can be recorded because the two ventricles tend to function as a single unit. If ventricular septal defect and pulmonary stenosis (tetralogy of Fallot) are present, phonocardiography reveals either a single second sound (large septal defect) or a normal aortic component followed by a small, late, pulmonary component (A-P) (marked pulmonary stenosis and small ventricular septal defect).

Abnormal Third and Fourth Sounds and the Gallop Rhythms

Triple and Quadruple Rhythms. *Triple rhythms* are due to: (1) accentuation of the third sound (*sound III*) (*diastolic* or *ventricular* type); (2) accentuation of the fourth sound (*sound IV*) (*presystolic* or *atrial* type); and (3) accentuation of sounds III and IV, with fusion of them into a new sound ("summation" type). *Quadruple rhythms* are due to accentuation of sounds III and IV, which remain distinct.

In the ventricular type of triple

rhythm, the third sound is unusually *large* and prolonged; this often occurs in conditions of severe diastolic overload (whether absolute or relative), and the sound commonly is followed by several aftervibrations (*diastolic* rumble). This is typical in *mitral insufficiency*. A loud, snapping, early third sound is frequently found in cases of constrictive or calcific pericarditis (pericardial knock); the diastolic sound coincides with the abrupt halting of right ventricular filling. The atrial type of triple rhythm is often observed in cases with ischemic or hypertensive heart diseases, and it is common in myocarditis, hyperthyroidism, and heart failure. It is observed particularly in conditions with systolic overload, as in pulmonary or *aortic stenosis*, and pulmonary or systemic hypertension. A triple rhythm of the summation type is usually evidence of heart failure in the presence of tachycardia, whereas a

quadruple rhythm generally indicates heart failure in the presence of a normal rate or of bradycardia.

Opening Snap. The *opening snap* is a high-pitched sound, best heard and recorded in the *third* and fourth *left interspaces*. The diagnostic importance of the opening snap has somewhat decreased, owing to the fact that a similar snap has been described in conditions other than *mitral stenosis*. A tricuspid opening snap may be observed in tricuspid stenosis and in atrial septal defect. A mitral opening snap may occur in left atrial tumors, mitral insufficiency without stenosis, patent ductus arteriosus, and ventricular septal defect.

Ejection Click. The ejection sound (see page 78) or ejection click represents the accentuation of a normal vibration, which can be found at the end of the first sound (*sound I*) and follows the opening of the aortic

(Continued on page 80)

valve. In aortic stenosis or dilatation of the ascending aorta, this vibration is larger, more delayed, and high-pitched. A similar vibration can be heard and recorded in cases of pulmonary stenosis or dilatation of the pulmonary artery over the pulmonary and right ventricular areas. The ejection clicks originate in the walls of either of the great vessels.

Midsystolic or Late Systolic Snap. Another snap can be recorded in subjects with a history of left-side pleurisy, or pericarditis, or with no history of disease. It is a midsystolic or *late systolic* vibration of a *high frequency*.

Murmurs

Phonocardiography has confirmed the "shape" and "phase" of *murmurs* which had previously been only surmised by means of auscultation (see page 74).

Systolic. These murmurs are of several types: (1) early systolic in decrescendo, in mitral or tricuspid insufficiency, unimportant inflow-tract murmur, and ventricular septal defect (muscular type); (2) *pansystolic,* in mitral or tricuspid insufficiency and ventricular septal defect; (3) late systolic in crescendo, in mitral insufficiency, patent ductus arteriosus (with pulmonary hypertension), ventricular aneurysm, adhesive pericarditis, muscular subaortic stenosis, and pulmonary stenosis; and (4) diamond-shaped (*crescendo-decrescendo*), in aortic or pulmonary stenosis, flow murmur of the *left* or right *outflow tract, mitral insufficiency* (see page 74), and ventricular septal defect.

Diastolic. These murmurs are of two types: (1) early and middiastolic (blowing) in decrescendo, *aortic* or pulmonary *insufficiency* (organic or relative) and (2) early, mid, and late diastolic (presystolic) rumble, in mitral or tricuspid stenosis (*inflow-tract murmurs* [see page 74] due to a functional mechanism).

Continuous. This type characterizes patent ductus arteriosus, AV fistula (systemic, pulmonary, or coronary), anastomotic vessels, coarctation, certain aneurysms of the aorta, and rupture of an aneurysm of the sinus of the aorta (Valsalva).

Inflow-Tract Flow or Stenotic Murmurs (Diastolic Rumbles). MITRAL STENOSIS. In cases with sinus rhythm, the *diastolic rumble* (see page 74) has two phases of greater loudness: an early diastolic that starts with the *opening snap* and coincides with a slow and prolonged duration of filling (middiastolic rumble), and a presystolic (*PM*) that coincides with the powerful contraction of the hypertrophied left atrium. In cases with atrial fibrillation, the middiastolic rumble is the only evidence of the stenosis. It is a murmur of low pitch and small amplitude, and it may have a decrescendo quality which fades in middiastole if the diastole is long. On the contrary, it may be larger and have a crescendo quality (simulating a *presystolic murmur*) when the diastole is short.

The presystolic murmur has a higher pitch than the previous phase of diastolic rumble, and it terminates with the delayed first sound. Relative or functional mitral stenosis occurs in pure mitral insufficiency, aortic insufficiency, patent ductus arteriosus, myocarditis, myocardial infarct, and severe left heart failure.

TRICUSPID STENOSIS. Tricuspid stenosis gives rise to a diastolic rumble and a presystolic murmur which are heard and recorded best over the third left, fourth left, or fourth right interspace, or over the xyphoid; thus, they may be confused with similar murmurs caused by mitral stenosis. The presystolic murmur, being related to right atrial contraction (which occurs before the left), is better separated from the first sound and has no crescendo configuration. An *opening snap* of the tricuspid valve may be detected. Both the murmur and the snap are increased by inspiration.

Relative or functional tricuspid stenosis occurs in atrial septal defect, partial anomalous pulmonary venous return or right heart failure, occasionally in pulmonary stenosis, primary pulmonary hypertension, constrictive pericarditis, and severe right heart failure.

Inflow-Tract Regurgitant Murmurs (Blowing Systolic Murmurs). MITRAL INSUFFICIENCY. The murmur may be from grade I to grade V and is *blowing, soft,* or moderately harsh. It is well recorded over the *left ventricular area* (see page 74) and even better over the left atrial (left axilla, left interscapulovertebral area, or within the esophagus); it is occasionally recorded along the left or right sternal borders or at the base (giant left atrium, deformity of the posterior cusp, or lesion of the posterior papillary muscle). Four patterns can be recognized: (1) The most typical is a high-pitched *pansystolic* murmur. (2) Less common is a high-pitched *systolic* murmur in *crescendo.* (3) There may be a systolic murmur in *decrescendo.* (4) The least common is a *diamond-shaped murmur,* which is caused by a lesion of the posterior mitral cusp. Relative mitral insufficiency usually produces a small or moderately loud murmur which frequently has a decrescendo type. However, severe mitral insufficiency owing to marked dilatation of the mitral orifice may cause a grade-II to grade-III murmur, having either a decrescendo or a pansystolic configuration.

TRICUSPID INSUFFICIENCY. Tricuspid insufficiency usually causes a pansystolic murmur which is audible over the third left, third right, or fourth right interspace. The murmur of tricuspid insufficiency usually lasts through the aortic sound to the pulmonary component of the second sound. It is increased by inspiration (in contrast to the murmur of mitral insufficiency).

Outflow-Tract Flow or Stenotic Murmurs (Harsh Systolic Murmurs). AORTIC STENOSIS. *Aortic stenosis* can be due to narrowing of the ascending aorta (supravalvular stenosis), the aortic valve (valvular stenosis), or the outflow tract of the left ventricle (subvalvular stenosis). The majority of cases present a prolongation of the *isovolumic* (see page 75) period and of the total duration of systole. A systolic murmur is typical of aortic stenosis. This is usually best recorded in the *third left interspace* (III) (see page 74), but it may be larger over interspace IV or V, especially in cases of subaortic stenosis. It is recorded well over the area of the ascending aorta (right interspace II) and at the suprasternal notch, especially in cases of valvular stenosis. The murmur is usually of grade III to grade V and is harsh; it may cover the pulmonary component of the second sound (the latter is often paradoxically split), and it is typically *diamond-shaped* (crescendo-decrescendo). Usually, it is well separated from the first sound, because it starts at the beginning of ejection and is initiated by an ejection sound. Its peak occurs after the anacrotic notch of the carotid pulse and is often more delayed if the stenosis is severe. In hypertrophic subaortic stenosis, the murmur usually starts later than in valvular stenosis. It may even begin at midsystole, when infundibular narrowing becomes greater, and it may have a crescendo type or, if diamond-shaped, a late occurrence of the

peak. The murmur is usually made up of vibrations of various frequencies.

Relative aortic stenosis occurs when the *outflow tract* (see page 74) of the left ventricle and the aortic valve is normal, while the ascending aorta is dilated. It is found in cases with aortitis, atherosclerosis of the aorta, Marfan's syndrome, or severe aortic insufficiency. The murmur is diamond-shaped but has an early peak. The second sound has a large aortic component, and splitting is consistent with the age of the patient (single sound in elderly patients, normal splitting in young subjects).

PULMONARY STENOSIS. A diamond-shaped systolic murmur is a typical finding in pulmonary stenosis. In severe cases the peak of the murmur occurs after the middle of systole, so that one may gain the impression of a crescendo murmur. The vibrations are of various frequencies. The murmur is recorded best in left interspaces II and III, but it may have a wide diffusion, especially in children. It often radiates upward to the left clavicle, and, if loud, can be recorded at both sides of the spine. The vibrations of the murmur extend, in severe cases, to the pulmonary component of the second sound, which is small and delayed. As they "ride over" the aortic component, they may simulate the existence of an early diastolic murmur.

Outflow-Tract Regurgitant Murmurs (Blowing Diastolic Murmurs). AORTIC INSUFFICIENCY. The aortic diastolic murmur is usually of high frequency and can be recorded only with equipment which has a good response in the high-frequency range. The typical configuration is that of a *crescendo-decrescendo pattern* (see page 74) (short crescendo phase followed by a much longer decrescendo phase); however, a simple *decrescendo* pattern may be present. Musical diastolic murmurs (regular vibrations) may be present in cases with "everted aortic valve" (rheumatic or syphilitic heart disease) or bacterial endocarditis. Relative aortic insufficiency may occur in patients with severe systemic hypertension, who present a moderate blowing diastolic murmur that disappears when the blood pressure is lowered by means of hypotensive agents. The murmur is caused by dilatation of the aortic ring. It is recorded as a short series of vibrations in decrescendo, which starts soon after a large, snapping aortic component of the second sound.

PULMONARY INSUFFICIENCY. This condition may be the result of a congenital lesion or the stretching of the valvular ring by long-lasting pulmonary hypertension. The murmur is similar to that of aortic insufficiency, except that it starts immediately after the pulmonary component of the second sound. It is usually in decrescendo, only occasionally showing a short-crescendo–long-decrescendo pattern.

Murmurs Caused by Shunts. In atrial septal defect the most commonly recorded murmur is diamond-shaped over the pulmonary area, as a result of increased pulmonary flow. The second sound is widely split and is not modified by respiration.

In *ventricular septal defect* (see page 74) one observes a pansystolic murmur over left interspaces III and IV, as well as over right interspace IV. If there is pulmonary hypertension, the murmur tends to become diamond-shaped. If the defect is in the muscular septum, the murmur may even be late systolic.

In *patent ductus arteriosus* the murmur is *continuous* and has its maximum amplitude in late systole and early diastole. If there is pulmonary hypertension, the diastolic phase may disappear while the maximum of the murmur is still, often, in late systole.

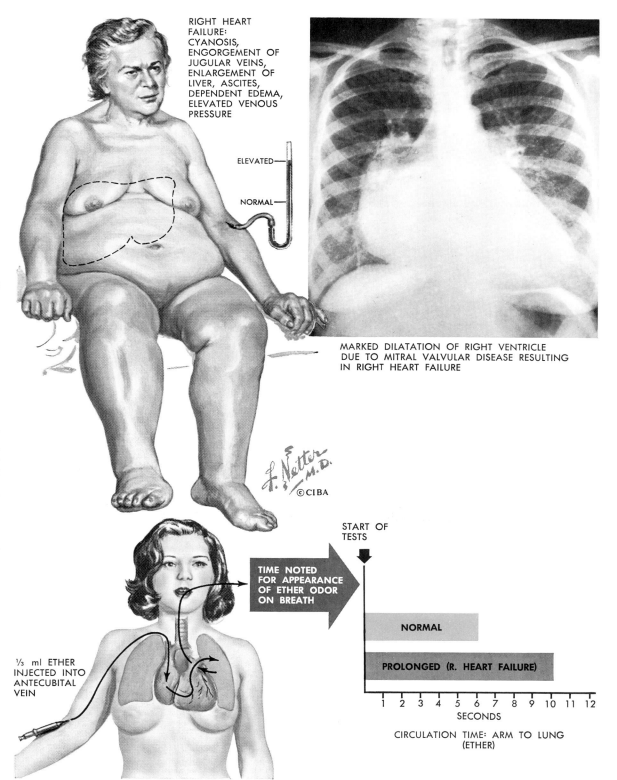

RIGHT HEART FAILURE: CYANOSIS, ENGORGEMENT OF JUGULAR VEINS, ENLARGEMENT OF LIVER, ASCITES, DEPENDENT EDEMA, ELEVATED VENOUS PRESSURE

ELEVATED

NORMAL

MARKED DILATATION OF RIGHT VENTRICLE DUE TO MITRAL VALVULAR DISEASE RESULTING IN RIGHT HEART FAILURE

RIGHT HEART FAILURE AND SYSTEMIC CONGESTION

⅓ ml ETHER INJECTED INTO ANTECUBITAL VEIN

START OF TESTS

TIME NOTED FOR APPEARANCE OF ETHER ODOR ON BREATH

NORMAL

PROLONGED (R. HEART FAILURE)

1 2 3 4 5 6 7 8 9 10 11 12
SECONDS

CIRCULATION TIME: ARM TO LUNG (ETHER)

Systemic congestion is commonly caused by right ventricular *failure,* which leads to an increase of the right ventricular diastolic pressure and of the right atrial and systemic *venous pressures.* As a result, the visible veins, and particularly the *jugular veins,* become *engorged* and actively pulsate. The *liver* becomes *enlarged* and tender. In severe or prolonged failure, *ascites* will develop. Finally, *cyanosis* and *dependent edema* are marked.

These manifestations are revealed by inspection and palpation. They are documented by chest X-ray (*dilatation* of the *right* heart), measurement of venous pressure (increase of venous pressure), and right-heart catheterization (increased right ventricular end-diastolic pressure).

It is not always understood that all these manifestations of so-called "backward failure" (venous congestion) are paralleled by the less obvious manifestation of "forward failure" (arterial depletion). Thus, the output of the right ventricle decreases (causing also a decrease of left ventricular output), the pulmonary circulation tends to become ischemic, and the chambers of the left heart are inclined to become smaller. *Circulation time is prolonged,* as revealed by both the *arm-to-lung (ether)* and the *arm-to-tongue (Decholin®) tests* (see page 82).

In the common circumstance in which *right heart failure* follows left heart failure, the lungs will become less congested, dyspnea and orthopnea will decrease, the liver will become severely engorged, the systemic veins will be turgid, and peripheral (dependent) edema will appear.

A common result of right heart failure is relative tricuspid insufficiency, caused by dilatation of the tricuspid ring and stretching of the papillary muscles of the right ventricle. This is revealed by large systolic pulsations of the jugular veins

and the liver (which appear in the respective graphic tracings as a systolic plateau) and by a right-side *pansystolic murmur* (see page 74). Right atrial distention is often followed by atrial fibrillation, with its typical absence of atrial waves in the jugular tracing and the electrocardiogram, and the well-known complete, nonperiodic irregularity of the ventricular complexes and of the radial pulse.

Similar manifestations can be related to chronic obstruction or impedance of the venous return, tricuspid passage, or right ventricular filling (see page 85). Cardiac catheterization may show, in the latter condition, a typical pattern (diastolic dip, diastolic plateau) which reveals the mechanical nature of the obstruction; if the tricuspid valve is narrowed, a diastolic gradient of pressure is observed between the right atrium and the right ventricle.

Dependent edema is a common result of right heart

failure. This is particularly obvious in the lower extremities and the sacrum. In an advanced stage the edema is diffuse and is associated with effusion in the serosa of various sites, particularly in the right pleural cavity and the peritoneal cavity (anasarca).

Another frequent result is a decrease in the amount of urine (oliguria), with greater excretion during the night (nocturia). The urine has a high specific gravity and contains protein, a few red cells, and epithelial casts.

Right ventricular failure is revealed by a rise of the diastolic pressure of the right ventricle. (The normal end-diastolic pressure is 0 to 5; abnormal, 8 to 20.) It frequently causes a relative tricuspid insufficiency, which can be recognized by the typical plateau pattern in the jugular and hepatic tracings and by the angiocardiogram of the right ventricle (reflux of radiopaque material into the right atrium).

ACUTE, SEVERE PULMONARY CONGESTION
DUE TO LEFT VENTRICULAR FAILURE

LEFT HEART FAILURE AND PULMONARY CONGESTION

Pulmonary congestion is commonly caused by *left heart failure,* which leads to an increase of the left ventricular diastolic pressure and of the left atrial and pulmonary venous pressures. As a result, the pulmonary capillaries become engorged. Exertional and positional *orthopnea* and, finally, continuous *dyspnea* occur, caused largely by reflexes arising in the pulmonary vessels and the left atrial wall, and there may be paroxysmal nocturnal dyspnea. These acute, occasional, or continuous disturbances can easily be ascertained by careful questioning and by observation of the patient in various positions (sitting versus lying supine).

The chest *X-ray* reveals a dilatation of the left heart chambers and an increased opacity of the pulmonary vasculature. Left-heart catheterization shows an increase in the diastolic pressure of the left ventricle as well as an increase of the left atrial, pulmonary "wedge," and pulmonary arterial pressures. The right ventricular pressure is elevated in systole, normal in diastole. This has been called a plateau pattern of pressure. The pattern of mitral insufficiency (relative) may be observed.

It is sometimes not realized that all these manifestations of so-called "backward failure" (pulmonary venous congestion) are paralleled by the less obvious manifestations of "forward failure" (arterial depletion). The output of the left ventricle decreases, causing also a decrease of the output of the right ventricle. Although this decrease is partly com-

5 ml DECHOLIN INJECTED INTO ANTECUBITAL VEIN

START OF TESTS

TIME NOTED FOR APPEARANCE OF BITTER TASTE ON TONGUE

NORMAL

PROLONGED (L. HEART FAILURE)

2 4 6 8 10 12 14 16 18 20 22 24
SECONDS

CIRCULATION TIME: ARM TO TONGUE (DECHOLIN)

pensated by peripheral vasoconstriction, so that no marked changes of blood pressure occur, the systemic circulation will tend to become ischemic. The most common results are weakness and oliguria. If some of the peripheral arteries are narrowed because of segmental lesions, ischemia becomes particularly obvious in those areas (cerebrum, heart, legs, etc.).

A common result of *left ventricular failure* is relative mitral insufficiency, caused by dilatation of the mitral valve and stretching of the papillary muscles of the left ventricle. This is revealed by an apical and left-side *pansystolic, blowing murmur* (see page 74) and, on fluoroscopy, by a systolic expansion of the left atrium. Atrial fibrillation is favored by this distention, and pulmonary congestion is markedly aggravated by it.

Only the *arm-to-tongue (Decholin®) time* is prolonged; the *arm-to-lung (ether) test* is still *normal* (see page 81).

Similar manifestations may be related to *chronic obstruction* at the level of the mitral valve or to *impeded left ventricular filling* (see page 83). In the former, a typical murmur is observed, and left-heart catheterization reveals the existence of a diastolic gradient of pressure between the left atrium and the left ventricle. In the latter, a typical pattern (diastolic dip, diastolic plateau) often reveals the mechanical nature of the left ventricular obstruction.

Left ventricular failure is revealed, on catheterization, by a rise of the end-diastolic pressure of the left ventricle. (The normal pressure is 3 to 6; abnormal, 10 to 25.)

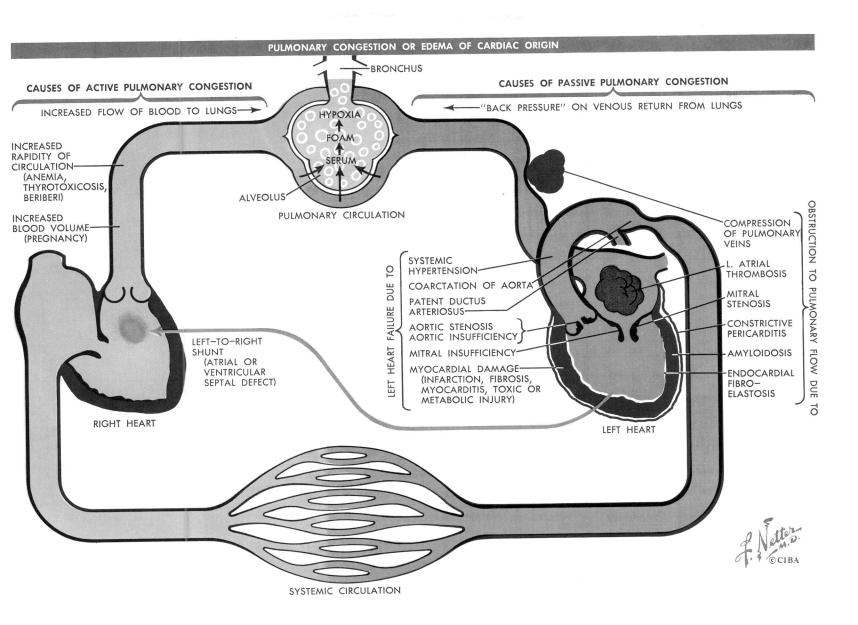

CAUSES OF ACTIVE PULMONARY CONGESTION

INCREASED FLOW OF BLOOD TO LUNGS →

CAUSES OF PASSIVE PULMONARY CONGESTION

← "BACK PRESSURE" ON VENOUS RETURN FROM LUNGS

INCREASED RAPIDITY OF CIRCULATION (ANEMIA, THYROTOXICOSIS, BERIBERI)

INCREASED BLOOD VOLUME (PREGNANCY)

BRONCHUS

HYPOXIA

FOAM

SERUM

ALVEOLUS

PULMONARY CIRCULATION

OBSTRUCTION TO PULMONARY FLOW DUE TO

COMPRESSION OF PULMONARY VEINS

L. ATRIAL THROMBOSIS

MITRAL STENOSIS

CONSTRICTIVE PERICARDITIS

AMYLOIDOSIS

ENDOCARDIAL FIBRO-ELASTOSIS

LEFT HEART FAILURE DUE TO

SYSTEMIC HYPERTENSION

COARCTATION OF AORTA

PATENT DUCTUS ARTERIOSUS

AORTIC STENOSIS AORTIC INSUFFICIENCY

MITRAL INSUFFICIENCY

MYOCARDIAL DAMAGE (INFARCTION, FIBROSIS, MYOCARDITIS, TOXIC OR METABOLIC INJURY)

LEFT-TO-RIGHT SHUNT (ATRIAL OR VENTRICULAR SEPTAL DEFECT)

RIGHT HEART

LEFT HEART

SYSTEMIC CIRCULATION

PULMONARY CONGESTION OR EDEMA OF CARDIAC AND OTHER ORIGINS

Pulmonary Congestion

Pulmonary congestion can be defined as an increase of the blood present in the vessels of the *lungs*. This can be due either to increased *pulmonary flow*, with or without an *arteriocapillary increase of pressure* (active congestion), or to *increased pulmonary venous capillary pressure* (passive congestion) (see page 84).

Active congestion of a moderate degree can be found in conditions associated with *increased rapidity of circulation* (anemia, thyrotoxicosis, beriberi heart) or *increased blood volume* (pregnancy). Severe active congestion, on the other hand, is found only in *left-to-right shunts,* where the output of the *right* ventricle may be from three to five times greater than that of the *left*.

Passive congestion is found in any condition in which there is *obstruction to flow*, at any point from the capillary bed of the lungs to the aortic valve and beyond. One typical cause of passive congestion is *chronic left ventricular failure*. This can be produced by: (1) extremely severe systolic overload of the left ventricle (*systemic hypertension, coarctation of the aorta, aortic stenosis*); (2) extremely severe diastolic overload of the left ventricle (*mitral insufficiency, patent ductus arteriosus, aortic insufficiency*); (3) *myocardial damage* and failure (*myocarditis*, myocardial *fibrosis*, myocardial *infarction*, *toxic* effects on the myocardium, *metabolic* alterations); and (4) formation of a left ventricular aneurysm, because this lesion decreases the efficiency of left ventricular contraction and increases the level of the diastolic pressure within the left ventricular chamber.

Another typical cause of passive congestion is obstruction to flow by: (1) impairment of left ventricular diastole because of *constrictive pericarditis* or *amyloidosis*; (2) impairment of mitral flow (mitral block) caused by rheumatic valvulitis (*mitral stenosis), left atrial thrombosis,* or *endocardial fibroelastosis*; and (3) *compression of the pulmonary veins* by a tumor or mediastinitis, or impedance to flow owing to venoconstriction.

Pulmonary Edema

Pulmonary edema is the infiltration of *serum* in the thin interalveolar septa, with immediate transudation into the *alveolar cavities*. This is followed by a churning of the fluid with air and by the formation of a bubbling *foam*, which may be eliminated through the air passages but which so impairs the process of respiration as to endanger life.

Pulmonary edema is found in association with a long list of disease states:

1. Of cardiovascular diseases, including all possible causes of active and passive pulmonary congestion as well as shock, the most common ones are mitral stenosis or insufficiency, aortic stenosis or insufficiency, coarctation of the aorta, systemic hypertension, acute myocarditis, thyrotoxic heart disease, and *myocardial infarct*.

2. Among diseases or *lesions* of (or surgery on) the central nervous system, the most typical causes are cerebrovascular accidents, including cerebral hemorrhage, cerebral thrombosis, sub-

(Continued on page 84)

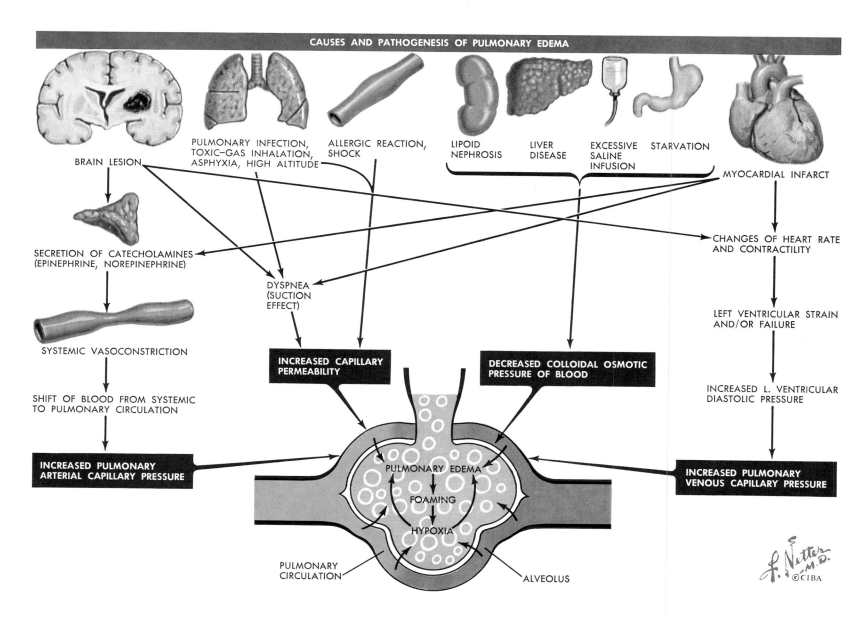

BRAIN LESION

PULMONARY INFECTION,
TOXIC–GAS INHALATION,
ASPHYXIA, HIGH ALTITUDE

ALLERGIC REACTION,
SHOCK

LIPOID
NEPHROSIS

LIVER
DISEASE

EXCESSIVE
SALINE
INFUSION

STARVATION

MYOCARDIAL INFARCT

SECRETION OF CATECHOLAMINES
(EPINEPHRINE, NOREPINEPHRINE)

DYSPNEA
(SUCTION
EFFECT)

CHANGES OF HEART RATE
AND CONTRACTILITY

SYSTEMIC VASOCONSTRICTION

**INCREASED CAPILLARY
PERMEABILITY**

**DECREASED COLLOIDAL OSMOTIC
PRESSURE OF BLOOD**

LEFT VENTRICULAR STRAIN
AND/OR FAILURE

SHIFT OF BLOOD FROM SYSTEMIC
TO PULMONARY CIRCULATION

INCREASED L. VENTRICULAR
DIASTOLIC PRESSURE

**INCREASED PULMONARY
ARTERIAL CAPILLARY PRESSURE**

PULMONARY EDEMA

FOAMING

HYPOXIA

**INCREASED PULMONARY
VENOUS CAPILLARY PRESSURE**

PULMONARY
CIRCULATION

ALVEOLUS

SECTION II—PLATE 45

PULMONARY CONGESTION OR EDEMA OF CARDIAC AND OTHER ORIGINS

(Continued from page 83)

arachnoid hemorrhage, and trauma to the skull. Poliomyelitis and tetanus may also lead to pulmonary edema.

3. Diseases or lesions of the lungs, including *pulmonary infections*, pulmonary embolism, *toxic gas inhalation*, and *asphyxia*, may cause pulmonary edema. Drowning, in either fresh or salt water, is also associated with pulmonary edema. A special condition is "*high-altitude* pulmonary edema."

4. Several toxic or *allergic* states may be factors, a special type being that associated with edema of the glottis.

5. Pulmonary edema may follow *excessive infusions*, particularly in surgical or obstetrical cases.

Three elements are important in the production of pulmonary edema:

1. *High pressure in the pulmonary capillaries* is favored by active and passive congestion, especially the latter. Whatever the cause, a most important favoring element is the rapid *shift of* a large mass of *blood* from the periphery to the lungs as a result of *systemic vasoconstriction* (narrowing of both the arterioles and the venules). This is often caused by sympathetic stimuli and is usually increased by sympathomimetic amines (*epinephrine* and *norepinephrine*). Typical examples of high pressure in the pulmonary capillaries are found in sudden left ventricular overload (paroxysmal hypertension) and in cases in which a sudden increase of venous return aggravates the effect of a mitral block (mitral stenosis) or that of a chronic *left ventricular failure*. It has been demonstrated that sympathetic stimuli cause a typical elevation of *left ventricular diastolic pressure* through modification of *left ventricular contractility*. This factor seems to be of great importance when related to blood shift with greater return to the left heart.

2. Apart from the increase related to capillary dilatation, certain conditions, such as *shock*, *allergic reaction*, inhalation of toxic gases, respiratory burns, asphyxia, and *hypoxia*, have been postulated as possible causes of an *increased permeability of the pulmonary capillaries*. It is possible that certain substances (still unidentified) contribute to the more common types of edema by increasing permeability. Of these, histamine would be the most likely.

3. A *decreased osmotic pressure of the blood* occurs after excessive saline infusions and in *lipoid nephrosis, starvation,* or *liver diseases*. As the effect of this factor is widespread, pulmonary edema due to decreased osmotic pressure is either part of a diffuse anasarca or is favored by mechanical factors (see 1) acting on the lungs.

It should be kept in mind that most elements of pulmonary edema are interrelated: Chemical and endocrine products may cause systemic arterial or pulmonary venous constriction and also may induce changes of permeability in the lungs; blood-pressure changes may cause a reflex release of hormones or chemicals; and neurogenic stimuli modify the caliber of the systemic vessels, cause the release of *catecholamines*, and influence the contractility of the heart.

Even though pulmonary congestion may be followed by pulmonary edema, the two conditions should not be confused.

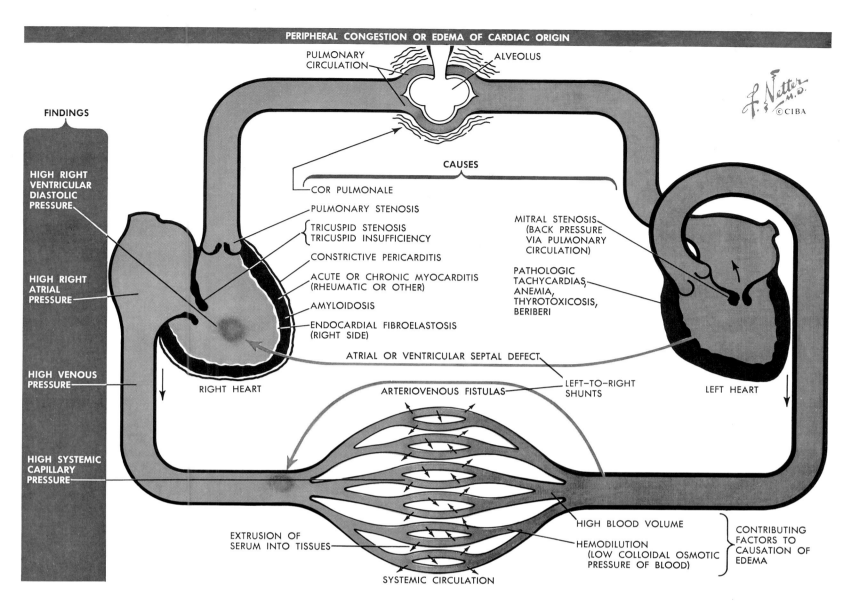

PULMONARY CIRCULATION — ALVEOLUS

FINDINGS

HIGH RIGHT VENTRICULAR DIASTOLIC PRESSURE

HIGH RIGHT ATRIAL PRESSURE

HIGH VENOUS PRESSURE

HIGH SYSTEMIC CAPILLARY PRESSURE

CAUSES

COR PULMONALE

PULMONARY STENOSIS

TRICUSPID STENOSIS
TRICUSPID INSUFFICIENCY

CONSTRICTIVE PERICARDITIS

ACUTE OR CHRONIC MYOCARDITIS (RHEUMATIC OR OTHER)

AMYLOIDOSIS

ENDOCARDIAL FIBROELASTOSIS (RIGHT SIDE)

ATRIAL OR VENTRICULAR SEPTAL DEFECT

ARTERIOVENOUS FISTULAS

LEFT-TO-RIGHT SHUNTS

MITRAL STENOSIS (BACK PRESSURE VIA PULMONARY CIRCULATION)

PATHOLOGIC TACHYCARDIAS, ANEMIA, THYROTOXICOSIS, BERIBERI

RIGHT HEART

LEFT HEART

EXTRUSION OF SERUM INTO TISSUES

HIGH BLOOD VOLUME

HEMODILUTION (LOW COLLOIDAL OSMOTIC PRESSURE OF BLOOD)

CONTRIBUTING FACTORS TO CAUSATION OF EDEMA

SYSTEMIC CIRCULATION

SECTION II—PLATE 46

Peripheral or Systemic Congestion or Edema of Cardiac Origin

Peripheral congestion or edema is caused by an *increase of systemic venous and capillary pressures.* Apart from a local increase (thrombophlebitis, varicose veins, or compression of the inferior vena cava by a pregnant uterus or by an abdominal mass), the most common cause of symmetrical and diffuse edema is to be found in the mediastinal organs, primarily the heart.

Right Ventricular Failure

Absolute right ventricular failure is found in *acute or chronic myocarditis,* like that of acute *rheumatic* fever, which causes inflammation of the right ventricular wall, altering contractility.

Relative right ventricular failure occurs in cardiac patients having severe overloading of the right ventricle due to valve lesions, shunts, or obstruction.

Overloading

Overloading due to *increased cardiac dynamics* happens in *pathologic tachycardias, anemia, thyrotoxicosis,* or *beriberi heart.* The heart beats faster, and cardiac output is increased. Relative failure may follow.

Diastolic or volume overloading occurs in congenital or acquired *shunts (atrial or ventricular septal defects, arteriovenous fistula)* and in Bernheim's syndrome. The increased volume of the right heart may be followed by right heart failure.

Systolic or pressure overloading occurs in pulmonary embolism with acute *cor pulmonale,* chronic cor pulmonale, *mitral stenosis,* or *pulmonary stenosis.* The increase in work may result in failure of the right ventricle.

Mechanical Impairment, Obstruction, or Imbalance

Mechanical impairment of *right ventricular diastole* develops in *constrictive pericarditis* or mediastinopericarditis, *amyloid* heart disease, or *endocardial fibroelastosis* of the *right* heart. Mechanical obstruction occurs in *tricuspid stenosis* (only the right atrium is distended and overloaded) and in Bernheim's syndrome. Mechanical imbalance occurs in *tricuspid insufficiency* in which both the *right ventricle* and the *right* atrium have to contend with *diastolic* overloading.

Consequences and Treatment

Certain *factors* increase the consequences of right heart failure or right heart obstruction:

1. An *increase in blood volume* is one of the common effects of right heart failure. This takes place through a pituitary-corticoadrenal-renal mechanism.

2. *Hemodilution* may be due to water retention or a hepatic disturbance.

While the chronically congested "cardiac liver" and renal insufficiency frequently add the element of hypoproteinemia to the picture of failure, nephrosis or Laennec cirrhosis of the liver may cause such a decrease of *colloidal osmotic pressure* that diffuse edema will occur. Although cardiac edema is associated with cyanosis and is influenced typically by gravity, hepatic or renal edema is usually associated with pallor and is more diffuse. The former is associated with elevated venous pressure; the latter is not.

Absolute right ventricular failure can be corrected by stimulating the myocardium or removing the cause. A decrease of the load may help temporarily. Relative right ventricular failure is best corrected by removing the cause, cardiac stimulants having only a secondary or collateral importance. Any obstruction to flow, causing congestion, is poorly aided by cardiac stimulants or drugs which decrease the blood volume; hence, corrective surgery is the treatment of choice.

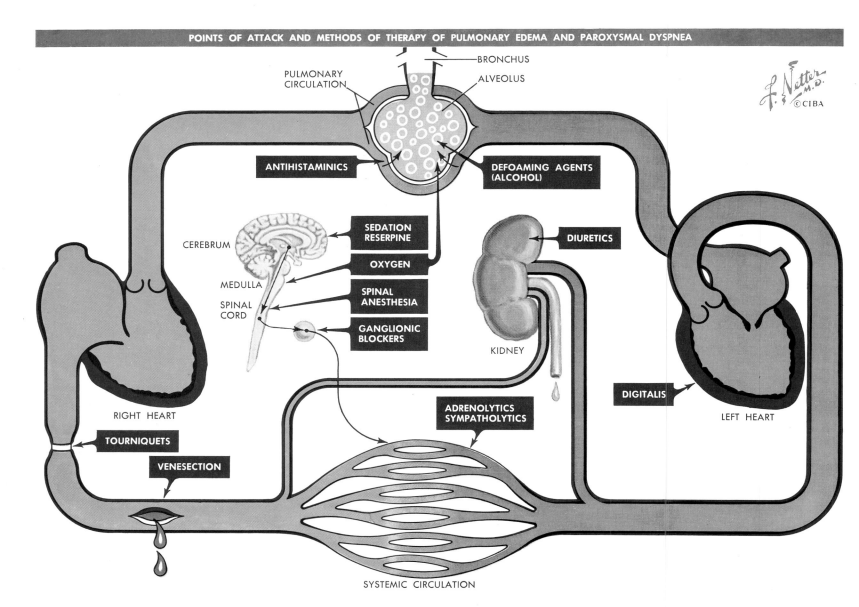

PULMONARY EDEMA AND PAROXYSMAL DYSPNEA—POINTS OF THERAPEUTIC ATTACK

The last stage of *pulmonary edema* is the process of foaming, which occurs in the bronchioles. This phenomenon is based on the interaction (churning) between air and transudate, and, in order for it to take place, a certain surface tension of the fluid is required.

Surface-Tension Changes

Modifications of surface tension can be obtained by the inhalation of *defoaming agents* (not to be confused with wetting agents). Both silicones and ethyl *alcohol* have been used with success, but the latter is more effective. Its administration is based on the bubbling of *oxygen* through a solution of pure alcohol* or by the employment of an atomizer.† Alcohol should be

*If administration is by mask (unconscious patients), alcohol is given in a 40 percent solution in water; if by nasal catheter (conscious patients), in a 95 percent solution in water.

†Alcohol is atomized as a 20 percent solution in water.

used intermittently; thus, only a local effect takes place, owing to the minimal amount absorbed, and no systemic (vasodilator) action ensues. (The latter is undesirable in certain cases.)

Clinical trials with *antihistamines* and anti-serotonins are still open to question.

Reduction of Congestion

Pulmonary congestion, whether active or passive, can be reduced in various ways, as follows:

1. The intravenous injection of rapidly acting *diuretics* reduces the blood volume.

2. The intravenous injection of *digitalis* glycosides (digoxin, ouabain) should decrease the level of left ventricular diastolic pressure, as a result of the stimulation of contractility of the left ventricle. Even in cases of mitral stenosis, a moderate improvement can be obtained by these drugs if they slow the rate and prolong diastole.

3. *Venesection* or the application of *tourniquets* will decrease venous return. The effect of pressure respiration is partly related to a similar mechanism; the intravenous injection of diuretics obtains the same result by decreasing the blood volume.

4. By causing a massive peripheral dilatation, blood can be shifted from the lungs to the periphery. This can be done by means of *sedatives*, narcotics, *sympatholytics, adrenolytics, ganglionic blockers*, or *spinal anesthesia*. Sympatholytics and adrenolytics are probably the most effective drugs.

Hypoxia

Hypoxia, an important element in pulmonary edema, can be combated by the administration of oxygen and, in certain cases, by intermittent positive-pressure respiration. Both methods can be associated with the use of defoaming agents.

Systemic-Pressure Maintenance

Reduction of venous return or massive systemic dilation may be dangerous in cases of mitral stenosis and shock; even though the pulmonary edema decreases, these patients may die from shock. Therefore, the methods listed above (1 through 4) should be employed with great care. Sympatholytics should be added to a venous infusion of plasma or saline in order to maintain an adequate level of systemic pressure. Digitalization should be cautious and not massive, especially in cases of recent myocardial infarct, where it may favor ventricular tachycardia.

Other Methods

Mechanical obstruction to blood flow is an indirect cause of pulmonary edema. A definite remedy for this can be obtained only by prophylactic surgery (aortic or mitral valvotomy, release of constrictive pericarditis, etc.).

Prophylaxis, in general, tends to the avoidance of pulmonary congestion by means of sedation (especially at night), digitalization, and the use of diuretics.

VALVULAR STENOSIS AND INSUFFICIENCY

Mitral Stenosis

Mitral stenosis, which may be "pure" or associated with insufficiency, is the most common valvular defect. It may be accompanied by lesions of the aortic valve and, more rarely, of the tricuspid valves.

Hemodynamics. Narrowing of the mitral valve impedes the free flow of blood from the left atrium to the left ventricle in diastole. This causes a persistent rise of *pressure* in the *left atrium* that, on catheterization, is revealed by a typical end-diastolic *pressure gradient.* Such a gradient is increased by a rapid heart rate (sinus or pathologic tachycardia), is greater for short diastoles (such as those repeatedly occurring with *atrial fibrillation),* and is accentuated by an increase in cardiac output, like that caused by exertion or excitement. A *fixed cardiac output* occurs in severe mitral stenosis, but minor involvement still allows for some increase in output. The high pressure in the left atrium is accompanied by comparatively *higher pressures* in the *pulmonary veins, capillaries,* and *arterioles.* Thus, "wedge" pressure (W) (see tabulated catheterization data) is raised in mitral stenosis. *Pulmonary-artery pressure* (PA) and right ventricular systolic pressure (RV) are proportionally increased by the stenosis. However, *pulmonary vasoconstriction* and/or *pulmonary arteriolar sclerosis* are often secondary phenomena. They result in a greater increase of pressure in the right heart, with the creation of a second pressure gradient between the large branches of the pulmonary artery and the pulmonary capillaries (or left atrial "wedge" pressure). An additional *pulmonary venous gradient,* caused by pulmonary venular constriction, has been reported. The pulmonary vascular changes can be partly decreased by oxygen inhalation or by drugs if the changes are functional, but not if they are related to sclerosis.

Clinical Features and Findings. The *signs and symptoms* of patients with mitral stenosis include palpitation, occasional exertional precordial pain, weakness, exertional *dyspnea,* orthopnea, and occasional paroxysmal dyspnea or *pulmonary edema. Hemoptysis* is more typical and is related to rupture of bronchial-pulmonary venous anastomoses. Oliguria, pain in the right upper

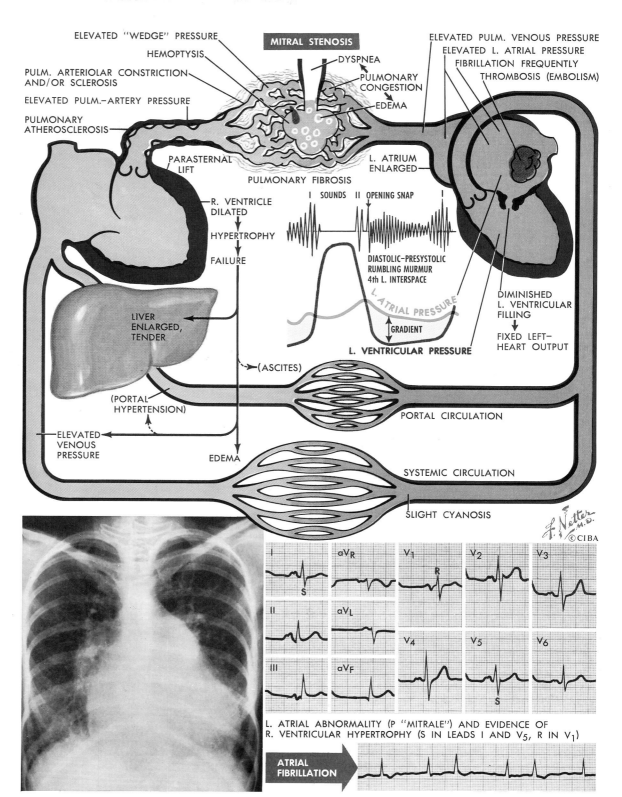

quadrant of the abdomen, and pitting *edema* are evidences of right heart failure. The patients often are pale. *Cyanosis* occurs in the advanced stage and is related to pulmonary arteriosclerosis, *heart failure,* or both.

Physical examination reveals a small, often irregular, pulse. There is a *parasternal lift* or a prominent retrosternal and epigastric pulsation. The cardiac dullness is usually more prominent at the right of the sternum. Often, there is a diastolic thrill in the *fourth* and fifth *left interspaces.* Auscultation may show several possible findings: (1) a *diastolic-presystolic rumbling murmur* in the fourth or fifth left interspace, well separated from *sound II* (the presystolic component disappearing if there is atrial fibrillation), and (2) an *opening snap,* audible over a wide area of the precordium, simulating a splitting of sound II. Other findings, which are incidental and sometimes confusing, include (3) a soft, blowing, early diastolic murmur in decrescendo at the second left intercostal space (aortic or pulmonic insufficiency); (4) a soft, blowing, pansystolic murmur at the center of the heart or the apex

(tricuspid or mitral insufficiency); and (5) a harsh, crescendo-decrescendo systolic murmur at the base (pulmonary-flow murmur or murmur of aortic stenosis). Small, crepitant rales may be heard at the base of the lungs. The liver edge may be palpable.

The *electrocardiogram* reveals that several arrhythmias may be present, the most common being *atrial flutter* or *fibrillation.* A right axis shift is frequently observed. Evidence of *right ventricular hypertrophy* is often present. If there is sinus rhythm, a grade-1 A-V block and evidence of *left atrial enlargement (left atrial abnormality* or *P "mitrale")* are often observed.

The data from auscultation are confirmed by the *phonocardiogram.*

The chest *X-ray* shows a vertical heart, enlarged to the right. The left main bronchus is raised. The left atrium may become prominent at the right side and is prominent in the oblique and lateral projections. A marked indentation separates it from the left ventricle. The pulmonary

(Continued on page 88)

VALVULAR STENOSIS AND INSUFFICIENCY

(Continued from page 87)

arc is prominent. The pulmonary vascular markings are increased in the early stage of the disease. In the late stage they become less visible, while, at the same time, the large branches of the pulmonary artery become further dilated. Kerley lines are visible in the lung fields. Calcification of the mitral ring or mitral valve is often noticed.

The *circulation time* of the arm-to-tongue interval (see page 82) is typically prolonged.

On *catheterization,* the most significant finding, obtained by simultaneous left ventricular (LV) and left atrial (LA) (or "wedge") tracings, is a difference between the end-diastolic pressure of the left atrium and that of the left ventricle. The pulmonary and right ventricular pressures are elevated and may be further raised by *pulmonary arteriolar constriction or sclerosis.*

The mitral-valve area can be measured by Gorlin's formula (see below) on the basis of flow and pressure. This formula is fairly accurate, in the absence of valvular insufficiency, and is based on the mitral-valve flow.

Complications. The most common complications include severe hemoptysis, pulmonary edema, *thromboembolic phenomena,* and the manifestations of right heart failure. Left atrial thrombosis (and the rarer ball-valve thrombus) may occur. Dysphonia, due to irritation of the left recurrent nerve by the large left atrium, is possible.

Mitral Insufficiency

Pure *mitral insufficiency* is probably the second most common valvular defect.

Hemodynamics. Valvular insufficiency causes the entry of a "regurgitant jet" into the *left atrium* during ventricular systole. Owing to the elastic distention of the atrial wall, the pressure rises more sharply in this chamber during the last part of systole and may reach its peak at the time of the second

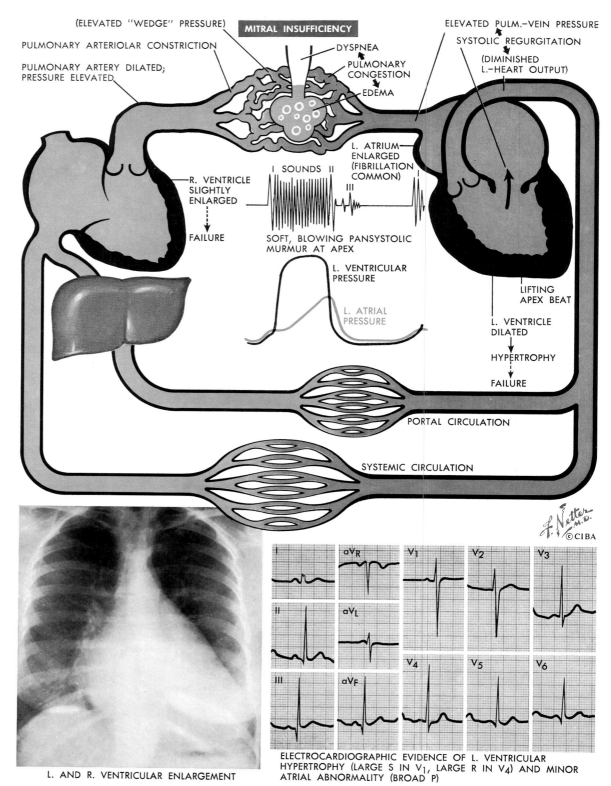

L. AND R. VENTRICULAR ENLARGEMENT

ELECTROCARDIOGRAPHIC EVIDENCE OF L. VENTRICULAR HYPERTROPHY (LARGE S IN V₁, LARGE R IN V₄) AND MINOR ATRIAL ABNORMALITY (BROAD P)

Mitral-valve flow (MVF) = $\dfrac{\text{Cardiac output (cc)}}{\text{Rate (min)} \times \text{average duration of diastole (sec)}}$

Mitral-valve area (MVA) = $\dfrac{\text{MVF}}{31 \sqrt{\text{average duration of diastole (sec)}}}$

The following are examples of catheterization data from two typical cases.

1. Minimal mitral stenosis without important pulmonary vascular changes:

	RA	RV	PA	W	LA	LV	Ao
Pressures	11	44/9	46/25 (39)*	(17)	(17)	107/13	115/80

Heart rate = 80
Cardiac output = 4.320 l/min; stroke volume = 53 cc
Cardiac index = 1.5 l/min/M²
Total pulmonary resistance = 721 dynes/sec/cm⁻⁵
Pulmonary arteriolar resistance = 380 dynes/sec/cm⁻⁵

Oxygen saturation in arterial blood = 96.8%
Functional mitral-valve area = 1.41 cm²
Mean mitral diastolic gradient = 9.27 mm Hg

2. Severe mitral stenosis with important vascular changes:

	RA	RV	PA	W	LA	LV	Ao
Pressures	10	93/7	101/45 (66)*	(23)	(23)	127/14	125/80

Heart rate = 60
Cardiac output = 3 l/min; stroke volume = 50 cc
Cardiac index = 2 l/min/M²
Total pulmonary resistance = 1,691 dynes/sec/cm⁻⁵
Pulmonary arteriolar resistance = 114 dynes/sec/cm⁻⁵
Oxygen saturation in arterial blood = 93%
Functional mitral-valve area = 0.65 cm²
Mean mitral diastolic gradient = 18.6 mm Hg

*Figures in parentheses represent mean pressures.

(Continued on page 89)

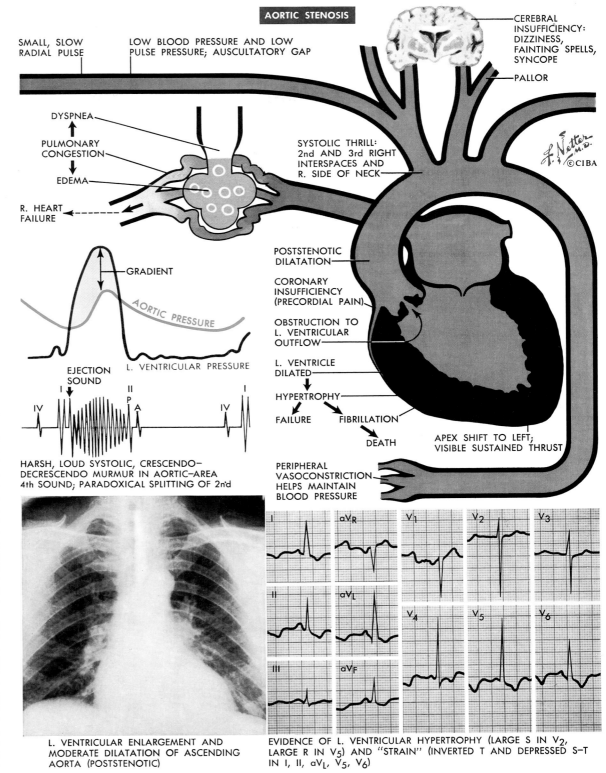

AORTIC STENOSIS

SMALL, SLOW RADIAL PULSE

LOW BLOOD PRESSURE AND LOW PULSE PRESSURE; AUSCULTATORY GAP

CEREBRAL INSUFFICIENCY: DIZZINESS, FAINTING SPELLS, SYNCOPE

PALLOR

DYSPNEA

PULMONARY CONGESTION

EDEMA

R. HEART FAILURE

SYSTOLIC THRILL: 2nd AND 3rd RIGHT INTERSPACES AND R. SIDE OF NECK

POSTSTENOTIC DILATATION

CORONARY INSUFFICIENCY (PRECORDIAL PAIN)

OBSTRUCTION TO L. VENTRICULAR OUTFLOW

L. VENTRICLE DILATED

HYPERTROPHY

FAILURE   FIBRILLATION

DEATH

APEX SHIFT TO LEFT; VISIBLE SUSTAINED THRUST

PERIPHERAL VASOCONSTRICTION HELPS MAINTAIN BLOOD PRESSURE

GRADIENT

AORTIC PRESSURE

EJECTION SOUND

L. VENTRICULAR PRESSURE

HARSH, LOUD SYSTOLIC, CRESCENDO-DECRESCENDO MURMUR IN AORTIC-AREA 4th SOUND; PARADOXICAL SPLITTING OF 2n'd

L. VENTRICULAR ENLARGEMENT AND MODERATE DILATATION OF ASCENDING AORTA (POSTSTENOTIC)

EVIDENCE OF L. VENTRICULAR HYPERTROPHY (LARGE S IN V_2, LARGE R IN V_5) AND "STRAIN" (INVERTED T AND DEPRESSED S-T IN I, II, aV_L, V_5, V_6)

Valvular Stenosis and Insufficiency

(Continued from page 88)

heart sound *(sound II)*. In diastole, the blood, which had passed through the mitral valve in systole, flows back to the left ventricle (in addition to the normal flow). This causes an increased filling of the *left ventricle*, resulting in *dilatation* of this chamber, with *hypertrophy* of its wall. Any increase of peripheral resistance would raise the level of *left ventricular systolic pressure* and thus the severity of *regurgitation*. Since the increase of pressure in the left atrium takes place only in systole (like a strong wave), the mean pressure in this chamber is only moderately elevated. However, peak pressures of 50 to 70 mm Hg can be observed in severe cases, and this will cause the left atrial mean pressure to rise by 15 to 23 mm Hg above the level of the left ventricular end-diastolic pressure. Thus, the pressure in the pulmonary vessels and the systolic pressure in the *right ventricle* will increase in proportion, though to a lesser degree than in mitral stenosis (see page 87). Volume overloading of the left ventricle causes several functional signs which are obvious on auscultation. Systolic distention of the left atrium can be revealed by roentgenological and other methods. Dilatation and hypertrophy of the left atrium and ventricle can be recognized by *roentgenological* and *electrocardiographic* studies.

Clinical Features and Findings. Among the *signs and symptoms*, palpitation, fatigability, and orthopnea are the most common. Paroxysmal *dyspnea* or *pulmonary edema* may occur, as may precordial pain. Physical examination shows a *lifting apex beat*, displaced downward and to the left, in the fifth or sixth left intercostal space. A systolic thrill at the apex is only exceptionally felt. Auscultation reveals the following: (1) a *soft*, *blowing*, *pansystolic murmur at the apex*, radiating toward the left axilla (the murmur may be late systolic in crescendo); (2) frequently, a large *sound III* (ventricular gallop) at the apex, which may be followed by a short rumbling murmur (functional diastolic rumble); and (3) occasionally, a mitral opening snap before sound III.

Unusual cases may have a maximal intensity of the murmur at the base; this murmur may have a crescendo-decrescendo character, simulating the murmur of aortic stenosis. This type of murmur seems to be caused by deformity of the posterior cusp or by shortening of its chordae tendineae, so that the "regurgitant jet" is directed toward the medial aspect of the atrium in the vicinity of the ascending aorta.

The *electrocardiogram* typically shows a left atrial abnormality (P "mitrale") and evidence of left ventricular hypertrophy.

The auscultatory data are confirmed by a *phonocardiogram*. There may also be evidence that methoxamine (a hypertensive drug) increases the murmur.

Chest *X-ray* shows an enlarged heart with a dilated pulmonary arch. Particularly enlarged are the left ventricle and the left atrium, so that no marked indentation exists between them, in the lateral projection. The left atrium may be extremely *enlarged* (giant left atrium) and bulge at the right of the right atrial border in the PA position.

Catheterization reveals the existence of mitral insufficiency through a typical systolic triangular wave in the left atrium (insufficiency wave or i wave; a misnomer is high systolic v wave). Quantitation of the insufficiency is best obtained by selective angiocardiography or an indicator-dilution curve, with injection into the left ventricle.

Complications. Atrial flutter and *fibrillation* often develop, though less frequently than in mitral stenosis. Hemoptysis may occur but is not common. Thromboembolic phenomena are rare, in contrast with mitral stenosis. Pulmonary edema is a definite possibility. Dysphonia may occur. The most common evolution is that of slowly increasing left and right heart *failure*.

Aortic Stenosis

Narrowing of the aortic valve may occur at any age: in children, as a result of a congenital lesion; in adults, following rheumatic endocarditis; and in mature and elderly people, because of calcification, possibly favored by previous rheumatic endocarditis. The hemodynamics and clinical picture are similar in the three groups; however, the typical rheumatic form may be associated with aortic insufficiency or mitral stenosis, whereas the senile form may or may not be associated with aortic insufficiency.

Hemodynamics. Narrowing of the aortic valvular orifice may be tolerated to an extreme degree, owing to the power of the *left ventricle*; an orifice of 0.5 cm² is still compatible with life. This is possible because of *hypertrophy* of the left ventricle, resulting in extreme systolic hypertension within the left ventricular cavity. At the same time, the decrease in cardiac output

(Continued on page 90)

VALVULAR STENOSIS AND INSUFFICIENCY

(Continued from page 89)

is partly compensated by reactive *vasoconstriction,* which *maintains* a moderately low pressure in the *aorta* and preserves a tolerable flow in the cerebral and coronary vessels, at the expense of other vascular districts. Some degree of diastolic hypertension within the left ventricle is due partly to a compensatory phenomenon and partly to decreased compliance; it will raise the pressure in the left atrium and pulmonary vessels and favor *pulmonary congestion* and *edema.* Coronary atherosclerosis is frequent and, together with the decrease in cardiac output, contributes to episodes of *coronary insufficiency. Cerebral insufficiency* is typical, not only during exertion but also at rest.

Clinical Features and Findings. The *signs and symptoms* include *dizziness* and *fainting* episodes, which are typical. *Precordial pain* (angina pectoris) is common. Exertional *dyspnea,* easy fatigability, and palpitation also occur frequently. There may be episodes of paroxysmal dyspnea or pulmonary edema. The patients are *pale.* They have a *small* (often rather *slow*) *radial pulse,* and their *blood pressure* is on the *low* side, with a reduced *pulse pressure.* The measurement of blood pressure reveals an *auscultatory gap* between the systolic and diastolic pressures. The *apex beat* is *sustained* and is somewhat displaced to the *left.* There is a *systolic thrill* over the *second and third interspaces* as well as over the *right side of the neck.* Auscultation reveals a *harsh, loud* (grade 3 to 6), *systolic, crescendo-decrescendo murmur,* preceded by a loud snapping sound (the *ejection sound*). This murmur is usually loudest at the base and on the right of the sternum and is audible over the right side of the neck, but it may be loudest over the center of the precordium or even at the apex. Reverse or *paradoxical splitting* of the second sound *(sound II)* frequently appears.

The *electrocardiogram* reveals marked evidence of *left ventricular hypertrophy.* There may be ventricular ectopic beats, left bundle-branch block, and grade-1 A-V block.

On the *phonocardiogram,* the first sound is small. After a short pause, one can see a large, high-pitched vibration (the ejection sound), which is followed by a diamond-shaped murmur (see page 79). The second sound shows a normal or large pulmonary component *(P)* followed by a small aortic component *(A)* (reverse splitting).

In the *carotid tracing* there are, typically, a slow rise, an anacrotic depression in the ascending limb, a series of indentations or a flat top, and a small dicrotic wave.

Chest *X-ray* shows that the cardiac shadow is only moderately enlarged, but there is increased curvature of the left ventricular border. The *ascending aorta* is dilated *(poststenotic dilatation).* There may be *moderate* dilatation of the left atrium and of the pulmonary vessels. Calcification of the aortic ring is often visible.

Simultaneous aortic and left ventricular *catheterizations* reveal a marked *gradient* of pressure across the aortic valve during systole. *Left ventricular* diastolic *pressure* is also somewhat elevated.

The following figures are from a typical case of rheumatic aortic stenosis in a man of 42 years.

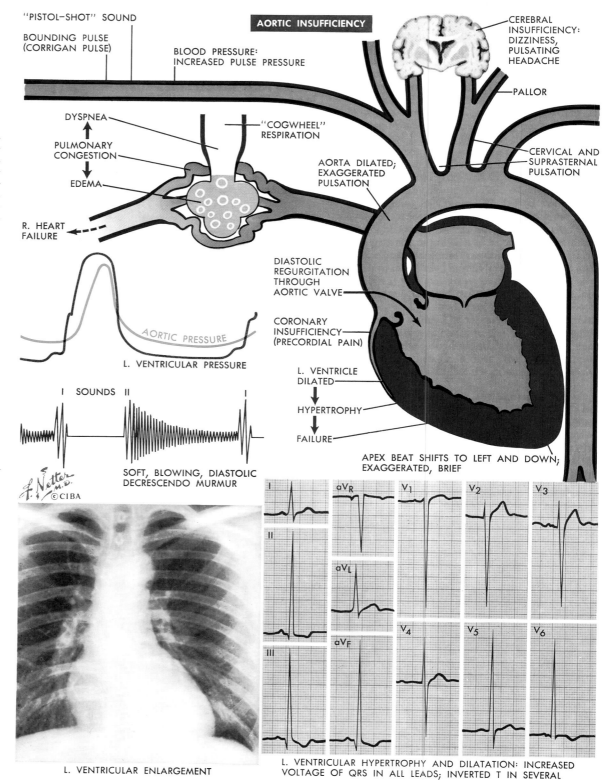

L. VENTRICULAR ENLARGEMENT

L. VENTRICULAR HYPERTROPHY AND DILATATION: INCREASED VOLTAGE OF QRS IN ALL LEADS; INVERTED T IN SEVERAL

RA	RV	PA	W	LA	LV	Ao
(9)*	20.4/2	14.5/5	(8.3)	(8.3)	185/4	90/60

Heart rate = 70
Cardiac output = 6.125 l/min; stroke volume = 85 cc
Cardiac index = 3.0 l/min/M²
Oxygen saturation in arterial blood = 93%
Functional aortic-valve area = 0.63 cm²
Mean aortic systolic gradient = 70.4 mm Hg

*Figures in parentheses represent mean pressures.

An *angiocardiogram* often permits one to localize the *obstruction* which, in rheumatic and senile cases, is at the level of the valve.

Complications. Sudden *death* occurs in a large percentage of cases — possibly as much as 30 percent. Pulmonary edema may also terminate life. Myocardial or cerebral infarcts are relatively common. Severe arrhythmias (ventricular tachycardia, complete A-V block, *ventricular fibrillation,* or cardiac arrest) may occur in the final stage, causing the demise of the patient.

Aortic Insufficiency

Rheumatic *aortic insufficiency* may be isolated or may be associated, to some degree, with aortic or mitral stenosis. Since relative mitral insufficiency, relative aortic stenosis, or relative mitral stenosis may frequently be present, the diagnostic problem may be particularly complicated. In the differential *diagnosis,* rheumatic aortic insufficiency will have to be distinguished from subacute bacterial, congenital (Marfan's and others), syphilitic, and atherosclerotic forms of this malady.

Hemodynamics. The left ventricular volume is increased by the "regurgitant jet." This causes a proportional increase in the stroke volume. As the ejection is made into a poorly filled aorta, there will be rapid ejection of a large mass of blood. In diastole, part of the blood will be

(Continued on page 91)

VALVULAR STENOSIS AND INSUFFICIENCY

(Continued from page 90)

pushed back into the left ventricle, decreasing the amount of effective flow in the periphery and increasing the filling of the left ventricle.

Clinical Features and Findings. The patients may have only minor *symptoms* for many years, and then abruptly become aware of several disturbing phenomena. These consist of exertional and paroxysmal *dyspnea*, *precordial pain* (angina pectoris), and occasional *dizziness*. On physical examination, the patients are *pale*. They have a *bounding pulse*, and several peripheral signs of hyperkinetic circulation are present. The *blood pressure* shows an *increase of pulse pressure*, unless cardiac output is severely decreased by associated mitral or aortic stenosis or by *left heart failure*. The *cervical* areas and the *suprasternal* notch show active *pulsations*, as do many peripheral arteries. The cardiac *apex* is displaced to the *left* and *downward*, and the apical thrust is lifting and *brief*. It is typical to hear a *soft, blowing*, prolonged *diastolic murmur in decrescendo*, which is maximal in the third left space and radiates downward. There may be associated phenomena, *i.e.*, a soft aortic component of the second sound, a third sound or a diastolic rumble at the apex (relative mitral stenosis, Flint's murmur), and a crescendo-decrescendo systolic murmur at the base (relative aortic stenosis). It is not uncommon to hear an aortic ejection sound.

The *electrocardiographic tracing* usually shows evidence of *left ventricular hypertrophy* and the so-called "strain pattern" which is the result of ventricular *dilatation*.

The *phonocardiogram* confirms the data of auscultation. The aortic component of the second sound *(sound II)* is usually smaller than normal. The diastolic murmur is of high frequency and often has a peak at the time of rapid filling in early diastole prior to its gradual decrease.

In the chest *X-ray* the cardiac shadow is severely *enlarged*, and the heart assumes an ovoid, oblong shape. The *aorta* is somewhat *dilated*. Fluoroscopy shows an *exaggerated pulsation* of the large arteries.

On *catheterization*, typical data are the increased systolic and decreased diastolic *pressures in the aorta*. Left ventricular diastolic *pressure* is raised by the "regurgitant stream" and may be above 20 mm Hg if there is severe *regurgitation*. This will elevate the pressure in the left atrium and the pulmonary vessels.

Angiocardiography affords the best evidence of the defect, if the contrast medium is injected at the root of the aorta, by showing retrograde filling of the *left ventricle*.

Complications. These patients may experience *coronary insufficiency* because of a hemodynamic mechanism plus early atherosclerosis. *Pulmonary edema* is a frequent complication and may prove fatal. Left heart *failure*, followed by right heart failure, occurs in the final stage.

Tricuspid Defects

Tricuspid defects are usually encountered in association with mitral stenosis.

Tricuspid Stenosis. *Tricuspid stenosis* decreases the output of the *right ventricle* and, thus, the pressure in the *pulmonary artery*. The pulmonary signs of mitral stenosis are decreased, so that the patient may

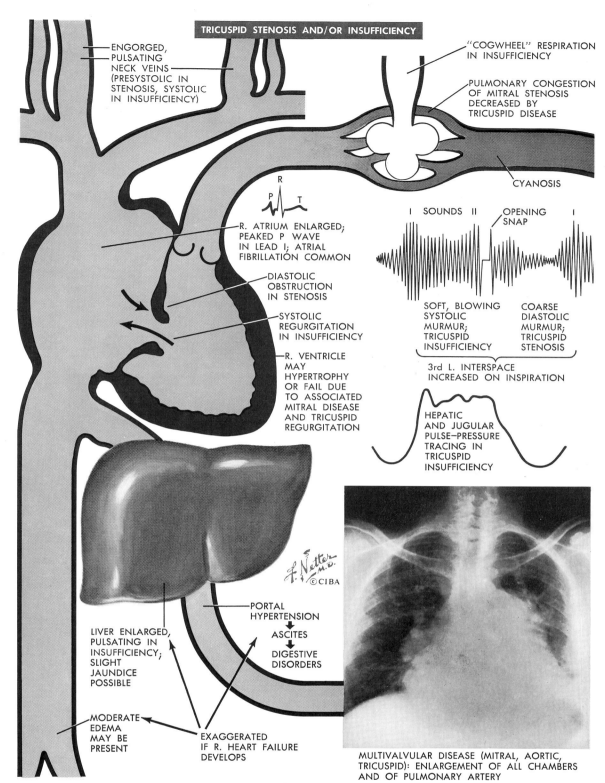

MULTIVALVULAR DISEASE (MITRAL, AORTIC, TRICUSPID): ENLARGEMENT OF ALL CHAMBERS AND OF PULMONARY ARTERY

lie supine without difficulty. On the other hand, the *neck veins* are *engorged* and show a *presystolic pulsation*. The liver is large and firm, and there may be *ascites*. The tricuspid *opening snap* and rumble are similar to those of mitral stenosis, but they may be recognized by graphic characteristics and because, typically, they increase during inspiration. A *diastolic* pressure gradient across the tricuspid valve is found through catheterization.

Tricuspid Insufficiency. *Tricuspid insufficiency* causes large *systolic* pulsations of the jugular veins and of the *enlarged liver*, and, at times, a typical balancelike motion of the precordium. A *soft, blowing, systolic murmur,* typically *increased on inspiration*, is heard over the *third* and *fourth left intercostal space*. Graphic *pulse-pressure tracings* (indirect *jugular* and *hepatic*, and direct *right atrial* on catheterization) show a typical systolic plateau, similar to a tracing of ventricular pressure.

The main *diagnostic* problem is differentiation between relative tricuspid insufficiency (common in mitral stenosis) and rheumatic tricuspid insufficiency. If both stenosis

and insufficiency of the tricuspid valve occur, the graphic tracings will show a slower rise and a slower descent of the plateau. However, pure or predominant rheumatic insufficiency of the tricuspid valve may occur, and then only long observation and the fact that digitalis fails to improve the picture will confirm the cause of the defect.

In general, people with tricuspid lesions seem sicker than they are and may be seen as ambulatory patients or may even continue their work for many years before reaching the final stage. Diuretics are generally more effective than digitalis.

Multivalvular Disease. The possible combinations are double (aortic and mitral) or triple (mitral, aortic, tricuspid) stenosis; aortic insufficiency plus mitral stenosis; mitral stenosis plus tricuspid stenosis or insufficiency; and aortic insufficiency plus mitral stenosis, with or without tricuspid involvement.

The *signs* are those of the various defects, though they are less striking unless one defect predominates. The *symptoms* are more severe than in single defects.

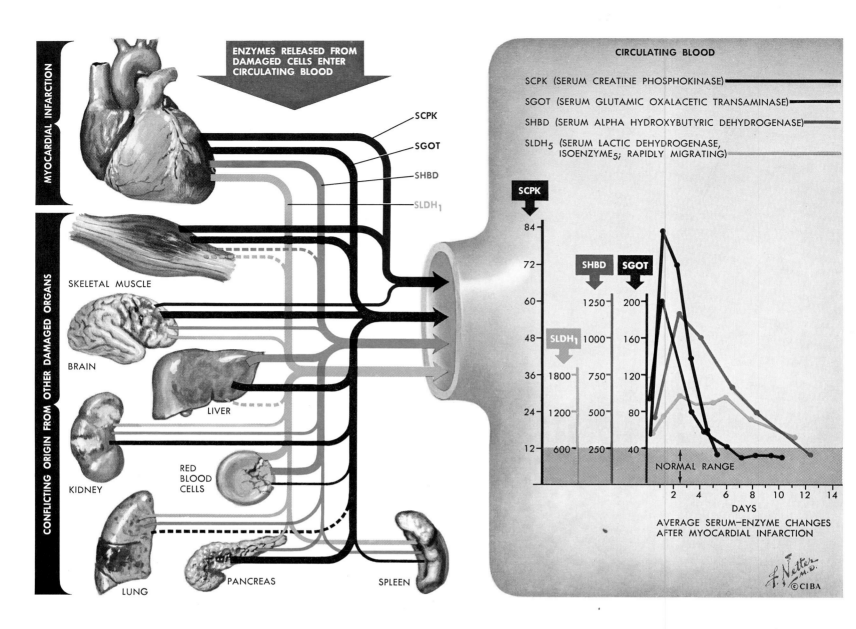

CIRCULATING BLOOD

SCPK (SERUM CREATINE PHOSPHOKINASE)
SGOT (SERUM GLUTAMIC OXALACETIC TRANSAMINASE)
SHBD (SERUM ALPHA HYDROXYBUTYRIC DEHYDROGENASE)
SLDH₅ (SERUM LACTIC DEHYDROGENASE, ISOENZYME₅; RAPIDLY MIGRATING)

AVERAGE SERUM—ENZYME CHANGES
AFTER MYOCARDIAL INFARCTION

SERUM ENZYMES IN MYOCARDIAL INFARCTION

The ability to measure *serum-enzyme activity* following *acute myocardial infarction* has increased our *diagnostic* accuracy, in both clinical and autopsy series, to 95 percent. The increased enzyme activity after acute injury to the heart muscle cell depends on the gradient between enzyme activity in the tissue and that in the serum. For example, the activity of glutamic oxalacetic transaminase (GOT) is 5000 times greater in human heart muscle than in the serum; that of lactic dehydrogenase (LDH), 3000 times. The release of muscle enzymes from damaged myocardium, with its high enzyme action, probably accounts for the major increase in serum activity following acute heart-cell injury.

Since the discovery of increased serum glutamic oxalacetic activity after acute myocardial infarction, the activity of many enzymes has been reported to increase also, but our discussion will be limited to a consideration of the four that have been best studied and are most widely used throughout the world. Unless there is acute damage of the organs depicted, the activities of these enzymes are not altered by infectious, degenerative, neoplastic, metabolic, or congenital disease states.

Demonstrated schematically is the *relative content* of enzyme activity in various organs. It can be seen that the *myocardium* is rich in all four; *skeletal muscle* in *SCPK, SGOT,* and *SHBD; brain* in SGOT and SCPK; *liver* in SGOT, but less in *SHBD* and *SLDH₁; kidney* in SGOT, with minimal activity of SHBD and SLDH₁; *red blood cells* high in SLDH₁ and SHBD; *lungs* richest in SHBD and SLDH₁; *pancreas* and *spleen* in SGOT with minimal concentrations of SHBD and SLDH₁.

These *relative concentrations* are important, since concomitant injury to tissues other than the heart or the skeletal muscles does not influence CPK activity, but it may increase the levels of SHBD and SLDH₁. Hemolysis, *e.g.,* may give very high false levels for these two enzymes, and liver-cell injury will primarily affect SGOT (SHBD and SLDH₁ less so). Hence, when interpreting these activities, one must consider possible damage to other organs also.

Table 1 lists the relative activities of these enzymes (together with SLDH) in most commonly encountered diseases in which enzyme alterations occur, and it emphasizes the specificity of CPK activity in acute myocardial infarction.

The changes in *serum activity* after myocardial infarction are depicted at the right. The activity of SCPK has been reported to be elevated in 60 to 100 percent of the patients after acute myocardial infarction, rising 4 to 6 hours after damage to the heart muscle cell, peaking at 12 to 36 hours, and falling to within normal limits in

2 to 7 days, depending on the size of the infarct.

The SGOT activity was elevated in 96 percent of the patients, after acute myocardial infarction, in 1255 cases reported in the literature. (This is the most thoroughly studied of all the enzymes.) Peak levels are seen 12 to 24 hours after infarction, and activity falls to normal limits within 2 to 7 days, again depending, in part, on the size of the infarction. Secondary SGOT elevations follow recurrent chest pain, owing to the extension or development of a new infarction.

The diagnostic accuracy of LDH after infarction was lower than the 96 percent reported from SGOT. Peak elevations developed after 3 to 4 days, falling to normal by day 8 to day 14 in 85 percent of the patients.

The SHBD activity rose in 90 to 100 percent of reported patients with myocardial infarction, peaking in 48 to 72 hours but persisting for 11 to 16 days. This longer half-life or slower clearing permits confirming infarction with serum drawn when SGOT and CPK activities may have normalized. The SHBD levels are high after muscle-cell injury but less affected by liver-cell injury. Hemolysis will give highly false levels.

The activity of SHBD closely parallels that of SLDH₁, since the rapidly migrating and relatively heat-stable LDH from the myocardium has a high SHBD activity. The slower but unstable LDH from the liver has a low SHBD activity. The analysis of SHBD activity is simpler and more accurate than that of SLDH₁ when done colori-

(*Continued on page 93*)

SERUM ENZYMES IN MYOCARDIAL INFARCTION

(Continued from page 92)

metrically or spectrophotometrically.

Electrophoretic studies have separated LDH into five components; the most rapidly migrating fractions are derived from the heart, red blood cells, and kidney, whereas the slower-moving components appear to come from the liver and skeletal muscles. Increased LDH activity following myocardial infarction is due primarily to the rapidly migrating components. This myocardial LDH is relatively heat-stable, thus permitting a partial differentiation between LDH activity which is due to liver-cell and skeletal-muscle damage and that which follows myocardial necrosis. Preliminary studies of these two methods, in the diagnosis of myocardial infarction, have been promising, but too few patients have been studied to permit a final evaluation of the role of *isoenzymes* in such diagnosis, despite reports that myocardial LDH remains elevated in the serum as long as 5 days after total SLDH activity has returned to normal.

The graph of enzyme activity shows that, in large infarctions, SCPK rises to proportionately higher levels: SCPK, seven times normal; SGOT, five times; SHBD, four times; and $SLDH_1$, two times normal. The duration of increased activity is two or three times greater for $SLDH_1$ and SHBD than for SCPK and SGOT. Smaller infarctions cause less peak activity, or shorter duration. It is important to remember that minimal hemolysis will produce significant increases in $SLDH_1$ and SHBD activities.

The $SLDH_1$ (probably identical to SHBD) increases after myocardial damage, but it is much less specific than SCPK. How tissue-specific the isoenzymes of LDH and even CPK will prove to be must await further study. Though the wide distribution of many enzymes is diminished in numerous cellular structures, this does not exclude the possibility of discovering enzymes in the serum that will reflect more specific sites of cellular abnormality and also give a more precise index of the degree of injury to heart muscle and other organs.

Unless the diagnosis of acute myocardial infarction is unequivocal, the activity of several enzymes should be measured. Since SGOT and SCPK levels increase most rapidly, they facilitate an *early* diagnosis. When studies are done 2 days or more after heart-muscle-cell damage, SLDH and SHBD activities will be higher and will persist for 4 to 16 days. When infarction is complicated by acute congestion of the liver, shock lasting 2 hours or more, liver disease, or pancreatitis, SCPK is the enzyme of choice, since its activity is not altered by these entities. Ideally, activity of all four enzymes should be determined; SCPK provides greater specificity, and $SLDH_1$ and SHBD improve a *late* diagnosis.

TABLE 1: DISEASE STATES ASSOCIATED WITH ALTERED ENZYME ACTIVITY

| | ENZYME ACTIVITY CHANGES | | | |
	SGOT	SLDH	SHBD (SLDH₁?)	SCPK
MYOCARDIAL				
ACUTE INFARCTION	+++	++	+++	++++
MYOCARDITIS	±	+	±	0
SEVERE PERICARDITIS	+	+	±	0
HEPATIC				
HEPATITIS	++++	++++	++++	0
CIRRHOSIS	±	±	±	0
OBSTRUCTIVE JAUNDICE	++	++	++	0
METASTATIC INVOLVEMENT	++	++	++	0
MONONUCLEOSIS	+	+	+	0
DRUG INJURY	+++	+++	+++	0
CHOLECYSTITIS	0	0	0	0
CENTRAL LOBULAR INJURY	++	++	++	0
SHOCK, 2+ HOURS	+++	+++	+++	0
ACUTE PASSIVE CONGESTION	+++	+++	+++	0
PERSISTENT RAPID ARRHYTHMIAS	+	+	+	0
MUSCLE—CELL DAMAGE				
INJURY AND BURNS	++	++	++	++
DERMATOMYOSITIS	++	++	++	+++
MUSCULAR DYSTROPHY	++	++	++	+++
MUSCULAR ATROPHY	0	0	0	0
CEREBRAL				
CEREBRAL VASCULAR ACCIDENTS	±	±	±	+
BRAIN TUMOR	±	±	±	±
DEGENERATIVE DISEASES	0	0	0	0
CONVULSIVE DISORDERS	0	0	0	0
MISCELLANEOUS				
INFARCTION; KIDNEY, SPLEEN, BOWEL	++	++	++	0
PANCREATITIS	+	+	+	0
DRUGS (OPIATES IN POSTCHOLECYSTECTOMY SYNDROME)	++	++	++	0
SEVERE PULMONARY INFARCTION	±	++	±	0
HEMOLYSIS	±	+++	+++	0

KEY

0 = NO CHANGE	+ + = MODERATE
± = VARIABLE	+ + + = MARKED
+ = MILD	+ + + + = SEVERE

© CIBA

TABLE 2: DISEASE STATES INFREQUENTLY ASSOCIATED WITH ALTERED ENZYME ACTIVITY

	SGOT	SLDH	SHBD (SLDH₁?)	SCPK
ANGINA PECTORIS	0	0	0	0
CORONARY INSUFFICIENCY WITHOUT INFARCTION	0	0	±	0
RHEUMATIC FEVER WITH CARDITIS	±	±	0	0
PULMONARY INFECTIONS	0	0	0	0
PERITONITIS	0	0	0	0
G.U. INFECTIONS	0	0	0	0
OTHER INFECTIONS	0	0	0	0
ARTHRITIS	0	0	0	0
OTHER BONE DISEASES	0	0	0	0
DERMATITIS	0	0	0	0
UREMIA	0	0	0	0
NEOPLASIAS WITHOUT LIVER INVOLVEMENT	0	±	±	0
LEUKEMIAS	0	±	±	0
ANEMIAS	0	0	±	0
METABOLIC DISEASES	0	0	0	0
ALLERGIC DISEASES	0	0	0	0
PREGNANCY	0	0	0	0

SHOCK

Cardiovascular "shock" may be defined as a pathologic process, hemodynamic and metabolic in nature, characteristically acute, produced by alterations of the vasopressor mechanisms, accompanied by severe and generalized circulatory failure, and characterized by a clinical syndrome in which the outstanding feature is arterial hypotension associated with signs of hyperactivity of the sympathetic nervous system. Hypotension may exist without shock, but shock cannot exist without hypotension. Autonomic nervous hyperactivity is an essential feature of shock.

Cardiocirculatory Insufficiency

Syncope, cardiac failure, shock, and cardiocirculatory arrest are four conditions which imply an inability of the cardiovascular system to supply blood adequately to the peripheral tissues, in relation to their needs.

In *syncope* the deficit is chiefly in the brain. Although acute, it is not severe; it is without metabolic repercussions, is not evolutive in character, is brief, and is rapidly reversible. It is usually self-limited but, if prolonged, may result, very infrequently, in cardiocirculatory arrest and death. This episode most frequently occurs without any underlying cardiocirculatory pathologic changes (functional syncope).

In *cardiac failure* the hypoperfusion is relatively slow in development and slight in magnitude, without clinically significant metabolic repercussions. There is time for compensatory mechanisms to come into play, and therefore it is tolerable and consistent with life for considerable periods of time.

In *shock* the tissue hypoperfusion is acute and severe. It leads to serious metabolic disturbances and is rapidly evolutive. The organism lacks either the time or the ability (or both) to bring compensatory mechanisms into play. In its early stages it is reversible, but, beyond a certain point, it enters the phase of a vicious cycle — hemodynamic and metabolic — and progresses inevitably to an irreversible phase which leads to cardiocirculatory arrest and death. This is a typical process.

Cardiocirculatory arrest implies a total

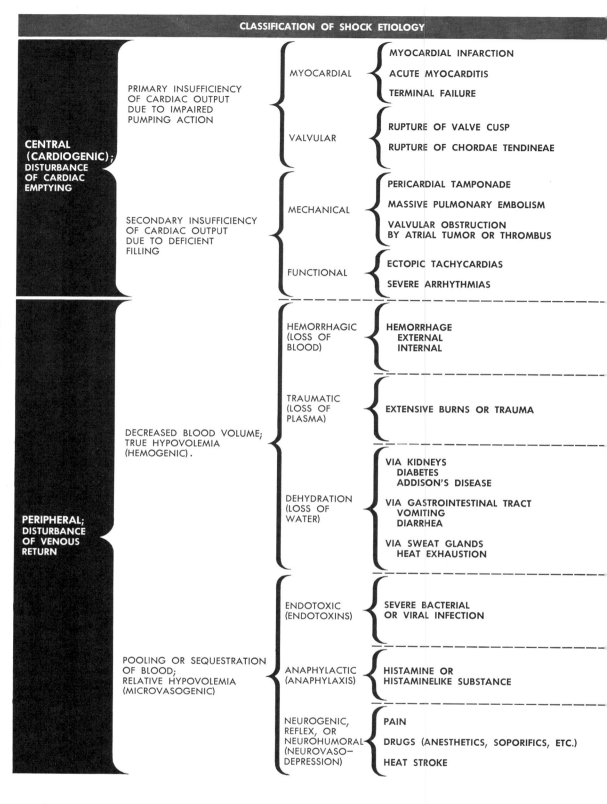

CLASSIFICATION OF SHOCK ETIOLOGY

CENTRAL (CARDIOGENIC); DISTURBANCE OF CARDIAC EMPTYING

PRIMARY INSUFFICIENCY OF CARDIAC OUTPUT DUE TO IMPAIRED PUMPING ACTION
- MYOCARDIAL
  - MYOCARDIAL INFARCTION
  - ACUTE MYOCARDITIS
  - TERMINAL FAILURE
- VALVULAR
  - RUPTURE OF VALVE CUSP
  - RUPTURE OF CHORDAE TENDINEAE

SECONDARY INSUFFICIENCY OF CARDIAC OUTPUT DUE TO DEFICIENT FILLING
- MECHANICAL
  - PERICARDIAL TAMPONADE
  - MASSIVE PULMONARY EMBOLISM
  - VALVULAR OBSTRUCTION BY ATRIAL TUMOR OR THROMBUS
- FUNCTIONAL
  - ECTOPIC TACHYCARDIAS
  - SEVERE ARRHYTHMIAS

PERIPHERAL; DISTURBANCE OF VENOUS RETURN

DECREASED BLOOD VOLUME; TRUE HYPOVOLEMIA (HEMOGENIC).
- HEMORRHAGIC (LOSS OF BLOOD)
  - HEMORRHAGE EXTERNAL INTERNAL
- TRAUMATIC (LOSS OF PLASMA)
  - EXTENSIVE BURNS OR TRAUMA
- DEHYDRATION (LOSS OF WATER)
  - VIA KIDNEYS DIABETES ADDISON'S DISEASE
  - VIA GASTROINTESTINAL TRACT VOMITING DIARRHEA
  - VIA SWEAT GLANDS HEAT EXHAUSTION

POOLING OR SEQUESTRATION OF BLOOD; RELATIVE HYPOVOLEMIA (MICROVASOGENIC)
- ENDOTOXIC (ENDOTOXINS)
  - SEVERE BACTERIAL OR VIRAL INFECTION
- ANAPHYLACTIC (ANAPHYLAXIS)
  - HISTAMINE OR HISTAMINELIKE SUBSTANCE
- NEUROGENIC, REFLEX, OR NEUROHUMORAL (NEUROVASO-DEPRESSION)
  - PAIN
  - DRUGS (ANESTHETICS, SOPORIFICS, ETC.)
  - HEAT STROKE

or almost total lack of blood flow to the peripheral tissues, because of the failure of the heart to pump blood and/or because of a tremendous atony and dilatation of the peripheral vascular beds. It is extremely acute and severe, leads rapidly to grave generalized metabolic disturbances, and is explosively evolutive. It is compatible with life for only a few minutes, unless resuscitation maneuvers are applied promptly and successfully. It could signify the terminal period of all diseases, or it could be an accident in a subject with a normal cardiocirculatory system.

Classification

The basic causes of shock may be *central* (i.e., at the heart level) or *peripheral* (i.e., at the vascular-bed level). Those patients belonging to the first group have an impairment in *cardiac emptying*, either *primary* because of a deficiency in the heart's *pumping* power, or *secondary* because of a *filling* deficiency, and both may be called *cardiogenic*. Those originating in the periphery of the circulatory system presuppose an *impairment in the venous return* of blood, due to two main causes: (1) decreased blood volume (true hypovolemia), which can be called *hemogenic*, because its genesis is in the blood components; or (2) pooling or sequestration of blood (relative hypovolemia), which can be called *microvasogenic* because of its genesis at the microcirculatory level.

Hemogenic shock can result from (1) hemorrhage (*hemorrhagic shock*), (2) loss of plasma following burns or tissue trauma (*traumatic shock* or *burn shock*), or (3) loss of water and electrolytes (*dehydration shock*).

Microvasogenic shock may be due to (1) endotoxins from severe infection, which may also cause

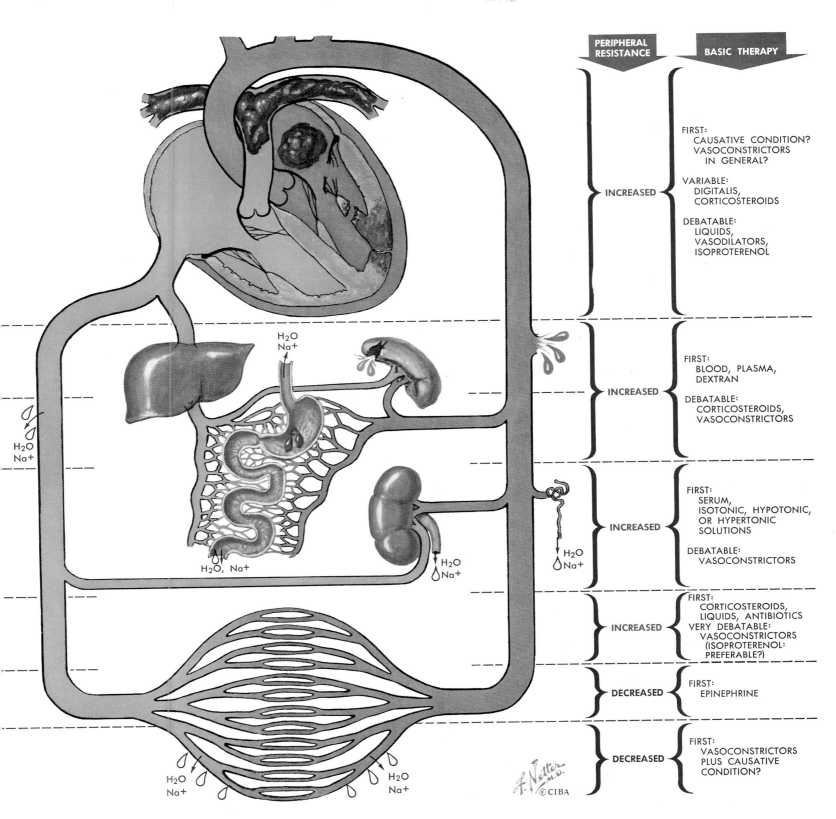

INCREASED

FIRST:
CAUSATIVE CONDITION?
VASOCONSTRICTORS
IN GENERAL?

VARIABLE:
DIGITALIS,
CORTICOSTEROIDS

DEBATABLE:
LIQUIDS,
VASODILATORS,
ISOPROTERENOL

INCREASED

FIRST:
BLOOD, PLASMA,
DEXTRAN

DEBATABLE:
CORTICOSTEROIDS,
VASOCONSTRICTORS

INCREASED

FIRST:
SERUM,
ISOTONIC, HYPOTONIC,
OR HYPERTONIC
SOLUTIONS

DEBATABLE:
VASOCONSTRICTORS

INCREASED

FIRST:
CORTICOSTEROIDS,
LIQUIDS, ANTIBIOTICS
VERY DEBATABLE:
VASOCONSTRICTORS
(ISOPROTERENOL:
PREFERABLE?)

DECREASED

FIRST:
EPINEPHRINE

DECREASED

FIRST:
VASOCONSTRICTORS
PLUS CAUSATIVE
CONDITION?

H_2O $Na+$ (left, upper)

H_2O $Na+$

H_2O, $Na+$

H_2O $Na+$

H_2O $Na+$

H_2O $Na+$

H_2O $Na+$

serious impairment of cardiac pumping action (*endotoxic shock*); (2) histamine or histamine-like substances (*anaphylactic shock*); or (3) neurogenic or reflex factors such as intense pain, drugs (anesthetics, barbiturates, etc.), or heat (heat stroke). All these can be aptly called "neurovasodepressor" shock and can interplay in its production.

Evolution

Although shock may be initiated by any one of the above factors, others may soon come into play, aggravating the situation and creating a vicious cycle. Thus, though shock may be precipitated by myocardial infarction with deficient cardiac output, the consequent peripheral hypoxia may result, later, in dilatation and an increased permeability of the peripheral vascular bed. Similarly, if shock is brought on by intense pain or by histamine liberation, resulting in peripheral vasodilatation, the consequent pooling of blood causes a decreased venous return and, thus, a diminished cardiac output, leading eventually to increased pooling and vascular permeability.

In shock precipitated by most of the listed causes, the peripheral resistance, paradoxically, is elevated initially, owing to compensatory constriction of the precapillary arterioles and postcapillary venules; however, in anaphylactic and in neurogenic or reflex shock ("neurovasodepressor"), resistance is initially decreased. This has an important bearing on *treatment*, particularly with regard to the administration of vasoconstrictors.

Clinical Features and Treatment

The *symptoms and signs* of shock may be classified as resulting from (1) a *hemodynamic disturbance* (arterial hypotension, filiform pulse, cyanosis, asthenia, oliguria), (2) *cellular hypoperfusion* (disturbance of consciousness, torpor, dyspnea, metabolic acidosis), and (3) *autonomic hyperactivity* (tachycardia, palpitation, pallor, cold sweat, tendency to paralytic ileus, hypersuprarenalism).

As the etiology of cardiovascular shock gradually becomes better understood, rational *treatment* of this condition improves. One should always think in pathophysiologic terms, thus enabling one, hopefully, to treat in specific syndromic rather than symptomatic terms. In any event, treatment as well as *diagnosis* should be prompt.

HEAD HYPEREXTENDED, NOSTRILS CONSTRICTED, CHIN DRAWN FORWARD IN PREPARATION FOR MOUTH–TO–MOUTH BREATHING

INTERMITTENT PRESSURE APPLIED WITH HEEL OF PALM OVER LOWER END OF STERNUM: MOUTH–TO–MOUTH BREATHING SIMULTANEOUSLY ADMINISTERED

HEART INTERMITTENTLY COMPRESSED BETWEEN STERNUM AND VERTEBRAE

CARDIOPULMONARY ARREST AND TREATMENT

External Resuscitation

Cardiopulmonary arrest, or sudden death, is the immediate and unexpected cessation of spontaneous circulation and respiration. It may occur in drowning, in asphyxia from any other cause, as an adverse reaction to drugs or anesthesia, in sudden and complete heart block, in electrocution, or after excessive vagal stimulation.

The etiology of *cardiopulmonary arrest* primarily may concern ventilatory insufficiency (as in those conditions resulting from asphyxia with cardiac arrest occurring from the resultant myocardial anoxia) or it may include cardiac malfunction, such as a mechanically ineffective arrhythmia (ventricular tachycardia, fibrillation, or asystole) following myocardial infarction.

There are three types of electrocardiographic patterns in cardiopulmonary arrest: (1) *cardiac asystole,* with a straight-line tracing; (2) *ventricular fibrillation* (see page 68), with an irregular, uncoordinated electrocardiographic pattern, resulting from asynchronous contraction of the various myocardial fibrils; and (3) *profound cardiovascular collapse* (also called downward displacement of the cardiac pacemaker), in which a coordinated electrical discharge may be recorded, but with no resultant effective mechanical action of the myocardium. Asystole usually results from some generalized cardiac hypoxia secondary to respiratory insufficiency or respiratory arrest. It may also occur after sudden and complete atrioventricular dissociation, profound drug overdosage, or marked vagal stimulation. Ventricular fibrillation is usually secondary to irritability of the ventricular myocardium. Profound cardiovascular collapse results from generalized myocardial depression or ischemia.

In treatment, emergency measures are directed toward artificial reinstitution of the circulation of blood oxygenated by artificial ventilation. The brain is the body tissue most sensitive to anoxia, and it will suffer irreversible cellular damage in as little as 4 to 6 minutes, depending on the antecedent physiological conditions. The emergency measures must be instituted within this brief period of time. Following the artificial reestablishment of the circulation of oxygenated blood, *definitive measures* are made to reestablish also the spontaneity of both ventilation and circulation. These measures consist of: (1) employment of pharmacologic agents to stimulate the myocardium and to improve the artificial circulation; (2) determination, by electrocardiography, of cardiac activity; (3) defibrillation of the heart from ventricular fibrillation or other arrhythmias, if present; and (4) further employment of

cardiac stimulatory or, if necessary, depressant pharmacologic agents. Following the successful reactivation of ventilation and circulation, the central nervous system must be protected from further insult by the prevention of cerebral edema.

External cardiopulmonary resuscitation is the simplest immediate emergency measure. Ventilation must be given at once and must be followed by external *cardiac compression.* The patient is placed supine on a hard surface, the mouth is cleared, and, with the *head in a hyperextended* position, expired air *(mouth-to-mouth) ventilation* is administered. With one hand, the resuscitator *pinches the nostrils* and uses them to hold the head in hyperextension. The other hand grasps the corner of the mandible and pulls it forward and upward, to open farther the oral airway. The resuscitator's mouth is opened widely, a deep breath is taken, and his mouth is applied to the patient's, to make a tight seal. Air is then puffed into the victim to make the chest rise. The resuscitator removes his head and lets the air exhale passively. Two or

three rapid breaths are given, and then the same or another resuscitator switches to external cardiac compression. The *heel of one hand* is placed *over the lower half of the sternum,* in a longitudinal fashion, and the opposite hand is placed over it. The resuscitator's full body weight is then utilized to *press the sternum posteriorly, to compress the heart against the vertebral column.* The sternum is depressed 4 to 5 cm, and the pressure is held for about ½ second and then is rapidly released. Pressure is reapplied approximately 80 times a minute. If there is only one resuscitator, he must switch back (approximately every 15 seconds) and give one or two very rapid ventilations. If two resuscitators are present, ventilation is effected between every fifth and sixth cardiac compression. Artificial ventilation and artificial circulation must be continued until spontaneity of these functions returns. This may entail definitive measures, as outlined subsequently.

The effectiveness of the circulation of oxygenated blood is evidenced by constriction of the pupils, pinkishness of

(Continued on page 97)

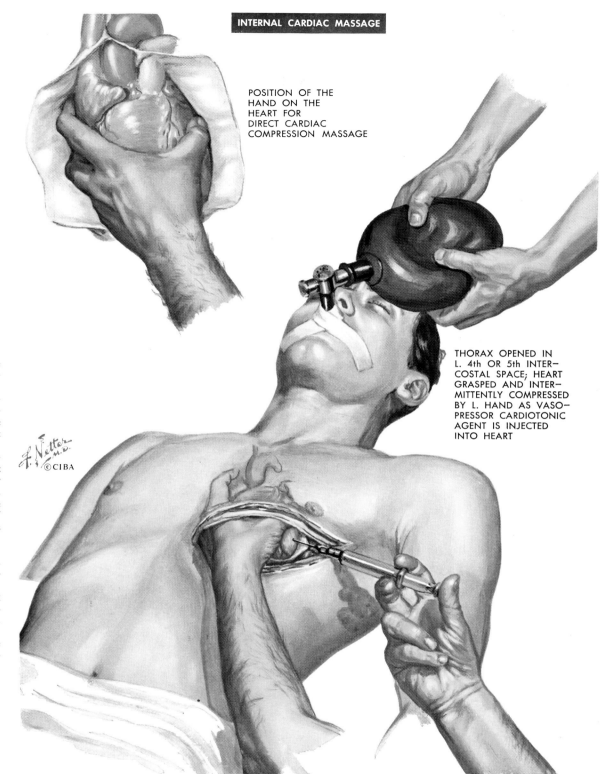

INTERNAL CARDIAC MASSAGE

POSITION OF THE HAND ON THE HEART FOR DIRECT CARDIAC COMPRESSION MASSAGE

THORAX OPENED IN L. 4th OR 5th INTER-COSTAL SPACE; HEART GRASPED AND INTER-MITTENTLY COMPRESSED BY L. HAND AS VASO-PRESSOR CARDIOTONIC AGENT IS INJECTED INTO HEART

CARDIOPULMONARY ARREST AND TREATMENT

(Continued from page 96)

the skin and mucous membranes, and, occasionally, spontaneous movements.

Internal Cardiac Massage

The recognition, by physicians of the midnineteenth century, that they were encountering sudden circulatory (cardiac) arrests in patients, because of an idiosyncratic reaction to anesthetics, led to experimental investigation and ultimate effective technics of cardiopulmonary resuscitation. It was in 1881 that Niehaus reported the first, but unsuccessful, attempt at cardiac resuscitation in man, utilizing the open-chest cardiac-compression technic developed by Schiff. The first successful use of Schiff's method occurred in 1901, but even before that, in 1885, Köenig described a method of external cardiac compression, and the details of two successful applications of this technic were reported by Maass in 1891. External cardiopulmonary resuscitation, however, was essentially not applied until it was rediscovered by Kouwenhoven et al., in 1960. Internal, or direct, cardiac massage, the prevailing procedure for cardiac arrest from 1901 to 1960, is still employed frequently and is specifically indicated when the cause of the sudden cardiac arrest may be within the thorax, such as following a crushing or penetrating wound of the chest. Also it is mandatory if external cardiac compression is impossible, because of the large size of the patient. When the chest already is open, as during a thoracic surgical procedure, and sudden cardiac arrest occurs, internal cardiac massage is the proper method.

In an emergency situation, a left anterior thoracotomy is rapidly carried out under unsterile conditions, opening the chest in the fourth or fifth intercostal space. The ribs are pulled apart manually, the left hand is introduced, and the heart is grasped, initially through the pericardium with the palm of the hand toward the apex of the ventricles. A milkinglike motion is then carried out, squeezing the heart from the apex toward the base. In this manner, blood is pumped out into both the pulmonary and the systemic circulation. The compression is held for approximately ⅓ to ½ second and then is totally released, to allow venous filling. It is repeated approximately 80 times per minute. The pericardium of the heart is opened anterior to the phrenic nerve, as soon as forceps and scissors are available. A better grasp of the heart is possible and better cardiac compression can be given once the pericardium is open.

As soon as it is available, a rib spreader is inserted (see page 98), and more sterile conditions are undertaken. Simultaneously

with the artificial circulation, the lungs must be ventilated by intubation of the trachea and positive-pressure insufflation with a self-expanding bag as depicted. The expired-air methods of ventilation are less effective with the chest open, although they can be employed.

With internal cardiac massage (compression) the status of heart action is readily identified: i.e., asystole is recognized by a totally quiet heart; ventricular fibrillation by a diffuse, irregular twitching or waving motion of the heart, but without any coordinated contraction; and profound cardiovascular collapse by the presence of weak ventricular contractions which obviously are not expelling any blood. It is very evident whether defibrillation is necessary or if only drug therapy is required.

With external cardiopulmonary resuscitation, the initial cardiotonic and vasopressor drugs are administered even before the type of cardiac arrest is known, since they are equally applicable in all situations. Generally, with internal cardiac massage, the same agents are employed immediately. Epinephrine, 0.5 mg, is given directly into the

bloodstream, either by an intracardiac injection or by an intravenous route, if available. This dose of epinephrine is repeated every 3 to 5 minutes for continuous stimulation of the heart and peripheral vasoconstriction, thereby causing more blood to be pumped to the brain and myocardium. Sodium bicarbonate (or another alkalizing agent) is also administered intravenously, in amounts approximating 44 mEq every 10 minutes, in order to prevent the development of severe metabolic acidosis. Generally, in cases of simple cardiopulmonary arrest, the utilization of either external or internal cardiac-massage technics, with cardiotonic-vasopressor and antacid agents, will result in reinstitution of cardiac activity from asystole or profound cardiovascular collapse. Ventricular fibrillation requires special treatment.

Defibrillation

Ventricular fibrillation is the incoordination of contrac-
(Continued on page 98)

DEFIBRILLATION

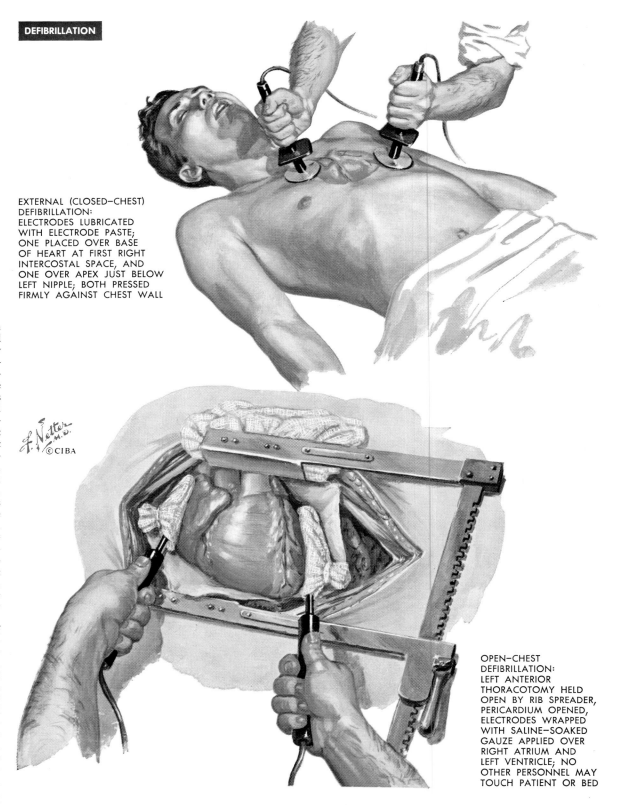

EXTERNAL (CLOSED–CHEST)
DEFIBRILLATION:
ELECTRODES LUBRICATED
WITH ELECTRODE PASTE;
ONE PLACED OVER BASE
OF HEART AT FIRST RIGHT
INTERCOSTAL SPACE, AND
ONE OVER APEX JUST BELOW
LEFT NIPPLE; BOTH PRESSED
FIRMLY AGAINST CHEST WALL

OPEN–CHEST
DEFIBRILLATION:
LEFT ANTERIOR
THORACOTOMY HELD
OPEN BY RIB SPREADER,
PERICARDIUM OPENED,
ELECTRODES WRAPPED
WITH SALINE–SOAKED
GAUZE APPLIED OVER
RIGHT ATRIUM AND
LEFT VENTRICLE; NO
OTHER PERSONNEL MAY
TOUCH PATIENT OR BED

CARDIOPULMONARY ARREST AND TREATMENT

(Continued from page 97)

tions of the heart muscle. It is due to an independent discharge of the electrical potential of the myocardial fibrils. It rarely reverts spontaneously to a sinus rhythm. Prevost and Battelli, in 1889, reported on investigations of electrical methods to terminate the fibrillation and reinstitute a spontaneous sinus rhythm. These studies were extended by Hooker, Kouwenhoven, and Langworthy, from 1928 to 1932, and were first applied successfully — using direct-contact electric shock — by Beck, in 1947. Kouwenhoven, and also Zoll, in the mid-1950's, developed an electric defibrillator which could be employed through the closed chest. This method revolutionized the indications and technics of applying electricity in the treatment of cardiac arrhythmias. Presently, with the direct-current defibrillator, it is possible not only to convert the dangerous ventricular fibrillations and ventricular tachycardias into a coordinated sinus rhythm but also to convert the less serious atrial flutter, atrial fibrillation, and other supraventricular rhythms, in patients who are adversely affected by their presence.

External (closed-chest) defibrillation of the heart, from either ventricular or supraventricular arrhythmias, is carried out by applying, to the chest wall, large insulated paddle *electrodes*, one of which is *placed over the apex of the heart (just below the left nipple)*, and the *other over the base of the heart (in the first right intercostal space)*. In utilizing the direct-current defibrillator, a point between 100 and 400 watt-seconds is selected, and the physician applies the current with a switch on the handle of one of the electrodes, but *only after* all other individuals have broken contact with the patient. If the initial shock is not successful in defibrillating the heart (as evidenced by observation of the electrocardiogram), then repeated shocks are necessary, possibly at a higher watt-second setting.

Internal or *open-chest defibrillation* is carried out through a *left anterior thoracotomy*. The *pericardium* must be *opened*. The *electrode* paddles, a special type with a concave surface, are *wrapped in gauze and soaked in saline*. One paddle is placed over the *right atrium* and the other over the *left ventricle*. Between 10 and 60 watt-seconds are then administered through the heart, *after all other individuals have removed contact from the patient*. The shock must be given under the control of the physician holding the paddles.

In order to obtain permanent defibrillation of the ventricle, it may be necessary to employ, intravenously, such cardiac depres-

sant drugs as lidocaine hydrochloride, 25 to 50 mg aliquots, quinidine gluconate, 100 to 200 mg aliquots, or procainamide hydrochloride, 100 to 200 mg aliquots. These pharmacologic agents depress irritable foci — the probable sites of origin of repetitive stimuli to ventricular tachycardia or fibrillation. In external (closed-chest) defibrillation, the status of the heart is interpreted from the electrocardiogram, but with open-chest defibrillation it can be determined by direct observation.

The quality of the myocardial fibrillations must be vigorous and coarse enough so that, following complete depolarization of the myocardium by massive electric shock, it will be possible for spontaneous coordinated discharge to occur. In the unoxygenated myocardium and when the fibrillations are of poor quality, defibrillation is not possible. The employment of epinephrine, 0.5 mg intravenously, will strengthen myocardial action and allow greater ease of defibrillation.

Once spontaneous cardiac action has been resumed, cardiac function is supported by vasopressor drugs, as

necessary. If the cardiac contractions are weak, calcium chloride, 0.5 to 1 gm, is given intravenously in repeated doses, every 5 minutes. Artificial ventilation is continued until good spontaneous ventilations are present.

After open-chest cardiac compression, the patient must be taken to the operating room for closure of the thorax. The pleural space and pericardium are irrigated with saline, and the pericardium is closed loosely. The ribs are approximated with catgut, and the chest wall is closed in layers, also with catgut. A wide-spectrum antibiotic is left in the pleural space, and the patient is given intravenous antibiotics, in large doses, for 1 week. Surprisingly, the infection rate is quite low, even though emergency cardiac open-chest massage is carried out under unsterile conditions.

With external cardiopulmonary resuscitation, no special operative procedures are necessary, but the patient is taken to the intensive-care unit for close observation. Any evidence of decreased cerebral function is treated by intravenous urea, hypothermia, and corticosteroids.

EXTRACORPOREAL CIRCULATION

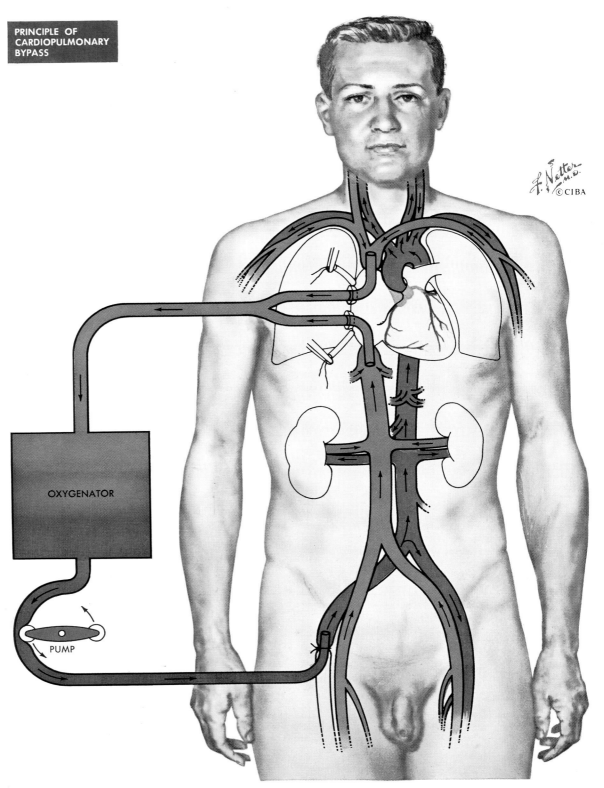

The Principle of Cardiopulmonary Bypass

The heart-lung machine makes it possible to operate within the heart under direct vision. This is necessary for the precise repair of cardiac valves, the replacement of valves by prostheses, or any intracardiac operation required for the correction of acquired or congenital abnormalities. This device also permits operations on the coronary arteries and the ascending arch of the aorta.

Before this apparatus was developed, all intracardiac operations had to be guided by the sense of touch, unaided by vision, or performed under total body hypothermia. The latter technic allowed about 8 minutes for operations within the bloodless heart; a *pump oxygenator,* on the other hand, allows intracardiac operations to be extended safely for a few hours.

During *cardiopulmonary bypass,* all venous blood ordinarily returning to the right atrium is diverted to an extracorporeal circuit. The blood is then passed through an artificial lung, where it takes up *oxygen* and gives off *carbon dioxide.* (Carbon dioxide elimination is an important function of an artificial lung, and hence the term "oxygenator" is not fully descriptive.) After passing through the artificial lung, the refreshed blood is pumped into the patient's arterial system. Thus, the heart and lungs contain no blood, except for that small quantity which enters the pulmonary vessels from the bronchial arteries. When the heart is opened, this blood is gently but continuously aspirated and returned, along with venous blood, to the heart-lung machine.

Two plastic cannulas, passed through the wall of the right atrium into the *venae cavae,* are usually used to lead venous blood away from the heart to the pump oxygenator. Cotton tapes are then placed around the cavae and their enclosed cannulas. Before these tapes are tightened, some vena caval blood continues to flow around the cannulas and through the patient's heart and lungs; thus, at this time, these organs are only partially bypassed. After the tapes have been tightened, all systemic venous blood is shunted to the extracorporeal circuit.

In certain instances, when operations are to be performed on the left side of the heart or aorta, a single large cannula may be placed in the right atrium or right ventricle. The pulmonary artery is then clamped, and all venous blood flows to the heart-lung machine.

The rate of flow of venous blood, from the patient to the extracorporeal circuit, can be increased either by elevating the patient's systemic venous pressure, by blood transfusions, or by reducing the pressure in the venous cannulas, by suction.

After passage of the venous blood through the pump oxygenator, where gaseous exchange takes place, the blood is returned to the patient through a cannula inserted into the *peripheral artery.* For this purpose, the common femoral or the external iliac artery is usually chosen. Occasionally, the cannula may be inserted through a stab wound in the ascending aorta or into the proximal left subclavian artery.

Adult patients under general anesthesia have a cardiac output of approximately 2.4 liters per square meter of body surface. This rate of blood flow must

(*Continued on page 100*)

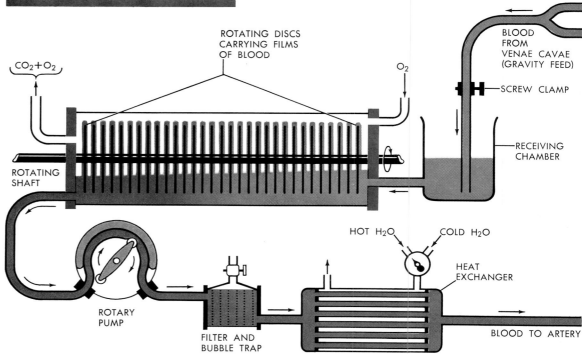

PRINCIPLE OF BUBBLE-TYPE OXYGENATOR

CO₂+O₂

DEFOAMING MATERIAL

OXYGENATING CHAMBER

BLOOD FROM VENAE CAVAE (GRAVITY FEED)

SCREW CLAMP

FILTER

O₂

HOT H₂O   COLD H₂O

HEAT EXCHANGER

ROTARY PUMP

BLOOD TO ARTERY

PRINCIPLE OF ROTATING-DISC OXYGENATOR

ROTATING DISCS CARRYING FILMS OF BLOOD

CO₂+O₂   O₂

BLOOD FROM VENAE CAVAE (GRAVITY FEED)

SCREW CLAMP

ROTATING SHAFT

RECEIVING CHAMBER

ROTARY PUMP

FILTER AND BUBBLE TRAP

HOT H₂O   COLD H₂O

HEAT EXCHANGER

BLOOD TO ARTERY

EXTRACORPOREAL CIRCULATION

(*Continued from page 99*)

be approximated through the extracorporeal circuit; metabolic acidosis will develop if lower flow rates are used.

Most heart-lung machines have two or more *pumps* incorporated into the extracorporeal circuit. Usually, *gravity drainage* alone provides adequate negative pressure to withdraw venous blood from the patient's body. A "coronary-sucker" pump is required to aspirate the small quantity of blood entering the cardiac chambers after diversion of the vena caval blood, as previously discussed. An "arterial" pump is required to deliver blood from the oxygenator to the patient's arteries. With certain types of artificial lungs—notably, the screen-type oxygenator—a third "recirculation" pump is used to maintain a constant flow of venous blood into the extracorporeal circuit. The purpose of this is to sustain a constant volume of blood in the artificial lung at all times. A change in the rate of flow over the screens of an oxygenator alters the thickness of the blood film on the screens and affects the volume of blood within the oxygenator. Such variations of blood volume in the extracorporeal circuit are undesirable, because they are accompanied by equal but opposite changes in the volume of blood in the patient's body.

Valveless pumps are commonly used in extracorporeal blood circuits. They produce less hemolysis and thrombosis and are easier to clean and sterilize than are pumps with internal valves. The valveless pump is, essentially, a piece of smooth, elastic tubing which is serially compressed by some external force, giving unidirectional flow to the fluid within the tubing. Backflow is prevented, because some portion of the tube is compressed at all times. The elastic recoil of the tubing, following compression, draws blood into the tubing in a forward direction. This sort of pumping is simply achieved by a roller passing over and compressing the tubing during the forward movement.

The Principle of the Bubble-Type Oxygenator

In this kind of *oxygenator*, oxygen is bubbled through a pool of venous blood. The bubble itself serves as the oxygenating surface. Since a sphere is the geometric form which encompasses the greatest volume within the smallest surface area, bubbles do not produce the greatest possible area of contact between gas and blood. Therefore, in order to be effective, the bubbles must be very small. However, the smaller the gas bubbles, the more difficult they are to remove from the blood, because of their buoyancy. Despite the use of *antifoaming agents,* there is danger of producing microscopic gaseous emboli. For this reason, the bubble oxygenator is not the ideal apparatus for use in long, total body perfusions. Foaming and turbulence and, hence, more hemolysis occur with this variety of oxygenator than with others, and there tends to be greater denaturization of plasma protein. On the other hand, the bubble-type oxygenator is manufactured commercially in a disposable form, with a sufficiently low priming volume so that it can be entirely filled with fluids other than blood. Thus, the bubble oxygenator has the advantage of always being readily available for emergency situa-

(*Continued on page 101*)

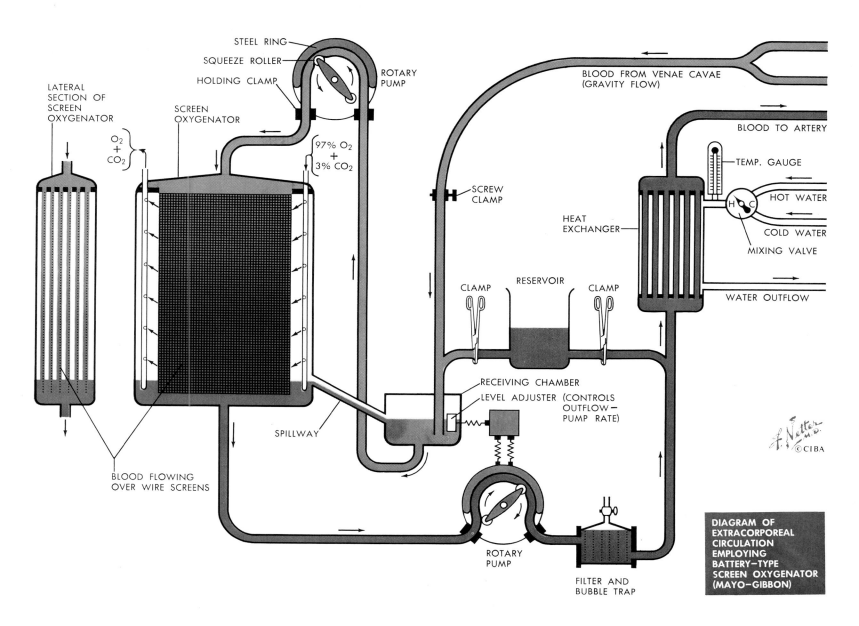

LATERAL SECTION OF SCREEN OXYGENATOR

STEEL RING
SQUEEZE ROLLER
HOLDING CLAMP
ROTARY PUMP

O₂ + CO₂

SCREEN OXYGENATOR

97% O₂ + 3% CO₂

BLOOD FROM VENAE CAVAE (GRAVITY FLOW)

BLOOD TO ARTERY

TEMP. GAUGE
HOT WATER
COLD WATER
MIXING VALVE
WATER OUTFLOW

SCREW CLAMP

HEAT EXCHANGER

BLOOD FLOWING OVER WIRE SCREENS

CLAMP   RESERVOIR   CLAMP

SPILLWAY

RECEIVING CHAMBER
LEVEL ADJUSTER (CONTROLS OUTFLOW— PUMP RATE)

ROTARY PUMP

FILTER AND BUBBLE TRAP

DIAGRAM OF EXTRACORPOREAL CIRCULATION EMPLOYING BATTERY–TYPE SCREEN OXYGENATOR (MAYO–GIBBON)

EXTRACORPOREAL CIRCULATION

(*Continued from page 100*)

tions. It has been shown to be safe to use for relatively short periods of total cardiopulmonary bypass.

The Principle of the Rotating-Disc Oxygenator

This oxygenator is composed of a series of *discs* mounted on an almost *horizontal* axle. The discs are turned by an external drive and are *rotated* through a pool of venous blood collected in a trough. The outer third of both sides of each disc becomes covered with a *thin film of venous blood*. It is then exposed briefly to the ambient gas mixture (*97 percent O₂ + 3 percent CO₂*) in the chamber above the trough. Dual gas exchange occurs, and the blood on the discs is returned once more to the bottom of the trough. Thus, venous blood flows into one end of the trough, and arterial blood is pumped from the opposite end. The rotating-disc oxygeazator is probably the type used most widely in this country. Because it creates less of a problem with bubble formation than does the bubble oxygenator, it can be safely used for longer perfusions.

It is relatively simple to cleanse and sterilize, and its priming volume falls somewhere between those of the bubble and the screen oxygenators. The mechanical agitation produced by the rotating discs through the pool of blood produces less hemolysis than does bubble oxygenation, but more than that which occurs with screen oxygenation.

The Principle of the Screen Oxygenator

This *oxygenator* consists of a battery of stainless-steel *screens* suspended *vertically* in a plastic, transparent chamber through which flows an *oxygen-rich gas mixture*. Venous blood flows from the *venae cavae* to a *receiving chamber*. This blood is then pumped by a "recirculation" *pump* from the *collecting chamber* into a small *reservoir* at the top of the oxygenator. The floor of this reservoir consists of stainless-steel bars separated from one another by narrow slits overlying each screen. The blood *filters* down through these slits, onto the screen, and is converted by *gravity descent* to a film of blood over the mesh. This thin film of blood on either side of the mesh is exposed to the gas within the oxygenator chamber. The *blood flow, over every horizontal wire of the screen*, produces sufficient turbulence, without foaming, to ensure that a constantly renewed surface of blood is exposed to the gas mixture during the descent. "Arterialized" (refreshed) blood collects at the bottom

of the oxygenator chamber and, from there, is pumped into the patient's *systemic arteries*. This kind of pump oxygenator ordinarily incorporates an automatic *level control*, which varies the arterial output of the machine according to the venous flow from the patient to the apparatus.

As with other varieties of pump oxygenators, a *heat exchanger* is usually incorporated in the arterial line. The heat exchanger can be used to maintain the blood at normal temperature, or lower, if desired. When the blood is cooled, it usually is carried down to the range of 28 to 32 degrees centigrade. At a body temperature of 30 degrees centigrade, the oxygen consumption by the tissues is decreased by approximately one half. Thus, using mild hypothermia, the output of the machine can be safely reduced. This, in turn, minimizes trauma to the blood. At this temperature, blood flow through the coronary arteries can be interrupted safely for short periods of time. Cardiac arrest ensues, and the surgeon has a motionless as well as a bloodless heart for the operation. This technic is commonly used in the repair of ventricular septal defects, where precise placing of sutures is required, and in operations upon the coronary arteries, where a motionless field is highly desirable.

The screen oxygenator has no moving parts, and there is little tendency toward foaming. Trauma to the formed elements of blood is minimized. Long perfusions are less dangerous to the patient with this apparatus than with the other two oxygenators described.

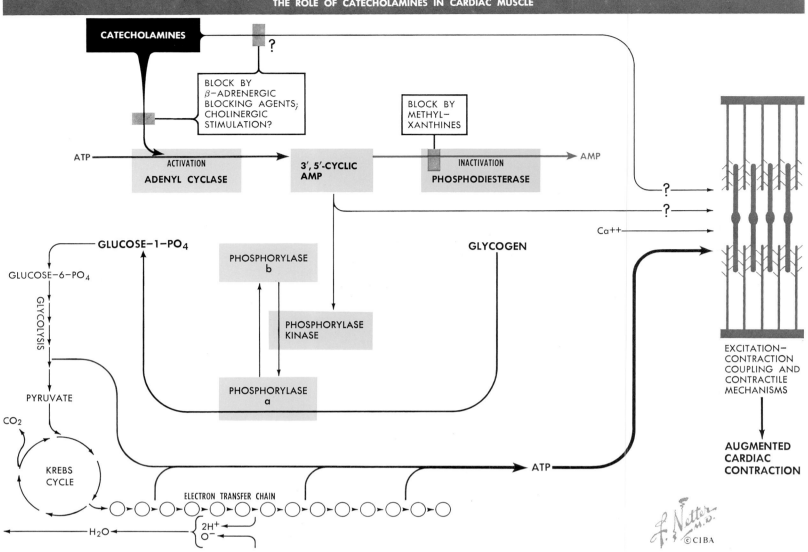

SECTION II—PLATE 62

DRUG ACTION ON HEART

Drugs influence profoundly the performance of the heart. They do so not by imparting new or unique properties to cardiac tissues but by modulating those physiological and biochemical events that are responsible for normal cardiac function. The important effects are the following: changes in heart rate (positive or negative chronotropic action), changes in force of contraction (positive or negative inotropic action), slowing or speeding of conduction, changes in automaticity and excitability, changes in the duration of the refractory period, and changes in blood flow through the coronary bed. A single drug can exert several of the above actions; therefore, an analysis of the total effects can become quite complex.

One of the most important mechanisms for the control of cardiac rate and output is the activity of the autonomic nerves (cardioaccelerator and vagus) which innervate the heart. The numerous and complex reflexes that influence the discharge rate of these nerves are discussed elsewhere (see pages 18, 19, and 42). The interruption of these reflex pathways can markedly affect cardiac function. Since all autonomic nerves have synapses at a ganglionic site before the nerve impulses reach the final neuroeffector junction, ganglionic blocking agents can achieve pharma-

cological denervation of the heart. Despite this, the automaticity of the denervated heart permits adequate function, but the patient being treated with ganglionic drugs cannot achieve rapid reflex adjustments in cardiac output.

Sympathomimetic Drugs

Practically all sympathomimetic drugs are congeners of the natural neurohumors released from sympathetic-nerve endings (norepinephrine) and the suprarenal medulla (epinephrine and norepinephrine). Their actions on the heart cannot be discussed adequately without a consideration of their actions on the peripheral circulation, especially the resistance vessels in the large vascular bed of striated muscle. This, in turn, requires a brief discussion of receptor mechanisms.

Sympathomimetic drugs are believed to act at special receptor sites in effector cells. These have been designated α and β. Activation of the α-receptors causes constriction of the resistance vessels of the peripheral vascular bed of the greater circulation, including the vessels of striated muscles. There are no important α-receptors in the heart. Activation of the β-receptors causes dilatation of the resistance vessels of the peripheral vasculature and is responsible, as well, for all the direct cardiac effects of sympathomimetic amines, since the heart contains essentially only β-receptors. These direct effects include a positive chronotropic and inotropic action, speeding of conduction, a marked increase in automaticity

along the conduction system and in cardiac muscle fibers, and coronary dilatation, and they result in an increase in cardiac rate, stroke volume, and cardiac output, as well as the possible appearance of cardiac arrhythmias ranging from premature systoles to ventricular tachycardia and ventricular fibrillation. At the same time, *phosphorylase b* is activated to *phosphorylase a*, resulting in the breakdown of *glycogen* which supplies energy to the heart via the glycolytic pathway and the *Krebs cycle* (see page 36). The increase in cardiac output is at the expense of a large increment in the utilization of energy and in oxygen consumption.

The mechanism by which sympathomimetic amines, that act on the β-receptors in the myocardium, activate phosphorylase is worthy of particular attention. The basic contributions of Sutherland and Rall, and their respective collaborators, have aroused great interest in the field. Briefly, the physiological events and pharmacological agents which cause β-receptor activity also *activate* the enzyme *adenyl cyclase,* the substrate of which is adenosine triphosphate (*ATP*). The compound that results from the reaction of enzyme and substrate is 3', 5'-cyclic adenosine monophosphate (*3', 5'-cyclic AMP*) which, in turn, mediates the conversion of inactive phosphorylase b to active phosphorylase a. The result is a rapid breakdown of glycogen and a greatly increased supply of energy to the cardiac muscle cell (see page 36); 3', 5'-cyclic AMP, in turn, is

(Continued on page 103)

DRUG ACTION ON HEART

(Continued from page 102)

rapidly *inactivated* by another enzyme, a specific *phosphodiesterase*. Thus, the duration of action of an activator of adenyl cyclase can be short. This series of reactions is depicted.

There is a very close relationship between the sympathomimetic amines with respect to their potency to exert positive inotropic and chronotropic actions in the heart, on the one hand, and their potency in activating adenyl cyclase, on the other. Thus, it has been proposed that, in the heart, adenyl cyclase may be the β-receptor or may be closely linked to the β-receptor. This theory could make pharmacodynamic events secondary to metabolic ones if phosphorylase activation were responsible, in some way, for the positive inotropic and chronotropic effects of sympathomimetic amines. Other theorists claim that the pharmacodynamic effects precede the metabolic effects. They ascribe a dual action to *catecholamines* — one to increase the work of the heart and the other to provide energy for the increased demands. There is evidence that both effects may be mediated by cyclic AMP. The problem could be resolved easily if it could be demonstrated that 3′, 5′-cyclic AMP mimics all the effects of catecholamines on the myocardium. Unfortunately, 3′, 5′-cyclic AMP does not cross cytostructural barriers.

Sympathomimetic amines differ markedly in their cardiac and peripheral actions and, consequently, their overall effect on the cardiovascular system. Consider the actions of *norepinephrine, epinephrine,* and *isoproterenol* as presented, in simplified form, in the following table.

Drug	Heart β-Receptors	Vascular-Bed α-Receptors	Vascular-Bed β-Receptors
Norepinephrine	+	+ +	−
Epinephrine	+ +	+	+ +
Isoproterenol	+ + +	−	+ + +

The overall cardiovascular actions of each drug can be reconstructed from the data in the table. *Norepinephrine* causes a marked *increase in peripheral resistance* and hence a *marked increase in systolic, diastolic,* and mean arterial pressure due to peripheral *vasoconstriction*. Compensatory reflexes, arising from the carotid sinus and the aortic arch, activate the *vagus* nerve and decrease the sympathetic tone to the heart. This may *result* in a *fall in heart rate* and *no change,* or an actual *fall, in cardiac output, despite moderate stimulation of the β-receptors*. Therefore, *peripheral blood flow* may be *decreased*. *Arrhythmias* may arise because of *increased automaticity*. *Epinephrine,* on the other hand, may actually cause a *fall in diastolic pressure* because of the predominant stimulation of the β-receptors and *dilatation* in certain peripheral blood vessels. The prominent chronotropic action on the heart results in an *increase in heart rate* that tends to *overcome* any *reflex vagal inhibition*. This, coupled with a positive inotropic action, results in a marked *increase in cardiac output* and a substantial *rise in systolic arterial pressure*. Compared to norepinephrine, mean arterial pressure is raised to a lesser extent, and *peripheral blood flow,* in most areas, is *increased* but in some areas, such as the *skin,* is markedly *decreased*. Finally, *isoproterenol* causes a *substantial fall in diastolic pressure* owing to *stimulation of the β-receptors in the peripheral vascular bed with no effect on α-receptors*. The marked positive chronotropic and inotropic effects greatly *increase*

cardiac output. Thus, *systolic pressure is maintained or elevated,* but *mean arterial pressure falls*. There is a *marked increase in peripheral blood flow*.

Certain sympathomimetic amines are devoid of β-receptor-stimulating properties. Examples are phenylephrine and methoxamine. The rise in blood pressure that they produce is totally dependent on the stimulation of the α-receptors, resulting in increased peripheral resistance. The cardiac responses are purely reflex in nature (primarily bradycardia). Nevertheless, the reflexes elicited may be useful in the treatment of cardiac arrhythmias (*e.g.,* supraventricular tachycardia).

Finally, there is a group of sympathomimetic amines that do not activate α- or β-receptors directly but exert their effects by releasing norepinephrine from the storage granules in *sympathetic*-nerve endings. The released neurohumor then acts at the receptor site. Examples are amphetamine and tyramine. They should not be relied upon as therapeutic agents for their cardiac action, but side actions on the heart should be kept in mind.

It is evident, from the above discussion, that the actions of the sympathomimetic amines, a group of congenerous agents, vary widely. The careful therapeutist selects the compound that is best suited to meet his needs. For example, in the treatment of cardiogenic shock, little more than manometric success would be achieved by a pure α-receptor stimulant that would increase peripheral resistance, decrease blood flow to vital organs (such as the kidney), and place an added burden on the heart. On the other hand, a pure β-receptor activator would greatly increase peripheral blood flow and cardiac output while maintaining adequate systolic and mean blood pressures. The dangers of arrhythmias can be minimized by careful regulation of the dosage.

α-**Adrenergic Blocking Agents.** Pure α-adrenergic blocking agents have no direct effect on the myocardium, nor can they block reflex sympathetic activity or the effects of sympathomimetic drugs on the heart. They are mentioned here because, when used as therapeutic agents, the responses elicited by their systemic actions (*e.g.,* a fall in blood pressure) may result in the reflex stimulation of cardiac β-receptors.

β-**Adrenergic Blocking Agents.** Effective and fairly specific β-adrenergic blocking drugs, such as propranolol, have been developed only recently, and their full potential as therapeutic agents is currently under active investigation. They have important cardiac actions in that they prevent the response of the β-receptors to sympathetic neurohumors and injected sympathomimetic amines. Thus, the sympathetic component of reflex responses of the myocardium and its conduction system is blocked, and a drug such as isoproterenol is essentially devoid of activity in the presence of β-receptor blockade.

As is the case with all agents that block the effects of neurohumors, the intensity of their pharmacodynamic action depends on the degree of tonic activity at the receptor site that is being blocked. Thus, when sympathetic tone to the heart is high, one would expect the β-adrenergic blocking agents to exert a negative inotropic and chronotropic action, decrease automaticity, prevent glycogenolysis, etc. These effects can be demonstrated in both experimental animals and humans.

At present, the main interest in the therapeutic usefulness of β-adrenergic drugs centers around their application in the treatment of angina pectoris and cardiac arrhythmias. The rationale for

their use in angina pectoris is both simple and sound. The increase in cardiac output and, thus, the work and the oxygen consumption of the myocardium that result from exercise or emotional stress are largely dependent on an increase of sympathetic tone to the heart. Thus, the individual with a reduced coronary blood flow can be protected from those exigencies by an effective blockade of the β-receptors. However, as is the case with many active drugs, an effective β-blocker is a double-edged sword. An individual with incipient heart failure and little cardiac reserve depends primarily on the positive inotropic and chronotropic effects of sympathetic-nerve stimulation of the myocardium to meet the demands of his daily activities. Deprivation of these important sympathetic reflex control mechanisms, by effective β-adrenergic blockade, can result in the precipitation of heart failure.

The concept that β-adrenergic blockade should have a favorable effect in the treatment of cardiac arrhythmias has a sound pharmacological basis. Since sympathetic-nerve impulses speed impulse formation, accelerate conduction, and markedly increase automaticity, a variety of arrhythmias should be favorably affected if these actions were attenuated by β-blockade. Actually, β-adrenergic blocking drugs have proved to be effective in a variety of arrhythmias, including those resulting from digitalis toxicity, paroxysmal atrial tachycardia, atrial fibrillation and flutter, and premature ventricular systoles. Surprisingly, these actions do not seem to result solely from β-adrenergic blockade. Rather, the β-blocking agents appear to share the properties of conventional antiarrhythmic agents such as quinidine and procainamide. (This will be discussed below.) Thus, their potential, in the treatment of cardiac arrhythmias, may result from a dual mechanism of action.

Other Mechanisms for Modulating Adrenergic Activity. During the past decade, knowledge of neurohumoral transmission has expanded greatly. Early in the 1950s, attention was centered primarily on the blockade of postsynaptic receptor cells, *e.g.,* the α- or β-receptor in the case of adrenergic nerves. More recently, a major effort has been directed toward research concerning the events that precede the release of a neurohumor by the *nerve action potential*. These events include the pathway of biosynthesis of the neurohumor, and the characteristics of the enzymes involved; the mechanisms of uptake and storage of the neurohumor, in combination with *ATP*, in special storage granules in the nerve endings; the mechanisms by which the nerve action potential effects the release of the stored neurohumor; and, finally, the mechanisms by which the action of the neurohumor, at the final postsynaptic receptor site, are terminated. The last-named event involves, in the case of *norepinephrine,* problems of diffusion, metabolic destruction, and reuptake by the nerve endings.

Many drugs have been discovered that can modulate the activity of the sympathetic nervous system by interfering with the complex sequence of events just described. Their main fields of usefulness are in the treatment of hypertension and in their actions on the central nervous system at which site adrenergic mechanisms play an important but ill-defined role. Their importance can be appreciated by the fact that drugs which can modulate central adrenergic mechanisms are useful in the treatment of schizophrenia and depression. As would be expected, these drugs have side actions in the heart. Only a few outstanding examples can be presented.

(Continued on page 105)

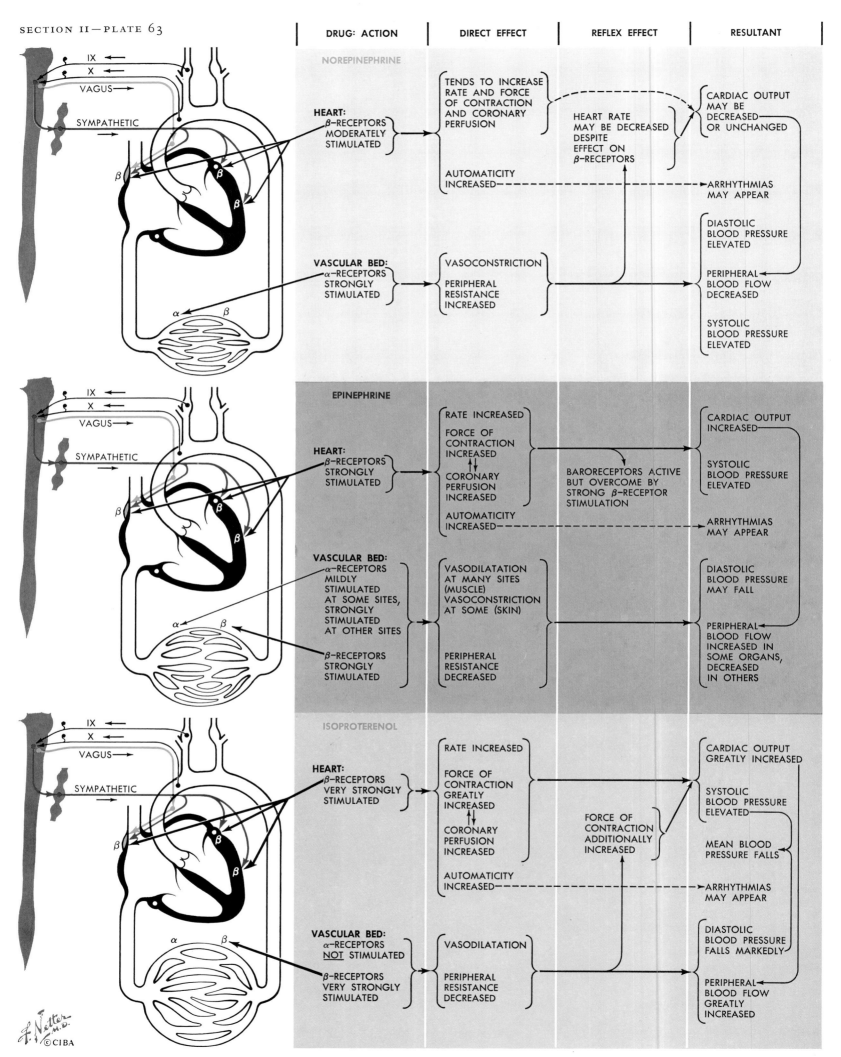

DRUG: ACTION	DIRECT EFFECT	REFLEX EFFECT	RESULTANT

NOREPINEPHRINE

HEART:
β–RECEPTORS MODERATELY STIMULATED

TENDS TO INCREASE RATE AND FORCE OF CONTRACTION AND CORONARY PERFUSION

HEART RATE MAY BE DECREASED DESPITE EFFECT ON β–RECEPTORS

CARDIAC OUTPUT MAY BE DECREASED OR UNCHANGED

AUTOMATICITY INCREASED

ARRHYTHMIAS MAY APPEAR

VASCULAR BED:
α–RECEPTORS STRONGLY STIMULATED

VASOCONSTRICTION

PERIPHERAL RESISTANCE INCREASED

DIASTOLIC BLOOD PRESSURE ELEVATED

PERIPHERAL BLOOD FLOW DECREASED

SYSTOLIC BLOOD PRESSURE ELEVATED

EPINEPHRINE

HEART:
β–RECEPTORS STRONGLY STIMULATED

RATE INCREASED

FORCE OF CONTRACTION INCREASED

CORONARY PERFUSION INCREASED

BARORECEPTORS ACTIVE BUT OVERCOME BY STRONG β–RECEPTOR STIMULATION

CARDIAC OUTPUT INCREASED

SYSTOLIC BLOOD PRESSURE ELEVATED

AUTOMATICITY INCREASED

ARRHYTHMIAS MAY APPEAR

VASCULAR BED:
α–RECEPTORS MILDLY STIMULATED AT SOME SITES, STRONGLY STIMULATED AT OTHER SITES

β–RECEPTORS STRONGLY STIMULATED

VASODILATATION AT MANY SITES (MUSCLE) VASOCONSTRICTION AT SOME (SKIN)

PERIPHERAL RESISTANCE DECREASED

DIASTOLIC BLOOD PRESSURE MAY FALL

PERIPHERAL BLOOD FLOW INCREASED IN SOME ORGANS, DECREASED IN OTHERS

ISOPROTERENOL

HEART:
β–RECEPTORS VERY STRONGLY STIMULATED

RATE INCREASED

FORCE OF CONTRACTION GREATLY INCREASED

CORONARY PERFUSION INCREASED

FORCE OF CONTRACTION ADDITIONALLY INCREASED

CARDIAC OUTPUT GREATLY INCREASED

SYSTOLIC BLOOD PRESSURE ELEVATED

MEAN BLOOD PRESSURE FALLS

AUTOMATICITY INCREASED

ARRHYTHMIAS MAY APPEAR

VASCULAR BED:
α–RECEPTORS NOT STIMULATED

β–RECEPTORS VERY STRONGLY STIMULATED

VASODILATATION

PERIPHERAL RESISTANCE DECREASED

DIASTOLIC BLOOD PRESSURE FALLS MARKEDLY

PERIPHERAL BLOOD FLOW GREATLY INCREASED

F. Netter M.D.
©CIBA

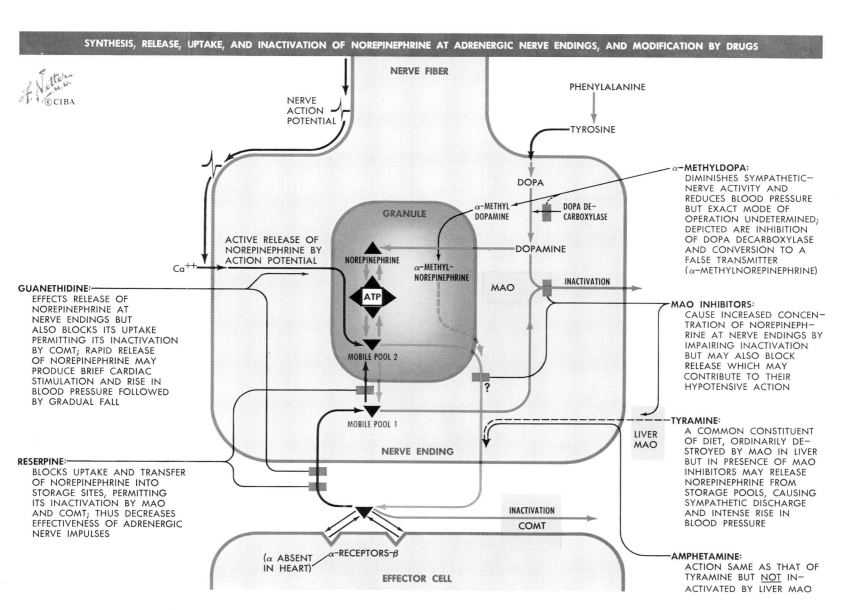

SECTION II—PLATE 64

DRUG ACTION ON HEART

(Continued from page 103)

RESERPINE. This drug, widely used in the treatment of hypertension, is also effective (but now largely replaced) in schizophrenia. It depletes adrenergic nerves of norepinephrine, primarily by *blocking* the *transport* of the *neurohumor into storage sites,* thus *permitting its inactivation by MAO and/or COMT.* As a consequence, cardiac *adrenergic nerve impulses become less effective* according to the dose employed. This may result in bradycardia, decreased cardiac output, impairment of the sympathetic component of compensatory cardiovascular reflexes, and lowered blood pressure.

GUANETHIDINE. This is a drug widely used in the treatment of hypertension and is another agent whose main site of action is predominantly on sympathetic-nerve endings. It is capable of effecting the *release of norepinephrine from storage sites in peripheral adrenergic nerves.* However, other mechanisms are involved, since the inhibition of responses to adrenergic nerve activity can be demonstrated before the depletion of catecholamines. There also is evidence that the *uptake of norepinephrine* by peripheral sympathetic-nerve endings *is impaired, permitting its inactivation by COMT.* The actions of *guanethidine* on the cardiovascular system are those

anticipated from marked inhibition of sympathetic activity. If the drug is given rapidly or in high dosage, there may be a *brief period of cardiac stimulation* and *elevation of blood pressure* owing to the *rapid release of stored neurohumor.* This is *followed by a gradual fall in blood pressure* as the response to sympathetic-nerve activity is decreased. Cardiovascular reflexes that depend on the activity of the sympathetic-nerve system are greatly depressed, and postural hypotension is commonly caused by the drug. Cardiac output may be reduced, and care must be exercised when a drug of this type is employed in patients with myocardial or renal insufficiency.

A unique feature of guanethidine is that it produces a pharmacological denervation hypersensitivity at the final sympathetic-effector site. Thus, a patient on guanethidine therapy is hypersensitive to epinephrine, norepinephrine, and all other sympathomimetic drugs that act directly on the receptor, and the effects of these agents on the heart are greatly exaggerated.

α-METHYLDOPA. This is another agent that attenuates *sympathetic nervous activity* by action on the peripheral *nerve fiber,* and it is thereby *useful in the treatment of hypertension.* Originally, it was thought to act by inhibiting *dopa decarboxylase* and thereby reducing the rate of synthesis and the store of norepinephrine in sympathetic-nerve endings. Although this is a provocative biochemical explanation for the mechanism of action, it does not fit the observed facts. At present, the mechanism of action of

α-methyldopa is an enigma. A possible explanation is that α-methyldopa follows the same anabolic pathway as *dopa.* The final product, α-*methylnorepinephrine,* is stored in the nerve endings and released by sympathetic-nerve stimulation. However, since it does not share the pharmacodynamic action of norepinephrine, it acts as a *false transmitter.* Even this attractive theory is not supported by a number of experimental observations.

The cardiovascular effects of α-methyldopa are complex. Sympathetic reflex activity is not severely affected, as it is with agents such as guanethidine, but the retention of salt and water, causing edema and congestive heart failure, is somewhat more common with α-methyldopa than with other hypotensive agents.

MONAMINE OXIDASE (MAO) INHIBITORS. Inhibitors of MAO, although used primarily as antidepressant drugs, have important cardiovascular actions that deserve brief discussion. The deamination of catecholamines by MAO is one of the main metabolic pathways for their inactivation. In the presence of an MAO inhibitor, the concentration of norepinephrine in the storage *granules* and nerve axoplasm is increased. Thus, drugs which indirectly cause the release of norepinephrine from peripheral nerve endings (e.g., *amphetamine* and *tyramine*) may cause a greatly exaggerated sympathetic discharge.

Tyramine is of little use as a drug but it is a common constituent of the diet. Since it is nor-

(Continued on page 106)

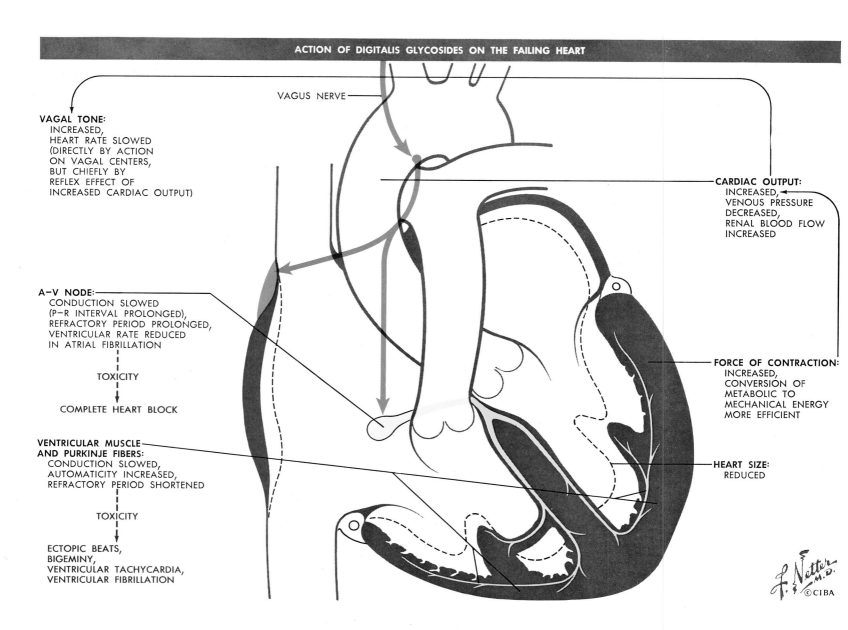

VAGUS NERVE

VAGAL TONE:
INCREASED,
HEART RATE SLOWED
(DIRECTLY BY ACTION
ON VAGAL CENTERS,
BUT CHIEFLY BY
REFLEX EFFECT OF
INCREASED CARDIAC OUTPUT)

CARDIAC OUTPUT:
INCREASED,
VENOUS PRESSURE
DECREASED,
RENAL BLOOD FLOW
INCREASED

A–V NODE:
CONDUCTION SLOWED
(P–R INTERVAL PROLONGED),
REFRACTORY PERIOD PROLONGED,
VENTRICULAR RATE REDUCED
IN ATRIAL FIBRILLATION

TOXICITY

COMPLETE HEART BLOCK

FORCE OF CONTRACTION:
INCREASED,
CONVERSION OF
METABOLIC TO
MECHANICAL ENERGY
MORE EFFICIENT

**VENTRICULAR MUSCLE
AND PURKINJE FIBERS:**
CONDUCTION SLOWED,
AUTOMATICITY INCREASED,
REFRACTORY PERIOD SHORTENED

TOXICITY

ECTOPIC BEATS,
BIGEMINY,
VENTRICULAR TACHYCARDIA,
VENTRICULAR FIBRILLATION

HEART SIZE:
REDUCED

SECTION II—PLATE 65

DRUG ACTION ON HEART

(Continued from page 105)

mally destroyed by the *monamine oxidase present in the liver,* it never reaches the peripheral circulation in a significant concentration. However, the patient under therapy with an MAO inhibitor has lost this protective hepatic function, and foods with a high tyramine content, such as cheese, can cause a general *sympathetic discharge.* The involvement of the cardiovascular system is prominent, and a precipitous increase in cardiac output and *rise in blood pressure* may result in fatal cerebral hemorrhage.

Paradoxically, MAO inhibitors cause a fall in blood pressure and find a limited usefulness as antihypertensive agents. Their mechanism of action is completely unknown.

Parasympathomimetic Drugs

These drugs have profound effects on the myocardium and are essentially catastrophic in nature, with little or no therapeutic application. They act at the S-A node to slow its rate of discharge, even to the point of cardiac arrest. They slow A-V conduction to the point of complete block. Whether they have a direct negative inotropic effect on cardiac muscle is debatable, but evidence for this is accumulating. In addition to actions on the heart, these agents can also cause a

marked decrease in peripheral resistance. These combined actions result in a profound fall in blood pressure. Although a parasympathomimetic drug such as methacholine may occasionally be useful in arresting an attack of paroxysmal tachycardia, it is probably lowest on the list of drugs of choice for the treatment of this condition.

Parasympathetic Blocking Agents. The important parasympathetic blocking agents of natural origin are atropine and scopolamine. However, this area has been a paradise for pharmaceutical chemists, and at least twenty-five synthetic agents of this class are available. The actions of these agents on the heart result from an inhibition of vagal tone at all peripheral-effector sites. Very small doses of atropine may cause a paradoxical bradycardia due to stimulation of the medullary vagal nuclei. However, the usual therapeutic doses cause tachycardia by blocking vagal effects on the S-A node. The response depends upon the dose and the degree of vagal tone. Atropine is also capable of blocking the effects of cholinergic nerve impulses and parasympathomimetic drugs on conduction. These blocking agents are of little therapeutic use in cardiovascular disorders, except rarely when the abnormality is due to increased vagal activity.

Xanthines

The xanthines, particularly theophylline, most commonly used for its cardiac effects in the form of aminophylline, exert prominent positive inotropic and chronotropic effects on the myocar-

dium. In the intact animal, the positive chronotropic action may be masked by central vagal stimulation. The xanthines also can increase automaticity in the myocardium and give rise to ectopic beats. The positive inotropic action of the xanthines is accompanied by an increase in oxygen consumption. Thus, the cardiac actions of the xanthines resemble those of the catecholamines but are much more prolonged, since the latter are rapidly inactivated in the body. This parallelism in action can be extended beyond the myocardium; *e.g.,* the xanthines relax smooth muscle, especially that of the bronchi, and also cause vasodilatation in the peripheral vascular bed. Thus they mimic, in many ways, the effects of catecholamines at β-receptor sites. At an enzymatic level, xanthines are potent inhibitors of the enzyme (phosphodiesterase) that destroys 3', 5'-cyclic AMP, discussed earlier with respect to its role in the actions of catecholamines on β-receptors (see page 102). It is conceivable that xanthines may act indirectly by potentiating the effect of sympathetic-nerve impulses.

Regardless of their mechanism of action, the positive inotropic effects of the xanthines are of great value in treating acute left heart failure. Here the xanthines can greatly increase cardiac output. The onset of action is almost immediate, following intramuscular administration, and the duration of action is sufficiently long so that more-lasting measures, such as intravenous digitalization, can be undertaken.

(Continued on page 107)

DRUG ACTION ON HEART
(*Continued from page 106*)

There is much controversial literature on the effects of the xanthines on coronary blood flow. There is little question that this flow is increased by the xanthines, but this could be either secondary to the increased metabolic activity or be a direct action. However, xanthines also increase the oxygen demand of the heart. Their usefulness in the treatment of coronary insufficiency is highly debatable.

Digitalis Glycosides

Digitalis glycosides and related cardiac glycosides are by far the most important drugs that act on the heart. The *actions of digitalis glycosides* on the heart can be separated into two major categories: (1) a positive inotropic action on the failing heart, and (2) a marked effect on the conduction system and cardiac automaticity.

The positive inotropic action of digitalis accounts for all the salutary effects of the drug in *congestive heart failure* uncomplicated by conduction defects. The *increased force of contraction* is accompanied by a *greater cardiac output,* a *decreased heart size,* a *fall in venous pressure,* and the mobilization of edema fluid as the *blood flow through the kidney is increased.*

The positive inotropic action of digitalis on the failing heart is unique in one very important respect. Despite the marked increase in cardiac work or output, there is no parallel increase in oxygen consumption. Thus digitalis is, in some way, able to increase the ability of the failing myocardial fiber to *convert metabolic to mechanical energy.* The mechanism by which this increased utilization of energy is achieved has intrigued investigators for decades. Numerous insufficiently supported theories have been proposed. A unique property of digitalis, at the enzymatic level, is its ability to inhibit the sodium- and potassium-stimulated adenosine triphosphatase (ATP-ase). It is thought that ATP-ase is intimately involved with the supply of energy for ion transport. During depolarization of the myocardial cell membrane, marked changes in ion permeability occur, and there is a rapid influx into the cell of those cations whose extracellular concentration is higher than the intracellular, principally Na^+ and Ca^{++}. The opposite occurs in the case of cations whose intracellular concentration is greater than the extracellular (see page 48). Thus, there is an outward diffusion of K^+. The restoration of this ionic imbalance requires the active transport of ions, the energy for which is, in some way, controlled by ATP-ase. Thus, the inhibition of ATP-ase by cardiac glycosides would change the cationic environment of the heart muscle fiber, namely by an increase in the net influx of Na^+ and Ca^{++} and an increment in the net efflux of K^+. An ion involved in the events that occur be-

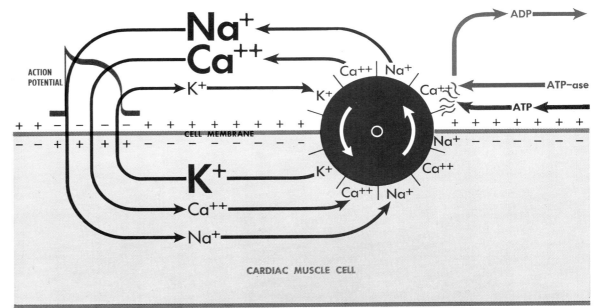

SODIUM- AND CALCIUM-ION CONCENTRATION IS GREATER OUTSIDE THE RESTING HEART MUSCLE CELL THAN WITHIN IT; THE REVERSE IS TRUE FOR POTASSIUM; DEPOLARIZATION PERMITS PASSIVE DIFFUSION OF Na+ AND Ca++ INTO THE CELL AND K+ OUT OF THE CELL. THIS SUDDEN INCREASE IN INTRACELLULAR Ca++ IS BELIEVED TO BE A CRITICAL EVENT

IN DEPOLARIZATION–CONTRACTION COUPLING. RESTORATION OF THE IONIC IMBALANCE TO THE RESTING STATE IS ACCOMPLISHED BY ACTIVE TRANSPORT, THE ENERGY FOR WHICH IS PROVIDED BY ATP; ATP–ase SOMEHOW RELEASES PHOSPHATE–BOND ENERGY FROM ATP WHICH THEN BECOMES ADP

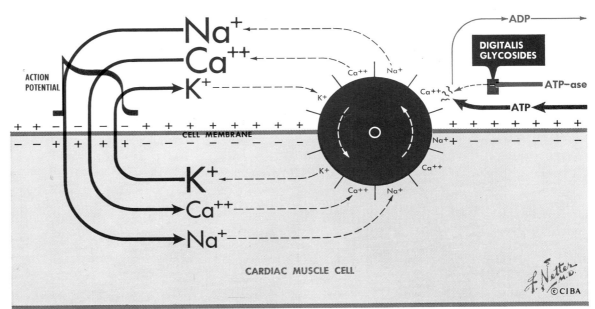

DIGITALIS GLYCOSIDES APPEAR TO INHIBIT ACTION OF ATP–ase, RESULTING IN GREATER NET INFLUX OF Ca++ AND Na+, WITH GREATER NET EFFLUX OF K+. THIS RESULTS IN GREATER INTRACELLULAR CONCENTRATION OF Ca++ AND Na+ AND LOWER CONCENTRATION OF K+. THIS IS

ONE OF MANY PROPOSED THEORIES TO EXPLAIN THE GREATER CARDIAC CONTRACTILITY PRODUCED BY DIGITALIS GLYCOSIDES. IT DOES EXPLAIN THE INCREASED SUSCEPTIBILITY OF THE DIGITALIZED HEART TO HYPOKALEMIA AND HYPERCALCEMIA

tween depolarization of the muscle fiber and the contractile process (depolarization-contraction coupling) is calcium. In its absence, depolarization can occur, but no contraction of the muscle ensues. Therefore, it is tempting to relate the positive inotropic action of digitalis to a net increment in calcium influx into the cardiac muscle cell, which, in some way, increases the efficiency of the contractile process.

The changes in the ionic composition of the myocardial cells and conduction system may also account for the marked changes in conduction and the many arrhythmias that can be produced by the cardiac glycosides. The changes that these glycosides produce in cardiac rate and rhythm are of clinical usefulness but, with overdosage, are responsible also for the serious nature of digitalis intoxication. Digitalis markedly *slows the heart rate* in patients with a sinus rhythm and a compensatory sinus tachycardia. The glycosides

are capable of stimulating the medullary *vagal center,* but this is an unimportant contribution to cardiac slowing. Rather, it is the increase in cardiac output which removes the need for compensatory tachycardia that restores the heart rate to normal after output becomes adequate to meet the oxygen demands of the body.

The digitalis glycosides have marked effects on conduction and these are so complex that only major features will be discussed. Conduction velocity in the atrium may be increased by low doses of digitalis but is slowed by higher doses. *Conduction through the A-V node* is markedly *slowed,* because of *increased vagal tone* and a *direct extravagal action* of the drug on the *node.* This is manifested by a *prolongation of the P-R interval* and can progress to partial or *complete A-V block.* With high doses of these glycosides,

(*Continued on page 108*)

conduction is also *depressed in the Purkinje fibers.* This occurs before *conduction in the muscle* is seriously *impaired.* Digitalis also affects the refractory periods of various cardiac tissues. Effects on the atrium are complex and depend, to a great extent, on the effects of the glycosides on vagal tone. The *refractory period of the A-V node* is markedly *increased,* and this is the main reason for the *reduction of ventricular rate,* following digitalization, in the patient with *atrial fibrillation.* Digitalis glycosides *shorten the ventricular refractory period,* as evidenced in the ECG by a shortened Q-T interval. The effect is not uniform throughout ventricular muscle and may contribute to the genesis of ectopic beats.

One of the most profound effects of digitalis, accounting for the many serious arrhythmias after high doses, is a marked increase in automaticity of the Purkinje fibers and the myocardial muscle fibers themselves. The arrhythmias produced by increased automaticity are, in order of their increasing seriousness, occasional *ectopic beats,* coupled beats *(bigeminy),* single-focus *ventricular tachycardia,* and multifocal ventricular tachycardia. As idioventricular activity increases, depression of conductivity in the ventricle also occurs, thus initiating *ventricular fibrillation.*

The described actions of digitalis have characteristic effects on the electrocardiogram that are of diagnostic importance (see page 69).

As mentioned earlier, the changes in force of contraction, conduction, and automaticity, which are the cardinal features of the action of digitalis on the heart, are presumed to be closely related to changes in the internal cationic environment of cardiac tissue cells. Therefore, abnormalities in electrolyte metabolism, in digitalized individuals, can accentuate the effects of the cardiac glycosides, particularly those related to conduction disturbances and increased automaticity. A negative K^+ balance markedly increases digitalis toxicity, and, since the cardiac glycosides are often prescribed in combination with diuretics that promote the renal loss of K^+, great care must be taken to maintain an adequate K^+ intake. If digitalis toxicity is accompanied by a negative K^+ balance, a correction of this imbalance will often ameliorate the signs and symptoms of the toxic effects. Conversely, hypercalcemia potentiates digitalis toxicity.

Digitalis represents one of the most useful drugs in the physician's armamentarium. However, it has been estimated that a potentially lethal dose is only twice that of a full therapeutic dose. This relatively low margin of safety can be augmented further by changes in the electrolyte composition of extracellular fluid. It is obvious that all digitalized patients require careful and individual supervision. Digitalis is perhaps the most misused of all drugs. Therefore the physician should have a full appreciation of the unique therapeutic and toxic potentialities of these most important cardiotonic agents. Finally, it should be emphasized that the only differences between the many available preparations of cardiac glycosides relate to their speed of onset of action and their duration of activity. None is superior with respect to the ratio between therapeutic and toxic effects.

Drugs in the Treatment of Angina Pectoris

The search for highly effective drugs in the treatment or prophylaxis of angina pectoris has provided vexing problems for the pharmacologist and therapeutist, with respect to both the usefulness of current agents and an explanation of their mechanism of action. There is little doubt that angina pectoris is due to a discrepancy between the demand for and supply of oxygen to the myocardium, leading to localized ischemia. This can be corrected by increasing the oxygen supply to the ischemic area or by decreasing the oxygen demand. It is only natural that attention has been directed toward powerful coronary vasodilating drugs in the treatment of angina pectoris. The fact that *nitroglycerin* is by far the most effective agent for the prophylaxis and treatment of angina pectoris, coupled with the knowledge that its primary pharmacological action is a nonspecific direct relaxation of vascular smooth muscle, has led, until recently, to the placid acceptance that an increase in coronary blood flow is responsible for the drug's effectiveness, especially since relaxation of coronary vessels can be demonstrated by a variety of technics, and an increase in coronary flow can be detected in preparations in which the elasticity of the coronary vascular bed is normal. Overlooked has been the fact that autoregulation of the coronary blood flow is one of its distinguishing physiological features, and probably no drug is capable of reducing coronary peripheral vascular resistance more than can the physiological stimulus of inadequate perfusion itself. Therefore, it may be that pharmacologists have been led up the primrose path in searching for more potent vasodilators, while our most valuable drug has been in use for almost 100 years. In other words, it has not been established that, in angina pectoris, peripheral coronary vasodilatation is the required drug action, or that some agents are effective through their vasodilating action.

It would be most gratifying, at this point, to make an apodictic statement as to the mechanism of action of nitroglycerin in the prophylaxis and treatment of angina pectoris, but one can speak with assurance only about its effectiveness. Countless studies have shown that nitroglycerin can increase exercise tolerance in anginal patients before myocardial hypoxia develops, as evidenced by ECG changes. Nitroglycerin, taken before a period of increased patient activity, will often prevent the attack that otherwise would be expected. Finally, an effective sublingual dose of this drug acts within 2 minutes to terminate anginal pain, and is especially effective if the patient can take the drug during the short period of premonitory tightness of the chest that may precede the onset of pain.

Yet, in most patients with a clear-cut anginal syndrome, nitroglycerin does not seem to increase coronary blood flow. In such patients the peripheral coronary vascular resistance appears to be "fixed," perhaps because of the potent vasodilating effects of myocardial ischemia, as cited above. Coronary blood flow also decreases as cardiac output and blood pressure fall, owing to a decreased venous return to the heart and a decrease in ventricular volume and cardiac output.

In 1867, Brunton, who introduced amyl nitrite for the treatment of angina pectoris, attributed the pain to "excess of work to be done over the power to do it." Undoubtedly, decreasing the heart's work load would be as effective as increasing the coronary perfusion, and this may well be the mechanism of action of nitroglycerin. However, it has been amply demonstrated that nitroglycerin increases the work capacity before anginal pain or ECG evidence of myocardial ischemia occur. Under conditions of enforced work, cardiac output does not fall, nor is the hypotensive effect of the drug obvious. It could be that the *nitrites* may act by redistributing coronary flow to the ischemic areas. The large coronary vessels do not participate in autoregulation, yet they are dilated by nitroglycerin. The large arteriosclerotic vessels probably do not respond, because of their diseased state. However, ischemic areas of the myocardium may receive part of their blood supply from collateral vessels arising from adjacent coronary arteries of normal elasticity. If these vessels are dilated by nitroglycerin, blood flow to the ischemic area could be increased by the diversion of blood through collateral channels. This may well represent an important mechanism of action.

Nitroglycerin has a duration of action of approximately 30 minutes. *Erythrityl tetranitrate,* administered sublingually, can increase exercise tolerance for a period of 2 hours, although its effects are not so predictable as those of nitroglycerin. The efficacy of the oral administration of the *long-acting organic nitrates* for the prophylaxis of anginal attacks is much more difficult to document. Experimental evidence of efficacy usually depends upon a record, kept by the patient, of the frequency of attacks and his dependence on nitroglycerin. Increased oxygen demands of the heart can arise from a variety of causes—primarily anxiety and emotional stress—that lead to sympathosuprarenal discharge and increased work of the heart. Thus, any medication given to the patient, with a reassurance by the physician as to its effectiveness, tends to allay anxiety and thus exert a favorable influence. Consequently, placebo effects, in the treatment of angina pectoris, may be as high as 50 percent. Under these circumstances, it takes a very carefully controlled study to establish the benefit of long-acting prophylactic preparations. Despite the absence of unequivocal evidence of efficacy, the long-acting organic nitrate preparations are widely employed and, in the absence of more effective compounds, represent an important part of the physician's therapeutic armamentarium.

A variety of compounds, other than the nitrites, have been employed for the treatment of angina pectoris. Other vasodilators have proved less effective than nitrites. It has been claimed that MAO inhibitors reduce the incidence of anginal attacks, but the rationale for their use is not clear, and well-controlled proof of efficacy is lacking. *Xanthines* can increase coronary blood flow but, as indicated above, they also increase the work of the heart and therefore have little or no therapeutic benefit in the control of anginal pain. The rationale for the use of *β-adrenergic blocking agents,* such as *propranolol,* was presented earlier, but its dangers may override its advantages. As an extreme measure, *thyroidectomy* or *antithyroid drugs* have been employed to reduce overall oxygen demand and thus decrease the demands on cardiac output. Furthermore, there is a synergistic action between the *thyroid hormones* and *catecholamine.* However, it is a rather drastic procedure to substitute one disease for another, unless the angina is incapacitating.

Drugs in the Treatment of Arrhythmias

In simplest terms, cardiac arrhythmias result from conduction disturbances, abnormal impulse formation, or a combination of both. In certain types of conduction disturbances, *e.g.,* complete heart block due to a lesion in the conduction system, drugs such as isoproterenol can only increase automaticity in the heart and increase

(Continued on page 109)

the rate of impulse formation at an ectopic site. In such conditions, drugs have largely been replaced by electronic pacemakers. However, other types of arrhythmias sometimes can be terminated by drugs, and their recurrence may be prevented by prophylactic therapy owing to the effects of the drugs on impulse formation, conduction velocity, and the refractory period. In the following discussion an attempt will be made to present briefly some of the current concepts of the pathological physiology of cardiac arrhythmias and the characteristic features of the drugs that are effective in their prophylaxis and treatment.

First, it should be recalled that many cells of the heart have inherent automaticity (automatic cells). These consist mainly of cells of the S-A node, certain cells of the atrium and A-V node, and those of the His-Purkinje system. All so-called automatic cells are potential sites of pacemaker activity. The transmembrane potentials recorded from an automatic cell differ, in one very important respect, from the potentials of most cells responsible for the contractile mechanisms of the heart. In the unipolar electrogram of a single cardiac fiber (see page 48), it will be observed that, following repolarization, the membrane remains polarized (diastolic polarization). It will not depolarize until the next impulse arrives and reduces the transmembrane potential from its resting diastolic-potential level to a threshold potential which initiates depolarization. In ordinary fibers the threshold potential is approximately -65 millivolts. In automatic fibers the unipolar electrogram differs in one important respect: after repolarization, the membrane does not remain polarized; instead, a slow spontaneous depolarization occurs. When this spontaneous depolarization reaches the threshold-potential level, the characteristic *action potential* is initiated and propagated. The rate of firing of any pacemaker site will be determined by three major factors: (1) the rate of spontaneous depolarization during phase 4 (see page 48); (2) the initial resting potential; (3) the threshold potential. The first is the most important. The faster or slower the rate of spontaneous depolarization, the sooner or later the threshold potential will be reached, and, thus, the faster or slower will be the rate of impulse formation. Assuming a constant rate of spontaneous depolarization, it will take longer to reach a threshold potential if the membrane is hyperpolarized than if it is partially depolarized. Also, a change in threshold potential can obviously change the rate of firing, all other events remaining constant.

Normally, automaticity is greatest in the S-A node, and the rate of impulse generation at this site determines the heart rate. Changes in heart rate are the result of changes in vagal or sympathetic-nerve activity (rate of acetylcholine or norepinephrine release). The neurohumors alter the electrical characteristics of the pacemaker exactly as expected and as described below.

Although normally the S-A node is the dominant spontaneous pacemaker, a number of physical and chemical alterations can occur in the myocardium and lead to increased automaticity. These are so numerous as to explain why every "normal" individual may experience premature systoles due to a localized increased automaticity in a potential pacemaker anywhere along the conduction system. Usually these are of little clinical importance; however, major and persistent changes in automaticity can occur, leading to pulsus alternans and serious tachycardias.

Among the physical mechanisms that can increase automaticity, the most important is stretch (see page 39). Thus, the dilated failing heart may exhibit ectopic pacemaker activity, and this may be corrected when compensation has been restored with digitalis, even though digitalis itself is capable of increasing automaticity. A decrease in pH, an increase in pCO_2, and a decrease in pO_2 can also increase automaticity. Among the various ions, changes in extracellular potassium concentration alter the maximum diastolic potential as well as the slope of phase 4; thus, hypopotassemia increases and hyperpotassemia decreases the likelihood of ectopic pacemaker activity. Calcium ions also exert a marked effect. An increase in ionized calcium displaces the threshold potential to a lower value, but a decrease in calcium not only has the opposite effect on threshold but also increases the slope of phase 4. Acetylcholine both decreases the slope of phase 4 and hyperpolarizes the membrane; therefore, it greatly decreases the rate of impulse formation. This is most prominent at the S-A node and the automatic fibers found in the atrium. Acetylcholine has little effect on the automaticity of fibers in the His-Purkinje system; therefore, an increase in reflex vagal activity is often effective in the treatment of supraventricular tachycardia, but it is of little value for correcting a tachycardia of ventricular origin. Increased sympathetic activity or injected catecholamines greatly augment automaticity by increasing markedly the slope of phase 4. This occurs throughout the entire conduction system and, normally, would result in pronounced sinus tachycardia. However, if reflex vagal activity decreases supraventricular automaticity, then single or multifocal ectopic pacemakers may arise in the ventricle, leading to severe, possibly fatal, arrhythmias. Digitalis markedly increases the automaticity in the His-Purkinje system. It also, in high dosage, causes A-V block. This accounts for the dangerous ventricular tachycardia that can occur with digitalis overdosage.

Reentry phenomena are also a major cause of arrhythmias. Reentry occurs when an impulse is forced to make a one-way transit around refractory cardiac tissue, regardless of the cause of refractoriness. If the course of the impulse is sufficiently long and the conduction velocity is sufficiently slow, the impulse, on returning to its original source, may find this source to be once more excitable; thus, a perpetual arrhythmia may be established. This may account for some cases of atrial flutter. Atrial fibrillation is believed to be caused by an ectopic focus firing at a frequency too high for the auricular muscle to follow, so that no organized beat occurs, or possibly by a circus movement as described above.

Reentry phenomena need not involve long pathways but can result from a current of injury. This occurs when adjacent fibers repolarize at different rates (*e.g.*, when one fiber is compromised by hypoxia, possibly due to coronary insufficiency, whereas a neighboring fiber is in a normal environment). The resulting potential difference may be sufficient to reexcite the first cell that becomes repolarized. Once the two cells are out of phase, the possibility of repetitive reciprocal activation between them would exist. This explanation could account for the severe arrhythmias that accompany myocardial infarction.

Finally, severe arrhythmias may result from altered conduction. Thus, if conduction proceeds normally in one branch of the Purkinje system and is slowed in another branch with unidirectional block, the latter impulse may reach the ventricular cells after they have recovered from the excitation caused by the normally conducted impulses, and they may contract again in response to the more slowly conducted impulse, resulting in a pulsus alternans.

Only four drugs are commonly used for the treatment of cardiac arrhythmias. Digitalis, as previously discussed, markedly slows A-V conduction and permits fewer impulses to pass through the A-V node. It is used as an antiarrhythmic agent almost exclusively in the treatment of supraventricular tachycardia and atrial flutter and fibrillation. It does not terminate the arrhythmia but does slow the ventricular rate. It will not be further discussed.

Other important antiarrhythmic drugs are quinidine, procainamide, and lidocaine hydrochloride. The last is used intravenously for acute arrhythmias; the former two are used for the treatment of acute arrhythmias and for prophylaxis. All share four properties in common that account for their antiarrhythmic activity and, in some cases, for arrhythmogenic properties: (1) a marked decrease in the automaticity of ectopic foci produced by a pronounced decrease in the slope of phase-4 spontaneous repolarization; (2) an increase in the threshold of excitability; (3) an increase in the "effective" refractory period, which may be due primarily to delayed repolarization during phase 2 or 3 of the electromyogram; and (4) a slowing of conduction velocity.

Automaticity. Changes in automaticity are probably responsible for the antiarrhythmic properties of quinidine and allied agents when these arrhythmias are caused by ectopic pacemaker activity. It is of interest that the effects of quinidine on spontaneous pacemaker activity are more pronounced at an ectopic site than at the normal pacemaker of the S-A node, probably because quinidine has a vagolytic action which would tend to increase automaticity of the S-A node.

Excitability. An increase in the threshold of excitability is observed only with high doses of quinidine and allied drugs. Theoretically, this property may exert a salutary effect on the arrhythmias owing to altered automaticity or to reentry phenomena due to a current of injury. However, the latter is probably much more susceptible to changes in the refractory period.

Refractory Period. The marked effect of quinidine and allied drugs on the refractory period is an important property of antiarrhythmic drugs that explains their effectiveness in arrhythmias involving reentry phenomena. For example, if auricular flutter or fibrillation is due to a circus movement, the latter's perpetuation requires reentry into excitable tissue. If the refractory period is prolonged, the impulse on reentry will find unexcitable tissues, and the fibrillation will be terminated. This also can pertain to reentry phenomena due to a current of injury.

Slowing of Conduction Velocity. This phenomenon has little to do with the antiarrhythmic effects of quinidine and allied drugs. For example, in the case of circus movement, if conduction is slowed more than the refractory period, the advancing wave of depolarization will always find excitable tissue in its path.

In this modern electronic age, termination of arrhythmias is not confined to the use of drugs. Electroshock therapy is being used more and more in the arrest of atrial flutter and fibrillation, supraventricular and ventricular tachycardia, and ventricular fibrillation. However, drugs will always play an important role in the prophylaxis of arrhythmias, and we can look forward to new and more effective agents in this field.

Section III

EMBRYOLOGY

by

FRANK H. NETTER, M.D.

in collaboration with

LODEWYK H. S. VAN MIEROP, M.D.
Plates 1-17

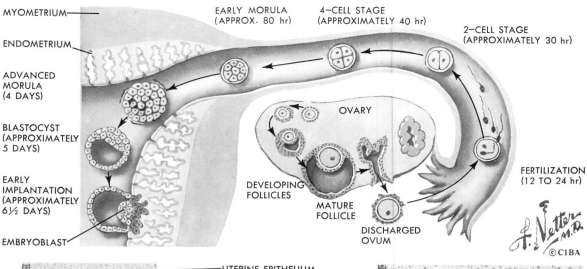

MYOMETRIUM

ENDOMETRIUM

ADVANCED MORULA (4 DAYS)

BLASTOCYST (APPROXIMATELY 5 DAYS)

EARLY IMPLANTATION (APPROXIMATELY 6½ DAYS)

EMBRYOBLAST

EARLY MORULA (APPROX. 80 hr)

4–CELL STAGE (APPROXIMATELY 40 hr)

2–CELL STAGE (APPROXIMATELY 30 hr)

OVARY

DEVELOPING FOLLICLES

MATURE FOLLICLE

DISCHARGED OVUM

FERTILIZATION (12 TO 24 hr)

AGE OF THE EMBRYO

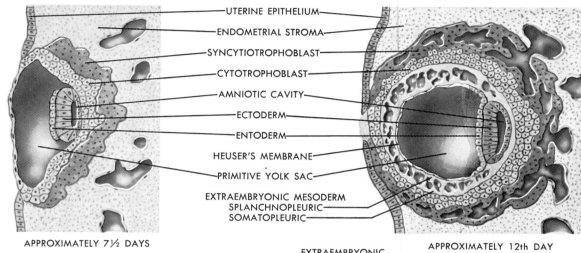

UTERINE EPITHELIUM

ENDOMETRIAL STROMA

SYNCYTIOTROPHOBLAST

CYTOTROPHOBLAST

AMNIOTIC CAVITY

ECTODERM

ENTODERM

HEUSER'S MEMBRANE

PRIMITIVE YOLK SAC

EXTRAEMBRYONIC MESODERM
SPLANCHNOPLEURIC
SOMATOPLEURIC

APPROXIMATELY 7½ DAYS

APPROXIMATELY 12th DAY

EXTRAEMBRYONIC MESODERM

PROCHORDAL PLATE

YOLK SAC

ENTODERM

ECTODERM

AMNIOTIC CAVITY

CONNECTING STALK

INTRAEMBRYONIC MESODERM

CYTOTROPHOBLAST

SYNCYTIOTROPHOBLAST

EXTRAEMBRYONIC CELOM

ENDOMETRIUM

EXOCELOMIC CYST

APPROXIMATELY 15th DAY

APPROXIMATELY 17th DAY

In most normal women, ovulation occurs approximately every 4 weeks. Usually, this event passes unnoticed; only in a small minority of women is it associated with lower abdominal pain, of varying intensity (Mittelschmerz), or some blood-tinged vaginal discharge.

Much more obvious is the phenomenon which takes place about 14 days after ovulation, if *fertilization* has not taken place. This phenomenon, occurring in both man and the higher primates, is called *menstruation*. The highly developed glandular and vascular *endometrium* breaks down and is largely shed, an event which is accompanied by a variable amount of bleeding and which generally lasts for about 4 to 5 days.

Because menstruation is obvious, and most women remember fairly accurately when they had their last "period," it is generally used as the basis for calculating the duration of pregnancy and the date of the expected confinement. This can be done with acceptable accuracy if

the periods are known to be regular, regardless of the duration of individual menstrual cycles, since, irrespective of the length of the latter, the interval between ovulation and subsequent menstruation is amazingly constant (14 ± 1 day). Longer or shorter periods are due to varying lengths of the endometrial-proliferation phase between the last day of menstruation and ovulation.

From the above discussion it is apparent that the age of an embryo can be given in two ways: (1) from the time of ovulation (ovulation age) or (2) from the time of the first day of the preceding menstrual period (menstrual age).

In obstetrical practice, menstrual age is usually used, but, because of its inherent inaccuracy, ovulation age is preferred in embryological studies. At pres-

ent, with a large and increasing amount of human and primate embryological material available, the ovulation age of human embryos can be estimated with considerable accuracy.

It is common practice, and desirable, to indicate the age of an embryo not only by its ovulation age but also by a more or less descriptive term. In the first 3 weeks, such a term generally describes the appearance of the whole embryo (*2-cell stage, morula, blastocyst,* etc.). At the end of the third week (20 to 21 days), the paraxial *mesoderm* begins to differentiate symmetrically and successively into paired blocks, called *somites,* in a craniocaudal direction, until about 44 pairs are formed. Between the 20th (1-somite) day and the 30th (28-somite) day, the number of

(Continued on page 113)

(Continued from page 112)

paired somites is usually given, in addition to the ovulation age, in days. Thereafter, counting somites becomes increasingly difficult, so a measurement of length is used. Generally, the distance between the vertex and breech, or the *crown-rump* (C-R) length (sitting height), is used. Additional measurements, such as the *crown-heel* length (standing height) and the weight, may be used during the fetal period, *i.e.,* from 3 months to term.

Early Embryonic Development

In man, as in most other primates, fertilization probably takes place in the proximal part of the uterine tube, near its fimbriated end, about *12 to 24 hours* after ovulation. The *ovum* is transported to the uterus by rhythmic contractions of the tube, aided by the action of the cilia of the epithelium. During this voyage, which takes about *4 days,* the ovum executes a number of cell divisions and, on reaching the uterus, consists of a clump of cells (*morula*) but has not increased appreciably in size.

After entering the uterus, the morula takes up fluid from its surroundings and enlarges until a *blastocyst* is formed. The wall of the blastocyst consists of a single layer of flattened cells, the *trophoblast,* and an eccentrically placed mass of cells, the inner cell mass or *embryoblast.* The trophoblast is responsible for the attachment of the blastocyst to the *uterine epithelium* and its subsequent *implantation* into the endometrium. Its cells soon differentiate into a *cyto-* and a *syncytiotrophoblast* and will eventually form the outer embryonic membrane (the *chorion*) and the fetal portion of the *placenta.* The embryo develops from the inner cell mass, which also contributes to the formation of the *amnion* and the *yolk sac.*

Soon after implantation, the cells of the inner mass differentiate into two layers — an inner layer of more or less flattened cells (the *entoderm*) and an outer layer of columnar cells (the *ectoderm*). Together, these two layers form the embryonic disc. At the same time, a space appears between the inner cell mass and the overlying trophoblast. This space, the *amniotic cavity,* is lined by the columnar ectodermal cells of the embryonic disc and by amniogenic cells derived from the trophoblast.

The cavity of the blastocyst becomes lined on the inside by entodermal cells migrating from the inner cell mass to form the *primitive yolk sac.* At the same time, or at least very soon thereafter, the entodermal cells of the primitive yolk sac are separated from the trophoblast by *extraembryonic mesoderm,* which assumes a loose reticular appearance. The embryo proper now is a disc made up of two layers of cells from which all the *intraembryonic* tissues will be derived: (1) the ectoderm, consisting of columnar cells in contact with (2) the cuboidal entodermal cells which form the roof of the primitive yolk sac. The remainder of the entodermal cells lining the yolk sac and in contact with the extraembryonic mesoderm form a membranous layer called *Heuser's membrane.**

The initially small cavities in the reticular extraembryonic mesoderm enlarge and become confluent (*extraembryonic celom*), except for a mesodermal stalk which connects the amnion to the trophoblast. This remaining mesodermal stalk later forms the *connecting* or *body stalk.*

With the formation of the extraembryonic celom, the extraembryonic mesoderm becomes separated into two layers — a parietal *somatopleuric* layer lining the trophoblast and part of the amnion, and a visceral *splanchnopleuric* layer covering the yolk sac.

At the same time, much of the primitive or primary yolk sac is pinched off, a process which results in the formation of the much smaller secondary yolk sac and a number of (*exocelomic*) cysts.

In the eventual cephalic end of the bilaminar disc, the entoderm thickens somewhat into the *prochordal plate.* Its appearance is the earliest indication of bilateral symmetry of the embryonic disc. At the opposite end of the disc, ectodermal cells begin to proliferate and migrate between the ectoderm and the entoderm to give rise to the third germ layer, the *intraembryonic mesoderm.* The exact manner in which this occurs, as well as the appearance and significance of such structures as *Hensen's node,* the *primitive streak,* and the *notochordal process* are topics which fall outside the scope of this book and will not be discussed here.

The mesodermal cells migrate laterally and cranially until, finally, ectoderm and entoderm are separated everywhere from each other by intraembryonic mesoderm, except at the prochordal plate, which remains bilaminar. This bilaminar part later becomes the *buccopharyngeal membrane* (see page 115). Laterally, all along the margin of the embryonic disc, the intraembryonic mesoderm is continuous with the extraembryonic mesoderm. The embryo, now trilaminar, becomes more elongated and pear-shaped when viewed from its dorsal (ectodermal) or ventral (entodermal) side. It is attached, at its narrow caudal end, to the extraembryonic portion of the ovum by the *connecting* or *body stalk* (see page 114).

The ovulation age of the embryo, at this stage of development, is about *20 days,* and its length is almost *1.5 mm.* The time is now rapidly approaching when simple physicochemical processes cannot adequately provide for the greatly increasing metabolic needs of the embryo, and a functional circulatory system becomes necessary.

---

*The origin of the mesotheloid cells forming Heuser's membrane is still uncertain. They may be derived from the entoderm (as in the macaque monkey) or they may differentiate locally from the cytotrophoblast. The primary or primitive yolk sac is also called the exocelomic cavity, a term which may be confused with extraembryonic celom.

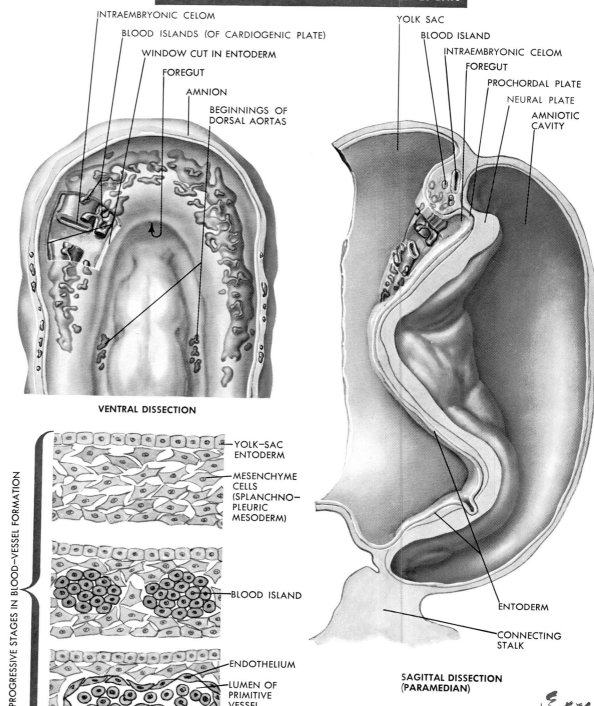

INTRAEMBRYONIC CELOM

BLOOD ISLANDS (OF CARDIOGENIC PLATE)

WINDOW CUT IN ENTODERM

FOREGUT

AMNION

BEGINNINGS OF DORSAL AORTAS

YOLK SAC

BLOOD ISLAND

INTRAEMBRYONIC CELOM

FOREGUT

PROCHORDAL PLATE

NEURAL PLATE

AMNIOTIC CAVITY

VENTRAL DISSECTION

YOLK–SAC ENTODERM

MESENCHYME CELLS (SPLANCHNO-PLEURIC MESODERM)

BLOOD ISLAND

ENDOTHELIUM

LUMEN OF PRIMITIVE VESSEL

PRIMITIVE BLOOD CELL

PROGRESSIVE STAGES IN BLOOD–VESSEL FORMATION

ENTODERM

CONNECTING STALK

SAGITTAL DISSECTION (PARAMEDIAN)

EARLY INTRAEMBRYONIC VASCULOGENESIS

Although the cardiovascular system is not the first organ system to make its appearance in the embryo, it reaches a functional state long before any of the others. It is further remarkable in that it does so while still in a relatively primitive state of development. The vascular system grows from a simple, bilaterally symmetrical plexus into an asymmetrical complex system of arteries, veins, and capillaries—a necessarily dynamic process involving the formation of new vessels and temporary detours, rerouting of the bloodstream, and the disappearance of previously dominant channels or even of entire vascular subsystems. It has to enlarge as the embryo grows; it must adapt itself to marked changes in the shape of the embryo and to the developmental changes taking place in the other organ systems. At the same time, while it is hard at work, the heart has to grow and differentiate from a simple tube into a complex four-chambered organ, possessing four sets of valves. Finally, because the very young embryo is tiny compared to the mass of extraembryonic (placental) tissue which the young heart also supplies with blood, this heart is relatively enormous as compared to the same organ in the adult.

Before describing the development of the cardiovascular system, it is necessary to relate briefly two processes which take place in the intraembryonic mesoderm; these are the appearance of the *intra-embryonic celom* and the formation of *somites*.

The intraembryonic celom or body cavity is formed by the confluence of small, initially isolated spaces, which appear in the lateral mesoderm. The resulting celomic cavities extend cranially and fuse with each other just anterior to the *prochordal plate*, resulting in a single horseshoe-shaped cavity. Somewhat later in development, a communication develops, on each side, between the caudal ends of the intraembryonic celom and the *extraembryonic celom* (see page 112).

The formation of the celom has sepa-

rated the mesoderm into two layers — the *parietal* or *somatopleuric mesoderm* in contact with the ectoderm, and the *visceral* or *splanchnopleuric mesoderm* in contact with the entoderm.

In the late *presomite* embryo, scattered masses of cells (*angiogenic cells*) appear in the mesenchyme derived from the splanchnopleuric mesoderm (*cardiogenic plate*) ventral to the anterior, horseshoe-shaped portion of the intraembryonic celom. From this anterior part of the celom will develop the *pericardial cavity* (see page 115). It lies, at this stage of development, anterior and lateral to the buccopharyngeal membrane or prochordal plate which separates it from the ectodermal neural plate.

The angiogenic cell clusters (*blood islands*) rapidly increase in number and size, acquire a *lumen*, unite, and form a plexus of vessels. From this plexus, which is, obviously, also horseshoe-shaped, the endocardial

tube will develop. The lateral portions of the plexus become simplified by coalescence into single *endothelial* tubes; initially, the central part of the plexus retains its plexiform condition.

Meanwhile, other clusters of angiogenic tissue have appeared bilaterally, parallel and rather close to the midline of the embryonic shield. These, too, acquire a lumen and form a pair of longitudinal vessels, the *dorsal aortas*. These vessels gain connections with the dorsocaudal aspect of the endothelial (*endocardial*) heart tubes, thereby establishing the arterial pole of the developing heart (see page 115). The caudal ends of the lateral endothelial heart tubes make contact with vessels arising in the yolk-sac mesoderm (*vitelline veins*) and, somewhat later, also with the developing *umbilical veins* (see page 116). Thus, the venous pole of the heart, still paired, is determined.

FORMATION OF THE
HEART TUBE

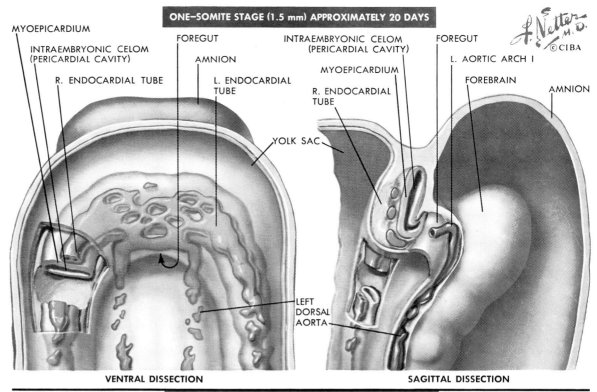

ONE-SOMITE STAGE (1.5 mm) APPROXIMATELY 20 DAYS

MYOEPICARDIUM

INTRAEMBRYONIC CELOM
(PERICARDIAL CAVITY)

R. ENDOCARDIAL TUBE

FOREGUT

AMNION

L. ENDOCARDIAL
TUBE

INTRAEMBRYONIC CELOM
(PERICARDIAL CAVITY)

MYOEPICARDIUM

R. ENDOCARDIAL
TUBE

FOREGUT

L. AORTIC ARCH I

FOREBRAIN

AMNION

YOLK SAC

LEFT
DORSAL
AORTA

VENTRAL DISSECTION

SAGITTAL DISSECTION

TWO-SOMITE STAGE (1.8 mm) APPROXIMATELY 21 DAYS

L. ENDOCARDIAL TUBE
COMMUNICATIONS
BETWEEN L. AND R.
ENDOCARDIAL TUBES
R. ENDOCARDIAL
TUBE

FOREGUT

AMNION

MYOEPICARDIUM
PERICARDIAL CAVITY
PERICARDIUM
ENTODERM

CARDIAC
JELLY

R. ENDOCARDIAL TUBE
BUCCOPHARYNGEAL MEMBRANE
FOREGUT

L. AORTIC ARCH I

AMNION

YOLK
SAC

L. AND R.
VITELLO-
UMBILICAL
VEINS

L. DORSAL
AORTA

VENTRAL DISSECTION

SAGITTAL DISSECTION

While the previously described, primitive, bilaterally symmetrical cardiovascular system makes its appearance, growth processes elsewhere profoundly influence the relative position of the cardiac portion of this system. The ectoderm of the anterior portion of the neural plate (the *forebrain*) grows rapidly, mainly in a cranial direction; it grows so swiftly that it successively carries with it, first, the adjacent part of the *buccopharyngeal membrane*, then more and more of this membrane, and, finally, all of it. In the same manner, the midcentral part of the cardiogenic plate and, to a lesser extent, the lateral parts of this plate are carried along simultaneously. This results in rotation of the buccopharyngeal membrane and the cardiac area, including the pericardial portion of the celom, along a transverse axis over approximately 180 degrees. This process, of course, is

much easier to illustrate than it is to describe.

Two other consequences of this growth process, which probably take place in a day or less, are: (1) acquisition by the *yolk sac* of an anterior diverticulum, the *foregut,* and (2) the *dorsal aortas* leaving the *endocardial tubes* at their now-cranial aspect, each aorta describing an arc along either side of the cranial end of the foregut. Thus, the first pair of *aortic arches* makes its appearance.

Similar, but less-pronounced, differential growth takes place all around the embryonic shield, particularly at its caudal end where the *hindgut* is formed in the same manner as the foregut. The originally flat embryonic shield curves in both an anteroposterior (craniocaudal) and a transverse direction. Its dorsal (ectodermal) surface becomes increasingly convex

and its ventral (*entodermal*) surface concave, while the secondary yolk sac assumes a dumbbell shape. The smaller part of the dumbbell comes to lie within the body of the embryo and may now be called the *midgut*. The larger part of the dumbbell is the definitive yolk sac; the narrow, intermediate portion becomes narrower and longer as growth progresses and is called the *vitelline duct*.

As a result of all these changes, the endothelial heart (endocardial) tubes have come to lie closer and parallel to each other, beginning with the arterial pole and progressing toward the venous pole.

Meanwhile, the splanchnopleure in the region of the cardiogenic plate overlying the heart tubes, now forming the dorsal wall of the *pericardial cavity,*

(Continued on page 116)

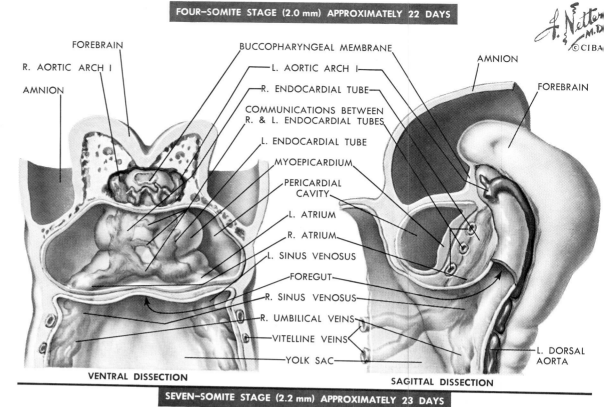

FOUR-SOMITE STAGE (2.0 mm) APPROXIMATELY 22 DAYS

FOREBRAIN
R. AORTIC ARCH I
AMNION
BUCCOPHARYNGEAL MEMBRANE
L. AORTIC ARCH I
R. ENDOCARDIAL TUBE
COMMUNICATIONS BETWEEN R. & L. ENDOCARDIAL TUBES
L. ENDOCARDIAL TUBE
MYOEPICARDIUM
PERICARDIAL CAVITY
L. ATRIUM
R. ATRIUM
L. SINUS VENOSUS
FOREGUT
R. SINUS VENOSUS
R. UMBILICAL VEINS
VITELLINE VEINS
YOLK SAC
AMNION
FOREBRAIN
L. DORSAL AORTA

VENTRAL DISSECTION   **SAGITTAL DISSECTION**

SEVEN-SOMITE STAGE (2.2 mm) APPROXIMATELY 23 DAYS

FOREBRAIN
R. AORTIC ARCH I
AMNION
BUCCOPHARYNGEAL MEMBRANE
L. AORTIC ARCH I
AORTIC SAC
BULBUS CORDIS
MYOEPICARDIUM
CARDIAC JELLY
PERICARDIAL CAVITY
VENTRICLE
R. ATRIUM
L. ATRIUM
R. SINUS VENOSUS
L. SINUS VENOSUS
FOREGUT
DORSAL MYOCARDIUM
DORSAL MESOCARDIUM
L. DORSAL AORTA
VITELLINE VEINS
R. UMBILICAL VEIN

VENTRAL DISSECTION   **SAGITTAL DISSECTION**

FORMATION OF THE HEART TUBE

(Continued from page 115)

becomes invaginated by the heart tubes and bulges more and more into this cavity. The plexiform, median portion of the original horseshoe, still separating the left and right heart tubes from each other, gradually disappears, resulting in a fusion of the heart tubes in a craniocaudal direction. Invagination of the posterior pericardium continues until the now-single straight heart tube, with its investing splanchnopleure, comes to lie completely within the *pericardial cavity* and is attached dorsally only by a fold of tissue, the *dorsal mesocardium*.

From the foregoing description, it is apparent that the human embryonic heart does not possess a *ventral* mesocardium at any time. Actually, only the bulboventricular part of the heart lies wholly intrapericardially, most of the atrial portion of the heart and all of the *sinus venosus* remaining out-

side the pericardium until later in development.

The splanchnopleuric mesodermal tissue surrounding the *endothelial heart (endocardial) tube* meanwhile has differentiated into three layers. The inner layer, immediately around the endothelium, is initially much thicker. In histologic sections it appears to be rather structureless, stains lightly, and contains very few nuclei. Because of its appearance, it has been called *cardiac jelly*. The next layer stains much darker and is densely nucleated, although, at first, it is only a few cell layers thick. The third (outer) layer consists of flat mesothelial cells which also line the remainder of the pericardial cavity. Only the bulboventricular part of the heart has a thick layer of cardiac jelly; in the atrial and sinus venosus regions it is almost nonexistent, except for

a ring around the junction of the *right* and *left atria*.

The second and third layers together are generally referred to as the *myoepicardial mantle*, since the *epicardium* and *myocardium* will develop eventually from these layers. The embryo now has 7 *somites*, is about 2.2 *mm* long, and is *approximately 23 days* old. About 3 days have elapsed, therefore, between the appearance of intraembryonic vasculogenesis and the formation of the endocardial tube. It is at about this time, or somewhat earlier, that the heart begins to beat. No known cardiac anomaly can be traced back and said to have been initiated during the developmental phases described thus far, with the possible exception of the rare and special cases of acardiac monsters seen infrequently in those twins with a common placental circulation.

F. Netter M.D. ©CIBA

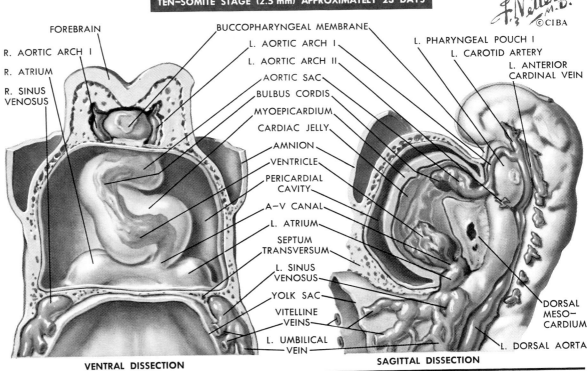

FOREBRAIN
R. AORTIC ARCH I
R. ATRIUM
R. SINUS VENOSUS
BUCCOPHARYNGEAL MEMBRANE
L. AORTIC ARCH I
L. AORTIC ARCH II
AORTIC SAC
BULBUS CORDIS
MYOEPICARDIUM
CARDIAC JELLY
AMNION
VENTRICLE
PERICARDIAL CAVITY
A-V CANAL
L. ATRIUM
SEPTUM TRANSVERSUM
L. SINUS VENOSUS
YOLK SAC
VITELLINE VEINS
L. UMBILICAL VEIN
L. PHARYNGEAL POUCH I
L. CAROTID ARTERY
L. ANTERIOR CARDINAL VEIN
DORSAL MESO-CARDIUM
L. DORSAL AORTA

VENTRAL DISSECTION   SAGITTAL DISSECTION

FORMATION OF THE HEART LOOP

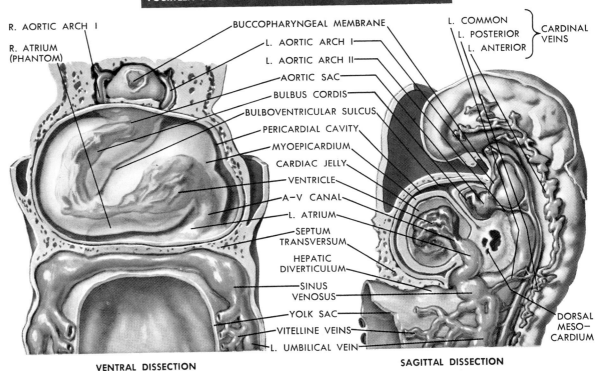

R. AORTIC ARCH I
R. ATRIUM (PHANTOM)
BUCCOPHARYNGEAL MEMBRANE
L. AORTIC ARCH I
L. AORTIC ARCH II
AORTIC SAC
BULBUS CORDIS
BULBOVENTRICULAR SULCUS
PERICARDIAL CAVITY
MYOEPICARDIUM
CARDIAC JELLY
VENTRICLE
A-V CANAL
L. ATRIUM
SEPTUM TRANSVERSUM
HEPATIC DIVERTICULUM
SINUS VENOSUS
YOLK SAC
VITELLINE VEINS
L. UMBILICAL VEIN
L. COMMON
L. POSTERIOR
L. ANTERIOR
CARDINAL VEINS
DORSAL MESO-CARDIUM

VENTRAL DISSECTION   SAGITTAL DISSECTION

At the beginning of the next phase of development, the bulboventricular part of the heart, as described earlier, is essentially a straight tube which lies free within the *pericardial cavity* and is attached posteriorly only by the *dorsal mesocardium*.

The cranial third of the tube is dilated and forms the *aortic sac*, from which originates the first pair of *aortic arches*. The caudal one third to one half is also slightly dilated. This is the early embryonic *ventricle*. The remaining, rather small, midportion will soon gain in importance and develop into the *bulbus cordis*.

The *atria* are still paired, only beginning to bulge into the pericardial cavity caudally and, therefore, lie extrapericardially embedded in the mesenchyme of the *septum transversum* and in a fixed position. While the embryo and the pericardial cavity show only a moderate increase in size during the next few days, the bulboventricular tube, particularly its midportion, continues to grow very rapidly in length. Because its two ends are fixed, the heart tube is forced to bend in order to adapt itself to the available pericardial space. At the same time, perforations appear in the dorsal mesocardium, leading to its disappearance as the openings increase in size.

Normally, the *bulboventricular loop* bends anteriorly and to the right. This has certain consequences: Externally, the originally straight left heart border becomes interrupted by an ever-increasing cleft, the *bulboventricular* (later, *conoventricuar*) *sulcus*. Since the bend-

ing of the tube involves all layers of its wall, the bulbo(cono)ventricular sulcus corresponds internally to a fold, the *bulbo(cono)ventricular* fold or *flange* (see page 120). Both the sulcus and the flange are very obvious and are well marked in fixed specimens. In living embryos, however, although the bend in the tube is pronounced, there is no actual kinking.

As a second consequence of the tube's bending, a certain amount of torsion occurs, since the ends of the tube are fixed. This twist is, at least in part, responsible for the position of the truncus and conus swellings, to be described later (see page 120).

Finally, the atrioventricular junction, which originally lies in the midline, is crowded laterally and comes to lie on the left side. At the same time, the early (*primitive*) embryonic *ventricle* (see page 118)

comes to lie in the left side of the pericardial cavity, and the right side of this cavity is now occupied by the tremendously elongated midportion of the original straight tube. This is the bulbus cordis.

While the foregoing events take place, the initial changes in the *endocardial* (heart) *tube* (see page 116) are concerned mainly with the development of local expansions throughout its length. The atrial portion of the heart, which, up to this point, consisted mainly of rather small *right* and *left primitive atria* (connected with each other by an equally small midportion), dilates considerably to form a large, almost common, atrium, the junction of the right and left atria being only slightly narrower than the atria themselves.

(Continued on page 118)

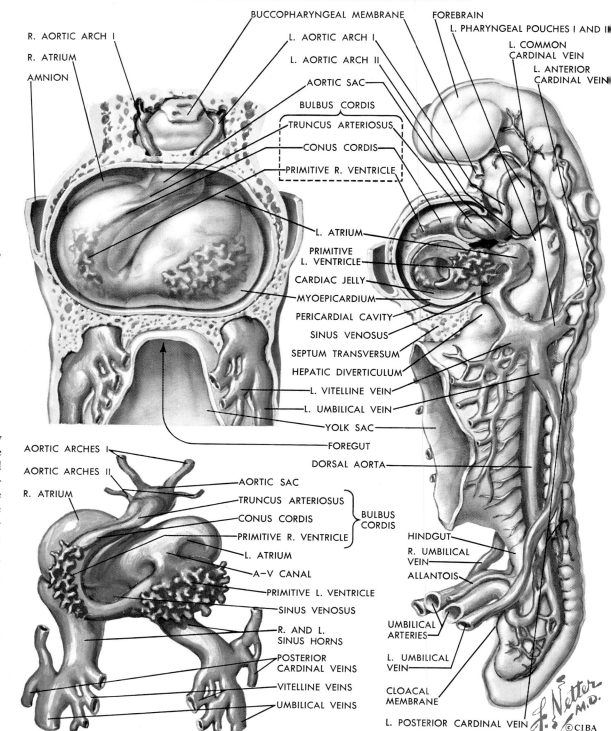

TWENTY-SOMITE STAGE (3.2 mm) APPROXIMATELY 25 DAYS

ENDOCARDIAL TUBE WITH MYOEPICARDIUM REMOVED

FORMATION OF THE HEART LOOP

(Continued from page 117)

This growth process takes place mainly in a dorsocranial direction, so that the atrium appears to "climb up" the dorsal pericardial wall, carrying with it the atrioventricular junction, which therefore assumes a more cranial position. The atrioventricular junction remains relatively narrow and may now be called the atrioventricular *(A-V) canal.* It forms the communication between the left side of the common atrium, *i.e.,* the *primitive left atrium* (see page 120), and the *primitive* embryonic *ventricle.* This ventricle also dilates and acquires a more capacious lumen which, as is true for the remainder of the heart, is still a rather smooth-walled structure. As with the atrioventricular canal, so also the junction of ventricle and *bulbus cordis* remains narrow. This junction, for reasons which will soon become apparent, may now be called the *primary interventricular foramen* (see page 124).

A further dilatation involves the proximal third of the bulbus cordis, the distal two thirds remaining relatively narrow for a time. At the venous end of the heart, growth proceeds to a point where the expanding common atrium has drawn the originally paired *sinus venosus* together until it consists, as did the atrium earlier, of a midportion and the *right* and *left sinus horns.* The wide sinoatrial junction lies in the midline, but, unlike the atria, the sinus horns will not normally form a large common chamber.

At the close of this phase of development, *diverticula* appear in two sharply defined areas along the ventral border of the endocardial tube just proximal to and

distal from the primary interventricular foramen, *i.e.,* in the early ventricle and in the proximal third of the bulbus cordis. These diverticula develop initially at the expense of the *cardiac jelly* and, later, of the *myoepicardium,* as the latter increases in thickness. They expand the capacity of the heart sections involved, giving them the densely trabeculated appearance so characteristic of young embryonic ventricles. The original, nontrabeculated, free lumen does not materially enlarge at first. Further developments will be taken up later.

At this point, although local elaborations have changed its appearance considerably, the heart still consists essentially of a single tube. Its external appearance, however, already strongly suggests its future four-chambered condition. This trabeculated,

early embryonic ventricle may be called the *primitive left ventricle,* since it will contribute the major portion of the definitive left ventricle. The proximal third of the bulbus cordis, also trabeculated, will become most of the future right ventricle and therefore may be called the *primitive right ventricle.*

The embryo is now about 3.2 *mm* long and *approximately 25 days* old, and it possesses 20 *somites.*

Abnormalities in the formation of the cardiac loop may be held responsible for such congenital cardiac malformations as ventricular inversion (usually associated with transposition of the great vessels and then known as corrected transposition), for juxtaposition of the atrial appendages (auricles), and probably also, at least in part, for the anomaly known as double-outlet right ventricle.

FORMATION OF THE CARDIAC SEPTA

At the close of the preceding phase of development, *i.e.*, in the 20-somite embryo, the heart completely occupies the *pericardial cavity*. The *primitive left ventricle* lies on the left and the *bulbus cordis* on the right, with the *primary interventricular foramen* (see page 124) connecting the two.

We have seen that the primitive left ventricle and the proximal third of the bulbus cordis become trabeculated along their ventral borders, owing to the formation of endocardial diverticula which invade the cardiac jelly and, later, the myocardium. Since the trabeculated part of the bulbus cordis will become most of the definitive right ventricle, it may now be called the *primitive right ventricle*. The adjacent third of the bulbus will form the outflow portions of both ventricles and may be indicated by the term *conus cordis*. (At times, the term "conus cordis" is confused with "conus arteriosus." The conus cordis is the *whole* segment of this particular part of the embryonic heart. As to partitioning into an anterolateral right ventricular portion and a posteromedial left ventricular portion, the term "conus arteriosus" [N.A.] is used for the anterolateral right ventricular portion *only*. "Conus cordis," an embryological term [Streeter], is therefore not equivalent to "conus arteriosus," which is an anatomical term.) The terminal third of the bulbus, after partition, develops into the proximal parts of the ascending aorta and the pulmonary trunk and therefore deserves the name *truncus arteriosus*. For reasons which will become apparent later, the most distal portion of the truncus arteriosus, together with the adjoining *aortic sac* from which the *aortic arches* (see page 118) arise, may be indicated by the term *truncoaortic sac*.

Further growth of the heart, particularly of the rapidly enlarging primitive atria, causes the truncoconal section of the bulbus cordis to shift from its far-lateral position in an embryo of about 3 mm (15 to 20 somites) to a more medial location, as seen in an embryo of about 5 mm. The result is that the truncus arteriosus comes to lie in a midsagittal position in a depression between the roofs of the *right* and *left primitive atria* (see page 120), and the conus cordis assumes an oblique position between the roof of the primitive left ventricle and the anteromedial wall of the right atrium.

The stage is now set for the septation of the heart. During this period, which lasts about 10 days (beginning in a *4-* to *5-mm* embryo, ovulation age *27 days*, and completed in a *16-* to *17-mm* embryo, age *37 days* [see pages 120 to 122]), no major changes in the external appearance of the heart take place. Its relative position, however, keeps changing because of the changing curvature of the embryo (particularly in the neck region) and the growth and development of neighboring organs. This makes it diffi-

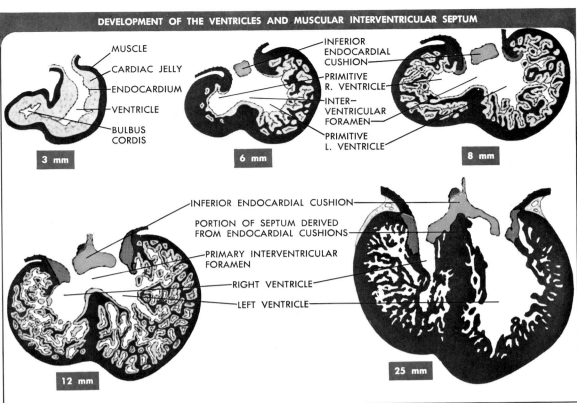

DEVELOPMENT OF THE VENTRICLES AND MUSCULAR INTERVENTRICULAR SEPTUM

MUSCLE
CARDIAC JELLY
ENDOCARDIUM
VENTRICLE
BULBUS CORDIS
3 mm

INFERIOR ENDOCARDIAL CUSHION
PRIMITIVE R. VENTRICLE
INTER-VENTRICULAR FORAMEN
PRIMITIVE L. VENTRICLE
6 mm   8 mm

INFERIOR ENDOCARDIAL CUSHION
PORTION OF SEPTUM DERIVED FROM ENDOCARDIAL CUSHIONS
PRIMARY INTERVENTRICULAR FORAMEN
RIGHT VENTRICLE
LEFT VENTRICLE
12 mm   25 mm

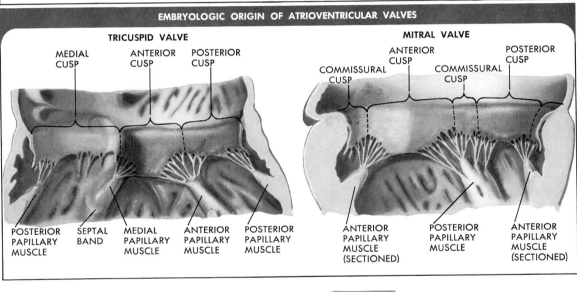

EMBRYOLOGIC ORIGIN OF ATRIOVENTRICULAR VALVES

TRICUSPID VALVE

MEDIAL CUSP   ANTERIOR CUSP   POSTERIOR CUSP

POSTERIOR PAPILLARY MUSCLE   SEPTAL BAND   MEDIAL PAPILLARY MUSCLE   ANTERIOR PAPILLARY MUSCLE   POSTERIOR PAPILLARY MUSCLE

MITRAL VALVE

ANTERIOR CUSP   POSTERIOR CUSP
COMMISSURAL CUSP   COMMISSURAL CUSP

ANTERIOR PAPILLARY MUSCLE (SECTIONED)   POSTERIOR PAPILLARY MUSCLE   ANTERIOR PAPILLARY MUSCLE (SECTIONED)

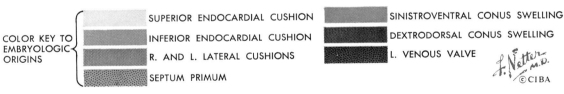

COLOR KEY TO EMBRYOLOGIC ORIGINS
- SUPERIOR ENDOCARDIAL CUSHION
- INFERIOR ENDOCARDIAL CUSHION
- R. AND L. LATERAL CUSHIONS
- SEPTUM PRIMUM
- SINISTROVENTRAL CONUS SWELLING
- DEXTRODORSAL CONUS SWELLING
- L. VENOUS VALVE

cult to appreciate spatial relationships. In the following discussion, therefore, the diaphragm (*septum transversum*) (see page 118) is assumed to maintain an approximately horizontal position, as in a standing person. The terms anterior (*front*), posterior, superior (*above*), and inferior are employed as indicated in the upper figure (see page 121).

The formation of the various cardiac septa takes place more or less simultaneously; for descriptive purposes, however, it is necessary to consider their development separately. This leads to a certain amount of unavoidable repetition which, in view of the complexity of the process of cardiac septation, may actually be an advantage.

Principles of Cardiac Septation

There are two fundamentally different ways in which a *septum* can be formed in a hollow organ such as the heart.

1. A relatively narrow segment of the organ, *e.g.*, the heart tube, does not increase in diameter or else does so relatively slowly; however, on both sides of the segment, rapid and expansive growth takes place. The portions of the walls of the expanded regions on each side of the narrow intervening segment come to face each other, appose, and may or may not fuse. If growth takes place more or less equally everywhere, the hollow organ at first assumes the shape of a dumbbell and, after fusion of the apposing walls, is transformed into an organ containing a diaphragm with a central opening. An example is the diaphragm which occasionally persists pathologically between the expanding common pulmonary vein and the primitive left atrium, resulting in a

(Continued on page 120)

FORMATION OF THE CARDIAC SEPTA

(Continued from page 119)

cardiac anomaly known as triatrial heart (see page 124).

Much more commonly, however, expansive growth takes place mainly in one direction, resulting in the formation of a septum with a very eccentrically placed communication between the two adjoining chambers. It is clear that a septum formed in this fashion is simply a reduplication of the wall of the organ. If fusion of the apposing walls occurs very early and keeps pace with the growth of the organ, the fact that the septum is a reduplication may never be very obvious, *e.g.,* the muscular ventricular septum in most birds and mammals. On the other hand, fusion may never occur, *e.g.,* the muscular ventricular septum in the manatee or sea cow.

It is clear that a septum formed passively, as described above, can never be complete; there is always an opening in it somewhere. Such an opening may be closed secondarily by a tissue contributed by neighboring structures, *e.g.,* closure of the *ostium primum* (see page 124) by extensions from the *endocardial cushions,* or by an adjacent septum, *e.g.,* closure of the foramen ovale by the *septum primum.*

Characteristically, passively formed septa are relatively thin even in the early phases of their development, their thickness being much less than their height.

2. The lumen of a hollow organ may be partitioned by the formation of two growing apposing masses of tissue which eventually touch each other and fuse. Such tissue masses have a very characteristic appearance in microscopic sections. They stain lightly, consist of rather undifferentiated mesenchymal cells, and contain relatively fewer nuclei than does the surrounding tissue. They are large and bulky and therefore are usually called *cushions* or *swellings.* Such actively formed septa are generally complete when fully developed. Characteristically, their thickness equals or exceeds their height in the early phases of their development; only secondarily do they become molded and transformed into thin septa.

The partition of the single heart tube into an organ consisting of four chambers, containing two pairs of valves and giving off two large arteries, is accomplished by the formation of seven septa.

Of these, three are formed passively (the *septum secundum* of the atrium, the muscular portion of the *ventricular septum,* and the *aorticopulmonary septum*). Three are formed actively (the *atrioventricular-canal septum,* the *conus septum,* and the *truncus septum*). One, the atrial *septum primum,* probably starts out as a passive formation but is completed by actively growing tissue (probably derived from the atrioventricular endocardial cushions) along its free margin.

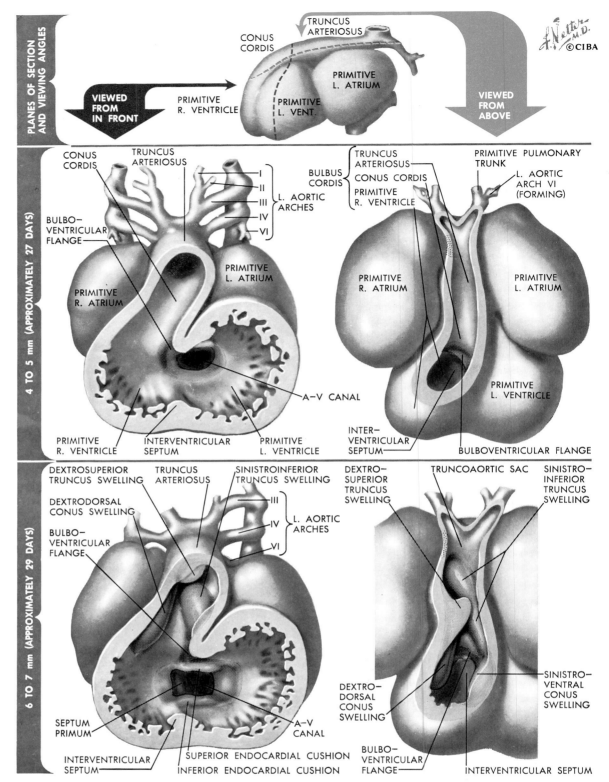

Development of the Ventricles and Cardiac Septa

The Ventricles

In the 20-somite embryo, the primitive right and left ventricles are little more than local widenings of the original cardiac tube. The formation of trabeculae in each has just begun, and they are connected to each other by a smooth-walled, relatively narrow channel, the *primary interventricular foramen* (see page 124).

In an embryo of about *4 to 5 mm* C-R (crown-rump) length, the atrioventricular (A-V) canal still leads into the primitive left ventricle, and blood can reach the primitive right ventricle only by way of the primary interventricular foramen. At this stage, the borders of the foramen are formed by the developing *interventricular septum* inferiorly and

anteriorly, and by the *bulbo(cono)ventricular flange* superiorly and posteriorly. The interventricular septum and the bulbo(cono)ventricular flange are continuous with each other; the distinction between the two is purely arbitrary but is useful for descriptive purposes.

Enlargement of the ventricles is accomplished by a centrifugal growth of the myocardium, always closely followed by increasing diverticulation and formation of trabeculae internally; this prevents the compact outer layer of the myocardium from becoming too thick and solid. It is interesting that the original free lumen of the ventricles retains its configuration for some time and enlarges at a relatively slow pace (see page 119). Typically, the ventricles of the embryonic heart consist of a tremendous mass of trabeculae enclosed by a rather thin outer layer of compact

(Continued on page 121)

FORMATION OF THE CARDIAC SEPTA

(Continued from page 120)

myocardium. In many lower animals, this condition persists, giving the ventricles a spongy appearance; in mammals, including man, most of the trabeculae eventually disappear. Of the trabeculae that remain, some coalesce to form larger structures, such as *papillary muscles,* the *moderator band,* and the *septal band;* others are reduced to thin fibrous strands, *e.g.,* the chordae tendineae of the atrioventricular valves.

Immediately adjacent to the atrioventricular orifices, the process of diverticulation takes place in a somewhat different manner. It leads to the formation of the atrioventricular valves and will be discussed in more detail later.

The medial walls of the growing and expanding ventricles appose and fuse, forming the major portion of the *muscular interventricular septum.* These fused medial walls also become trabeculated, particularly in their apical portions. On the right, a large trabecula, the septal band, appears early (in embryos of about 9 mm C-R length) and runs from the anteroinferior border of the primary interventricular foramen toward the apex, where it loses itself among apical trabeculae. One of these, the *moderator band* (septomarginal trabecula), is fairly constant and connects the septal band with the *anterior papillary muscle* and the parietal wall of the right ventricle (see page 122). It is of interest to note that in the manatee or sea cow the medial ventricular walls do not fuse, the two ventricles remaining almost completely separate. Lesser degrees of such nonfusion may occasionally be seen in human hearts, where it manifests itself as a more or less deep apical cleft (bifid apex).

The *primary interventricular (I-V) foramen* (see page 124), as we shall see, never closes but actually enlarges and, in the fully developed heart, gives access to the aortic vestibule. The enlargement of the foramen normally takes place at a much slower pace than does the growth of the ventricles. This gives the erroneous impression that the ventricular septum grows up from the apical portion of the ventricles.

The Atrioventricular Canal

Division of the *atrioventricular canal* into a right and a left atrioventricular orifice is executed by a pair of apposing masses of mesenchymal tissue which make their appearance at the superior and inferior borders of the canal in embryos of about 6 mm C-R length. Because of their histologic appearance, their position, and their origin, these masses have been called the atrioventricular endocardial cushions (pages 120 to 122). At this time, the atrioventricular canal and the truncoconal region of the heart have begun to realign themselves, and both have shifted medially from the far-lateral position (left and right, respec-

tively) seen in younger specimens. At 6 mm, this shift has not as yet been completed; the atrioventricular canal still gives access only to the *primitive left ventricle* and is separated from the *conus cordis* by the *bulbo(cono)ventricular flange.* With further development, this flange will have to recede and be effaced; only then can realignment of the *conus* and the atrioventricular canal progress to a point where blood can enter the *primitive right ventricle* directly from the *atrium.* In embryos of about 9 mm C-R length, the posterior extremity of the flange is seen to terminate almost midway along the base of the *superior endocardial cushion* and is much less prominent. In older embryos, both the shift to the left and the effacement continue until the flange eventually becomes unrecognizable as such. As a result, the plane of the *primary interventricular foramen* (see page 124) (the posterosuperior border of which is formed, as we have seen,

by the conoventricular flange) inclines more and more to the left from an originally vertical position. As a further result, direct access is gained from the primitive left ventricle to the *posteromedial portion of the conus cordis* (by way of the primary interventricular foramen) and therefore, as we shall see later, to the *aorta.*

Meanwhile, the atrioventricular canal has enlarged to the right, while the growing endocardial cushions project progressively into the lumen and approach each other. Similar, but much smaller, masses of tissue, the *lateral atrioventricular cushions,* appear on the right and left borders of the atrioventricular canal. The right and left extremities of both major cushions develop prominences — the right and left tubercles of the endocardial cushions.

In a *9-mm* embryo, the lumen of the atrioventric-

(Continued on page 122)

FORMATION OF THE CARDIAC SEPTA

(Continued from page 121)

ular canal, when seen from in front, is shaped like the classical dog's bone of the cartoonists. Shortly thereafter, the major cushions reach each other and begin to fuse, resulting in a complete division of the canal into *right* and *left atrioventricular orifices* in embryos of 10 to 11 mm (see page 124). At the same time, the cushions begin to bend and, after fusion, eventually form an arch which has its concavity directed anteriorly and toward the *left ventricle,* and its convexity posteriorly toward the atria. The free margin of the atrial *septum primum* meets the convex atrial side of the fused endocardial cushions about midway between their extremities and fuses with them. That portion of the endocardial cushions to the left of the septum primum eventually becomes the *anterior* or *aortic cusp* of the *mitral valve* and therefore does not participate in the formation of the cardiac septum.

With deepening of the endocardial-cushion arch or bay, the right halves of the fused endocardial cushions come to lie more and more in a sagittal plane, *i.e.,* at about the same plane but somewhat to the right of the *muscular interventricular septum* (see page 124). The communication still remaining between the *right* and *left ventricles,* the *secondary interventricular foramen,* is bordered at this point by the muscular ventricular septum inferiorly and anteriorly, the right tubercles of the fused endocardial cushions posteriorly, and the conus septum superiorly. The plane of the secondary interventricular foramen therefore inclines somewhat to the right, while that of the primary interventricular foramen, as we have seen, has come to deviate to the left. They share, however, the top of the muscular septum as part of their inferior borders. Before the closure of the secondary interventricular foramen can be discussed, it is necessary to direct our attention to the truncus arteriosus and the developments which have taken place there.

The Truncus Arteriosus

Septation of the truncoconal area of the *bulbus cordis* begins at about the 6-mm stage (see page 120), as in the A-V canal, with the appearance of two apposing masses of tissue in the midtruncus, the *truncus swellings.* In appearance, these closely resemble the atrioventricular *endocardial cushions.* One swelling is located on the dextrosuperior wall of the truncus (*dextrosuperior truncus swelling),* the other on the sinistroinferior wall (*sinistroinferior truncus swelling).* The former grows distally and to the left toward the *truncoaortic sac* along the roof of the truncus, the latter distally and to the right along its floor; *i.e.,* their directions of growth cross each other.

The swellings rapidly enlarge, soon touch each other over an increasing area,

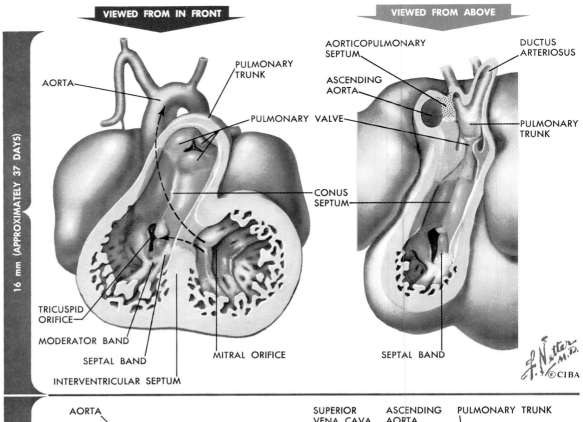

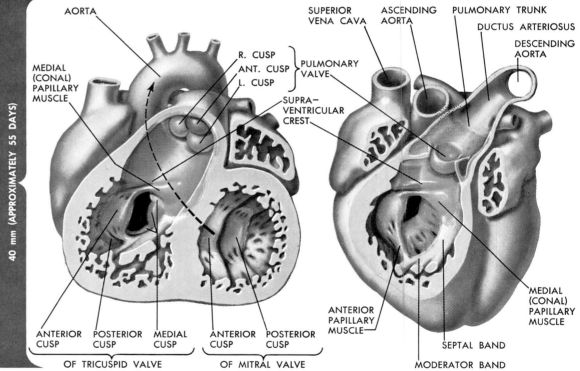

and fuse to form the truncus septum, thus dividing the truncus into an *aortic* and a *pulmonary channel* (see page 121). The truncus swellings (and therefore the truncus septum) are large and bulky, and, to accommodate them, the initially slender truncus area of the heart becomes quite bulbous.

Meanwhile, proximal extensions of the truncus swellings are meeting the distal extremities of a similar pair of mesenchymal masses developing in the conus cordis — the *conus swellings.* With further growth, the distal surface of the fused truncus swellings presents a front which faces the origin of the sixth aortic arches. The distal, still-undivided portion of the truncus, together with the adjacent aortic sac, dilates to form the truncoaortic sac. At the same time, the sixth arches move closer together and to the left, their most proximal portions possibly fusing for a short distance. The origins of the *fourth aortic arches*

(from the roof of the truncoaortic sac) (see page 120) shift somewhat to the right. As a result, the *sixth arches* become aligned with the pulmonary channel and the fourth arches with the aortic channel. At the same time, the dorsal wall of the truncoaortic sac, between the origins of the fourth and sixth arches, invaginates to form a short, rather thick, eventually vertically disposed septum, the *aorticopulmonary septum,* the leading edge of which approaches the distal face of the truncus septum and fuses with it.

Whereas the truncus swellings consist of typical, pale-staining, relatively cell-poor cardiac mesenchyme, the aorticopulmonary septum is composed of more densely nucleated tissue, histologically indistinguishable from the adjacent pretracheal tissues.

The partition of the truncoaortic area (and therefore the creation of the *pulmonary trunk* and the

(Continued on page 123)

FORMATION OF THE CARDIAC SEPTA

(Continued from page 122)

proximal *ascending aorta*) is now complete. The manner in which this occurs, as described above, accounts for most of the spiral course of the aorta and the pulmonary trunk around each other. Later growth, and particularly the considerable relative increase in diameter of these two vessels, accentuates this twist which is so characteristic of the fully developed normal heart.

The Conus Cordis

At about the time that the truncus swellings appear, another pair of endocardial mesenchymal masses can be seen. One of these is located on the dextrodorsal wall, the other on the sinistroventral wall, of the *conus cordis* (see page 120). They initially grow much more slowly than do their truncal counterparts; in a *9-mm* embryo, when the truncoaortic septum has been completed, the conus swellings have reached some prominence but are still widely separated from each other. The lumen of the truncocordal area, between the truncus septum distally and the conus swellings proximally, is oval in cross section. It is surrounded by cardiac mesenchyme which, although not equal in thickness along its circumference, does not project into the lumen as yet. Soon after the truncus septum has been completed, the conus swellings begin to grow rapidly toward each other and in a distal direction toward the truncus septum. The *dextrodorsal conus swelling* becomes continuous with the dextrosuperior truncus swelling, and the *sinistroventral conus swelling* with the sinistroinferior truncus swelling (see page 121). Fusion of the conus swellings presumably begins proximally, progressing rapidly in a distal direction to complete the partition of the truncoconal part of the heart. Theoretically, therefore, one would expect to find a stage where the proximal conus and the truncus are divided, but where the area in between is still patent. As yet, such a stage has not been observed in a human embryo. Apparently, the final phase of conotruncal partition takes place very rapidly and is completed in embryos of about *14 to 15 mm*. It is interesting, however, that in pig embryos of 20 to 25 mm, such an opening is still present, indicating an interesting species difference in the timing of cardiac partition, whereas the actual mechanism is the same or at least very similar.

The proximal extremity of the dextrodorsal conus swelling in a 7-mm embryo terminates to the right of the right lateral cushion of the atrioventricular canal and is separated from it by a groove. Growth of the primitive right ventricle, together with the enlargement and shift to the right of the atrioventricular canal, changes this relationship so that the dextrodorsal conus swelling comes to terminate at the superior border of the *right*

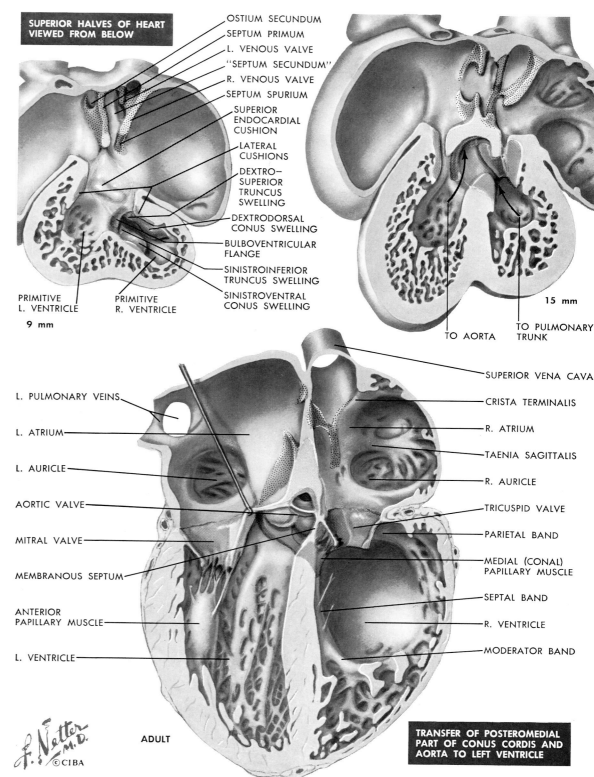

SUPERIOR HALVES OF HEART VIEWED FROM BELOW

OSTIUM SECUNDUM
SEPTUM PRIMUM
L. VENOUS VALVE
"SEPTUM SECUNDUM"
R. VENOUS VALVE
SEPTUM SPURIUM
SUPERIOR ENDOCARDIAL CUSHION
LATERAL CUSHIONS
DEXTRO-SUPERIOR TRUNCUS SWELLING
DEXTRODORSAL CONUS SWELLING
BULBOVENTRICULAR FLANGE
SINISTROINFERIOR TRUNCUS SWELLING
SINISTROVENTRAL CONUS SWELLING

PRIMITIVE L. VENTRICLE
PRIMITIVE R. VENTRICLE
9 mm

15 mm
TO AORTA
TO PULMONARY TRUNK

L. PULMONARY VEINS
L. ATRIUM
L. AURICLE
AORTIC VALVE
MITRAL VALVE
MEMBRANOUS SEPTUM
ANTERIOR PAPILLARY MUSCLE
L. VENTRICLE

SUPERIOR VENA CAVA
CRISTA TERMINALIS
R. ATRIUM
TAENIA SAGITTALIS
R. AURICLE
TRICUSPID VALVE
PARIETAL BAND
MEDIAL (CONAL) PAPILLARY MUSCLE
SEPTAL BAND
R. VENTRICLE
MODERATOR BAND

ADULT

TRANSFER OF POSTEROMEDIAL PART OF CONUS CORDIS AND AORTA TO LEFT VENTRICLE

atrioventricular (tricuspid) orifice (see page 122). To the right it then blends with the right lateral cushion, and to the left with the right tubercle of the superior endocardial cushion.

The sinistroventral conus swelling extends proximally along the right side of the upper anterior part of the muscular *interventricular septum,* growing downward over the upper part of the septal band and blending with it. Completion of the conus septum divides the conus into an anterolateral and a posteromedial portion. Together, the primitive right ventricle and the anterolateral portion of the conus form the definitive *right ventricle*. The posteromedial part of the conus, with the effacement of the conoventricular flange and the formation of the arch or bay by the fused atrioventricular *endocardial cushions,* becomes continuous with the primitive left ventricle, thus forming the aortic vestibule and establishing the

definitive left ventricle. In this way the aorta is transferred to the left.

With completion of the conus septum, the originally large interventricular communication (foramen) becomes much reduced in size, and, in a 15- to 16-mm embryo, the remaining *secondary interventricular foramen* is bordered, as we have seen, by the conus septum, the top of the muscular ventricular septum, and the right tubercles of the endocardial cushions. Final closure of the secondary interventricular foramen is accomplished by tissue derived mainly from an extension of the *inferior endocardial cushion*, which grows along the top of the ventricular septum, and fusion of this extension with the abutting part of the conus septum and the left aspect of the right limb of the fused endocardial cushion. This region, after complete closure of the secondary interventricular

(Continued on page 124)

FORMATION OF THE CARDIAC SEPTA

(Continued from page 123)

foramen, is initially quite thick, and only much later, and with the formation of the *septal (medial) cusp* of the *tricuspid valve,* does an area of variable extent become thin and fibrous; this is the *interventricular part of the membranous septum.* That part of the endocardial-cushion arch or bay between the junction with the *septum primum* and the ventricular septum also becomes much thinner, eventually, to form the *atrioventricular portion of the membranous septum.*

The Sinus Venosus

The cardiovascular system in the early-somite embryo is paired and symmetrical, as we have seen. At about the 4-somite stage, the paired endothelial heart tubes, ventral to the foregut, fuse with each other, a fusion which begins in the bulboventricular region and gradually progresses toward the venous pole of the heart. The *sinus venosus* maintains its paired condition longer; in fact, it never loses it completely. Thus, in a 4-mm (30-somite) embryo, one may distinguish a central, unpaired part, the transverse portion of the sinus venosus, and the *right* and *left sinus horns.*

The sinus venosus, at this stage, receives three pairs of veins. Most medially, at the junction of the sinus horns and the transverse portion, the *vitelline (omphalomesenteric) veins* enter the floor of the sinus; lateral to these, the *umbilical (allantoic) veins* enter the sinus horns coming in from below, with the *common cardinal veins* coming in from above. At first, the sinus venosus is not well demarcated from the atrium; *i.e.,* there is a wide, centrally located communication between the two. Later, however, the left horn and the transverse portion of the sinus venosus become more and more separated from the left side of the atrium by the development of a deep fold. The proximal portions of the umbilical veins soon disappear. Owing to the development of anastomotic channels between the right and left systemic veins and the preferential flow of blood to the right side, the right sinus horn and the proximal cardinal and vitelline veins gain in importance, whereas their left counterparts become greatly reduced in size. At the same time, the right sinus horn attains a more vertical position and becomes incorporated into the right atrium. The communication between the sinus venosus and the atrium is now limited to this horn. The transverse portion and the proximal left sinus horn become the *coronary sinus;* the distal left sinus horn and the left common cardinal vein usually obliterate (ligament of Marshall) (see pages 5 and 130).

On the right side, the cardiac wall at the sinoatrial junction folds in, as it does also on the left, but to a lesser extent. In a 20-somite embryo, this reduplication already is present and forms the *right*

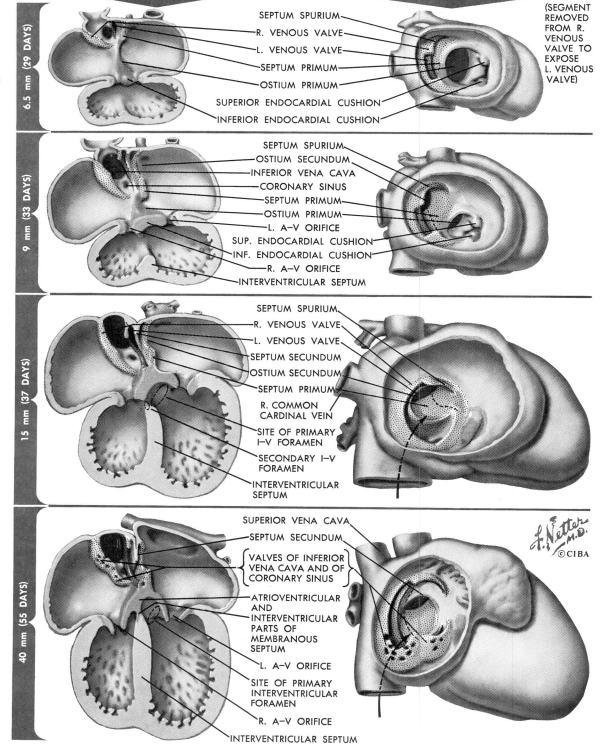

INFERIOR HALVES OF HEART VIEWED FROM ABOVE

OPENED AND VIEWED FROM RIGHT SIDE

(SEGMENT REMOVED FROM R. VENOUS VALVE TO EXPOSE L. VENOUS VALVE)

6.5 mm (29 DAYS)
SEPTUM SPURIUM
R. VENOUS VALVE
L. VENOUS VALVE
SEPTUM PRIMUM
OSTIUM PRIMUM
SUPERIOR ENDOCARDIAL CUSHION
INFERIOR ENDOCARDIAL CUSHION

9 mm (33 DAYS)
SEPTUM SPURIUM
OSTIUM SECUNDUM
INFERIOR VENA CAVA
CORONARY SINUS
SEPTUM PRIMUM
OSTIUM PRIMUM
L. A–V ORIFICE
SUP. ENDOCARDIAL CUSHION
INF. ENDOCARDIAL CUSHION
R. A–V ORIFICE
INTERVENTRICULAR SEPTUM

15 mm (37 DAYS)
SEPTUM SPURIUM
R. VENOUS VALVE
L. VENOUS VALVE
SEPTUM SECUNDUM
OSTIUM SECUNDUM
SEPTUM PRIMUM
R. COMMON CARDINAL VEIN
SITE OF PRIMARY I–V FORAMEN
SECONDARY I–V FORAMEN
INTERVENTRICULAR SEPTUM

40 mm (55 DAYS)
SUPERIOR VENA CAVA
SEPTUM SECUNDUM
VALVES OF INFERIOR VENA CAVA AND OF CORONARY SINUS
ATRIOVENTRICULAR AND INTERVENTRICULAR PARTS OF MEMBRANOUS SEPTUM
L. A–V ORIFICE
SITE OF PRIMARY INTERVENTRICULAR FORAMEN
R. A–V ORIFICE
INTERVENTRICULAR SEPTUM

venous (sinus) valve. Another smaller fold, the *left venous (sinus) valve,* appears somewhat later on the left side of the sinoatrial junction, so that, in a 4- to 6-mm embryo, the vertically disposed, slitlike sinoatrial orifice is flanked on each side by a valvelike structure. Superiorly, the venous (sinus) valves join each other to form a single fold, the *septum spurium.* The venous (sinus) valves are of relatively enormous size in a 16-mm embryo, but later they become much smaller. The left venous (sinus) valve eventually fuses with the atrial septum. The superior cranial part of the *right venous (sinus) valve* and the *septum spurium* usually disappear altogether. The inferior part of the right vienous (sinus) valve, in its lower portion, fuses locally with the *sinus septum;* the latter develops between the orifice of the right vitelline vein (which forms the terminal posthepatic portion of the *inferior vena cava*) and the orifice of the coronary

sinus. Thus, the inferior part of the right venous (sinus) valve is divided into a larger *inferior vena caval valve* and a smaller *coronary-sinus valve.*

The Atria, Atrial Septum, and Pulmonary Veins

In a 20-somite embryo, expansion of the atrial portion of the heart is well on its way. Owing to the presence of the *truncus arteriosus,* however, a depression is formed in the roof of the common atrium. As expansion proceeds, the depression deepens, corresponding internally to a more or less sickle-shaped crest. This is the first passively formed portion of the *septum primum.* Its free edge is directed toward the *atrioventricular canal,* and the foramen between the left and right primitive atria, which it borders, is

(Continued on page 125)

FORMATION OF THE CARDIAC SEPTA

(Continued from page 124)

the *ostium primum*. Extensions from the *superior* and *inferior endocardial cushions* grow along the edge of the septum primum. Proliferation of this tissue, with the concomitant fusion of the endocardial cushions, brings about the closure of the ostium primum, a process which is completed in embryos of about 10 to 11 mm C-R length. Before this happens, however, in 7- to 8-mm embryos, perforations appear in the septum primum posterosuperiorly. These rapidly coalesce to form the *ostium secundum,* thus ensuring continued communication between the right and left primitive atria.

The part of the primitive right atrium between the septum spurium and the *left venous (sinus) valve* on the one hand, and the septum primum on the other, is called the *interseptovalvular space.* Its dome-shaped roof is easily visible externally between the grooves which indicate the positions of the septum primum and the septum spurium.

The single embryonic *pulmonary vein,* present in a 5- to 6-mm embryo, develops as an outgrowth of the posterior left atrial wall near the atrial floor and just to the left of the septum primum. It gains connections with the splanchnic plexus of veins in the region of the developing lung buds. Later in development, the vein itself and parts of its first four branches expand tremendously and become incorporated into the left atrium to form the larger, smooth part of the adult atrium. In the fully developed heart, the original embryonic left atrium is represented by little more than the trabeculated atrial appendage. The intrapulmonary part of the splanchnic venous plexus ultimately loses its connections with the systemic veins and drains exclusively by way of the pulmonary veins.

On the right side, the right sinus horn is similarly incorporated into the right atrium; it enlarges mainly in its vertical diameter, *i.e.,* the relative distance between the common cardinal vein (proximal *superior vena cava*) and the *inferior vena cava* increases. In addition, the area just to the right of the right venous (sinus) valve becomes trabeculated, grows, and expands as new trabeculae (*pectinate muscles*) are added. This new addition to the atrium becomes the lateral wall and the largest part of the definitive right atrium; the original embryonic right atrium becomes the *right auricle* (atrial appendage), containing the earliest-appearing pectinate muscles, including the *taenia sagittalis* (see page 123). A large trabecula, running from the right side of the superior vena caval orifice downward just to the right of the right venous (sinus) valve, is called the *crista terminalis.* The intercaval part of the right atrium, derived from the right sinus horn, remains smooth-walled.

The growth and expansion of the atria, as just described, have a number of consequences: (1) The *right common*

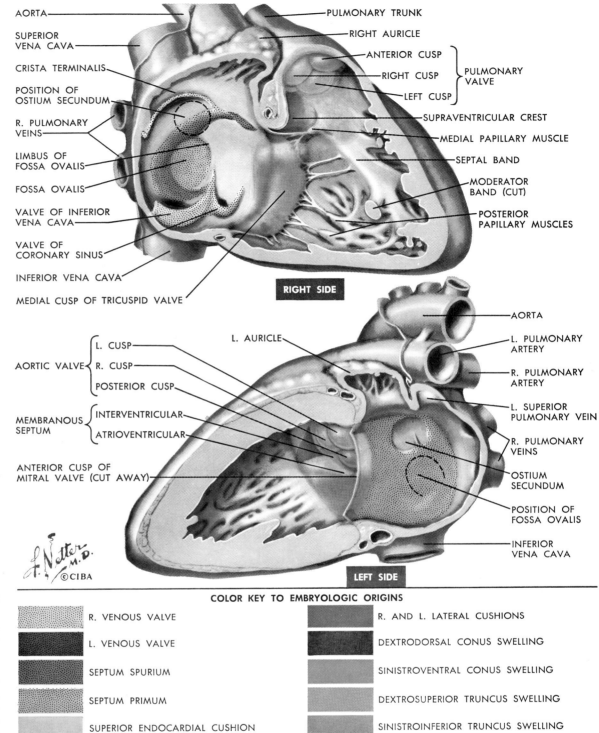

RIGHT SIDE

AORTA — PULMONARY TRUNK — RIGHT AURICLE — ANTERIOR CUSP / RIGHT CUSP / LEFT CUSP PULMONARY VALVE — SUPRAVENTRICULAR CREST — MEDIAL PAPILLARY MUSCLE — SEPTAL BAND — MODERATOR BAND (CUT) — POSTERIOR PAPILLARY MUSCLES

SUPERIOR VENA CAVA — CRISTA TERMINALIS — POSITION OF OSTIUM SECUNDUM — R. PULMONARY VEINS — LIMBUS OF FOSSA OVALIS — FOSSA OVALIS — VALVE OF INFERIOR VENA CAVA — VALVE OF CORONARY SINUS — INFERIOR VENA CAVA — MEDIAL CUSP OF TRICUSPID VALVE

LEFT SIDE

L. AURICLE — AORTA — L. PULMONARY ARTERY — R. PULMONARY ARTERY — L. SUPERIOR PULMONARY VEIN — R. PULMONARY VEINS — OSTIUM SECUNDUM — POSITION OF FOSSA OVALIS — INFERIOR VENA CAVA

AORTIC VALVE { L. CUSP / R. CUSP / POSTERIOR CUSP }
MEMBRANOUS SEPTUM { INTERVENTRICULAR / ATRIOVENTRICULAR }
ANTERIOR CUSP OF MITRAL VALVE (CUT AWAY)

COLOR KEY TO EMBRYOLOGIC ORIGINS

R. VENOUS VALVE — R. AND L. LATERAL CUSHIONS
L. VENOUS VALVE — DEXTRODORSAL CONUS SWELLING
SEPTUM SPURIUM — SINISTROVENTRAL CONUS SWELLING
SEPTUM PRIMUM — DEXTROSUPERIOR TRUNCUS SWELLING
SUPERIOR ENDOCARDIAL CUSHION — SINISTROINFERIOR TRUNCUS SWELLING
INFERIOR ENDOCARDIAL CUSHION — INTERCALATED VALVE SWELLINGS

cardinal vein initially enters the heart posteriorly, and the ostium secundum is located in the posterosuperior portion of the septum primum. Both move in a supero-anterior direction, until the *common cardinal vein* (superior vena cava) comes to enter the heart superiorly, and the ostium secundum finally is located anterosuperiorly. Their position relative to each other does not change much. (2) The roof of the interseptovalvular space is folded in more and more, resulting in the formation of a septum, the *septum secundum,* the free edge of which is directed inferiorly and posteriorly bordering a foramen, the *foramen ovale.* This process obliterates the lumen of the interseptovalvular space, and the septum secundum comes to overlap the ostium secundum. The left venous (sinus) valve approaches the right side of the septum secundum and finally fuses with it. Similarly, the septum primum approaches the left aspect of the septum secundum

but does not fuse with it completely until after birth.

Postnatally, after fusion of the septum primum and the septum secundum, the foramen ovale becomes the fossa ovalis, and the free edge of the septum secundum is called the *limbus fossae ovalis.*

In about 20 percent of the cases, fusion of the septum primum and the septum secundum remains incomplete, leaving an oblique potential passage between the two atria, a condition which is referred to as "probe patency" of the foramen ovale.

The Atrioventricular Valves

In an embryo of about 10 to 12 mm C-R length, when the atrioventricular canal has been divided into right and left atrioventricular orifices, both orifices come to be surrounded by young mesenchymal tissue.

(Continued on page 126)

Medially, the tubercles of the endocardial cushions are found; laterally, the lateral cushions. A section through the atrioventricular-canal area, at this stage of development, initially appears to be identical to a transverse section of the truncus arteriosus in a somewhat younger embryo, the *truncus swellings* being analogous to the *atrioventricular endocardial cushions,* and the *intercalated valve swellings* to the *lateral cushions.*

It would not be correct to state that the atrioventricular valves are derived from the mesenchyme surrounding the atrioventricular orifices. This is true only for most of the *anterior* (aortic) *cusp* of the *mitral valve* and the major part of the *anterior cusp* of the *tricuspid valve* (see page 122). A major component of the other *atrioventricular-valve* cusps is derived from the ventricular muscle and is liberated from the ventricular wall by the process of diverticulation and undermining described earlier. In principle, a skirt of ventricular muscle, partly covered on its atrial side by endocardial-cushion-type tissue, is formed at each atrioventricular orifice, originating from the atrioventricular junction and attached to the apices of the ventricles by trabeculae retained for this purpose (see page 119). On the left side, the skirt is incompletely divided into four compartments: two anteriorly (derived largely from the left halves of the endocardial cushions and therefore containing very little muscle initially) and two posteriorly (containing more muscle on their ventricular surface). All are thick and fleshy at first; only later do they become thin and fibrous.

Each half of each component, together with the adjoining half of the next component, forms a cusp, and each half forms its own *papillary muscle* and *chordae tendineae.*

In principle, then, the *mitral valve* is a quadricuspid valve; eventually, however, two of the cusps become much larger than the others, and the papillary muscles fuse in pairs, forming an *anterior* and a *posterior papillary muscle.* Their dual origin is still, however, often recognizable in adult hearts; usually, they have a bifid apex or are even, occasionally, completely separated though close together.

The two small cusps are usually identifiable in the adult and are called *commissural cusps* (see page 119).

As in the case of the cusps themselves, the chordae tendineae are initially thick, muscular, and few in number; only later are they transformed into delicate fibrous strands. The papillary muscles remain muscular. The mitral valve is formed comparatively early in development (embryos of about 15 to 16 mm C-R length).

The *tricuspid valve* is formed in a similar manner, but there are a few irregularities: (1) The *superior endocardial cushion* contributes to only a very small part of the valve, and (2) the conus septum forms a *medial (conal* or *septal) papillary muscle,* its chordae tendineae, and the most medial portion of the *anterior cusp.*

Furthermore, the primordium of the lateral and larger portion of the anterior cusp is formed very early (long before the other cusps have begun to make their appearance) and already, in a 15- to 16-mm embryo, is free from the ventricular wall. This is probably the reason that its origin is normal in cases of Ebstein's anomaly of the tricuspid valve (see page 143). The small portion of the septal (*medial*) *cusp,* which, in the adult, overlies the *membranous septum,* is formed last. In fact, occasionally it is not formed at all, and a small gap, usually of no functional significance, remains in the tricuspid valve.

The Semilunar Valves

The primordia of the semilunar valves are already visible as small tubercles in a 9-mm embryo (see page 121), just after partitioning of the truncus has been completed. Each *truncus swelling* carries a tubercle on the extremity of its distal face. One of each pair is assigned to *pulmonary* and *aortic channels,* respectively. On the walls of both aortic and pulmonary channels, opposite the fused truncus swellings, a third small cushion appears. These two *intercalated valve swellings* form the third tubercle of each arterial-valve primordium. Starting at the tubercles, the semilunar-valve cusps and the sinuses of Valsalva (see page 12) are formed by a process of excavation of the truncus and intercalated valve swellings in a proximal direction. This process is already well advanced at the 16-mm stage and virtually completed in the 40-mm embryo. It explains the "migration" of the arterial valves, which at first lie far distally, to a much more proximal position as found in the fully developed heart. Both the aortic and the pulmonary roots, consisting of the sinuses of Valsalva and the semilunar valves, therefore are derived from the truncus and intercalated valve swellings.

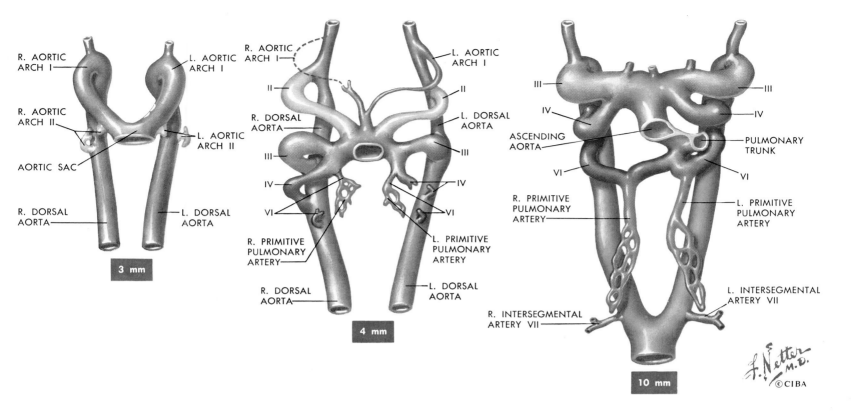

Labels in figure (left panel, 3 mm):
R. AORTIC ARCH I — L. AORTIC ARCH I
R. AORTIC ARCH II — L. AORTIC ARCH II
AORTIC SAC
R. DORSAL AORTA — L. DORSAL AORTA
3 mm

(middle panel, 4 mm):
R. AORTIC ARCH I — L. AORTIC ARCH I
II — II
R. DORSAL AORTA — L. DORSAL AORTA
III — III
IV — IV
VI — VI
R. PRIMITIVE PULMONARY ARTERY — L. PRIMITIVE PULMONARY ARTERY
R. DORSAL AORTA — L. DORSAL AORTA
4 mm

(right panel, 10 mm):
III — III
IV — IV
ASCENDING AORTA — PULMONARY TRUNK
VI — VI
R. PRIMITIVE PULMONARY ARTERY — L. PRIMITIVE PULMONARY ARTERY
R. INTERSEGMENTAL ARTERY VII — L. INTERSEGMENTAL ARTERY VII
10 mm

DEVELOPMENT OF THE MAJOR BLOOD VESSELS

The early embryonic vascular system is plexiform. Preferential flow related to the development of the various organ systems, however, leads to enlargement of certain channels in the plexus. This expansion is brought about in part by the fusion and confluence of adjacent smaller vessels and partly by the enlargement of individual capillaries. Thus, a number of vascular systems develop. As the embryo grows, new organs appear, while others are transient and disappear. The various vascular systems are also continuously modified and adapted to satisfy changing needs.

Initially, the arteries and veins consist simply of endothelial tubes and cannot be distinguished from each other histologically. In later development, typical vessel walls are differentiated from the surrounding mesenchyme.

The final pattern of the vascular system is genetically determined and varies with the animal species. Variations are, however, extremely common in both arterial and venous patterns, and local modifications occur in cases of abnormal development of organs.

Only the development of the aortic-arch system and the major systemic veins will be discussed here. The development of the pulmonary veins has been alluded to earlier (see page 124).

The Aortic-Arch System

The major arterial conduits in an early-somite embryo are represented by a pair of vessels, the *dorsal aortas,* which run with the long axis of the embryo and form the continuation of the endocardial heart tubes. Because of the changing position of the cardiogenic plate containing the heart tubes, the cranial portions of the dorsal aortas come to describe an arc on both sides of the foregut, thus establishing the *first pair of aortic arches* (mandibular arches).

Primitively, six pairs of aortic arches appear in vertebrates, in conjunction with the development of the corresponding pharyngeal or visceral arches. With the appearance of jaws phylogenetically, the first two pairs of pharyngeal arches become highly modified to form elements of the mouth and middle ears.

In gill-bearing vertebrates, the third to sixth (occasionally more or less) pharyngeal arches bear gills, or branchiae, and are called branchial arches.

In lung-breathing amniotes, including man, the branchial arches are present, as such, only in early embryonic life; they become greatly modified later, or they retrogress altogether. Certain of the branchial-arch arteries are retained to form the large arteries of the neck and thorax.

In an embryo of about 3 *mm,* the first pair of arches is large; the second pair is just forming. The junction of the truncus arteriosus and the first pair of arches is somewhat dilated and is called the aortic sac. It is from this aortic sac that subsequent aortic arches originate, new arches being added as the heart and the aortic sac undergo a relatively caudal displacement. A true ventral aorta is not present in embryos of the higher mammals. Distally, the dorsal aortas fuse to form a single vessel; this fusion progresses in a cranial direction, in both an absolute and a relative sense.

In a *4-mm* embryo, the *first arch* has largely disappeared as such, but part of it persists as a portion of the maxillary artery. The *second arch* is also on its way out; all that remains of it, eventually, is the tiny stapedial artery. The *third arch* is well developed and large. The *fourth* and *sixth arches* are being formed as ventral and dorsal sprouts. The ventral portion of the sixth arch already has as its major branch the *primitive pulmonary artery,* even though the arch itself has not yet been completed.

In a *10-mm* embryo, the first two aortic arches have disappeared as such; the third, fourth, and sixth arches are large. The truncoaortic sac has been divided so that the sixth arch is now continuous with the *pulmonary trunk.* Of the *intersegmental arteries,* the seventh cervicals will play

an important role in the formation of the subclavian arteries. They are located at about the level where the dorsal aortas join each other.

In a *14-mm* embryo, the aortic-arch system has largely lost its original symmetrical pattern. The dorsal aortas between the *third* and *fourth* arches (the *carotid ducts*) have disappeared, and the third arches begin to elongate as the heart descends farther. This descent has also caused a relative shortening of the paired portion of the dorsal aorta. The dorsal portion of the right *sixth arch* has disappeared; its counterpart on the left persists, until birth, as the *ductus arteriosus.* The very small and transient fifth arch, present somewhat earlier (in embryos of about 11 to 13 mm), can no longer be found. The *seventh intersegmental arteries* have migrated craniad.

The aortic sac has been "pulled out" on both sides: on the *right,* it forms the *brachiocephalic* (innominate) *trunk;* on the *left,* it becomes part of the definitive *arch of the aorta,* up to the origin of the left third arch (*common carotid artery*).

In a *17-mm* embryo, the right dorsal aorta, between its junction with the left dorsal aorta and the origin of the right seventh intersegmental artery, has become very attenuated and soon disappears. The remainder of the right dorsal aorta persists as part of the *proximal subclavian artery.*

After birth, the distal part of the left sixth aortic arch, the *ductus arteriosus,* normally also obliterates (*ligamentum arteriosum*), and the adult *aortic-arch* system is established. The ultimate fate of the various components of the embryonic aortic-arch system may be tabulated as follows:

1. Truncus arteriosus:	Proximal portions of ascending aorta and *pulmonary trunk.*
2. Aortic sac:	Distal portion of *ascending aorta,* brachiocephalic (innominate) artery, and aortic arch up to origin of left common carotid artery.
3. First arches:	Parts persist as components of maxillary arteries.

(*Continued on page 128*)

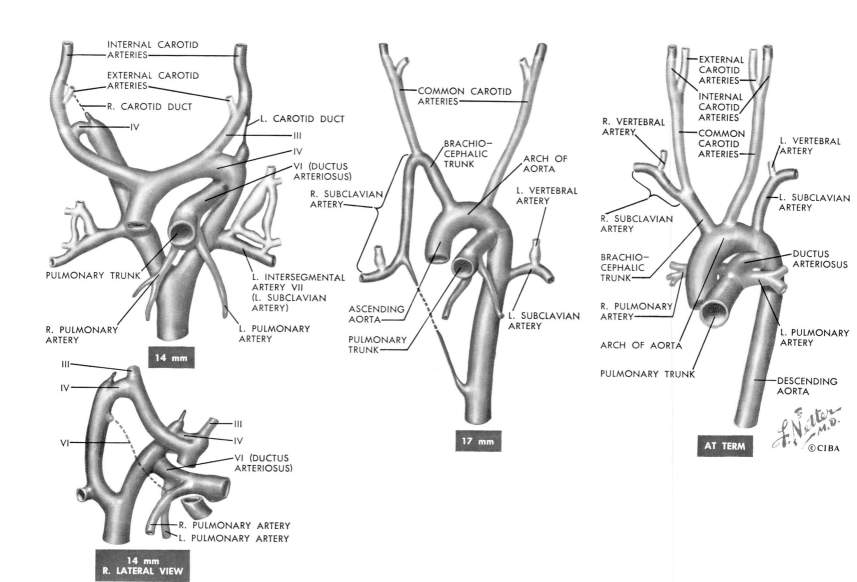

DEVELOPMENT OF THE MAJOR BLOOD VESSELS

(Continued from page 127)

4. Second arches: Parts persist as stapedial arteries.

5. Third arches: *Common carotid arteries* and proximal segment of *internal carotid arteries.*

6. Fourth arches: Right: Most-proximal segment of *right subclavian artery.* Left: Aortic-arch segment between *left common carotid* and *left subclavian arteries.*

7. Fifth arches: No known derivations. Transient and never well developed.

8. Sixth arches: Right: Proximal part becomes proximal segment of *right pulmonary artery;* distal part disappears early. Left: Proximal part becomes proximal segment of *left pulmonary artery;* distal part persists, until birth, as ductus arteriosus.

9. Right dorsal aorta: Cranial portion becomes part of *right subclavian artery;* remainder disappears.

10. Left dorsal aorta: Distal aortic arch.

11. Right seventh intersegmental artery: Part of right subclavian artery.

12. Left seventh intersegmental artery: *Left subclavian artery.*

The Major Systemic Veins

The development of the great systemic veins is a complex—but also a very interesting—process and, from a clinical point of view, of considerable importance. Few organ systems in the body are so subject to variations and anomalies in their final, fully developed state. Although such variations and anomalies are generally of little functional importance to the individual, they do, at times, cause confusion in carrying out diagnostic angiocardiographic studies, and may bring about potentially disastrous accidents when surgical correction of cardiac anomalies is attempted.

In the very young embryo, the major veins develop, from an initially plexiform bed, as a number of channels which run mainly in a longitudinal direction. In a *4-mm* embryo (see page 120), three main groups of veins may be distinguished: (1) The *vitelline venous system,* consisting of *right* and *left vitelline (omphalomesenteric) veins,* carries the blood from the yolk sac and enters the *sinus venosus.* (2) The

umbilical venous system collects the blood from the chorionic villi (later the placenta) and carries it, by way of the *right* and *left umbilical veins,* to the embryo. The right and left umbilical veins may unite to form a single vein in the body or connecting stalk, but, within the embryo, they become paired again and enter the sinus venosus lateral to the vitelline veins. (3) The *cardinal venous system* is entirely intraembryonic. The *anterior cardinal veins* drain the cranial region of the embryo. The *posterior cardinal veins* arise somewhat later as longitudinal vessels running in the dorsolateral portion of the urogenital fold. They drain the body of the embryo, including the large *mesonephroi,* and also, initially, the anterior extremities. The anterior and posterior cardinal veins join to form the short *common cardinal veins* which enter the *right* and *left sinus horns* just lateral to the umbilical veins.

Soon after the posterior cardinal veins have been established, a new venous system develops as a pair of veins, the *subcardinal veins,* which run medially in the urogenital fold. Their main function is to drain the urogenital system of the developing embryo: at first, the mesonephroi and the gonads; later, the *metanephroi* (kidneys), *gonads,* and *suprarenal glands.* Cranially, they empty into the posterior cardinal veins.

In an embryo of about *10 mm* C-R length, the cardinal venous system is symmetrical and equally well developed bilaterally. The vitelline

(Continued on page 129)

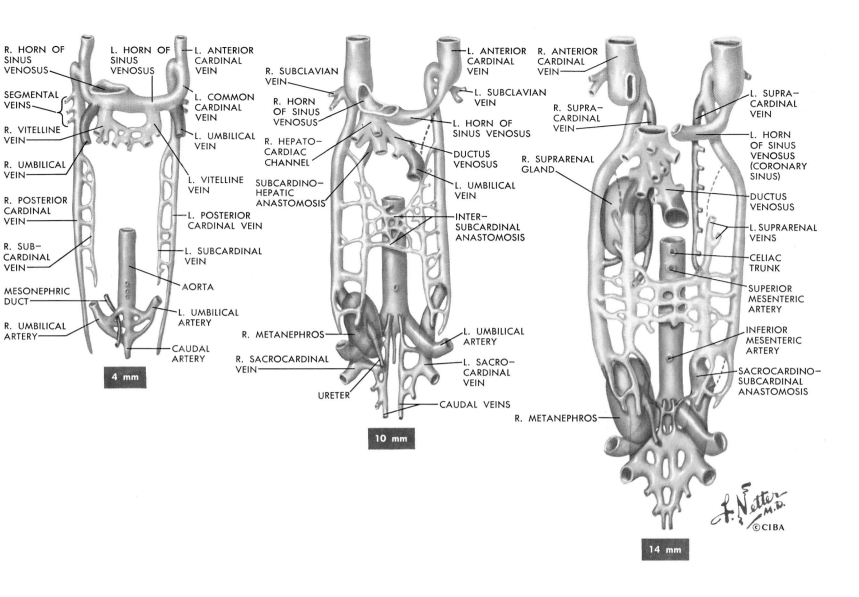

R. HORN OF SINUS VENOSUS
L. HORN OF SINUS VENOSUS
L. ANTERIOR CARDINAL VEIN
SEGMENTAL VEINS
R. VITELLINE VEIN
R. UMBILICAL VEIN
R. POSTERIOR CARDINAL VEIN
R. SUB-CARDINAL VEIN
MESONEPHRIC DUCT
R. UMBILICAL ARTERY
L. COMMON CARDINAL VEIN
L. UMBILICAL VEIN
L. VITELLINE VEIN
L. POSTERIOR CARDINAL VEIN
L. SUBCARDINAL VEIN
AORTA
L. UMBILICAL ARTERY
CAUDAL ARTERY

4 mm

R. SUBCLAVIAN VEIN
R. HORN OF SINUS VENOSUS
R. HEPATO-CARDIAC CHANNEL
SUBCARDINO-HEPATIC ANASTOMOSIS
R. METANEPHROS
R. SACROCARDINAL VEIN
URETER
L. ANTERIOR CARDINAL VEIN
L. SUBCLAVIAN VEIN
L. HORN OF SINUS VENOSUS
DUCTUS VENOSUS
L. UMBILICAL VEIN
INTER-SUBCARDINAL ANASTOMOSIS
L. UMBILICAL ARTERY
L. SACRO-CARDINAL VEIN
CAUDAL VEINS

10 mm

R. ANTERIOR CARDINAL VEIN
R. SUPRA-CARDINAL VEIN
R. SUPRARENAL GLAND
L. SUPRA-CARDINAL VEIN
L. HORN OF SINUS VENOSUS (CORONARY SINUS)
DUCTUS VENOSUS
L. SUPRARENAL VEINS
CELIAC TRUNK
SUPERIOR MESENTERIC ARTERY
INFERIOR MESENTERIC ARTERY
SACROCARDINO-SUBCARDINAL ANASTOMOSIS
R. METANEPHROS

14 mm

SECTION III—PLATE 16

DEVELOPMENT OF THE MAJOR BLOOD VESSELS

(Continued from page 128)

veins, in the region of the *septum transversum* (see page 118) and around the duodenum, have broken up into an anastomosing plexus. Of the parts of the two main vessels remaining between the plexus and the sinus venosus — the *hepato-cardiac channels* — the left one has disappeared, but the right one becomes greatly enlarged and persists as the terminal posthepatic portion of the inferior vena cava. Further developments concerning the vitelline venous system will not be elaborated here.

The right umbilical vein has disappeared; the left umbilical vein has gained connections with the vitelline venous plexus, after which its proximal portion also disappears. All the umbilical venous blood now enters the vitelline venous (liver) plexus. A direct route, the *ductus veno-sus,* is created between the left umbilical vein and the *right hepatocardiac channel* by the enlargement and confluence of the plexal channels between them, allowing most of the umbilical venous blood to enter directly into the right atrium.

The *subcardinal veins* have gained in importance, and numerous anastomoses with the posterior cardinal veins have been established. The

growing mesonephroi have brought the *left* and *right subcardinal veins* closer together, and an anastomosing plexus of veins has developed between them (*intersubcardinal anastomosis*). The right subcardinal vein has become connected to the right hepatocardiac channel by a plexus which rapidly is transformed into a large channel, the *subcardinohepatic anastomosis* (hepatic segment of the inferior vena cava).

A new venous system has appeared bilaterally in the caudal region of the embryo. Its two main channels, the *sacrocardinal veins* (Grünwald, P., Z. mikr. anat. Forsch., 43:275, 1938), run more dorsally than the posterior cardinal veins. They ascend behind and arch over the umbilical arteries to empty into the posterior cardinal veins.

Two smaller longitudinal veins, the *caudal veins,* occupy a more ventral position and are connected to the *sacrocardinal veins* by numerous *anastomoses.*

Caudal to the mesonephroi, the *metanephroi* (kidneys) have made their appearance.

In a *14-mm* embryo, the *left posterior cardinal vein* has begun to dwindle, and the left horn of the sinus venosus, the future *coronary sinus,* has become attenuated.

The subcardinal veins, particularly on the right, and the subcardinohepatic anastomosis have enlarged considerably and are rapidly becoming the principal venous channels to the heart. At this time, they have lost their cranial connections with the posterior cardinal veins, and some of the cranial tributaries are

now draining the developing suprarenal glands.

The intersubcardinal anastomoses consist of fewer but larger channels. Anastomoses have developed between the subcardinal and sacrocardinal veins. These *sacrocardinosubcardinal anastomoses* enlarge rapidly, while the connections between the sacrocardinals and posterior cardinals are interrupted. Extensive anastomoses have appeared between the right and left sacrocardinal and caudal veins.

Yet another new venous system has made its appearance, dorsolateral to the aorta, in the form of two longitudinal channels, the *supracardinal veins.* Cranially, they empty into the terminal portion of the posterior cardinal veins; caudally, they anastomose with the subcardinal veins. They drain the body wall by way of the intercostal veins, taking over this function from the posterior cardinal veins.

In a *17-mm* embryo, the upper limbs are drained by veins which empty into the *anterior cardinal veins.* The *left horn of the sinus venosus* has attenuated further.

With the rapidly decreasing importance of the mesonephroi and the transfer of the function of the posterior cardinals to the subcardinal veins, major portions of the posterior cardinal veins have disappeared. Eventually, only the terminal portions, beyond the junction with the supracardinal veins, will persist to form, on the right, the arch of the *azygos vein* and, on the left, a portion of the *superior intercostal vein.*

(Continued on page 130)

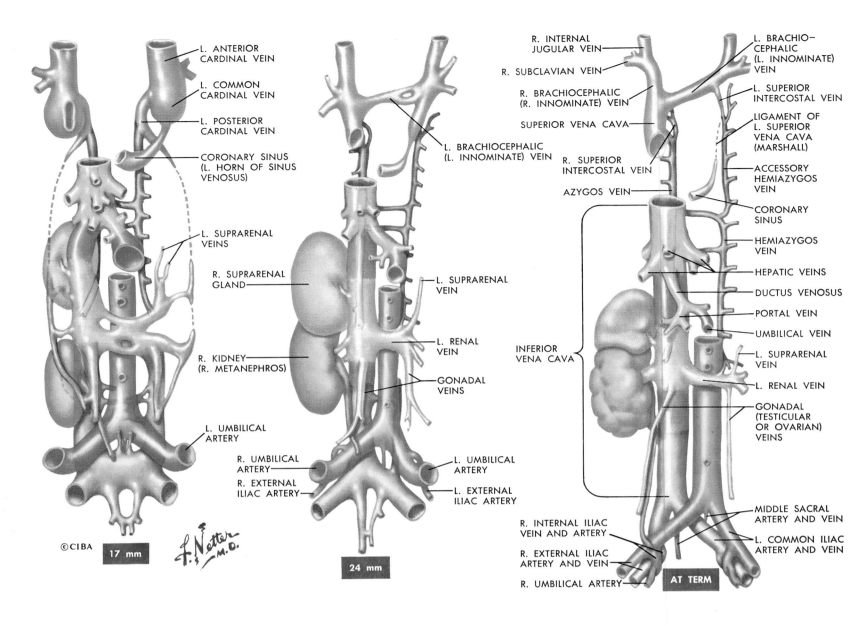

L. ANTERIOR CARDINAL VEIN

L. COMMON CARDINAL VEIN

L. POSTERIOR CARDINAL VEIN

CORONARY SINUS (L. HORN OF SINUS VENOSUS)

L. SUPRARENAL VEINS

R. SUPRARENAL GLAND

R. KIDNEY (R. METANEPHROS)

L. UMBILICAL ARTERY

©CIBA   17 mm

R. INTERNAL JUGULAR VEIN

R. SUBCLAVIAN VEIN

R. BRACHIOCEPHALIC (R. INNOMINATE) VEIN

SUPERIOR VENA CAVA

R. SUPERIOR INTERCOSTAL VEIN

AZYGOS VEIN

L. BRACHIOCEPHALIC (L. INNOMINATE) VEIN

L. SUPRARENAL VEIN

L. RENAL VEIN

GONADAL VEINS

R. UMBILICAL ARTERY

R. EXTERNAL ILIAC ARTERY

L. UMBILICAL ARTERY

L. EXTERNAL ILIAC ARTERY

24 mm

L. BRACHIO-CEPHALIC (L. INNOMINATE) VEIN

L. SUPERIOR INTERCOSTAL VEIN

LIGAMENT OF L. SUPERIOR VENA CAVA (MARSHALL)

ACCESSORY HEMIAZYGOS VEIN

CORONARY SINUS

HEMIAZYGOS VEIN

HEPATIC VEINS

DUCTUS VENOSUS

PORTAL VEIN

UMBILICAL VEIN

L. SUPRARENAL VEIN

L. RENAL VEIN

GONADAL (TESTICULAR OR OVARIAN) VEINS

INFERIOR VENA CAVA

MIDDLE SACRAL ARTERY AND VEIN

L. COMMON ILIAC ARTERY AND VEIN

R. INTERNAL ILIAC VEIN AND ARTERY

R. EXTERNAL ILIAC ARTERY AND VEIN

R. UMBILICAL ARTERY

AT TERM

SECTION III—PLATE 17

DEVELOPMENT OF THE MAJOR BLOOD VESSELS

(Continued from page 129)

The right sacrocardinal and subcardinal veins, together with the subcardinohepatic anastomosis and the hepatocardiac channel, have become the main drainage pathways for the lower body of the embryo. A large channel has developed in the anastomotic plexus between the sacrocardinal veins. This will become the proximal part of the *left common iliac vein*. The left sacrocardinal vein proximal to this anastomosis and the left sacrocardinosubcardinal anastomosis have begun to dwindle and will eventually disappear as a major channel.

The intersubcardinal anastomosis consists of a few large channels. The subcardinal veins caudal to the anastomosis become attenuated and drain mainly the gonads but, at first, the kidneys also. As the kidneys migrate craniad, however, they continually acquire new venous (and arterial) channels until their final position, approximately at the level of the intersubcardinal anastomosis, has been reached.

Anastomotic veins have developed between the supracardinal veins in front of the spine.

In a 24-mm embryo, an anastomosis has appeared between the anterior cardinal veins. It will become the major venous channel draining

the left side of the head and the left upper extremity, and it is known, in the adult, as the *left brachiocephalic (innominate) vein*. The *left common cardinal vein* and the adjacent distal part of the left sinus horn have become attenuated further and ordinarily become atretic (*ligament of left superior vena cava* or *ligament of Marshall*). The terminal portion of the left proximal posterior cardinal vein and the part of the anterior cardinal vein between it and the left brachiocephalic vein are retained as a small vessel, the *left superior intercostal vein,* which receives blood from the second and third intercostal spaces. (The first intercostal space drains its blood on both sides into the brachiocephalic or the vertebral vein.) A similar vessel on the right, the *right superior intercostal vein,* empties into the azygos vein.

The fourth to eleventh right intercostal veins empty into the right supracardinal vein which, together with the terminal portion of the posterior cardinal vein, forms the azygos vein. The left fourth to seventh (or eighth) intercostal veins run into the corresponding portion of the left supracardinal vein (*accessory hemiazygos vein*) which, in turn, empties into the azygos vein by way of one or more prevertebral anastomoses. Similarly, the left eighth (or ninth) to eleventh intercostal veins join the caudal portion of the left supracardinal or *hemiazygos vein*. The portions of the left supracardinal vein between the third and fourth and between the seventh and eighth intercostal veins may or may not

become interrupted. Variations in this region are extremely common.

The *inferior vena cava* has become established as the main venous channel of the lower body. Its composition, from bits and pieces of embryonic venous systems, is as follows:

1. Terminal part of the right vitelline vein (hepatocardiac channel): Posthepatic segment
2. Subcardinohepatic anastomosis: Hepatic segment
3. Part of right subcardinal vein: Renal segment
4. Sacrocardinal vein and sacrocardinosubcardinal anastomosis: Prerenal segment

The persisting parts of the subcardinal veins not included in the inferior vena cava have become the *gonadal* (spermatic or ovarian) *veins* and *suprarenal veins*.

The intersubcardinal anastomosis has become the part of the *left renal vein* between the entrance of the left suprarenal and gonadal veins and the vena cava. The remainders of the left renal vein and the right renal vein are newly elaborated metanephric veins which drain into the subcardinal veins. After birth, the left *umbilical vein* and the *ductus venosus* obliterate and are represented postnatally as *ligamentum teres hepatis* and *ligamentum venosus*. Again, it is not surprising, considering the complex developmental history of the systemic veins, that variations and anomalies are extremely common.

Section IV

DISEASES — CONGENITAL ANOMALIES

by

FRANK H. NETTER, M.D.

in collaboration with

RALPH D. ALLEY, M.D. and LODEWYK H. S. VAN MIEROP, M.D.
Plates 3, 6, 8, 10, 18, 24

LODEWYK H. S. VAN MIEROP, M.D.
Plates 1, 2, 4, 5, 7, 9, 11-17, 19-23, 25-32

ANOMALIES OF THE GREAT SYSTEMIC VEINS

Anomalies involving the large systemic venous trunks are not uncommon. This is not surprising, in view of the complex embryogenesis and the tremendous variability of the venous system in general. Since such abnormal channels almost always empty into other systemic veins, they rarely cause functional changes disturbing to the patient; thus, they usually are discovered accidentally at postmortem examination or in the course of cardiovascular diagnostic or surgical procedures. They may occur as isolated malformations but, more commonly, are associated with other cardiovascular anomalies. Their presence, if unsuspected, may lead to troublesome or even dangerous situations in those surgical cases where total cardiopulmonary-bypass technics are employed.

Left Superior Vena Cava

By far the most common clinically significant anomaly is a *persistence of the left superior vena cava.* This vein, after being formed by the confluence of the left jugular and the subclavian veins, descends into the chest parallel to the *right superior vena cava,* anterior to the left-lung hilus, and always enters the markedly dilated *coronary sinus* along a course ordinarily occupied by the ligament and vein of Marshall. This topographical position is to be expected since, embryologically, a persistent left superior vena cava represents a retention of the left anterior and common cardinal veins and the left sinus horn. Anatomically, the *hemiazygos vein* resembles the normal right-side *azygos vein* and may approximate the latter in size.

The right superior vena cava is usually present as well, but it may be absent. The two venae cavae may be equal in size, or one (generally the left) may be smaller than its counterpart. The left innominate vein, if present, is smaller than normal or may be more or less plexiform.

The coronary-sinus ostium is very large, as a result of the increased flow of blood through it. Occasionally, a defect is present in the wall between the sinus and the left atrium. Generally, such a defect results in a left-to-right shunt; i.e., left atrial blood enters the coronary sinus and is carried to the right atrium. Hemodynamically, therefore, it resembles an atrial septal defect. If the defect is very large, and particularly if the coronary-sinus ostium is small or atretic, the left superior vena cava is said to enter the left atrium, although (from a developmental point of view) this is, strictly speaking, not correct.

Patients with this anomaly present a typical *clinical picture* consisting of moderate central cyanosis without other symptoms. There is no murmur, and the heart is normal in size. The *electrocardiogram* generally shows signs of left ventricular hypertrophy. Similar, but

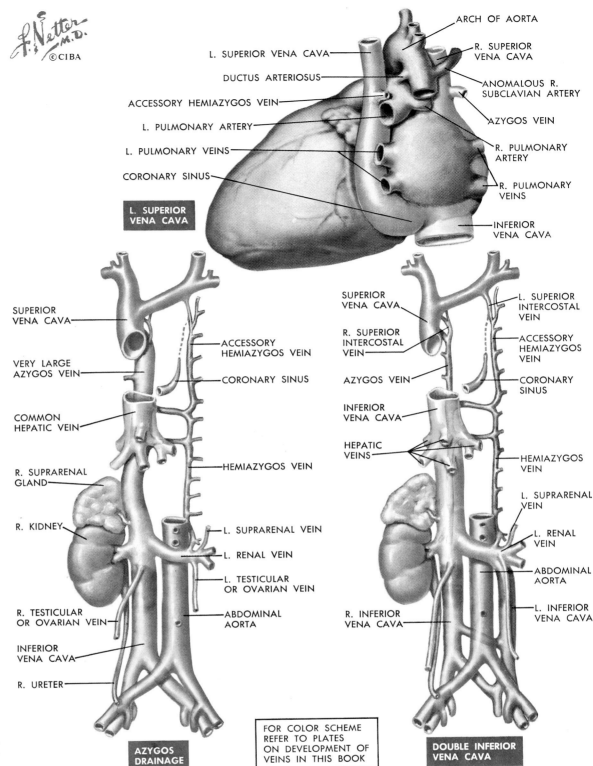

somewhat more pronounced, findings have been described in the very rare cases of isolated drainage of the inferior vena cava into the left atrium.

Azygos Drainage of the Inferior Vena Cava

Absence of the hepatic segment of the inferior vena cava is an uncommon anomaly in which the prehepatic portion of the inferior vena cava drains into the right atrium by way of an enormously enlarged azygos vein (*azygos drainage of the inferior vena cava*). The *hepatic veins* empty into the right atrium by way of a short common stem which normally forms the most proximal part of the inferior vena cava. Azygos drainage of the inferior vena cava may occur rarely as an isolated lesion; usually, however, it is associated with other serious cardiac anoma-

lies, e.g., the *asplenia* (see page 136) or polysplenia syndrome.

Double Inferior Vena Cava

Other systemic venous anomalies, such as the *double inferior vena cava* illustrated, generally involve the inferior vena caval bed and are of more importance to general surgeons and urologists than to cardiologists and cardiac surgeons.

Patients with significant cardiac anomalies associated with various types of partial inversion of the thoracic or abdominal viscera are particularly prone to harbor anomalies of the great systemic venous trunks. Because such anomalies may cause difficulties at surgery, their presence or absence should be clearly established as part of the diagnostic work-up. This is most easily done by *angiocardiography.*

Anomalous Pulmonary Venous Connection

In cases of *anomalous pulmonary venous connection (APVC)*, some or all of the *pulmonary veins* fail to communicate with the *left atrium* and discharge their blood, instead, either into major systemic veins or directly into the *right atrium*. Only the isolated forms of APVC will be considered here. When they occur with other cardiac malformations, the clinical and hemodynamic features are usually modified or are chiefly determined by the complicating defect.

In *partial APVC*, one or more pulmonary veins empty into the proximal *superior vena cava*, close to the right atrium, or into the sinus portion of the right atrium itself. The involved veins almost always drain part or all of the right lung; the others empty normally into the left atrium. An atrial septal defect is generally present. Particularly common is the one referred to as the *sinus venosus type of atrial septal defect (ASD)*. The *clinical picture* closely resembles that seen in other forms of ASD and will not be discussed here (see page 137).

In *total APVC* (*TAPVC*), all the pulmonary venous blood enters the systemic venous system or the right atrium. An atrial septal defect or a patent foramen ovale is always present. Several types are distinguished, depending upon the manner in which the pulmonary venous blood enters the systemic circuit.

Embryologically, the intrapulmonary veins are derived from the venous plexus around the foregut and, in early embryonic life, anastomose freely with the systemic veins. After the embryonic main pulmonary vein has made its appearance as an outgrowth of the primitive left atrium and has established connections with the pulmonary venous plexus, the systemicopulmonary venous anastomotic channels normally obliterate. If the embryonic pulmonary vein does not develop at all or if it obliterates secondarily, some of the anastomotic channels are retained, and the result is TAPVC.

Total Anomalous Pulmonary Venous Connection to Left Superior Vena Cava

By far the most common form of *TAPVC* is that *to a persistent left superior vena cava*, illustrated as seen from behind. In this type, the right pulmonary veins converge to form a single vessel which runs behind the small left atrium to join the left pulmonary veins. From the junction of the pulmonary veins, a large single vessel, representing a persistence of the distal left superior vena cava, carries the pulmonary venous blood by way of a dilated *left brachiocephalic (innominate) vein* and the right superior

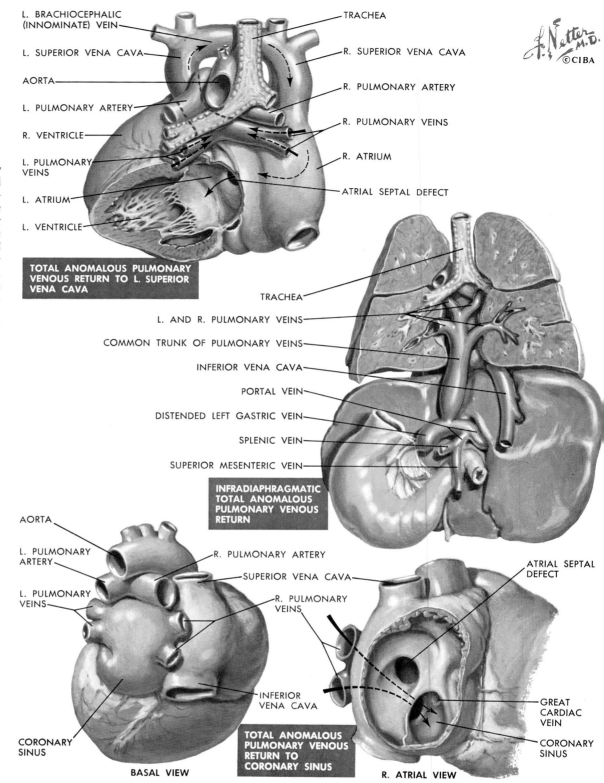

TOTAL ANOMALOUS PULMONARY VENOUS RETURN TO L. SUPERIOR VENA CAVA

INFRADIAPHRAGMATIC TOTAL ANOMALOUS PULMONARY VENOUS RETURN

TOTAL ANOMALOUS PULMONARY VENOUS RETURN TO CORONARY SINUS

BASAL VIEW

R. ATRIAL VIEW

vena cava to the right atrium. An atrial septal defect or, more commonly, a widely patent foramen ovale allows part of the right atrial blood to enter the left atrium. Tremendous right atrial and right ventricular enlargement develop early and rapidly.

Symptoms generally appear shortly after birth. These consist, initially, of rapid respirations followed by dyspnea, feeding difficulties, failure to thrive, and frequent respiratory infections. As a rule, there is no obvious cyanosis, at least at first, a reflection of the fact that a large amount of oxygenated pulmonary venous blood is mixed with a relatively much smaller amount of systemic venous blood. Cyanosis becomes more pronounced if there is bronchopneumonia or congestive failure. Failure almost always appears within the first 6 months of life, and the great majority of these infants die during their first year. For some reason, a small number of the patients improve,

and even a very few of these may reach adult age.

Cyanosis and clubbing of the digits are common only in older children and adults. The heart is enlarged. There is no thrill, as a rule, but a lower left parasternal "heave" is usually present. A systolic murmur, of mild to moderate intensity, is present at the left upper sternal border or, sometimes, somewhat lower. The pulmonary second sound is usually loud and often split. A diastolic tricuspid-flow murmur may be present along the right lower sternal border or over the xiphoid.

The *roentgenographic features* in older children and adults are characteristic. The dilated left and right superior venae cavae cause a rounded shadow in the upper mediastinum. Together with the rounded and enlarged heart shadow, a typical "figure-eight" or snowman" appearance is created. The pul-

(Continued on page 135)

ANOMALOUS PULMONARY VENOUS CONNECTION

(*Continued from page 134*)

monary vascularity is greatly increased.

The *electrocardiogram* almost invariably shows right axis deviation and severe right atrial and right ventricular hypertrophy.

At *cardiac catheterization,* the oxygen content of the right superior vena caval blood is found to be very high, indicating a massive L→R (left-to-right) supracardiac shunt, and the blood oxygen content is nearly uniform in all cardiac chambers.

The *diagnosis* can be confirmed easily by selective injection of a contrast medium into the *pulmonary trunk.* After passage of the dye through the lungs, the anomalous veins opacify quite satisfactorily.

Total Anomalous Pulmonary Venous Connection to Coronary Sinus

In *TAPVC to the coronary sinus,* the pulmonary veins join to form a very short, wide, common vessel which empties into the hugely dilated coronary sinus. The *clinical picture* and *electrocardiographic findings* are similar to those described above. The *radiographic appearance* is different, in that the upper mediastinum is not widened. The right atrium may be huge. There are cardiomegaly and plethora of the lung fields. *Cardiac catheterization* fails to show the high oxygen content of the superior vena cava; otherwise, the findings are similar to those observed in TAPVC to the left superior vena cava. *Angiocardiography* is much less helpful, and the anomaly may be difficult to demonstrate with certainty.

Other types of TAPVC, *e.g.,* to the right atrium or to several different sites, are much more uncommon as isolated malformations, but they may be seen in association with other severe cardiac defects.

Infradiaphragmatic Total Anomalous Pulmonary Venous Connection

In an unusual but interesting form of TAPVC, generally occurring as an isolated anomaly, the pulmonary veins drain into the portal venous system. This is commonly referred to as *infradiaphragmatic TAPVC,* all the others being grouped under the heading of *supradiaphragmatic TAPVC.* In the infradiaphragmatic type, the pulmonary veins join to form a long single vessel which descends in front of the esophagus and runs with it through the esophageal hiatus, to enter somewhere in the proximal portal venous system, generally the *left gastric vein.* Usually, there is a stenotic

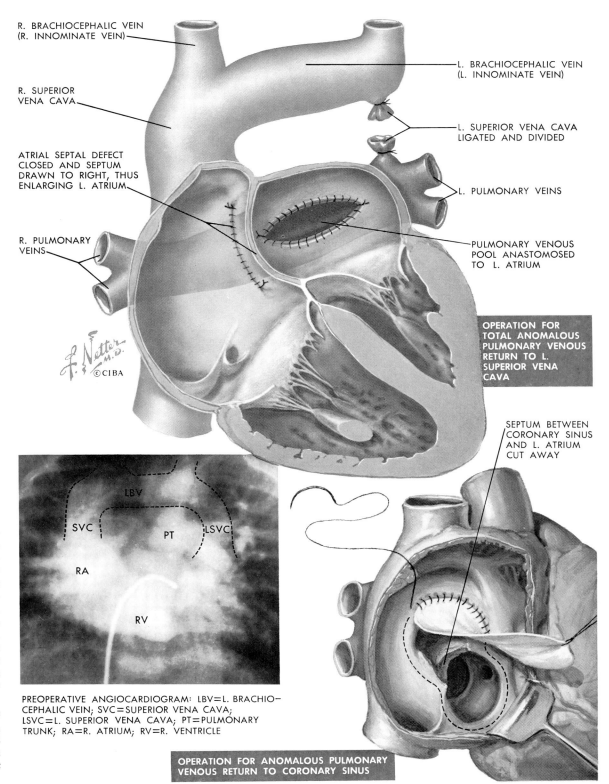

R. BRACHIOCEPHALIC VEIN (R. INNOMINATE VEIN)

L. BRACHIOCEPHALIC VEIN (L. INNOMINATE VEIN)

R. SUPERIOR VENA CAVA

L. SUPERIOR VENA CAVA LIGATED AND DIVIDED

ATRIAL SEPTAL DEFECT CLOSED AND SEPTUM DRAWN TO RIGHT, THUS ENLARGING L. ATRIUM

L. PULMONARY VEINS

R. PULMONARY VEINS

PULMONARY VENOUS POOL ANASTOMOSED TO L. ATRIUM

F. Netter M.D.
©CIBA

OPERATION FOR TOTAL ANOMALOUS PULMONARY VENOUS RETURN TO L. SUPERIOR VENA CAVA

SEPTUM BETWEEN CORONARY SINUS AND L. ATRIUM CUT AWAY

PREOPERATIVE ANGIOCARDIOGRAM: LBV=L. BRACHIO-CEPHALIC VEIN; SVC=SUPERIOR VENA CAVA; LSVC=L. SUPERIOR VENA CAVA; PT=PULMONARY TRUNK; RA=R. ATRIUM; RV=R. VENTRICLE

LBV
SVC
PT
LSVC
RA
RV

OPERATION FOR ANOMALOUS PULMONARY VENOUS RETURN TO CORONARY SINUS

area in the preesophageal vein just before it enters the portal venous bed. This stenosis, plus the fact that the pulmonary venous blood has to traverse the hepatic capillary bed before it can enter the right atrium by way of the hepatic veins, causes severe pulmonary venous hypertension and is responsible for the characteristic *clinical picture* and laboratory findings, which are quite different from those seen in the various supradiaphragmatic types. The illustration shows the anomaly as seen from the back.

Severe *symptoms* appear soon after birth, and almost all infants die within a very few days or weeks. The symptoms include a clear-cut and persistent cyanosis, marked dyspnea, and serious feeding difficulties. Cardiac failure becomes evident very early, and it is almost impossible to treat it successfully. In spite of the fact that the infants are obviously very sick, there are no abnormal cardiac findings. The heart

is not enlarged, and a murmur, if present, is faint.

The *electrocardiogram* is normal or nearly so. The *roentgenogram* is characteristic but not pathognomonic, since it is also seen in other anomalies in which pulmonary venous obstruction occurs. There is evidence of severe pulmonary venous hypertension: The hilar markings are pronounced and fuzzy, and the lungs show a curious reticulated appearance.

The *treatment* of TAPVC is *surgical.* A communication is created between the pulmonary venous junction and the left atrium; any coexisting *atrial septal defect is closed,* and all extracardiac anomalous connections with the systemic venous system are interrupted. In older children and adults, this can be accomplished with generally good results. In the very sick, small infant, surgical correction is difficult and may require two stages. The salvage rate, at present, is low, particularly in the infradiaphragmatic type.

ANOMALIES OF THE ATRIA

Juxtaposition of the Atrial Appendages

In *juxtaposition of the atrial append-ages (auricles)*, the main bodies of the atria are essentially normally located, but there is levoposition of the right atrial appendage; *i.e.,* instead of being to the right of the arterial trunks, the right atrial appendage crosses behind them to appear on their left, interposing itself between the great arteries and the left atrial appendage.

Juxtaposition of the atrial appendages has no functional significance, since it does not, itself, cause any hemodynamic disturbance. Its presence, however, always indicates the coexistence of other major cardiac anomalies. Transposition of the great vessels and a ventricular septal defect are invariably present, and atresia of the tricuspid valve is common. Also depicted is a double aortic arch.

Cor Triatriatum

Cor triatriatum is rare; a fibromuscular septum divides the left atrium into a pos-terosuperior part, receiving the *pulmo-nary veins,* and an anteroinferior part giving access to the *mitral valve* and left atrial appendage. This defect is probably due to incomplete incorporation of the embryonic common pulmonary vein into the left atrium. The original pulmonary venous ostium is represented by an open-ing of variable size. Rarely, the septum is imperforate, in which case the distal pul-monary venous compartment drains by way of a defect into the right atrium, or an anomalous vessel into the systemic venous system. Usually, the fossa or fora-men ovale is located between the antero-inferior compartment and right atrium.

The severity of *symptoms* depends upon the size of the opening between the two compartments of the left atrium. Respiratory difficulties and dyspnea may be marked, and cardiac failure develops early. If the ostium is very small, death occurs within the first year of life; if it is larger, symptoms appear later and closely resemble those seen in mitral stenosis, *i.e.,* chronic cough, dyspnea, fatigability, chest pain, and hemoptysis. Cyanosis may be present, and there is marked cardiomegaly. A mild or moderate systolic murmur is usually heard, but a diastolic murmur is seldom present.

The *electrocardiogram* usually simu-lates that of right ventricular hypertrophy.

The *diagnosis* of cor triatriatum is diffi-cult to establish with certainty, so most afflicted infants still die untreated. *Surgi-cal repair* in older patients is feasible, and, by open-heart technics, relatively simple; the anomalous membrane is excised.

Asplenia Syndrome

Congenital absence of the spleen rarely occurs alone. In most cases, other visceral anomalies are present. In about

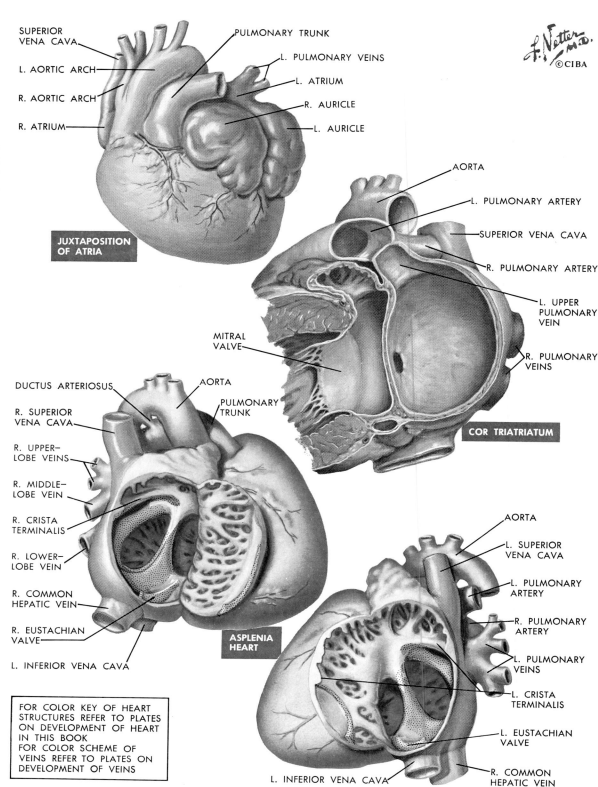

FOR COLOR KEY OF HEART STRUCTURES REFER TO PLATES ON DEVELOPMENT OF HEART IN THIS BOOK
FOR COLOR SCHEME OF VEINS REFER TO PLATES ON DEVELOPMENT OF VEINS

60 percent of these, the typical *asplenia syndrome* is found, of which the most important and interesting feature is the tendency for normally asymmetrical organs, such as the liver and the lungs, to develop more or less symmetrically. The stomach may be located on either side or, rarely, in the midline. Both lungs are usually trilobed and resemble a normal right lung. The heart is generally severely malformed. Usu-ally, a single or common ventricle is present, and an endocardial-cushion defect of the complete type is fre-quently found. Transposition of the great vessels is the rule, and this is usually associated with pulmonary stenosis. The atrial septum is usually reduced to a peculiar triangular band of muscle which crosses the common atrioventricular orifice. In typical cases, both the right and left atria morphologically resemble a nor-mal right atrium (isomerism of the atria); this means that both sinus horns have been incorporated into

their corresponding atria. A coronary sinus is therefore absent. Total anomalous pulmonary venous connec-tion is customary. The great systemic veins also tend to develop symmetrically, there being, at times, a bilat-eral *superior vena cava* and a large vein entering on each side of the atrial floor, representing a bilateral persistence of the proximal vitelline veins. One of these drains one lobe of the liver (*common hepatic vein*), the other the opposite lobe, and the remainder of the inferior vena caval bed. Obviously, in these cases, the situs of the viscera is impossible to determine (situs ambiguus).

The *diagnosis* of asplenia syndrome should be sus-pected in any infant with congenital heart disease associated with some form of partial visceral hetero-taxy, particularly if cyanosis is present. Howell-Jolly and Heinz bodies are typically present in the peripheral-blood smear. The *prognosis* is poor.

DEFECTS OF THE ATRIAL SEPTUM

The atrial septum normally consists of two overlapping, closely adjacent components. Each forms an incomplete partition. The right-side component, corresponding to the embryonic septum secundum, is muscular and firm and has a posteroinferior oval-shaped opening — the *foramen ovale*. The left-side component, derived from the embryonic *septum primum,* is fibrous and thin and has a somewhat round opening anterosuperiorly — the *ostium secundum.* Together, the two components act as a one-way flap valve, allowing the flow of blood from right to left (normal prior to birth) but not from left to right. After birth, with the establishment of pulmonary circulation, the increased amount of blood entering the left atrium elevates the pressure in that chamber, thereby closing the flap valve. In most cases, this functional closure is eventually followed by anatomical closure; *i.e.,* the two components of the septum fuse. In the minority of cases where fusion fails, an increase in the right atrial pressure due to congenital cardiac anomalies, or any other condition which elevates right ventricular and right atrial pressure, causes the right atrial blood to flow again into the left atrium. Such a *probe-patent foramen ovale,* however, should not be considered a form of atrial septal defect. By itself, it causes no hemodynamic abnormalities.

In *true atrial septal defect* (ASD), there is an abnormal opening in the atrial septum allowing blood to flow either way. Ordinarily, a predominantly left-to-right shunt exists. In the presence of associated anomalies or other conditions tending to increase right atrial pressure, the shunt is always from right to left (as in tricuspid-valve atresia), or an initially left-to-right shunt reverses (*e.g.,* after pulmonary vascular changes with pulmonary hypertension).

Ostium Secundum Defect

Of the two main kinds of ASD, the so-called *secundum type* is more common and is one of the most frequently seen congenital cardiac anomalies. The normal resorptive process which leads to the formation of the ostium secundum in the embryo is exaggerated, and most of the *septum primum* disappears. Most ASDs of this type are large. Consequently, the resulting left-to-right shunt is generally substantial, causing a severalfold increase in pulmonary blood flow. Both the right atrium and the right ventricle dilate and hypertrophy, and the pulmonary arteries enlarge considerably. Even though pulmonary venous return and, therefore, blood flow in the left atrium are increased, the latter chamber does not enlarge, since it can readily "bleed off" through the defect into the more distensible right atrium. Systemic blood flow is generally at a low-normal rate or, occasionally, diminished.

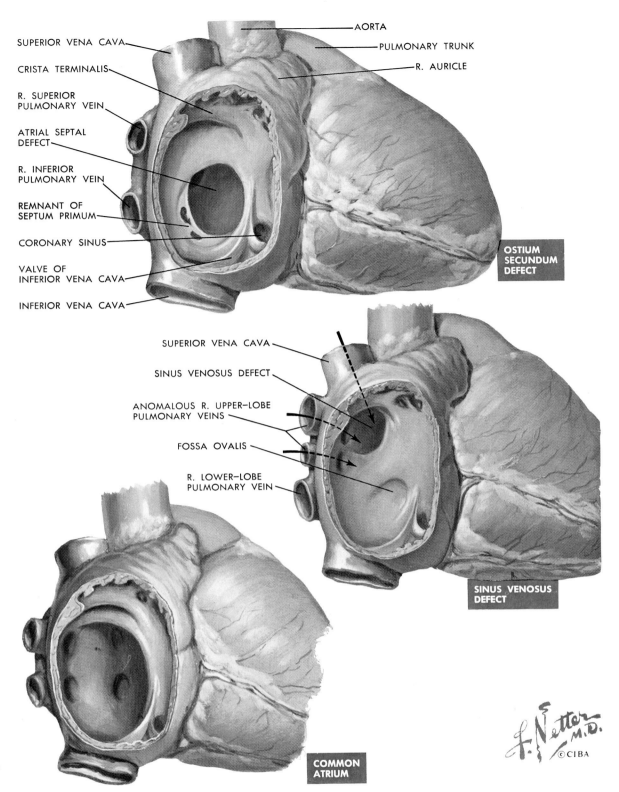

Labels: AORTA · PULMONARY TRUNK · R. AURICLE · SUPERIOR VENA CAVA · CRISTA TERMINALIS · R. SUPERIOR PULMONARY VEIN · ATRIAL SEPTAL DEFECT · R. INFERIOR PULMONARY VEIN · REMNANT OF SEPTUM PRIMUM · CORONARY SINUS · VALVE OF INFERIOR VENA CAVA · INFERIOR VENA CAVA · **OSTIUM SECUNDUM DEFECT**

SUPERIOR VENA CAVA · SINUS VENOSUS DEFECT · ANOMALOUS R. UPPER-LOBE PULMONARY VEINS · FOSSA OVALIS · R. LOWER-LOBE PULMONARY VEIN · **SINUS VENOSUS DEFECT**

COMMON ATRIUM

The *clinical features* are not remarkable, considering the size of the defect and the magnitude of the shunt. Only rarely are infants with ASD symptomatic; in fact, this anomaly is so well tolerated that disabling symptoms usually do not occur until adulthood, when it is the most common congenital cardiac defect. In children and young adults, the only symptoms are mild fatigability and dyspnea following exertion. Many patients are not even aware of the significance of these conditions, recognizing them for what they were only in retrospect, after the defect has been corrected surgically and the subjects have more energy and breathe more easily. Growth and development are generally normal. The heart is only slightly or moderately enlarged, and a thrill is extremely uncommon in isolated ASD. A left lower parasternal "heave" is often present, but a precordial bulge is seen only in patients with marked cardiomegaly. The mur-

mur heard in ASD is not loud; it is systolic, medium-pitched, and of the ejection type. It is best heard at the base to the left of the sternum. It is caused not by the left-to-right shunt itself but by the increased amount of blood passing through the otherwise-normal pulmonary valve. A similar mechanism is thought to cause the faint, short, diastolic murmur heard in the tricuspid-valve area (tricuspid-flow murmur). Characteristically, the second sound at the upper left sternal border is split, and the splitting is fixed; *i.e.,* the time interval between the aortic and pulmonic components of the second sound remains constant with all phases of respiration, unlike the variable splitting which is heard in normal children. The pulmonic or second component of the second sound is often louder than its aortic counterpart. An ejection click is rare in children but may be present in adults,

(*Continued on page 138*)

DEFECTS OF THE ATRIAL SEPTUM

(Continued from page 137)

indicating the presence of pulmonary hypertension.

The classic *roentgenographic features* are mild to moderate cardiomegaly; a prominent right heart border, due to right atrial enlargement; evidence of right ventricular enlargement; a prominent pulmonary-artery segment at the left upper heart border, due to dilatation of the *pulmonary trunk;* and marked hypervascularity of the lung fields. On fluoroscopy, distinct hilar pulsations can easily be seen. The left atrium is never enlarged, and the barium-filled esophagus is therefore not displaced posteriorly.

The *electrocardiographic features* are usually unmistakable. Right axis deviation is the rule, although, in some cases, the axis may be normal or, rarely, even oriented to the left. Prominent, peaked P waves may be seen in leads II and aV$_F$ and in the right precordial leads. Most cases show an rSr' or an rSR' pattern over the right precordium, indicating a mild to moderate right ventricular enlargement. An rR', an Rs, and particularly a qR pattern, not commonly seen in children, indicate more severe degrees of right ventricular hypertrophy, as seen with the development of pulmonary vascular changes and hypertension.

At *cardiac catheterization,* it is usually easy to enter the left atrium through the defect, particularly when this is carried out from "below" by way of the saphenous vein. A distinct increase in oxygen content of the right atrium and an early opacification of the right atrium, on selective left atrial *angiocardiography,* demonstrate the presence of an ASD. Right ventricular and pulmonary-artery pressures are normal or only slightly elevated in most children and young adults. Pulmonary hypertension may be present occasionally in early infancy or late in the course of the disease. A slight (10 to 15 mm Hg) pressure gradient across the pulmonary-artery valve is common and does not, as a rule, indicate organic pulmonary-valve stenosis, since it disappears after surgical closure of the defect.

Generally, the clinical, roentgenographic, and electrocardiographic findings are so characteristic that many cardiologists do not hesitate to refer ASD patients to a surgeon, without catheterization or angiocardiographic studies.

Medical treatment is unimportant. In children, cardiac failure does not occur, except (rarely) in infants with very large defects. Bacterial endocarditis, the bane of many types of congenital heart disease, is extremely rare in uncomplicated ASD. *Surgical treatment* ensures complete cure; it is so easily done, employing a cardiopulmonary bypass, and carries so little risk that it should always be advised. It is almost always possible to close the defect by *direct suture.* Because the defect is so well tolerated, one can comfort-

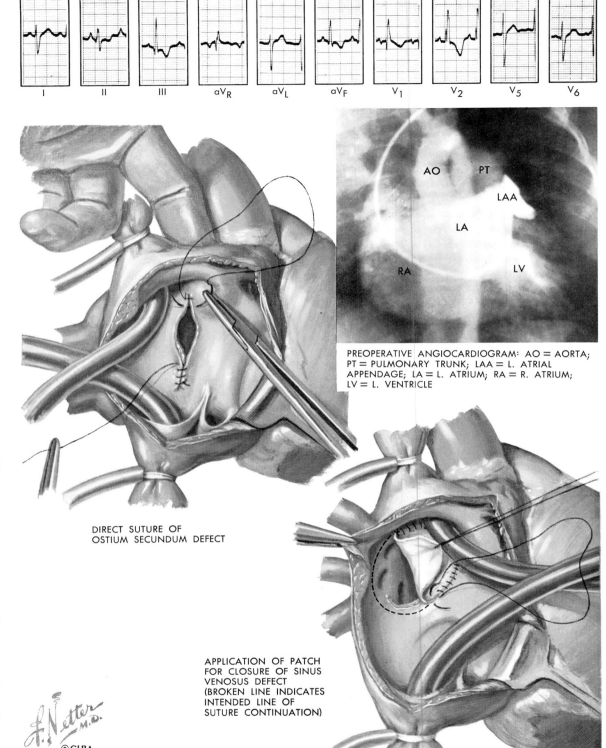

DIRECT SUTURE OF
OSTIUM SECUNDUM DEFECT

PREOPERATIVE ANGIOCARDIOGRAM: AO = AORTA; PT = PULMONARY TRUNK; LAA = L. ATRIAL APPENDAGE; LA = L. ATRIUM; RA = R. ATRIUM; LV = L. VENTRICLE

APPLICATION OF PATCH FOR CLOSURE OF SINUS VENOSUS DEFECT (BROKEN LINE INDICATES INTENDED LINE OF SUTURE CONTINUATION)

©CIBA

ably postpone surgery until the child is 8 to 10 years of age, or older.

Common Atrium

Very large secundum defects, involving practically all the septum and referred to as *common atrium,* are seldom seen. The *symptoms* tend to be more pronounced, and slight arterial desaturation may be present, owing to easy mixing of blood at the atrial level. A prosthesis, consisting of a free pericardial graft, is usually necessary to close the defect.

Sinus Venosus Defect

In the *sinus venosus type of ASD,* the region of the *fossa ovalis* is normal, the defect being located high in the septum at the ostium of the *superior vena cava,* which tends to straddle the defect. Partial anomalous pulmonary venous return is almost always present.

Such anomalous veins usually drain the right upper lobe and the middle lobe. The embryology of this much rarer kind of atrial septal defect is not clear. The *clinical picture* and the *roentgenographic* and *electrocardiographic findings* are similar to those described above.

Surgical correction of this defect may require the use of a *pericardial patch* to reroute the anomalous venous return to the left atrium and simultaneously close the ASD without compromising the lumen of the superior vena cava or the pulmonary veins.

A third variety of anomalous interatrial communication is the so-called *ostium primum defect.* Although it resembles other types of ASD in some of its clinical features, it differs significantly in others, and, strictly speaking, it is not a defect of the atrial septum proper. It is due to a developmental anomaly of the embryonic atrioventricular endocardial cushions (see page 139).

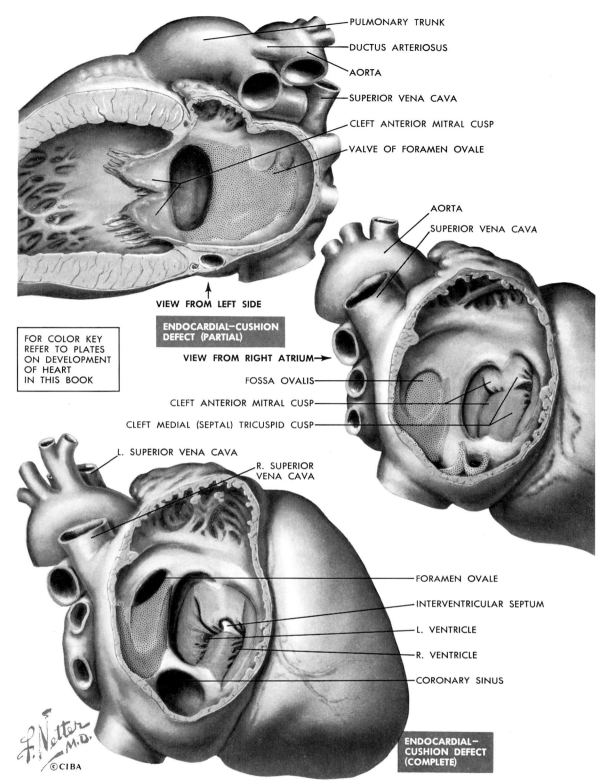

PULMONARY TRUNK

DUCTUS ARTERIOSUS

AORTA

SUPERIOR VENA CAVA

CLEFT ANTERIOR MITRAL CUSP

VALVE OF FORAMEN OVALE

VIEW FROM LEFT SIDE

ENDOCARDIAL–CUSHION DEFECT (PARTIAL)

FOR COLOR KEY REFER TO PLATES ON DEVELOPMENT OF HEART IN THIS BOOK

VIEW FROM RIGHT ATRIUM→

FOSSA OVALIS

CLEFT ANTERIOR MITRAL CUSP

CLEFT MEDIAL (SEPTAL) TRICUSPID CUSP

AORTA

SUPERIOR VENA CAVA

L. SUPERIOR VENA CAVA

R. SUPERIOR VENA CAVA

FORAMEN OVALE

INTERVENTRICULAR SEPTUM

L. VENTRICLE

R. VENTRICLE

CORONARY SINUS

ENDOCARDIAL–CUSHION DEFECT (COMPLETE)

ENDOCARDIAL-CUSHION DEFECTS

This group of anomalies is of extreme interest not only to the cardiologist but also to the embryologist, the pathologist, and the surgeon. As the name indicates, all types are primarily due to a developmental defect of the atrioventricular endocardial cushions. Normally (see pages 119-126), the endocardial cushions fuse with each other and bend to form an arc, the convexity of which is toward the atrial side. The atrial septum fuses with the apex of the arc, thus dividing it into two approximately equal parts. The right half contributes to the ventricular septum, the atrioventricular septum, and the medial or septal cusp of the tricuspid valve. The left half of the fused cushions forms the aortic or anterior cusp of the mitral valve. In *endocardial-cushion defects (ECD)*, the cushions fuse only in part or not at all, and the arc is usually not formed. This results in the pathological features so characteristic of ECDs, which are shared by all types to a varying degree:

1. The *aortic cusp of the mitral valve is cleft,* and its origin is *concave* instead of *convex,* as in the normal heart.

2. The *interventricular septum* has a peculiar, scooped-out appearance.

3. The left ventricular-outflow tract is narrower and longer than normal.

4. The superior-inferior diameter of the *ventricles* is increased at the base.

5. A large, very characteristic, interatrial communication, a ventricular communication, or both, may be found.

If fusion of the cushions fails completely, the atrioventricular ostia form a large, single ostium (*complete type of endocardial-cushion defect,* also called *persistent common atrioventricular canal*), and there is a large, central septal defect which allows free communication between all four chambers. The common atrioventricular valve consists of the normal left mural (posterior) mitral-valve cusp, the anterior and posterior tricuspid-valve cusps, and two large cusps which cross the defect and which have developed from the unfused endocardial cushions. Either or both of these cusps may be attached to the top of the ventricular septum by *short chordae tendineae.* The specimen illustrated here also has a persistent *left superior vena cava.*

If the cushions fuse only centrally, there is a division of the atrioventricular canal into right and left atrioventricular

ostia, but the *mitral valve,* and often the *septal cusp of the tricuspid valve,* is cleft (*partial endocardial-cushion defect*). Several types are distinguished, depending largely upon whether there is an interventricular and/or an interatrial communication. The partial form, with only an interatrial communication, is known as the *ostium primum type of ASD.* This is a rather unfortunate term, since the communication does not really correspond to the embryonic ostium primum, its position being similar to that of the atrioventricular septum of the normal heart. It must be emphasized that the atrial septum in ECDs typically is normally developed and complete, although associated ASDs are not uncommon. The cleft mitral valve is usually (but not always) incompetent. Even in cases of complete ECD, the valve may be competent.

The *clinical manifestations* of the ostium primum type of ECD resemble, in many ways, those seen in

uncomplicated ASD. Symptoms tend to appear earlier in life, however, and growth retardation, fatigability, dyspnea, and the occurrence of respiratory infections are often more pronounced. Pulmonary vascular changes, resulting in right ventricular and pulmonary-artery hypertension, are more common and are likely to occur earlier. A thrill is not uncommon, and, on auscultation, one again finds the systolic murmur at the left upper sternal border and the fixed splitting of the second sound, as in ASD. In addition, however, in somewhat over half of the cases, a high-pitched, blowing, systolic murmur of mitral insufficiency is present at or within the apex and transmitted to the axilla.

Roentgenographically, the heart tends to be somewhat larger than in cases of atrial septal defect, and it may assume a configuration of left ventricular

(*Continued on page 140*)

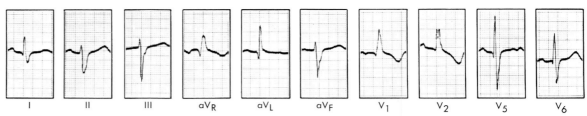

| I | II | III | aV_R | aV_L | aV_F | V_1 | V_2 | V_5 | V_6 |

SUTURE OF CLEFT
IN MITRAL VALVE

ENDOCARDIAL-CUSHION DEFECTS

(Continued from page 139)

enlargement, with the apex turned down and out in cases where there is significant mitral insufficiency. Even in the presence of mitral insufficiency, however, there is no left atrial enlargement unless the interatrial communication is small or absent. Other features are similar to those seen in atrial septal defect.

The *electrocardiogram* almost always shows a left deviation of the QRS axis in the frontal plane, usually ranging between 0 and −60 degrees, but sometimes more to the left. In the complete type of endocardial-cushion defect, the QRS axis may be located in the right upper quadrant. The precordial leads are similar to those seen in ASD, but the evidence for right ventricular enlargement tends to be more pronounced, and the left precordial leads may show a pattern of left ventricular hypertrophy owing to the presence of mitral incompetence. The left axis deviation seen in ECD is apparently not related to any left ventricular hypertrophy that might be present, but it seems to be due to an abnormal anatomical position of the conduction system.

Cardiac-catheterization findings are similar to those in ASD and usually are not helpful in differentiating the two entities. *Angiocardiography*, on the other hand, is an extremely valuable tool, since a selective left ventricular angiogram shows a configuration not observed in any other cardiac anomaly. The scooped-out ventricular septum and the long, narrow, left ventricular outflow are readily apparent during diastole, whereas during systole, the two halves of the cleft mitral-valve cusp are seen to bulge into the left atrium, with a notch indicating the position of the cleft. Mitral insufficiency, if present, is, of course, also readily demonstrated.

The *complete type of endocardial-cushion defect* usually causes severe problems early in infancy (repeated respiratory infections, feeding difficulties, growth retardation or serious failure to thrive, dyspnea, and congestive heart failure). Most of these children die within the first 2 years of life. Cyanosis is rare unless there is an associated obstruction of the right ventricular-outflow tract, respiratory infection, or heart failure. Cardiomegaly develops rapidly after birth. In general, the larger the ventricular component, the sicker the child; if

ENDOCARDIAL-
CUSHION DEFECT

PREOPERATIVE ANGIOCARDIOGRAM (SYSTOLE): ARROW INDICATES CLEFT IN ANTERIOR CUSP OF MITRAL VALVE

DEMONSTRATION USING PAPER, ILLUSTRATING THAT SUTURE OF MITRAL-VALVE CLEFT MAY IMPAIR OPENING IN SOME CASES

NORMAL:
VALVE ATTACHMENT
CONVEX UPWARD

OSTIUM PRIMUM DEFECT:
VALVE ATTACHMENT
CONCAVE UPWARD

SCOTCH TAPE

VALVE CLOSED

VALVE CLOSED

VALVE OPENED;
VALVE SEGMENTS
(PAPERS) OVERLAP

VALVE OPENED;
VALVE SEGMENTS
(PAPERS) SEPARATE

PATCH APPLIED TO
OSTIUM PRIMUM
DEFECT

this component is small, the *clinical manifestations* resemble those of the partial ostium primum type. There is a well-documented common association between endocardial-cushion defects (particularly the complete type) and mongolism, or Down's syndrome. Among all cases of complete endocardial-cushion defects, the *incidence of mongolism is about 35 to 40 percent*.

The *treatment* of ECDs consists of open *surgical correction* of the malformation, always employing a cardiopulmonary bypass. Although technically much more difficult than closure of a simple ASD, the procedure can be carried out, at present, with an acceptably low mortality rate if the anomaly is of the partial type. The interatrial communication is accurately closed by employing a prosthesis of appropriate size. Direct suture should not be done, in most cases, since it may cause distortion of the left atrioventricular

ostium and thereby aggravate mitral insufficiency. Traditionally, the cleft in the anterior cusp of the mitral valve has been sutured, in an effort to create a more or less normal cusp and reduce insufficiency when it was present or prevent the development of insufficiency when it was not. Although suture of the cleft in cases with marked mitral incompetence seems justified, the wisdom of carrying out such a procedure in cases with a competent valve is highly debatable. In fact, suture of a competent cleft may well be contraindicated, since it will interfere with the ability of the cusp to open freely and completely.

Correction of the complete forms of endocardial-cushion defect is technically more difficult — in some cases, impossible. In addition, the children thus afflicted are generally smaller and much more disabled, and, in many, the associated Down's syndrome may present a sensitive and difficult ethical problem.

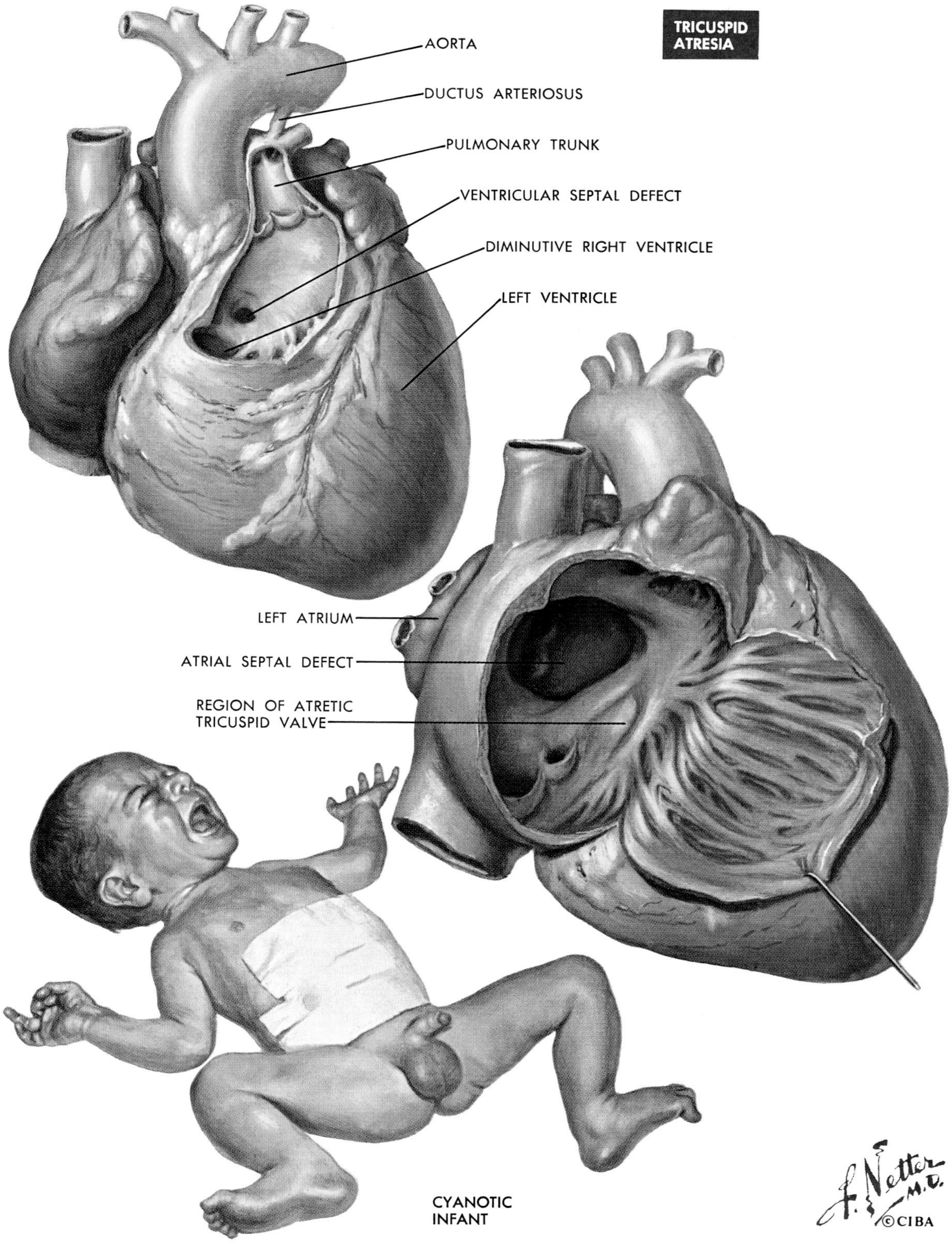

AORTA

DUCTUS ARTERIOSUS

PULMONARY TRUNK

VENTRICULAR SEPTAL DEFECT

DIMINUTIVE RIGHT VENTRICLE

LEFT VENTRICLE

TRICUSPID ATRESIA

LEFT ATRIUM

ATRIAL SEPTAL DEFECT

REGION OF ATRETIC TRICUSPID VALVE

CYANOTIC INFANT

ANOMALIES OF THE TRICUSPID VALVE

Of the congenital tricuspid-valve anomalies, only two—*tricuspid-valve atresia* and *Ebstein's anomaly* — are of real clinical significance. *Tricuspid insufficiency* and *stenosis* occurring as isolated lesions are extremely rare. Some forms of septal defects, such as endocardial-cushion defects or ventricular septal defects may involve the tricuspid valve's medial cusp, rendering this cusp insufficient or allowing for a direct shunt from the left ventricle to the right atrium. Tricuspid-valve stenosis is the usual accompaniment of pulmonary atresia or severe stenosis, in cases where the ventricular septum is intact. Actually, the tricuspid valve, in these cases, although small and often with thickened cusps, is normally formed, and the stenosis is really a secondary hypoplasia.

Tricuspid Atresia

Tricuspid atresia, although not a common anomaly, is seen often enough to have considerable clinical importance. Next to transposition of the great arteries, it is the most common cause of pronounced cyanosis in the neonatal period, and the degree of cyanosis is usually more marked than in cases of transposition.

Only rarely is there a recognizable, small tricuspid annulus, which then forms the rim of an imperforate membrane. Usually, there is a mere dimple, or no indication at all of a tricuspid valve, in the floor of the right atrium. Several subtypes are distinguished, based largely on whether there is an associated transposition of the great vessels (with or with-

out pulmonary stenosis) and whether the *ventricular septal defect*, which is almost always present, is large or small. Of these various kinds, tricuspid atresia, without transposition and with a relatively small ventricular septal defect, is by far the most common. Unfortunately, it also carries one of the worst prognoses, the great majority of afflicted infants dying during the first year and usually within weeks or months. The right atrium, in these cases, is dilated, and either the foramen ovale is patulous or there is an *atrial septal defect*. The mitral valve is large, as is the left ventricle. Usually, there is no trace of a right ventricular-inflow portion, and the infundibulum generally is present and thin-walled. Pulmonary-valve stenosis may be associated, but this is uncommon.

Outstanding among the *clinical features* is the

early appearance of moderate to marked *cyanosis*, progressing with time and increasing with *crying*. Cerebral hypoxic spells, similar to those seen in tetralogy of Fallot and consisting of a sudden deepening of cyanosis, crying, lethargy, and, at times, unconsciousness, are seen occasionally. They usually last only a few minutes but may lead to the death of the infant. The mechanism of these spells is not known.

Clubbing of the digits takes time to develop and is never present at birth. Generally, it is not well marked until the infant is about 3 months of age. In the few children who live for any length of time, there usually are dyspnea on exertion (or even at rest) and fatigability. Occasionally, a youngster may squat, but this is not an outstanding feature, as it is in tetralogy

(*Continued on page 142*)

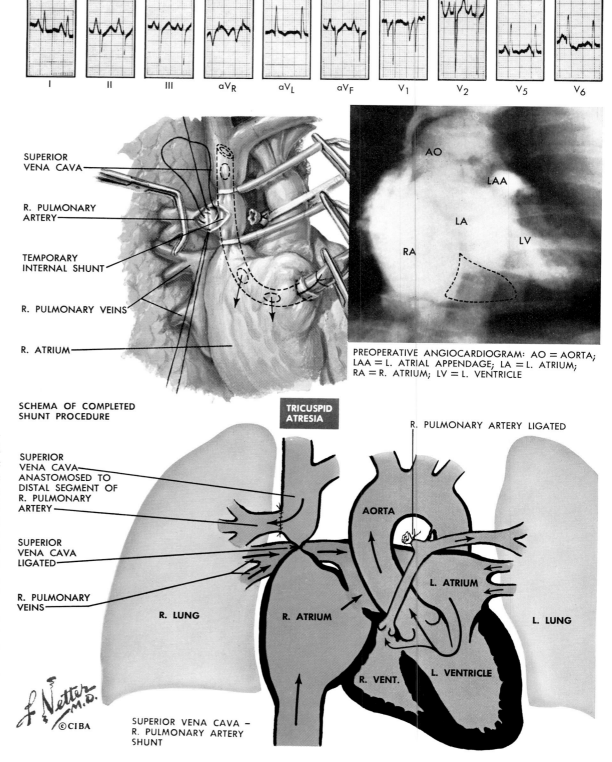

I   II   III   aV$_R$ aV$_L$ aV$_F$ V$_1$ V$_2$ V$_5$ V$_6$

SUPERIOR
VENA CAVA

R. PULMONARY
ARTERY

TEMPORARY
INTERNAL SHUNT

R. PULMONARY VEINS

R. ATRIUM

PREOPERATIVE ANGIOCARDIOGRAM: AO = AORTA;
LAA = L. ATRIAL APPENDAGE; LA = L. ATRIUM;
RA = R. ATRIUM; LV = L. VENTRICLE

AO   LAA   LA   LV   RA

ANOMALIES OF THE TRICUSPID VALVE

(Continued from page 141)

SCHEMA OF COMPLETED
SHUNT PROCEDURE

TRICUSPID ATRESIA

R. PULMONARY ARTERY LIGATED

SUPERIOR
VENA CAVA
ANASTOMOSED TO
DISTAL SEGMENT OF
R. PULMONARY
ARTERY

SUPERIOR
VENA CAVA
LIGATED

R. PULMONARY
VEINS

AORTA

L. ATRIUM

R. LUNG   R. ATRIUM   L. LUNG

L. VENTRICLE

R. VENT.

SUPERIOR VENA CAVA –
R. PULMONARY ARTERY
SHUNT

of Fallot. Cardiomegaly is typically absent in cases of tricuspid atresia, and there is no precordial bulge. A systolic thrill is rare. The apical heart sounds are unremarkable. The second sound at the base is normal or slightly increased and single, the pulmonary component being markedly diminished or absent, as a result of the greatly reduced pulmonary blood flow. Typically, there is a harsh systolic murmur of moderate intensity, best heard at about the third left interspace parasternally.

Roentgenographically, the heart is either normal in size or only very slightly enlarged. The right heart border is prominent owing to the enlarged right atrium; the left border may have a peculiar angulated or squared-off appearance, and the pulmonary-artery segment is reduced or absent. In the left anterior oblique position, the anterior heart border may be flattened. The vascularity of the lung fields is diminished.

The *electrocardiogram* is much more helpful in arriving at a diagnosis than are the X-ray plates. Left axis deviation, left ventricular hypertrophy, and right atrial hypertrophy are invariably present. These are so typical for tricuspid atresia, and so unusual in other types of cyanotic congenital heart disease, that any cyanotic baby showing left axis deviation and left ventricular hypertrophy in the electrocardiogram, and without cardiomegaly, should be considered to have tricuspid atresia. The P waves are generally tall and peaked (often very tall), indicating right atrial hypertrophy.

Cardiac catheterization for the purpose of obtaining hemodynamic data generally should not be done. It contributes little to what is already known or suspected on clinical grounds, merely adding another not-innocuous procedure which the very sick infant must undergo. A simple venous *angiocardiogram* or a selective right atrial angiocardiogram confirms the *diagnosis.* Opacification of the right atrium is rapidly followed by visualization of the *left atrium, left ventricle,* and *great vessels.* Generally, there is a typical, more or less triangular, filling defect between the opacified right atrium and the left ventricle. This area is normally occupied by the inflow portion of the right ventricle. A left ventricular injection in the lateral position shows the diminutive right ventricular-outflow portion to be filling by way of the ventricular septal defect.

Treatment is *surgical* and, obviously, can be only palliative. It is aimed at increasing pulmonary blood flow, which can be accomplished either by a side-to-side anastomosis of the *ascending aorta* to the *pulmonary artery* or by the creation of a subclavian artery–pulmonary artery *shunt (Blalock-Taussig operation).* In older children, an *anastomosis between the superior vena cava* and the *distal right pulmonary artery (Glenn procedure)* is preferred. In this operation, the *proximal pulmonary-artery stump* is *ligated* as is the *superior vena cava,* between the *anastomotic site* and the *right atrium.* This operation has the considerable advantage of bringing blood directly from a large systemic vein to the *right lung,* thus entirely bypassing the right heart. Unfortunately, it is not suitable in very small subjects (who are the sickest

(Continued on page 143)

ANOMALIES OF THE TRICUSPID VALVE

(Continued from page 142)

EBSTEIN'S ANOMALY: HEART VIEWED FROM RIGHT SIDE

ANGIOCARDIOGRAM: PT = PULMONARY TRUNK; RA = R. ATRIUM; RV = R. VENTRICLE; ARV = "ATRIALIZED" R. VENTRICLE

DISPLACED "ORIGIN" OF TRICUSPID VALVE

SUPERIOR VENA CAVA

PULMONARY VALVE

CRISTA TERMINALIS

OSTIUM OF SUPERIOR VENA CAVA

FORAMEN OVALE (ATRIAL SEPTAL DEFECT)

ORIFICE OF CORONARY SINUS

"ATRIALIZED" PORTION OF R. VENTRICLE

ATRIOVENTRICULAR JUNCTION

INFERIOR VENA CAVA

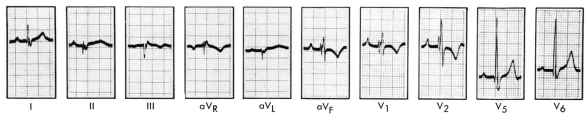

I   II   III   aV$_R$ aV$_L$ aV$_F$ V$_1$ V$_2$ V$_5$ V$_6$

and comprise the majority of cases of tricuspid atresia), because the low-pressure shunt between the small infant vessels has a strong tendency to thrombose, with disastrous consequences. This is also characteristic, but to a lesser extent, of the Blalock-Taussig operation.

Of the other (much rarer) forms of tricuspid atresia, those with a moderately large ventricular septal defect and a normal to slightly increased pulmonary vasculature carry a much better *prognosis* and do not require *treatment,* since the situation cannot be improved upon with present-day knowledge. Another form which has a fairly good prognosis is that which is associated with transposition and a mild to moderate subpulmonic stenosis. A very few cases of such patients reaching adult age have been reported.

Ebstein's Anomaly of the Tricuspid Valve

Ebstein's anomaly of the tricuspid valve, as an isolated malformation, is less common than tricuspid atresia. It is, however, of considerable clinical importance, since most patients reach childhood, adolescence, or even adulthood. The anomaly must therefore be much better tolerated than is tricuspid atresia.

In principle, Ebstein's anomaly consists of a *downward displacement of the tricuspid-valve "origin"*; i.e., the valve cusps, with the exception of the medial two thirds of the anterior cusp, appear to originate from the right ventricular wall — often as low as the junction of the inflow and outflow portions of the right ventricle — instead of from the tricuspid

annulus. The valve tissue is almost always redundant and wrinkled, and the chordae tendineae are poorly developed or absent.

Embryologically, the anomaly can be considered an abnormality in the undermining process of the right ventricular wall, which normally leads to a liberation of the inner layer of ventricular muscle. This process should continue until the *atrioventricular junction* is reached. Much of the apical portion of the valve "skirt" thus formed is normally resorbed, until only papillary muscles and narrow strands remain. The latter become fibrous (chordae tendineae), as do the valve cusps themselves. In Ebstein's anomaly, the process of undermining apparently is incomplete and does not reach the annulus. Individual cases vary greatly in this respect, and, instead of cusps, chordae

tendineae, and papillary muscles, there often are sheets of valve tissue with few or no chordae tendineae incorporating the papillary muscles. The anterior cusp is "liberated" very early in embryonic life, which may be the reason why this cusp always originates normally. The actual valve opening, located close to the crista supraventricularis, is usually much smaller than the normal tricuspid ostium; in addition, the valve is almost always incompetent.

The downward displacement of the valve divides the right ventricle into two parts: (1) an "atrialized" part between the normal annulus and the abnormal valve origin and (2) the normal outflow portion of the right ventricle. The size of the *"atrialized" portion of the right ventricle* varies greatly, and its wall may

(Continued on page 144)

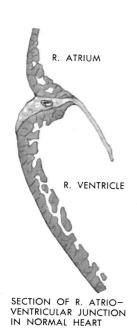

R. ATRIUM

R. VENTRICLE

SECTION OF R. ATRIO-
VENTRICULAR JUNCTION
IN NORMAL HEART

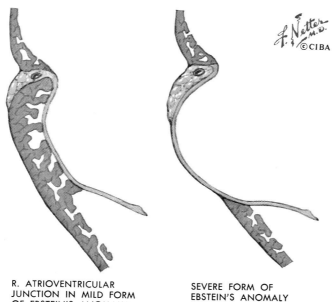

R. ATRIOVENTRICULAR
JUNCTION IN MILD FORM
OF EBSTEIN'S ANOMALY

SEVERE FORM OF
EBSTEIN'S ANOMALY

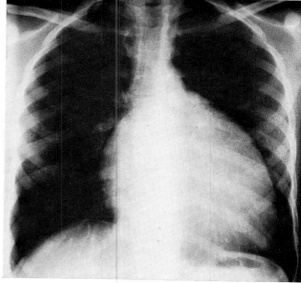

X-RAY: EBSTEIN'S ANOMALY IN A 10-YEAR-OLD GIRL

ANOMALIES OF THE TRICUSPID VALVE

(Continued from page 143)

be fibrous and paper-thin or muscular and fairly normally formed. Very rarely, the valve is imperforate, or its free portion is practically nonexistent. The *pulmonary valve* may be stenotic or, rarely, atretic.

The *clinical features* are highly diverse, an expression of the considerable variability of the pathology. In general, the larger and thinner-walled the "atrialized" portion of the right ventricle, the smaller will be the remaining normally developed part of the ventricle; and the greater the insufficiency of the tricuspid valve, the more serious the hemodynamic situation. In severe cases, symptoms, consisting of cyanosis, dyspnea, and feeding difficulties, may begin in the neonatal period. The early occurrence of heart failure is an ominous sign and is usually followed by death within weeks. In milder cases, symptoms may not appear until later in childhood. Occasionally, the degree of malformation is slight and is compatible with a fairly active and normal life. Cyanosis and clubbing are usually present in older children, and these youngsters tend to be underdeveloped and thin. Cyanosis in infancy often subsides temporarily, only to reappear later. Fatigue is a prominent symptom, as are exercise intolerance and dyspnea on effort. Cardiac arrhythmias are very common, usually consisting of some form of supraventricular tachycardia.

There is almost always considerable cardiomegaly, to both the left and the right (owing to enlargement of the right atrium and the "atrialized" right ventricle), and the peripheral pulses are weak. The apical impulse is diffuse and poorly felt. A precordial bulge and thrill are unusual. The first heart sound is of normal intensity and often is split, the second component being peculiarly loud. The second sound is generally normal. A loud, early diastolic third sound is heard along the left lower sternal border, and a

fourth sound may be present. A systolic murmur, of mild to moderate intensity, is usually present along the left lower sternal border and may, at times, be accompanied by a diastolic murmur. The systolic murmur sometimes may have a curious scratchy quality, resembling that of a pericardial friction rub.

Roentgenograms of the chest show moderate to marked cardiomegaly, and the heart is often box-shaped or funnel-shaped, mainly because of a tremendous right atrial enlargement and of displacement and dilatation of the right ventricular-outflow tract. The pulmonary vascular markings are decreased, and the main pulmonary-artery segment is small or absent. Left atrial enlargement is never seen in this anomaly. Rarely, the heart may be almost normal in size and shape, indicating a mild degree of the deformity.

The characteristic *electrocardiogram* displays right axis deviation, low voltage, and widened QRS complexes in the limb leads and the right precordial leads, and, in the latter, a right bundle-branch-block pattern with "splintering" of the complexes. A pattern of right ventricular hypertrophy is rarely seen, and left ventricular hypertrophy is invariably absent. Tall, peaked P waves are usually seen in leads II, aV_F, and V_1 to V_3, and the P-R interval is commonly prolonged. The Wolff-Parkinson-White syndrome (see page 61), relatively common in Ebstein's anomaly, is usually of the type-B variety.

Cardiac catheterization once carried the stigma of being fraught with danger in Ebstein's malformation, because several deaths were reported as having occurred during or following the procedure. Although it is true that there is a distinct tendency for arrhythmias to occur during cardiac catheterization, the early fears have not been fully justified, and the procedure should be used to establish the *diagnosis* and determine the degree of severity. The catheter has a tendency to coil in the right atrium and thus outlines its tremendous size. The pressure in the "atrialized" portion of the right ventricle is low and, in general, resembles that measured in the right atrium. Right ventricular pressures are normal, except in the rare case with associated pulmonary stenosis and consequent elevation of the right ventricular

pressure. If an electrode catheter is employed, pressure tracings and intracavitary *electrocardiograms* can be recorded simultaneously. Placement of the catheter in the distal portion of the right ventricle will show typical right ventricular electrocardiographic and pressure tracings. On pulling back into the "atrialized" portion of the right ventricle, the former do not change significantly, whereas the pressure drops. On further withdrawal into the right atrium, the electrocardiographic complexes assume a right atrial configuration with large P waves, and the pressure tracings show no further change.

On selective right atrial *angiocardiography* in the supine position, the contrast medium opacifies successively the smooth-walled right atrium, the "atrialized" portion of the right ventricle, and (often after some delay) the trabeculated right ventricular-outflow portion. The diaphragmatic border of the right heart may have a trilobed, scalloped appearance. Injection into the right ventricular outflow outlines the "incomplete" right ventricle and regurgitation across the tricuspid valve.

Medical treatment is indicated mainly in cases with congestive heart failure or paroxysmal supraventricular tachycardia. It consists of the usual anticongestive measures (digitalis, diuretics, oxygen, sedation, bed rest, and reduced salt intake) and the administration of antiarrhythmic drugs (digitalis, quinidine, or Pronestyl®) to control the tachycardia.

Surgical treatment is not simple and is usually palliative. The choice of procedure depends on whatever pathology is present. In general, surgery should be advised only for patients who are definitely symptomatic and incapacitated. A *superior vena cava*–pulmonary artery shunt, as described for tricuspid atresia, has resulted in variable, usually disappointing, clinical improvement. Rehabilitation of incapacitated patients has been achieved by prosthetic replacement of the anomalous valve and, in suitable cases, by resection or plication of the nonfunctioning "atrialized" portion of the right ventricle. An *atrial septal defect*, if present, should probably be closed at the same time, to achieve the full benefit of the procedure.

DEFECT OF MEMBRANOUS
VENTRICULAR SEPTUM
(VIEWED FROM RIGHT
VENTRICLE)

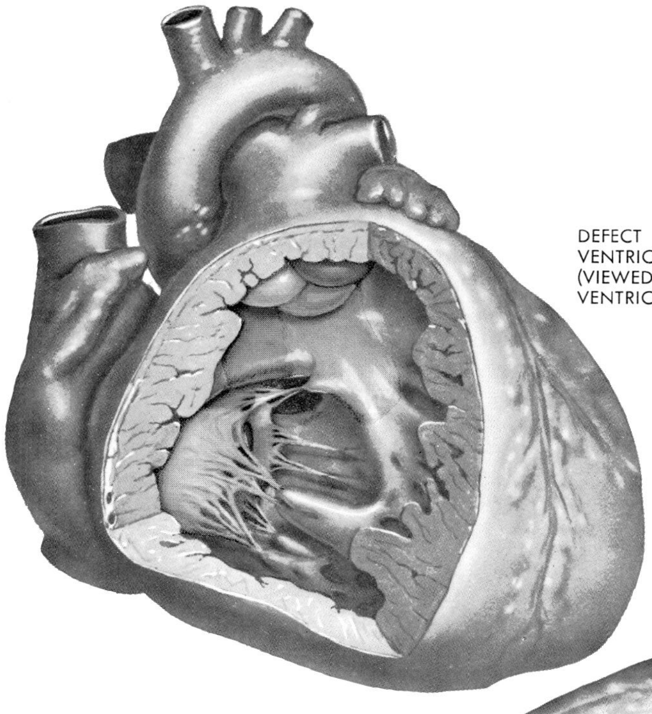

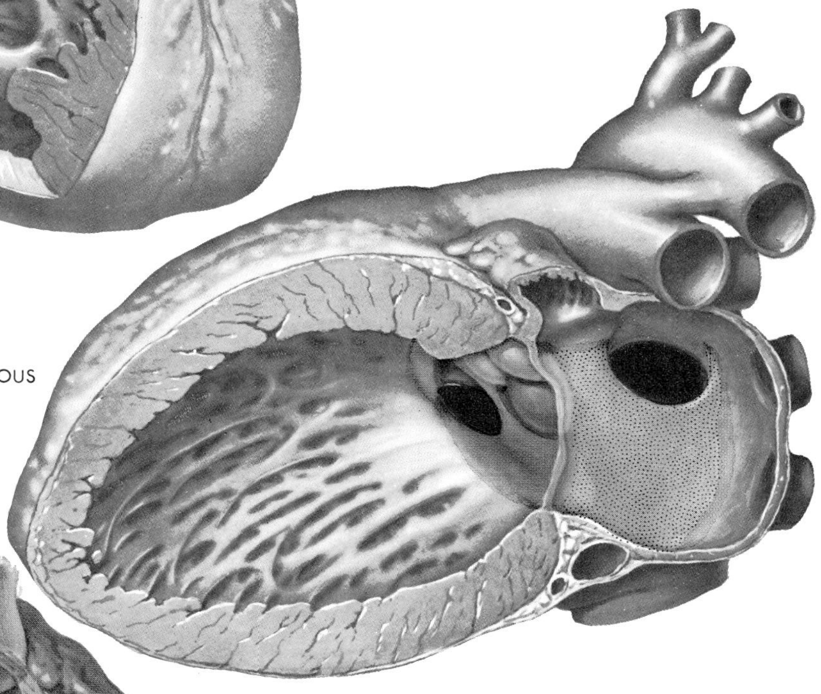

DEFECT OF MEMBRANOUS
VENTRICULAR SEPTUM
(VIEWED FROM LEFT
VENTRICLE)

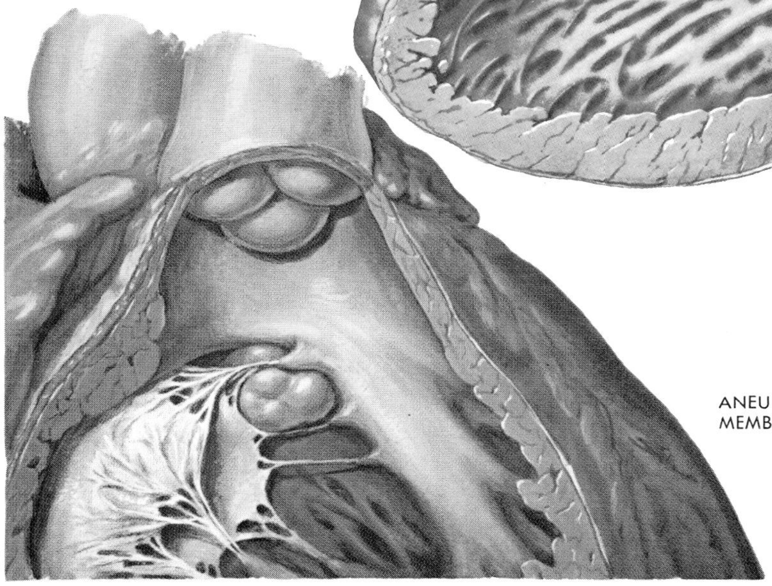

ANEURYSM OF
MEMBRANOUS SEPTUM

ANOMALIES OF THE VENTRICULAR SEPTUM

Of the anomalies involving *ventricular septal defects* (VSD), those located beneath the aortic valve, *i.e.*, the membranous ventricular septal defects, are by far the most common. Not only are they very frequently seen in association with other cardiac anomalies, but, even when occurring as isolated lesions, they constitute the most important and commonest type of congenital heart disease. This is not surprising, considering the complex embryological history of the subaortic portion of the ventricular septum. It is the last part of the septum to close, a closure which is effected by the fusion of components from the embryonic muscular septum, the endocardial cushions, and the conal swellings. Anomalous development of any one or several of these contributors will lead to a defect of the septum. It is therefore obvious that, though located in the same general area, these defects may vary considerably in position and size. Some are found immediately beneath the right and posterior aortic-valve cusps. These probably are due chiefly to a deficiency of the conus septum and, because of lack of support for the aortic-valve cusps, may lead to prolapse of one or the other or both of the cusps, causing aortic insufficiency. Others, due mainly to a deficiency of the right limb of the endocardial cushions or to the failure of fusion of otherwise normally developed endocardial cushions with the ventricular septum and/or conus septum, are located a few millimeters away from the aortic valve, leaving a rim of muscular or fibrous tissue.

Because all the above-mentioned defects are located in the general area where, in the normal heart, the *membranous septum* is found, they are usually rather loosely referred to as "membranous septal defects."

The *clinical features* vary, as might be expected in an anomaly with a diverse pathologic anatomy. Children who have

small defects and shunts are well developed and asymptomatic, and the *electrocardiogram* (see page 146) is normal. Chest *roentgenograms* (see page 146) also are generally normal though, occasionally, the vascular pattern may be slightly increased, and there may be evidence of some left atrial enlargement. Such cases are commonly referred to as having "maladie de Roger." A harsh systolic murmur, often well localized and, at times, quite loud, is heard best over the lower left parasternal area or (sometimes) somewhat higher up. A thrill may be palpable.

Treatment is generally not indicated unless the anomaly is complicated by endocarditis, which, fortunately, occurs only rarely.

Large defects may cause *symptoms* in early infancy. Growth failure is usual in such cases; weight gain

may be distressingly slow, and the children are pale, delicate-looking, and scrawny. Feeding difficulties, respiratory infections, and congestive failure are common, and the infants may spend more time in the hospital than at home. There is cardiomegaly, and a loud, harsh, holosystolic murmur audible over the left lower sternum, accompanied by a thrill, is almost invariably present. A soft, apical diastolic rumble, ascribed to torrential blood flow across the mitral valve, is often also heard.

The chest *roentgenogram* shows cardiomegaly, mainly due to biventricular and left atrial enlargement; marked hypervascularity of the lungs, with a prominent pulmonary trunk and main pulmonary arteries; and a relatively small aorta.

(Continued on page 146)

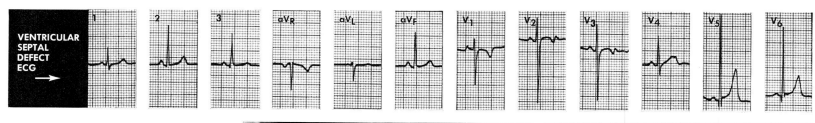
SECTION IV—PLATE 14

Anomalies of the Ventricular Septum

(Continued from page 145)

Electrocardiographically, one generally finds right axis deviation and evidence of biventricular enlargement. This often takes the form of large biphasic QRS complexes in the midprecordial leads (Katz-Wachtel phenomenon).

Cardiac catheterization readily demonstrates a marked increase in the oxygen content of the right ventricular blood samples, and the catheter may enter the left ventricle or aorta through the defect. The right ventricular and pulmonary-artery pressures are elevated and may reach systemic levels. The pulmonary hypertension is due, in part, to some increase in vascular resistance, but probably mostly to the tremendously increased pulmonary blood flow, which may be several times that of the systemic blood flow. The injection of a radiopaque medium selectively into the pulmonary trunk, after passage through the lungs, demonstrates the interventricular shunt. A selective left ventricular *angiogram* will give even clearer pictures of the shunt.

Therapeutically, these infants may present quite a problem. Every effort should be made to carry the little patients through the first year, after which many improve greatly, probably because of the relative decrease in size of the VSD. If *medical treatment* is unsuccessful, a pulmonary banding procedure may be carried out. In this *operation,* a plastic band is placed around the pulmonary trunk, just above the valve, and tightened until the diameter of the vessel is reduced by about two thirds, and the pressure distally has dropped nearer to normal. Usually, there is a concomitant rise in aortic pressure, indicating a more favorable ratio between pulmonary and systemic blood flows. The results of the operation may, at times, be excellent, but there are many failures as well. In any case, it is a temporary procedure and is followed by closure of the defect some

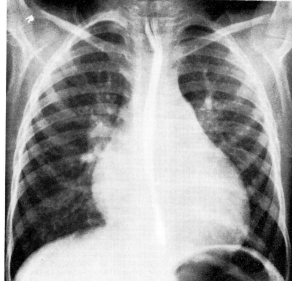

X—RAY: VENTRICULAR SEPTAL DEFECT IN A 5—YEAR—OLD BOY

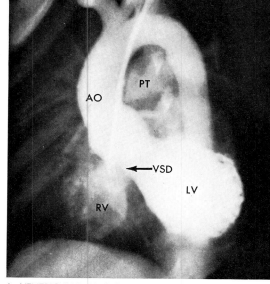

L. VENTRICULAR ANGIOCARDIOGRAM: AO=AORTA; PT=PULMONARY TRUNK; LV=LEFT VENTRICLE; RV=RIGHT VENTRICLE; VSD=VENTRICULAR SEPTAL DEFECT   ©CIBA

years later, at which time the band is removed.

Fortunately, most children with *moderately sized ventricular septal defects* do not have the stormy infancy described above, although respiratory infections are very prevalent, and many patients are rather small for their age. Dyspnea on exertion is also common, but congestive heart failure occurs only very rarely in older children; when it does, one should always consider the possibility of a complicating lesion, such as prolapse of an aortic-valve cusp causing aortic regurgitation, or bacterial endocarditis. A harsh, rather loud, holosystolic murmur, accompanied by a thrill, is generally best heard along the lower left sternal border. An apical diastolic murmur of moderate intensity (mitral-flow murmur) is commonly audible at the apex.

Clinically and *roentgenographically,* there is usually moderate cardiomegaly; the pulmonary vasculature is distinctly increased, and the left atrium is enlarged.

The *electrocardiogram* typically shows a normal or right axis deviation with a pattern of so-called left ventricular diastolic overloading, consisting of deep Q waves, very tall R waves, and (often) tall, peaked T waves, in the left precordial leads. Evidence for biventricular enlargement is also common.

Cardiac-catheterization findings are similar to those described above; however, the right ventricular and pulmonary-artery pressures are generally only slightly or moderately elevated and show little tendency to rise during childhood. A left ventricular *angiogram* is easily done in this age group, and it will clearly demonstrate the size and position of the defect.

Treatment is *surgical* and consists of closure of the defect, either by direct suture or by means of a prosthesis and employing a cardiopulmonary bypass. The risk of the operation, at present, is well below 10 percent, and heart block due to injury to the atrioventricular bundle — a dreaded surgical compli-

cation — has become rather uncommon as experience has increased.

Some patients with ventricular septal defects either always have had, or develop as young adults, very marked pulmonary hypertension owing to vascular changes in the lungs. The pulmonary vascular resistance equals or exceeds the systemic resistance, and the shunt across the defect is, or becomes, bidirectional or mainly from right to left, causing cyanosis and digital clubbing. In some cases, a murmur is only barely audible — an expression of the presence of equal pressures in the two ventricles and little net shunt. The pulmonary second sound is loud and snapping, and the pulmonary valve may become incompetent, resulting in a diastolic murmur at the left upper sternal border.

Roentgenographically, there is little or no cardiomegaly. The pulmonary trunk may be hugely dilated. The peripheral lung fields are clear and appear hypovascular, and the main hilar vessels are large. The *electrocardiogram* reveals a right axis deviation and marked right ventricular hypertrophy, as evidenced by R or qR waves in the right precordial leads and rS waves on the left.

Surgical closure of the defect carries a prohibitive mortality (nearly 100 percent) and is contraindicated.

Aneurysm of Membranous Septum

Aneurysms of the membranous septum (see page 145) are being *diagnosed* with increasing frequency as selective left ventricular *angiocardiography* is carried out more and more routinely. Such an aneurysm may be intact or may contain one or more perforations. It does not, in itself, produce *symptoms,* unless it is large enough to cause right ventricular-outflow obstruction, or unless an aortic cusp prolapses into it — both very rare complications.

(Continued on page 147)

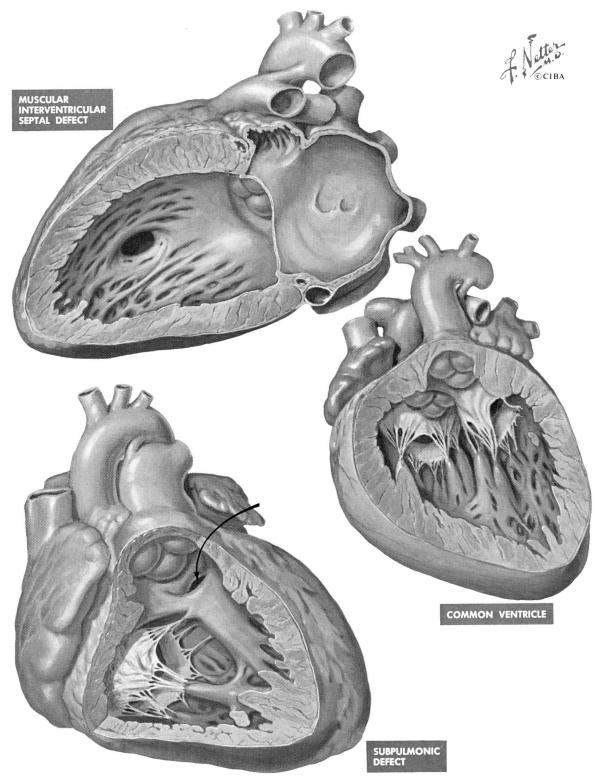

ANOMALIES OF THE VENTRICULAR SEPTUM

(Continued from page 146)

Muscular Interventricular Septal Defects

Defects of the muscular interventricular septum may occur anywhere in the septum. They may be single or multiple, and of any size. If located in the trabeculated apical part of the septum, they may escape notice. The *symptoms* and signs depend on the combined size of the defects. *Treatment* is *surgical* and generally is simple.

A special form of muscular defect is located beneath the two arterial valves. It is due to malalignment of the truncus and conus septa which do not meet each other and therefore cannot fuse. The truncus septum is deviated to the left, and the pulmonary artery overrides the anteriorly located defect. The murmur tends to be located somewhat higher than usual and may sound superficial.

Common Ventricle

In a *common ventricle,* the entire septum is absent except for a low ridge usually present along the posteroinferior ventricular wall. Both atrioventricular valves enter the common chamber, and both resemble, structurally, the normal mitral valve. The two posterior papillary muscles, together with the muscular ridge referred to above, may form a single muscle mass. The two great arteries are almost always transposed, and both may originate from the common chamber, or one (usually the aorta) may spring from a small outflow chamber separated from the main ventricular body by a muscular septumlike ridge. Associated pulmonary stenosis is frequent and generally, if not too severe, improves the *prognosis.* Ventricular inversion is common and is present in the specimen illustrated here.

The *clinical features* depend largely on whether pulmonary stenosis is present; if present, such cases resemble those with tetralogy of Fallot (see page 148). If there is no stenosis, the *symptoms* and signs are

those of a large ventricular septal defect, except that the thrill and the loud systolic murmur are not present. A soft systolic murmur at the base is probably due to a large pulmonary blood flow across the normal pulmonary valve. As in ventricular septal defect, an apical diastolic rumble may be heard. Vascular changes in the lung develop early, resulting in a high resistance to blood flow and in pulmonary hypertension.

Roentgenographically, the heart is normal in size if pulmonary stenosis is present, and the pulmonary vasculature is diminished. In cases without pulmonary stenosis, cardiomegaly may be present, and is associated with an increase in the vascular pattern. In patients with severe pulmonary hypertension as a result of the intrapulmonary vascular changes, cardiomegaly is mild or absent; the hilar vessels are

large, but, peripherally, the markings are diminished.

There is no characteristic *electrocardiogram* associated with the common ventricle, and there is a tremendous variation in the QRS axis and precordial-lead patterns. *Selective angiocardiography* establishes the *diagnosis.*

The *treatment,* at present, can be only palliative, since total correction is not possible, for both anatomic and hemodynamic reasons. Cases with mild to moderate pulmonic stenosis require no *surgical treatment* and may do fairly well for many years. If there is severe pulmonary stenosis, a Blalock-Taussig shunt or an anastomosis from the superior vena cava to the pulmonary artery may be made. In young children without pulmonary stenosis, a pulmonary-artery banding procedure may be considered.

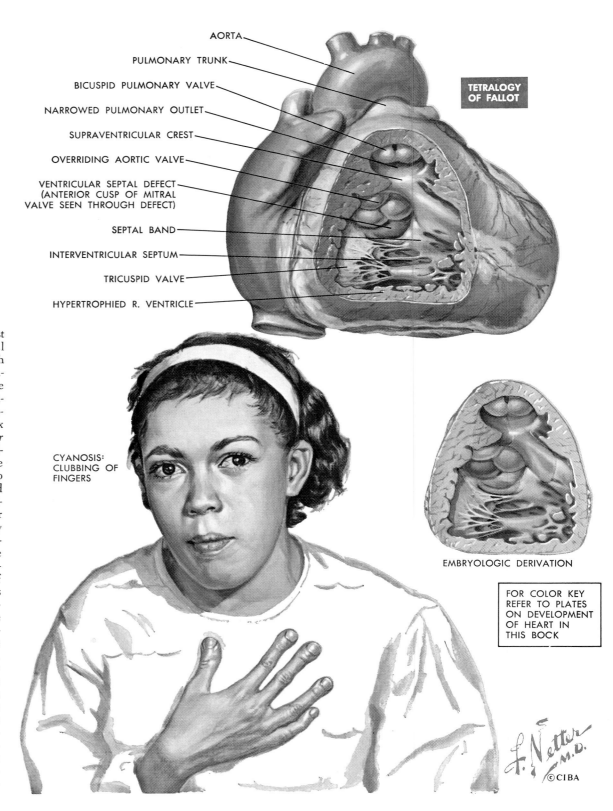

AORTA

PULMONARY TRUNK

BICUSPID PULMONARY VALVE

NARROWED PULMONARY OUTLET

SUPRAVENTRICULAR CREST

OVERRIDING AORTIC VALVE

VENTRICULAR SEPTAL DEFECT
(ANTERIOR CUSP OF MITRAL
VALVE SEEN THROUGH DEFECT)

SEPTAL BAND

INTERVENTRICULAR SEPTUM

TRICUSPID VALVE

HYPERTROPHIED R. VENTRICLE

TETRALOGY
OF FALLOT

CYANOSIS:
CLUBBING OF
FINGERS

EMBRYOLOGIC DERIVATION

FOR COLOR KEY
REFER TO PLATES
ON DEVELOPMENT
OF HEART IN
THIS BOCK

ANOMALIES OF THE RIGHT VENTRICULAR-OUTFLOW TRACT

Tetralogy of Fallot

This cardiac anomaly is by far the most common form of cyanotic congenital heart disease which is compatible with life for any length of time. Cases reaching adulthood, though not common, are by no means exceptionally rare. Classically, as described by Fallot, the four abnormalities which constitute the complex are *right ventricular-outflow stenosis or atresia, ventricular septal defect, overriding of the aorta* (the aorta straddles the ventricular septal defect and seems to originate from both ventricles), and *right ventricular hypertrophy.* Anatomically, there is always right ventricular infundibular stenosis, but the *pulmonary valve,* though frequently *bicuspid,* is stenotic in only about 40 percent of the cases. Nonstenotic valves may be hypoplastic, as part of a general hypoplasia of the *pulmonary trunk.* Stenotic valves may be bicuspid, tricuspid, or domeshaped, without well-defined cusps. The degree of infundibular stenosis is extremely variable, ranging from complete atresia to a barely detectable condition. The ventricular septal defect is usually large, offering little or no resistance to blood flow, and involving not only the area of the membranous septum but also the adjacent more-anterior portions of the ventricular septum. The "aortic override," though variable, is always unmistakable, and, commonly, the aorta appears to originate mostly from the right ventricle. The right ventricle is always markedly hypertrophied, a reflection of the fact that, during life, the right ventricular pressure is high and is identical to that of the left ventricle.

From a developmental point of view, tetralogy of Fallot is a simple anomaly caused by a single embryologic error. The conus septum is located too far anteriorly, particularly in its lower portion, dividing the conus into a smaller, anterior, right ventricular portion (hence the infundibular stenosis) and a larger posterior part. It cannot form the *crista supraventricularis* and participate in the closure of the *interventricular septum,* which, in turn, makes it impossible for the *aortic valve* to seat itself in its normal position; thus, its free edge is so far removed from the *tricuspid valve* that it cannot contribute to the formation of that valve. This explains

why, in tetralogy, the medial papillary muscle is absent and the tricuspid valve is abnormally formed. The truncus septum is also usually displaced anteriorly, thus (in part, at least) accounting for the small pulmonary trunk and the disproportionately large ascending aorta.

The *clinical picture* depends mainly on the degree of right ventricular-outflow obstruction. Usually, it is moderate, at least initially, and the shunt across the ventricular septum is mainly from left to right. Therefore, many children with tetralogy of Fallot are not clinically cyanotic during the first few months of life, but they become so as they grow and as the stenosis becomes relatively more severe. More venous blood enters the aorta directly from the right ventricle, and the pulmonary blood flow decreases in a relative sense. At first, *cyanosis* is obvious only with exertion or crying, but soon (generally within the first few

years of life) the children become cyanotic even at rest, and *clubbing of the fingers and toes* develops. Occasionally, the infundibular stenosis is so mild that cyanosis never develops ("pink" tetralogy). These children, particularly in infancy, may behave more like patients with a ventricular septal defect with large left-to-right shunts.

At the other extreme are those cases where the infundibulum, the pulmonary valve, or both are atretic or severely stenosed. Such infants are generally cyanotic from birth, although the severity of the condition may sometimes be masked by a short-lived patency of the ductus arteriosus, which temporarily maintains a fairly good pulmonary circulation. The ductus usually (and unfortunately) closes, however, within the first 2 weeks of life, often causing rapid deterioration of the infant's condition, so that *surgical*

(Continued on page 149)

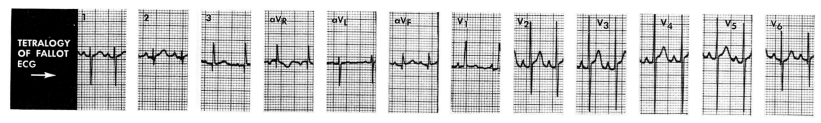

ANOMALIES OF THE RIGHT VENTRICULAR-OUTFLOW TRACT

(Continued from page 148)

intervention, aimed at increasing the pulmonary blood flow, becomes imperative.

A worrisome phenomenon occurs, at times, in young children with tetralogy of Fallot. This is the so-called hypoxic or blue spell. A period of crying suddenly leads to a marked increase in cyanosis, dyspnea, and unconsciousness, sometimes with convulsions. Such spells may occur only occasionally or as often as several times a day, and they may last for minutes or hours. They tend to be associated with bowel movements or feeding and to be more common in the early part of the day, but they can happen at any time and for no apparent reason. Hypoxic spells are serious and may be followed by death. They have been ascribed to a sudden spasm of the right ventricular infundibulum and a corresponding decrease in pulmonary blood flow. Though more common in frankly cyanotic infants, they may also occur in the less severe forms of tetralogy.

Squatting is a posture characteristically assumed by children with cyanotic tetralogy of Fallot who have reached walking age. Assumption of this pose usually follows some degree of physical exertion, which may consist simply of walking. The posture rapidly restores arterial oxygen saturation (by a mechanism not completely understood). Dyspnea and hyperpnea on exertion are common, as in all forms of cyanotic congenital heart disease. Usually, the children are underdeveloped, and there is clubbing of the fingers and toes, except in the first few months of life. There is usually no prominence of the left chest, and a thrill is palpable at the lower left sternal border, in most cases.

On auscultation, the first heart sound is normal. The aortic component of the second sound is loud, but P_2 is diminished or absent. In acyanotic or mildly cyanotic forms of tetralogy, a pulmonic component may be present, and the second sound may then be widely split. The systolic murmur is usually loud and of the stenotic crescendo-decrescendo type, ending before or at aortic closure. In general, the more severe the tetralogy, the shorter the murmur; occasionally, no murmur is heard at all. Likewise, during a hypoxic spell the murmur may be less

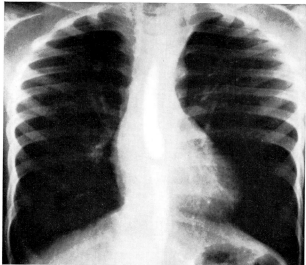

X-RAY: TETRALOGY OF FALLOT IN A 6-YEAR-OLD BOY

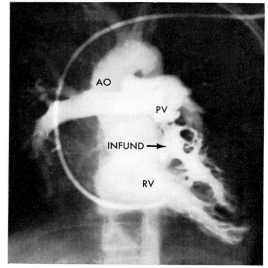

R. VENTRICULAR ANGIOCARDIOGRAM: AO=AORTA; PV=PULMONARY VALVE; RV=RIGHT VENTRICLE; INFUND=INFUNDIBULUM ©CIBA

obvious or may disappear altogether, only to return upon recovery.

The *radiographic appearance* of the heart characteristically shows it to be normal in size. The apex is elevated, and the pulmonary segment is small or concave (boot-shaped heart). The aortic knob is prominent, and the pulmonary vasculature is diminished. The aortic arch is located on the right side in a high percentage of cases (about 25 percent).

The *electrocardiogram* characteristically shows right axis deviation and right ventricular hypertrophy of the systolic-overload type, with tall R waves in the right precordial leads. Transition is usually early and rather sudden in V_2 or V_3 and is an expression of the small size of the heart. Additional evidence of left ventricular hypertrophy may be present in the left precordial leads in "pink" tetralogies, where the ventricular shunt is mainly or exclusively from left to right.

On *cardiac catheterization,* the pressures in the ventricles are found to be equal and at systemic levels; the right and left ventricular-pressure tracings are identical and of a normal, squared-off configuration. There is evidence of bidirectional shunting across the ventricular septal defect, the right-to-left component usually being dominant. Arterial oxygen saturation varies considerably from case to case. The aorta is often entered easily from the right ventricle, and the pressure in the pulmonary artery, if it can be determined, is low.

Angiocardiography is of extreme value, particularly to the surgeon, in delineating the anatomy of the right ventricular outflow and determining the size and position of the pulmonary artery.

The *prognosis* depends upon the severity of obstruction of the right ventricular outflow. Infants who are cyanotic at or shortly after birth seldom survive the first year, unless an operation is performed. Individuals with the lesser forms of the anomaly may live for many years and, though handicapped in many ways, are usually alert and do well intellectually. The more common and dreaded complications are bacterial endocarditis, cerebral vascular accidents due to thrombosis or severe hypoxia, and brain abscess. Central-nervous-system symptoms appearing in patients over

2 years of age with cyanotic congenital heart disease almost always indicate the presence of a brain abscess. It is extremely rare in infants. On the other hand, cerebral vascular accidents hardly ever occur in patients over 2 years of age.

Treatment is both *medical* and *surgical.* Failure is extremely uncommon beyond infancy, but it may occur in babies and should be treated in the usual manner. Hypoxic spells are often dramatically relieved by the administration of morphine and oxygen. Cyanotic children with normal or nearly normal hemoglobin levels can usually be shown to be relatively anemic, and they should be given iron therapy until the hemoglobin has increased to 15 to 17 gm%. Venesection, at one time, was popular in cases with high hematocrit levels, but this has been found commonly to increase the symptoms and signs of hypoxia. It should be carried out in small increments and with caution, and then only in symptomatic patients with very high (80 or more) hematocrit levels.

Surgical treatment is much more important. Any cyanotic infant or child too young for total correction, but with significant symptoms, should have the benefit of some type of palliative procedure. An end-to-side *subclavian artery–pulmonary artery shunt (Blalock-Taussig operation)* is the procedure of choice in patients *beyond* the age of infancy. It is technically relatively simple to carry out, and there is little danger of creating too large a shunt, which might lead to heart failure. In infants, with their small vessels, it is much less satisfactory. The shunt often thromboses immediately, or the infant rapidly outgrows his shunt, necessitating a second operation on the opposite side. Creation of a direct side-to-side *ascending aorta–pulmonary artery shunt* is preferable. The older *Potts procedure* (anastomosis from descending aorta to pulmonary artery) has been found so difficult and so dangerous to undo, when total correction is carried out at a later age, that it has been abandoned. An alternate operation, which may be done in young infants and may be preferred by some surgeons for older children as well, is the *Brock procedure.* This consists of removing at least some of the stenosing

(Continued on page 150)

OBSTRUCTING TISSUE AT PULMONARY OUTFLOW EXCISED TO RELIEVE SUBPULMONIC STENOSIS

CORRECTIVE OPERATION FOR TETRALOGY OF FALLOT

STENOTIC PULMONARY VALVE OPENED

PATCH APPLIED TO CLOSE VENTRICULAR SEPTAL DEFECT AND DIRECT BLOOD FROM L. VENTRICLE TO AORTA

ANOMALIES OF THE RIGHT VENTRICULAR-OUTFLOW TRACT

(Continued from page 149)

infundibular muscle tissue through a right ventricular stab wound, and cutting the *pulmonary valve* also if it is stenotic. The operation is carried out blindly, is difficult to do adequately, and is not without danger, particularly to the *aortic valve*.

The results of total correction of tetralogy of Fallot are dramatic and spectacular, but, unfortunately, this procedure still carries such a high surgical risk that it should be performed only in older children, and then only following a temporary shunting procedure, unless the patient has a very mild form of the anomaly. It is essential that the right ventricular (pulmonary)-*outflow obstruction* be adequately relieved. This entails *excision* of as much obstructing muscle *tissue* as possible, and it may involve the use of a so-called outflow patch to widen the infundibulum and, at times, also the pulmonary root and trunk. The VSD is closed, employing a second patch of appropriate size.

In the severest forms of the anomaly, where there is atresia or near atresia of the right ventricular outflow, total correction may not be possible. In such cases, a permanent superior vena cava–right pulmonary artery shunt often gives excellent palliative results.

Eisenmenger Complex

In this anomaly, there is a large *ventricular septal defect* (VSD) similar to that seen in tetralogy of Fallot, and the aorta overrides the defect. The *crista supraventricularis,* however, is not significantly displaced but is hypoplastic and, occasionally, nearly absent. As in tetralogy of Fallot, the tricuspid valve is abnormally formed. Since there is no right ventricular-outflow obstruction, the pulmonary artery is large. The anomaly is rare, and there still is considerable controversy as to whether it exists as an anatomical entity. The term "Eisenmenger syndrome" has crept into usage to designate situations where a left-to-right shunt, regardless of its level, has changed gradually to a predominantly right-to-left shunt, with severe pulmonary hypertension due to pulmonary vascular changes and a concomitant rise in pulmonary vascular resistance. Pathologically, the Eisenmenger complex may be differentiated from a simple VSD by noting the

R. COMMON CAROTID ARTERY

R. SUBCLAVIAN ARTERY

R. PULMONARY ARTERY

R. LUNG

AORTA

PULMONARY TRUNK

BRACHIOCEPHALIC TRUNK (INNOMINATE ARTERY)

R. BLALOCK SHUNT

PARIETAL BAND

PULMONARY VALVE

AORTIC VALVE

BROCK OPERATION

anomalous *tricuspid valve.* In a simple VSD, the valve is normally formed, and a medial papillary muscle is present. At times, differentiation of the Eisenmenger complex from acyanotic tetralogy of Fallot is difficult, since, in the latter, as in all forms of tetralogy, the crista may not only be displaced but also be hypoplastic. Embryologically, the anomaly is due to hypoplasia of the conus septum.

In young children, the *clinical picture* is that of a VSD with a large left-to-right shunt and right ventricular and pulmonary-artery hypertension. As might be expected, the pulmonary component of the second sound is very loud, and an ejection click is usually present. Pulmonary vascular changes develop early, and older children become increasingly cyanotic.

Radiographically, there are, in young children, cardiomegaly and increased pulmonary vascularity. In older patients, the heart is only slightly enlarged or

of normal size, and the vascular pattern of the peripheral lung fields is attenuated, while the main pulmonary arteries remain large.

Initially, the *electrocardiogram* usually shows biventricular enlargement; in older patients, it resembles more and more the pattern seen in tetralogy of Fallot. At *cardiac catheterization,* the right ventricular and pulmonary-artery pressures are very high and equal to the systemic pressure, and, even in acyanotic patients with a predominant left-to-right shunt, some systemic arterial desaturation may be detectable by oximetry. *Angiocardiography* occasionally demonstrates the hypoplastic crista.

Pulmonary banding should be carried out early, in an effort to prevent the development of pulmonary vascular changes. Once there is an established right-to-left shunt, *surgery* is contraindicated.

(Continued on page 151)

FOR COLOR KEY REFER TO PLATES ON DEVELOPMENT OF HEART IN THIS BOOK

ANOMALIES OF THE RIGHT VENTRICULAR-OUTFLOW TRACT

(Continued from page 150)

Double-Outlet Right Ventricle

In this anomaly, both the aorta and the pulmonary artery originate from the *right ventricle*. The pulmonary artery is normally located; the aorta springs from the ventricle to the right of and posterior to the pulmonary artery. Pulmonary valvar with infundibular stenosis, usually severe, is a frequent accompaniment. A muscular band of varying width (derived from the bulboventricular flange, see below) separates the *aortic valve* from the *mitral valve*. A ventricular septal defect is always present, forming the sole outlet for the *left ventricle*. Embryologically, the anomaly is probably due to a persistent bulboventricular flange, which keeps the aortic and mitral valves separated and prevents the normal transfer of the aorta to the left ventricle. Since the conus septum cannot develop in its normal relation to the right A-V valve, it cannot contribute to the formation of this valve.

The *clinical picture* and *roentgenographic findings* resemble those of the Eisenmenger complex. The *electrocardiogram* shows biventricular or predominantly right ventricular enlargement, and the QRS axis is commonly oriented to the right and superiorly. When pulmonary stenosis is present, the anomaly may be mistaken for tetralogy of Fallot. *Cardiac catheterization* demonstrates systemic pressures in the right ventricle and may, even in acyanotic children, show mild systemic arterial desaturation. The aortic blood always has a higher oxygen saturation than does the pulmonary-artery blood. *Angiocardiographically,* the aorta is seen to be far to the right, the aortic valve is too "high," and the aorta and pulmonary artery are almost in the same frontal plane.

Treatment is *surgical*. As in the Eisenmenger complex, pulmonary banding should be done early in patients without pulmonary stenosis. Total correction is feasible (in those who do not have prohibitive pulmonary vascular changes) by connecting the VSD and the adjacent right-side aorta by a half-shell-shaped patch. Occasionally, enlargement of the VSD will be required. Where pulmonary valvar with infundibular stenosis is present, outflow-tract enlargement with a prosthesis is usually also necessary, not

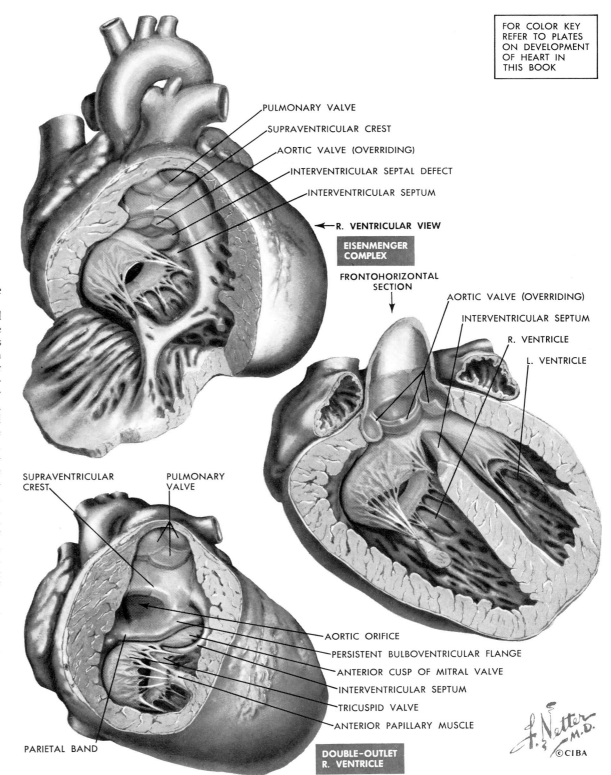

PULMONARY VALVE
SUPRAVENTRICULAR CREST
AORTIC VALVE (OVERRIDING)
INTERVENTRICULAR SEPTAL DEFECT
INTERVENTRICULAR SEPTUM

R. VENTRICULAR VIEW

EISENMENGER COMPLEX

FRONTOHORIZONTAL SECTION

AORTIC VALVE (OVERRIDING)
INTERVENTRICULAR SEPTUM
R. VENTRICLE
L. VENTRICLE

SUPRAVENTRICULAR CREST
PULMONARY VALVE

AORTIC ORIFICE
PERSISTENT BULBOVENTRICULAR FLANGE
ANTERIOR CUSP OF MITRAL VALVE
INTERVENTRICULAR SEPTUM
TRICUSPID VALVE
ANTERIOR PAPILLARY MUSCLE

PARIETAL BAND

DOUBLE-OUTLET R. VENTRICLE

F. Netter M.D. ©CIBA

only because of the severity of the pulmonary stenosis but in consequence of the obstructive effect of the anterior bulge of the subjacent tunnel patch. A major right coronary conal artery, which is commonly present, should be taken into account in placing the ventriculotomy, as its position may render inoperable some cases with pulmonary stenosis.

A special form of double-outlet right ventricle, in which the VSD is located anteriorly, beneath the pulmonary valve, is known as the *Taussig-Bing complex*. The pulmonary valve overrides the defect, and, at *cardiac catheterization,* the saturation of the pulmonary-artery blood is higher than that of the aorta. Corrective *surgery* consists of completing the transposition of the pulmonary artery to the left ventricle by patch closure of the VSD, and intraatrial venous transposition, as described by Mustard. Though the result is a hemodynamic improvement, whether the

right ventricle can sustain the systemic circulation for a normal life span remains conjectural. Again, the degree of pulmonary vascular resistance must be taken into account in selecting patients for surgery.

Right Ventricular-Outflow Obstruction with Intact Ventricular Septum

This anomaly is not uncommon. In the great majority of cases, the obstruction is due to *stenosis of the pulmonary valve.* "Pure" subvalvular (infundibular) stenosis is rare and may be the result of an abnormality in the architecture of the right ventricular-outflow musculature, or it may be part of the myocardial-dysplasia syndrome and be associated with idiopathic subaortic hypertrophic stenosis. The pathologic anatomy of the pulmonary-artery root and valve varies in

(Continued on page 152)

PULMONARY VALVAR STENOSIS
WITH INTACT SEPTUM:
HYPERTROPHY OF RIGHT VENTRICLE

PULMONARY VALVAR
STENOSIS AND ATRESIA

STENOTIC PULMONARY VALVE VIEWED
FROM ABOVE: POSTSTENOTIC DILATATION
OF PULMONARY TRUNK

COMPLETE ATRESIA OF
PULMONARY VALVE

BICUSPID PULMONARY VALVE

ANOMALIES OF THE RIGHT VENTRICULAR-OUTFLOW TRACT

(Continued from page 151)

isolated or pure pulmonic-valve stenosis. Commonly, the valve is more or less dome- or cone-shaped, with the valve ostium located at the apex of the dome. Rudimentary and fused commissures are present near the base of the dome, and the sinuses of Valsalva are hypoplastic. In other cases, the valve cusps are fairly normally formed but thickened, and the commissures are fused for a variable distance or, occasionally, completely obliterated (pulmonary-valve atresia). The valve may be bicuspid or tricuspid. A bicuspid (but not stenotic) pulmonary valve causes little or no functional disturbance and has little clinical significance. Unlike the aortic valve, calcification does not occur in later life. Even in relatively mild cases of pulmonary-valve stenosis, hypertrophy of the right ventricle (RVH) is present. If the stenosis is very severe, the degree of hypertrophy becomes immense, and the tricuspid valve is often somewhat hypoplastic and thickened and may be incompetent.

The clinical features vary considerably, depending upon the degree of stenosis present. Children with mild or moderate stenosis are well developed or even chubby, are not cyanotic, and are asymptomatic except, perhaps, for some fatigue and dyspnea on exertion. In youngsters with very severe stenosis, cyanosis is common and is usually due to a right-to-left shunt, at the atrial level, through a patent foramen ovale. A tricuspid regurgitant murmur may be present in these children. Heart failure is rare but may occur, generally in infancy. A forceful precordial heartbeat may be palpable, and a thrill is usually felt at the base, to the left of the sternum, in the suprasternal notch. In the same areas, a typical diamond-shaped, loud, systolic murmur is audible, often preceded by an ejection click if the stenosis is mild or moderate. If both components of the second sound are present, they are clearly split in proportion to the severity of the stenosis. There is fairly good correlation between the electrocardiographic findings and the degree of stenosis. The ECG may be normal in very mild cases, but, usually, clear-cut evidence of RVH is present. In general, the more severe the stenosis, the more the QRS axis shifts to the right, and the taller the R waves become in the right precordial leads. The T waves are usu-

ally inverted in the right precordial leads, but they may be upright, even if the corresponding QRS complex looks unimpressive. In severe cases, the sequence of R and S waves may be reversed in the precordial leads.

Radiographically, the heart is normal or only slightly enlarged, except in severe cases where a considerable enlargement may be seen, particularly in the presence of failure. The vasculature is normal or somewhat diminished, and there is poststenotic dilatation of the pulmonary trunk and left pulmonary artery, except when the stenosis is subvalvar or of extreme degree.

At cardiac catheterization, the right ventricular pressure is found to be elevated (up to 200 mm Hg or more in severe cases). Understandably, the pulmonary-artery pressure is normal or decreased. The arterial blood is desaturated in severe cases in which a

right-to-left shunt is present. Selective right ventricular angiocardiography is helpful in outlining the particular anatomy present.

No treatment is indicated in patients with mild pulmonic-valve stenosis. In the more severe cases, the treatment is surgical and consists of relieving the obstruction, employing open cardiopulmonary-bypass technics. Closed transventricular pulmonary valvotomy is indicated as an emergency procedure in infants with severe stenosis who are cyanotic, have syncopal episodes, or are in heart failure. In infants, it is advisable to relieve the stenosis, at least partially, by the transventricular approach, if the right ventricular pressure is 100 mm Hg or higher. Even if no clear-cut symptoms are present, this is done in an effort to prevent the development of massive RVH, which may make the operation difficult and hazardous in somewhat-older children.

ANOMALIES OF THE LEFT VENTRICULAR-OUTFLOW TRACT

Bicuspid Aortic Valve

Aortic-valve anomalies are common. A *bicuspid* (but not stenotic) *aortic valve* causes no symptoms in children or young adults, and the only finding is a systolic murmur in the aortic area. Later in life, however, such valves almost invariably become thickened and calcified, with resultant significant stenosis. In a bicuspid aortic valve, the cusps are almost always unequal in size, and the larger member of the pair is approximately equally divided by an abortive raphe. A truly bicuspid valve is uncommon.

Aortic Valvar Stenosis

Stenotic aortic valves are usually also bicuspid. Only occasionally is a fairly well-developed tricuspid valve seen in which the commissures are partially fused. Poststenotic dilatation of the ascending aorta is common. Stenotic aortic valves almost invariably calcify later in life.

The *clinical picture* varies with the degree of stenosis. Severe aortic stenosis may cause cardiac failure and death early in infancy. More often, however, aortic valvar stenosis is well tolerated, and the patients, both children and even young adults, are usually asymptomatic and well developed. Symptoms consist of fatigue, chest pains, and syncope. Cardiac failure is very rare in children. Obvious cardiomegaly is uncommon, but a precordial or apical "heave" is usually present. A loud, typically stenotic murmur, preceded by an ejection click and often accompanied by a thrill, is best heard at the second interspace, to the right of the sternum, and is transmitted well to the apex and along the neck vessels. A suprasternal thrill is always palpable.

Roentgenographically, the heart is normal in size or only mildly enlarged, with a rounded left heart border in most cases. A poststenotic dilatation of the ascending aorta may be present. The *electrocardiogram* is normal in mild or even in moderately severe cases. *Normal X-rays and ECGs do not necessarily indicate mild stenosis.* On the other hand, clear-cut evidence of left ventricular hypertrophy (LVH) on the electrocardiogram generally indicates a very significant degree of obstruction. The *vectorcardiogram* is somewhat more sensitive in this condition, since the QRS forces in the horizontal plane are found to be directed far posteriorly. The only accurate means of evaluating the severity of the condition is to carry out *cardiac catheterization* and determine the pressure gradient across the valve. *Angiocardiography* is useful in distinguishing valvar aortic stenosis from other forms of left ventricular-outflow obstruction. It will also indicate whether the aortic root is hypoplastic, making *surgical treatment* difficult or impossible.

The *prognosis,* during childhood and adolescence, is good. Sudden death — the only major complication other than bacterial endocarditis — does occur, but its incidence is not so high as formerly was thought, and it is minimal in cases with normal electrocardiograms. Nevertheless, aortic stenosis of other than a mild degree is the only congenital cardiac anomaly in which the patient's

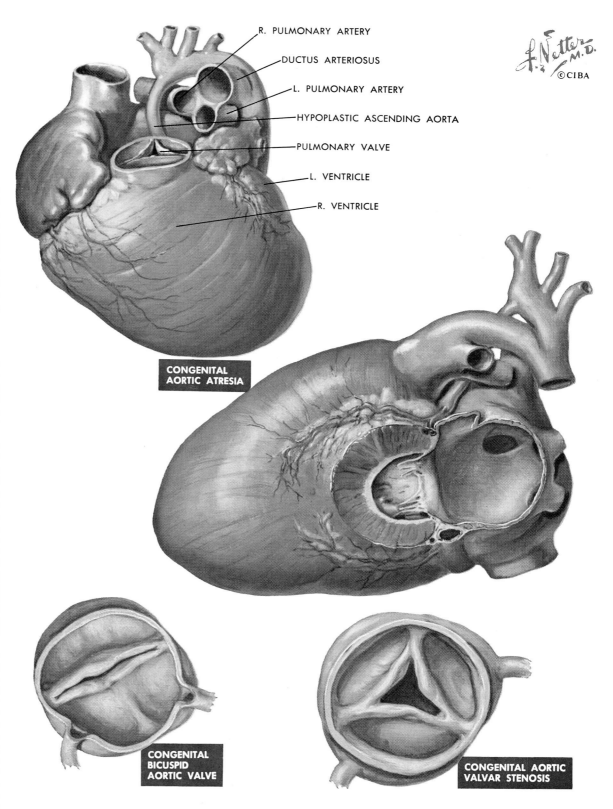

R. PULMONARY ARTERY
DUCTUS ARTERIOSUS
L. PULMONARY ARTERY
HYPOPLASTIC ASCENDING AORTA
PULMONARY VALVE
L. VENTRICLE
R. VENTRICLE

CONGENITAL AORTIC ATRESIA

CONGENITAL BICUSPID AORTIC VALVE

CONGENITAL AORTIC VALVAR STENOSIS

activities, particularly participation in competitive athletics, should be restricted. The early optimism concerning *surgery* has been dampened somewhat; even if the stenosis can be relieved adequately, the long-term prognosis is prejudiced by the likelihood of calcification and restenosis of the valve. Moreover, the risk of bacterial infection remains. Hence surgery, at present, is postponed as long as possible and reserved for patients who are symptomatic, show deterioration on the electrocardiogram, or have high pressure gradients across the valve.

Aortic Atresia

Aortic atresia is not so rare as was originally thought. The aortic valve is completely atretic or very severely stenotic, and the *ascending aorta is markedly hypoplastic*. It serves merely to bring blood to the coronary arteries. The aorta is always fed by a widely patent *ductus arteriosus*. The ventricular septum is generally intact, and the *left ventricle* is diminutive or, occasionally, absent. Its endo-

cardium is markedly fibroelastic, thickened, and pearly white, resembling enamel. The mitral valve usually is tiny but normally formed; rarely, it is atretic or absent. Left atrial blood shunts across an atrial septal defect or, more commonly, across a foramen ovale whose valve has prolapsed to the right into the right atrium.

The *prognosis* is extremely poor. Severe congestive failure develops in an otherwise-well-developed baby within days or, at best, a very few weeks after birth. The infant becomes seriously dyspneic and is grayish-cyanotic. The peripheral pulses everywhere are feeble or absent, or they rapidly become so. Cardiomegaly develops within days after birth, and it generally is already marked when the first chest X-ray is taken, at which time the lungs are seen to be decidedly hypervascular. As may be expected, the *electrocardiogram* shows noticeable right atrial and right ventricular hypertrophy. Most infants die within the first 2 weeks of life. No satisfactory *treatment* is available at present.

(Continued on page 154)

ANOMALIES OF THE LEFT VENTRICULAR-OUTFLOW TRACT

(*Continued from page 153*)

Fibrous Subaortic Stenosis

In this uncommon anomaly, a partial or complete *ring* of fibrous tissue is located just below the aortic valve. This tissue extends, at times, into the base of the aortic sinuses of Valsalva, and the aortic-valve cusps may be abnormally formed. Occasionally, the aortic valve is stenotic or *incompetent*. The fibrous ring causes a subaortic stenosis of varying degree. The embryology of this anomaly is not clear but probably is due to malformation of the proximal extremity of the truncus septum where it joins the conus septum.

The *clinical picture* and the *roentgenographic* and *electrocardiographic* findings resemble those of the more common valvar aortic stenosis (see page 153).

At *cardiac catheterization*, it is usually possible to enter the left ventricle retrograde from the aorta. The ventricular pressure is elevated to a varying degree, depending on the amount of stenosis present. On drawing the catheter back into the aorta, the ventricular systolic pressure drops sharply as soon as the subaortic ring has been passed; usually, no further drop is seen on withdrawal beyond the valve. Thus, the infundibular nature of the stenosis is demonstrated. Selective left ventricular *angiocardiography* may visualize the stenotic ring.

The *treatment* is *surgical* and consists of transaortic removal of the ring, assisted by a cardiopulmonary bypass. Since this ring is predominantly a crescent across the anterior two thirds of the outflow tract, damage to the aortic cusp of the mitral valve must be avoided. As the aortic-valve cusps are usually normal, the long-term surgical result is more favorable than in valvar stenosis.

Idiopathic Hypertrophic Subaortic Stenosis

In this anomaly, no discrete stenosis of the left ventricular-outflow tract is demonstrable anatomically. It represents one manifestation of a condition characterized by enormous hypertrophy of the ventricular musculature. Most commonly, this involves the left ventricular wall, particularly the *septum,* but the right ventricle may also be hypertrophied, as in the specimen shown. The illustration depicts the anterosuperior half of the heart as seen from below and behind. It is not known why the ventricles are so tremendously hypertrophied or whether the condition represents a true anatomical anomaly. Several members in a family may be affected.

Clinically, the patients are asymptomatic initially, and most live into late childhood or early adult life. Sudden death is common. The clinical picture resembles that in other forms of aortic stenosis, but there are important differences. Usually, there is a systolic murmur, which is heard best at the lower left sternal border rather than in the aortic area. An ejection click is not present. Mitral insufficiency may be associated and tends to be maximal rather late in systole. The peripheral pulses are usually easily palpable and may seem brisk, because the initial phase of ventricular ejection is normal, giving the typical rapid rise in arterial pressure. With further contraction, the left ventricular outflow is suddenly severely narrowed, and the arterial pressure drops while

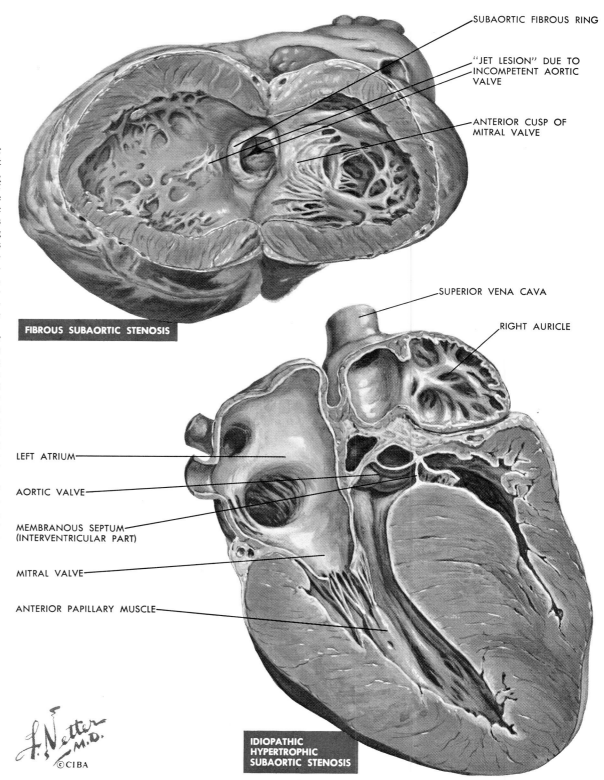

SUBAORTIC FIBROUS RING

"JET LESION" DUE TO INCOMPETENT AORTIC VALVE

ANTERIOR CUSP OF MITRAL VALVE

FIBROUS SUBAORTIC STENOSIS

SUPERIOR VENA CAVA

RIGHT AURICLE

LEFT ATRIUM

AORTIC VALVE

MEMBRANOUS SEPTUM (INTERVENTRICULAR PART)

MITRAL VALVE

ANTERIOR PAPILLARY MUSCLE

IDIOPATHIC HYPERTROPHIC SUBAORTIC STENOSIS

the proximal ventricular pressure rises. Finally, as the outflow portion of the left ventricle relaxes again, the remainder of the blood can be discharged into the aorta. This causes a second hump in the arterial-pressure tracing.

Roentgenographically, the heart is mildly to moderately enlarged, with a rounded left heart border. The pulmonary vasculature is normal. The *electrocardiogram* shows left ventricular hypertrophy, even in those cases where little or no pressure gradient is demonstrable. If a gradient is present at *cardiac catheterization,* it may be localized in the body of the ventricle, at the level of the apices of the hypertrophied *papillary muscles,* or in the subaortic area. It may vary considerably in severity from day to day and is increased, or induced when not present initially, by exercise or by the infusion of isoproterenol. *Angiocardiographically,* the left ventricle is thick-walled and has a peculiar and characteristic appearance in systole. Mitral incompetence is commonly present.

Surgical treatment is developmental. Variable degrees of relief of the left ventricular-outflow gradient, by resec-

tion of the hypertrophied septal muscle mass, have been reported. Various approaches, such as aortotomy and left, transmitral, and right ventriculotomy, presently have their adherents.

Supravalvar aortic stenosis is an interesting form of left ventricular-outflow obstruction in which there is a waist-like narrowing of the ascending aorta just above the aortic valve. The ascending (or even entire) aorta may be hypoplastic, and the sinuses of Valsalva often are aneurysmal. Coarctations and hypoplasia of the pulmonary arteries are common. The lesion is often part of a syndrome, the other manifestations of which are mental retardation, peculiar faces with wide nasal bridges, abnormally formed ears, recessed chins and narrow jaws with irregularly placed teeth, and hypercalcemia in early childhood. The *diagnosis* can be established best by *aortography* and pulmonary *arteriography*.

Surgical treatment consists of incising the ascending aorta longitudinally across the narrow area, followed by interposition of a Teflon® prosthetic patch.

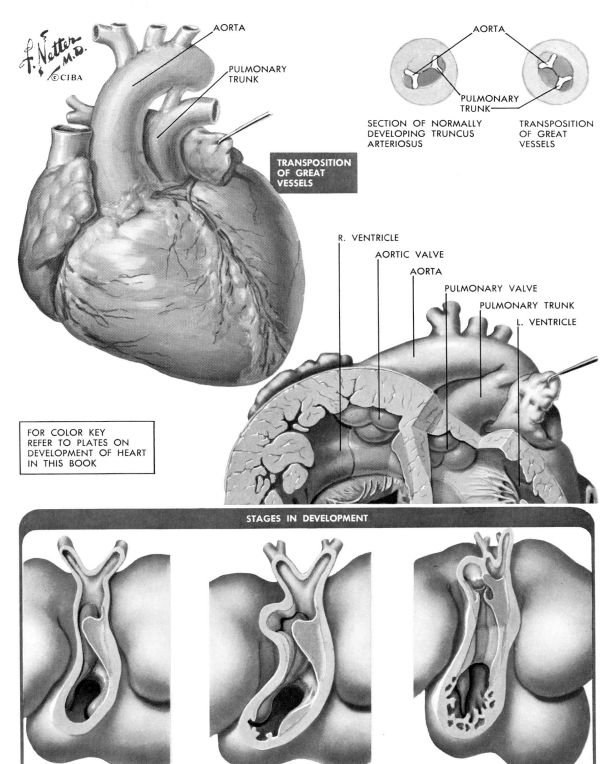

AORTA

PULMONARY TRUNK

TRANSPOSITION OF GREAT VESSELS

AORTA

PULMONARY TRUNK

SECTION OF NORMALLY DEVELOPING TRUNCUS ARTERIOSUS

TRANSPOSITION OF GREAT VESSELS

R. VENTRICLE

AORTIC VALVE

AORTA

PULMONARY VALVE

PULMONARY TRUNK

L. VENTRICLE

FOR COLOR KEY REFER TO PLATES ON DEVELOPMENT OF HEART IN THIS BOOK

STAGES IN DEVELOPMENT

6 TO 7 mm

8 to 9 mm

16 mm

TRANSPOSITION OF THE GREAT VESSELS

An abnormal anteroposterior relationship of the two arterial trunks, with one or both vessels arising from the wrong ventricle, is extremely common and often forms a component of complex cardiac anomalies. In simple, complete *transposition of the great vessels*, the *aorta* arises anteriorly from the *right ventricle* and the *pulmonary trunk* posteriorly from the *left ventricle,* the two arterial trunks running parallel to each other. Only this type of transposition, without associated anomalies other than a septal defect, patent ductus arteriosus, or pulmonary stenosis, will be considered here.

The anteroposterior relationship between the aorta and the pulmonary artery varies somewhat, but, most commonly, the pulmonary artery lies posterior and to the left of the aorta. In uncomplicated cases, the ventricles are normally formed. The *aortic valve,* however, lies slightly more to the right of the *pulmonary valve* than in a normal heart. In somewhat less than half the cases, the ventricular septum is intact, and no other anomalies are present.

The great morphologic similarity of hearts which have isolated transposition of the great vessels suggests that the anomaly is a simple one, *i.e.,* due to a single embryological error. Furthermore, since the ventricles are normally formed, the error probably takes place in the *truncus arteriosus.* It may be recalled that, normally, two pairs of truncus swellings develop. Of these, the major pair executes the partitioning of the truncus, and the other (the intercalated valve swellings) merely forms a pair of arterial cusps (see pages 119-126). It is possible that transposition is the result if the wrong truncus swellings become the major pair. In that case, the pulmonary and aortic intercalated valve swellings form the truncus septum and align themselves, respectively, with the sinistroventral and dextrodorsal conus swellings. The result is that the aorta arises from the right ventricle anteriorly, the pulmonary artery from the left ventricle posteriorly. The conus septum develops normally, and therefore its derivatives (the crista supraventricularis, the medial

portion of the tricuspid valve, and the medial papillary muscle) are normal.

Transposition of the great vessels, the most frequent cause of cardiac failure in early infancy (particularly in cases with an intact septum), shows the following *clinical features:* If a ventricular septal defect is present, failure occurs usually after a few weeks or months. If there is pulmonary stenosis in addition, it may be delayed much longer or may occur only late, as a terminal event. Cardiomegaly is absent at birth but is usually already marked within the first 2 weeks of life. The anteroposterior diameter of the chest is increased, and a left precordial bulge is common. Cyanosis may be present from birth or may appear within the first few days or weeks of life. It appears earlier, is more intense, and progresses more rapidly if associated anomalies, which provide for mixing between the circulations, are absent. Con-

versely, children with large atrial or ventricular septal defects may not become cyanotic for many months or even, in exceptional cases, for a few years. Cyanosis increases on crying, but this intensification is not so pronounced, as a rule, as in cardiac anomalies where venoarterial shunting is associated with diminished pulmonary blood flow (*e.g.,* tetralogy of Fallot). Although the birth weight is usually normal, weight gain is poor, and infants who survive for some time become progressively more underweight. Dyspnea and rapid, shallow respirations are usually present.

The second heart sound at the base is loud because of the close proximity of the aortic valve to the chest wall. It may appear single, owing to poor transmission of the pulmonary component of the second sound because of the far-posterior location of the pulmonary valve. In cases with an intact ventricular septum, a

(Continued on page 156)

TRANSPOSITION OF THE GREAT VESSELS

(Continued from page 155)

murmur is usually absent or, if present, is not loud. If a ventricular septal defect is present, a murmur is almost always audible and may be quite loud but, often, not harsh and pansystolic. A diastolic mitral-flow murmur may be present. In patients with associated pulmonary stenosis, a moderately loud systolic murmur, often accompanied by a thrill, is audible at the base.

The *roentgenologic findings* are usually typical. The heart is enlarged and characteristically egg-shaped, and the upper mediastinum is narrow, because the aorta and the pulmonary artery lie almost in the same sagittal plane. The pulmonary vasculature is increased, with corresponding left atrial enlargement. In cases with pulmonary stenosis, there is little or no cardiomegaly, and the vasculature is normal or diminished.

The *electrocardiogram* typically shows right axis deviation, right atrial hypertrophy, and right ventricular hypertrophy. In the newborn period, it may be difficult to detect abnormalities in the electrocardiogram unless qR complexes are present in the right precordial leads. Additional evidence for left ventricular hypertrophy is usually seen in cases with a large ventricular septal defect or a patent ductus arteriosus.

Although the *diagnosis* usually can be made on clinical grounds, confirmation by *angiocardiography* may be required, especially when the picture is obscured by associated anomalies. A peripheral venous angiocardiogram can be carried out simply and is indicated in very sick infants, but selective angiocardiography is more precise and is to be preferred.

The *prognosis* in simple transposition of the great vessels is extremely poor, and the great majority of infants die within the first 3 months of life. It is considerably better if an atrial septal defect or a ventricular septal defect with pulmonary stenosis is also present.

Medical treatment is useful only in combating cardiac failure, and *surgery* is usually carried out at a very early age. In infants, this consists of the creation of an *atrial septal defect (Blalock-Hanlon procedure)*, which gives very satisfactory

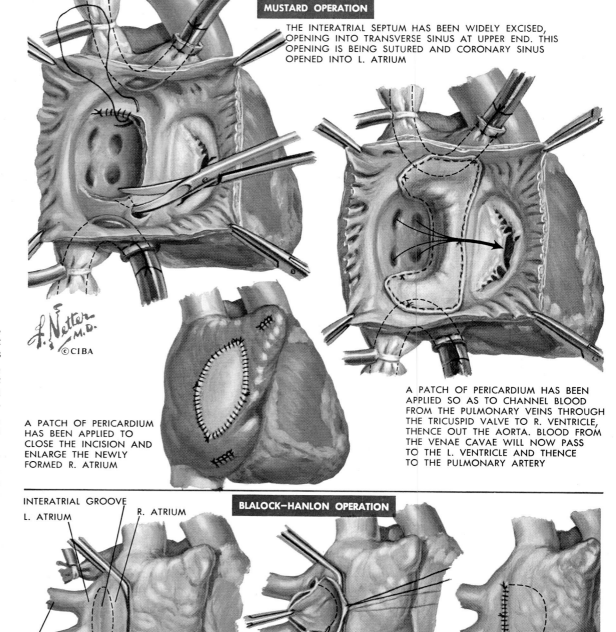

MUSTARD OPERATION

THE INTERATRIAL SEPTUM HAS BEEN WIDELY EXCISED, OPENING INTO TRANSVERSE SINUS AT UPPER END. THIS OPENING IS BEING SUTURED AND CORONARY SINUS OPENED INTO L. ATRIUM

A PATCH OF PERICARDIUM HAS BEEN APPLIED TO CLOSE THE INCISION AND ENLARGE THE NEWLY FORMED R. ATRIUM

A PATCH OF PERICARDIUM HAS BEEN APPLIED SO AS TO CHANNEL BLOOD FROM THE PULMONARY VEINS THROUGH THE TRICUSPID VALVE TO R. VENTRICLE, THENCE OUT THE AORTA. BLOOD FROM THE VENAE CAVAE WILL NOW PASS TO THE L. VENTRICLE AND THENCE TO THE PULMONARY ARTERY

BLALOCK–HANLON OPERATION

INTERATRIAL GROOVE

L. ATRIUM

R. ATRIUM

L. PULMONARY VEINS

LINE OF INCISION

CLAMP HAS BEEN APPLIED SO AS TO EXCLUDE THE INTERATRIAL GROOVE AND R. PULMONARY VEINS

CLAMP HAS BEEN MOMENTARILY LOOSENED TO PERMIT INTERATRIAL SEPTUM TO BE DRAWN OUT AND EXCISED

ATRIAL SEPTAL DEFECT

A LARGE ATRIAL SEPTAL DEFECT HAS THUS BEEN CREATED

palliation in patients who survive the operation. At present, it is also possible to create an atrial septal defect "medically" (Rashkind procedure). A balloon-tipped catheter, introduced via the femoral vein, is passed through the foramen ovale into the left atrium. After inflation of the balloon with dilute radiopaque fluid, the catheter is withdrawn forcefully, thus tearing the thin valve of the foramen ovale. This procedure can be carried out even in small, sick infants, and it may be lifesaving. Various methods of anatomical, or at least functional, correction have been devised in the past decade. Of these, the *Mustard operation* has been found to give the best results and has superseded the older technics. With the aid of a cardiopulmonary bypass, the atrial septum is removed, and a *pericardial graft* is sutured into the atrium in such a way that the *pulmonary* venous blood is directed toward the *right ventricle* and the

systemic venous blood toward the *left ventricle*. This operation is most successful in children over 2 years of age in whom the ventricular septum is intact and the only associated lesion is a naturally occurring or artificially created atrial septal defect. If pulmonary stenosis or a ventricular septal defect or both are present, total correction is much less satisfactory, and the surgical mortality is high. Children with transposition and a ventricular septal defect rapidly become inoperable, in consequence of the early development of pulmonary vascular changes resulting in a very high pulmonary vascular resistance. Relief of the stenosis of the posteriorly positioned pulmonary-artery valve is technically difficult and often is impossible to carry out satisfactorily. In patients with a ventricular septal defect and marked pulmonary stenosis, the creation of a palliative superior vena cava-pulmonary artery shunt is preferred (see page 142).

TRANSPOSITION OF THE GREAT VESSELS WITH INVERSION OF THE VENTRICLES (CORRECTED TRANSPOSITION OF THE GREAT VESSELS)

As in simple, complete transposition of the great vessels, the ascending *aorta* is situated anterior and parallel to the *pulmonary trunk,* but it arises anteriorly from the left-side ventricle, and the pulmonary trunk originates posteriorly from the right-side ventricle. So, the transposition is, at least functionally, corrected; *i.e.,* the aorta receives arterial blood and the pulmonary artery gets venous blood. In addition to the reversed anteroposterior relationship of the great vessels, the left-right relationship of the ventricles is also reversed. The right-side ventricle morphologically resembles a normal left ventricle, and its atrioventricular valve is a mitral valve. The left-side ventricle structurally resembles a right ventricle and contains a tricuspid valve. The morphology and position of the atria are normal.

The left atrioventricular valve is usually abnormal and incompetent. Ebstein's anomaly of the left-side tricuspid valve is common. Other often-associated defects are ventricular septal defect, pulmonary stenosis, and double-inlet (right-side) left ventricle with a rudimentary left-side (right ventricular) outflow chamber from which the aorta arises.

Corrected transposition can be thought of as being due to a single embryologic error. If very early the cardiac tube bends to the left rather than the right, and the bulboventricular loop internally develops normally (but in *mirror image*), then all structures derived from the bulboventricular part of the heart (*e.g.,* the atrioventricular valves, the ventricles, and the proximal great arteries) will become inverted. Only the intrapericardial, freely movable part of the embryonic heart can participate in the inversion; the fixed, extrapericardial portions (the atria, sinus venosus, and truncoaortic sac) cannot. Hence, the atria develop normally and are normally located. Development of the truncoaortic sac itself proceeds normally, but, since partitioning of the inverted *truncus arteriosus* takes place in mirror image, the end result is transposition of the great vessels, with the aorta arising anteriorly from a left-side right ventricle and the pulmonary trunk posteriorly from a right-side left ventricle.

The *clinical features* are determined largely by the character and severity of associated anomalies. Conduction disturbances, with varying degrees of heart block, are common and may occur in the absence of ventricular septal or other gross defects. In the rare uncomplicated cases, the second sound at the base to the left of the sternum is loud because of the anterior location of the aortic valve. A soft systolic murmur, of uncertain origin, may

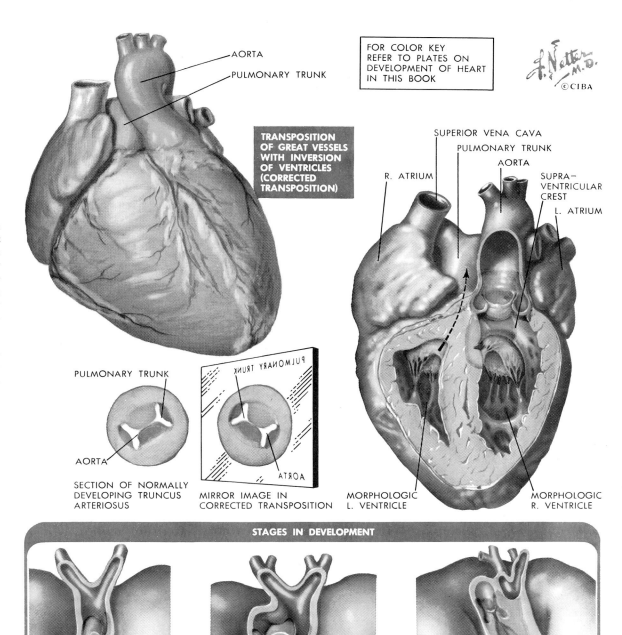

AORTA

PULMONARY TRUNK

FOR COLOR KEY REFER TO PLATES ON DEVELOPMENT OF HEART IN THIS BOOK

TRANSPOSITION OF GREAT VESSELS WITH INVERSION OF VENTRICLES (CORRECTED TRANSPOSITION)

SUPERIOR VENA CAVA
PULMONARY TRUNK
AORTA
SUPRA-VENTRICULAR CREST
R. ATRIUM
L. ATRIUM

PULMONARY TRUNK

PULMONARY TRUNK

AORTA

AORTA

SECTION OF NORMALLY DEVELOPING TRUNCUS ARTERIOSUS

MIRROR IMAGE IN CORRECTED TRANSPOSITION

MORPHOLOGIC L. VENTRICLE

MORPHOLOGIC R. VENTRICLE

STAGES IN DEVELOPMENT

6 TO 7 mm

8 TO 9 mm

16 mm

be audible at the base. Other auscultatory findings may also vary.

Chest *roentgenograms* may show features which suggest corrected transposition. The vascular pedicle may be narrow, as in simple, complete transposition. Of more significance is an indentation of the left side of the barium-filled esophagus, caused by the posteriorly located, enlarged pulmonary trunk. The left upper heart border may be unusually straight, or even convex, owing to the anterior and leftward position of the ascending aorta. Other roentgenographic features vary greatly and are determined by whatever associated lesions are present.

The *electrocardiogram* often shows differing amounts of heart block, and the presence of congenital complete heart block, in an otherwise asymptomatic child, should always raise the possibility of corrected transposition. Reversal of the initial ven-

tricular activation is evident in the electrocardiogram by the absence of a Q wave in leads I, aV$_L$, and the left precordial, and a qR or QS pattern in the right precordial leads. Associated defects obviously will modify the electrocardiogram to a varying extent.

At *cardiac catheterization,* the *diagnosis* may be suspected because of the unusually medial and posterior position of the tip of the venous catheter if it can be made to enter the pulmonary trunk, and the anterior and far-leftward position of the arterial catheter if it is passed into the ascending aorta. *Angiocardiography* is more valuable than cardiac catheterization and easily establishes the diagnosis.

The *prognosis* of the very rare, uncomplicated cases without conduction disturbances should be good. In complicated cases, it depends on the severity of the associated anomalies. The latter also determine what type of *surgery,* if any, is indicated.

ANOMALIES OF THE TRUNCUS SEPTUM

Persistent Truncus Arteriosus

In this defect, a large single vessel arises from the heart, giving off the coronary and pulmonary arteries and the aortic arch with its usual branches. The truncal valve is generally tricuspid but may be *quadri-* or bicuspid. A large *ventricular septal defect* is always present and located anteriorly. Several types are known, depending upon the manner in which the pulmonary arteries arise from the common trunk. In the most common form, there is a short main stem which bifurcates into a *right* and a *left pulmonary artery*. More rarely, these arteries arise independently from the trunk, or the pulmonary arteries, as such, are absent.

The *clinical features* in the common type depend largely on the pulmonary vascular bed. If the resistance in this bed is high, pulmonary blood flow will be equal to, or less than, systemic. The child is markedly cyanotic and has polycythemia, clubbing of the fingers, dyspnea on exertion, and easy fatigability. If the pulmonary vascular resistance is still fairly low (usually in infants and very young children), pulmonary blood flow is increased enormously. Cyanosis is only mild or absent, but the infants are dyspneic and have feeding difficulties, frequent respiratory infections, and growth failure. Congestive heart failure is common. With the development of a high pulmonary vascular resistance in the few surviving children, the left-to-right shunt gradually diminishes, and the heart decreases in size. The patient's general condition improves, but cyanosis appears and, generally, is progressive. Some patients remain practically acyanotic for many years; others are among the most deeply cyanotic individuals ever seen.

A systolic murmur is best heard at the third or fourth intercostal space to the left of the sternum and is preceded by an ejection click. The first sound is normal. The second sound is very loud and may be followed by a diastolic murmur. Usually, such a murmur is due to incompetence of the truncal valve. A continuous, machinery-type murmur, so characteristic of patent ductus arteriosus, is unusual.

The *roentgenographic findings* vary. In children with large left-to-right shunts, the heart is large (at times with an upturned apex), and the vascularity is much increased. The left upper heart border is usually concave, and the aortic knob is large. As the magnitude of this shunt diminishes with an increase of pulmonary vascular resistance, the cardiomegaly and pulmonary plethora also decrease.

The *electrocardiogram* shows a normal or, more commonly, a right axis deviation and either right ventricular hypertrophy or, in cases with large left-to-right shunts, biventricular or (rarely) only left ventricular hypertrophy. Tall, peaked P waves are common. *Cardiac catheteriza-*

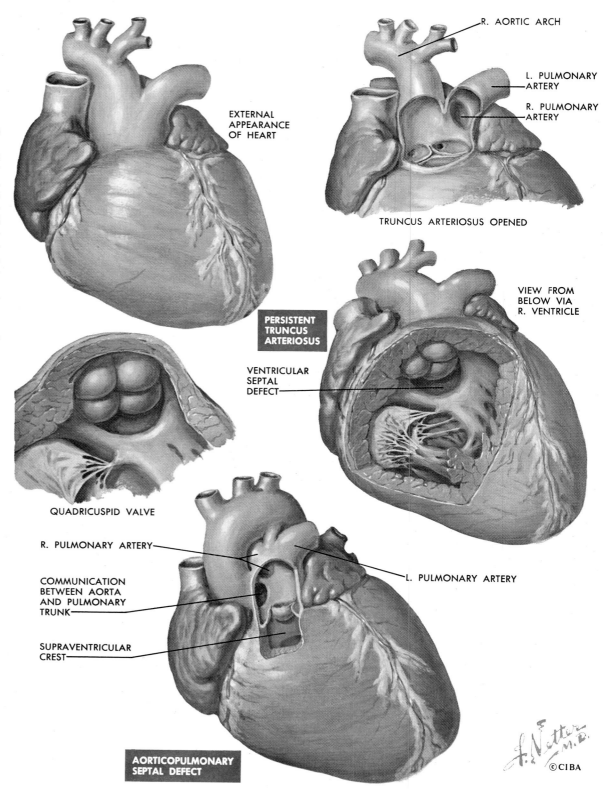

EXTERNAL APPEARANCE OF HEART

R. AORTIC ARCH

L. PULMONARY ARTERY

R. PULMONARY ARTERY

TRUNCUS ARTERIOSUS OPENED

PERSISTENT TRUNCUS ARTERIOSUS

QUADRICUSPID VALVE

VIEW FROM BELOW VIA R. VENTRICLE

VENTRICULAR SEPTAL DEFECT

R. PULMONARY ARTERY

COMMUNICATION BETWEEN AORTA AND PULMONARY TRUNK

L. PULMONARY ARTERY

SUPRAVENTRICULAR CREST

AORTICOPULMONARY SEPTAL DEFECT

tion is not very helpful and may give confusing data. *Angiocardiography,* particularly retrograde *aortography,* establishes the *diagnosis.*

Treatment is symptomatic only; at present, no satisfactory *surgical procedure* is available to correct the anomaly. The *prognosis* generally is poor, particularly in infants with excessive pulmonary blood flow, most of whom die within the first year. The mildly cyanotic patient with high pulmonary vascular resistance and almost normal pulmonary blood flow has the best prognosis and may reach the third or even the fourth decade.

Aorticopulmonary Septal Defect

This is a rare congenital anomaly, usually characterized by the presence of a large defect between the ascending aorta and the pulmonary trunk.

Initially, the *clinical features* are those of a large left-to-right shunt at the ventricular or arterial level and are roughly intermediate in severity between those of persistent truncus arteriosus and patent ductus arteriosus.

The *electrocardiogram* usually shows a pattern of biventricular hypertrophy, at least in childhood, and the *roentgenograms* resemble those seen in a large patent ductus arteriosus. Retrograde *aortography* is *diagnostic.*

The *prognosis* without *surgical treatment,* though more favorable than that of truncus arteriosus, is still rather poor, and the mortality during the first year of life is significant. Fortunately, surgical repair of the defect, employing a cardiopulmonary bypass, can be carried out rather easily, but it should be done at a fairly early age, before an increase in the pulmonary vascular resistance renders the patient inoperable.

ANOMALOUS LEFT CORONARY ARTERY AND ANEURYSM OF THE SINUS OF VALSALVA

The anomalous origin of both coronary arteries from the pulmonary artery is extremely rare and is not compatible with postnatal life. A similar, equally rare anomaly involving the right coronary artery does not cause symptoms at all.

Anomalous Left Coronary Artery

More common (but still infrequently seen) is the *anomalous origin of the left coronary artery from the pulmonary artery*. Since, before birth, pressures in the aorta and pulmonary artery are equal, and oxygen saturation of the blood in these vessels is not very different, the anomaly is of no consequence prenatally.

After birth, with the normally occurring fall in pulmonary-artery pressure, perfusion of the anomalous left coronary artery is greatly reduced, resulting in myocardial ischemia. Given time, the normally present, but small, intercoronary anastomoses expand. The normal right coronary artery and its branches become dilated and tortuous, but the left coronary artery remains rather small and thin-walled. The potential benefit for the left ventricular myocardium from the developing large intercoronary anastomoses is, however, largely lost, owing to a runoff of the blood into the low-pressure pulmonary artery, so that little blood reaches the myocardium itself. The left ventricle dilates greatly, and its myocardium becomes fibrotic, particularly in its anterolateral and apical portions. The endocardium is thickened and fibroelastotic, and calcifications may be present.

In infants, the main *clinical features* are congestive heart failure with episodes of distress, characterized by pallor, restlessness, slight cyanosis, dyspnea, and sweating. Sometimes, the legs are drawn up as if in pain, and the infant's cry is high-pitched. The attacks may be precipitated by feeding or straining and are thought to be anginal in nature. Between episodes, the child is happy and asymptomatic until the onset of congestive heart failure. The heart is considerably enlarged, but any murmur is insignificant. Symptoms usually do not appear until the babies are 4 to 6 weeks old, and most die within the next few weeks. Occasionally the child's condition improves, and the cardiomegaly recedes. A minority of cases are asymptomatic in early childhood and may present themselves later with signs of mitral insufficiency. Sudden death is common.

There are no characteristic *roentgenographic findings*. There is marked general cardiomegaly in infants, and the pulmonary vasculature is normal, or there may be evidence of pulmonary venous con-

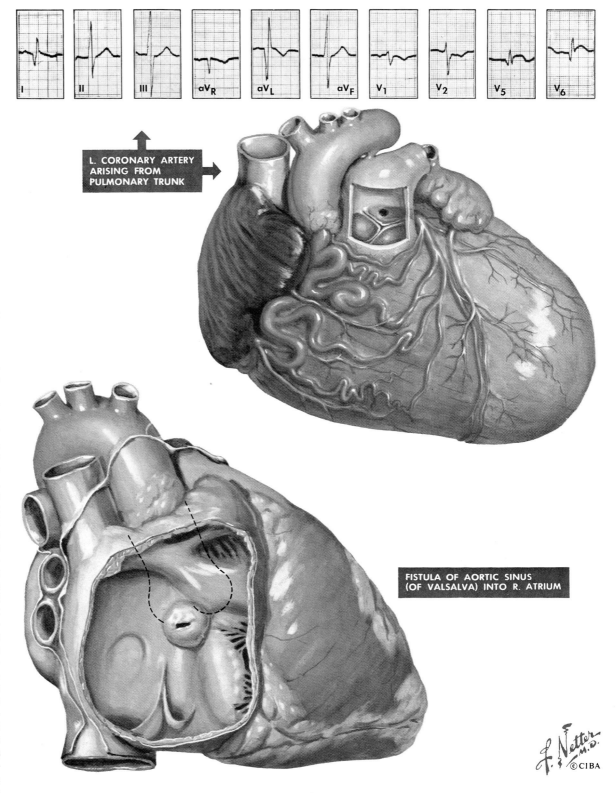

L. CORONARY ARTERY ARISING FROM PULMONARY TRUNK

FISTULA OF AORTIC SINUS (OF VALSALVA) INTO R. ATRIUM

gestion. In older individuals, the heart is normal in size or only moderately enlarged. The *electrocardiogram*, in symptomatic infants, typically shows the pattern of anterolateral myocardial infarction and, usually, also of left ventricular hypertrophy. In older children and adults, the electrocardiogram, as a rule, indicates only left ventricular hypertrophy. *Cardiac catheterization* is not helpful, but *retrograde aortography* confirms the *diagnosis*.

Treatment is *surgical*, i.e., ligation of the defective artery at its origin, to prevent further runoff.

Aneurysm of an Aortic Sinus of Valsalva

This condition is due to a congenital weakness of the bottom of the right coronary or, less commonly, the noncoronary sinus. By itself, it does not usually cause symptoms. Rarely, conduction disturbances,

including complete heart block, are present. Rupture of a congenital aortic-sinus aneurysm, occurring usually in young adults, is virtually always into a cardiac chamber, generally the right ventricle or the right atrium. The sudden onset of an often-large aortocardiac shunt may precipitate congestive heart failure or be rapidly fatal. Therefore, the *clinical features* are often quite dramatic — dyspnea, chest pain, bounding pulses, and a machinery-type murmur accompanied by a thrill over the lower precordial area.

Chest *roentgenograms* are normal in intact aneurysms; after rupture, cardiomegaly usually develops rapidly, and the vasculature is increased. The *electrocardiogram* is not specific. *Retrograde aortography* establishes the *diagnosis*.

Treatment is *surgical* and consists of removal of the aneurysm and transaortic closure of its orifice, employing a cardiopulmonary bypass.

ANOMALIES OF THE AORTIC-ARCH SYSTEM

Patent Ductus Arteriosus

As an isolated anomaly, this is one of the most common and, in general, one of the most benign types of congenital heart disease. It represents a continued patency of a channel — the ductus arteriosus — which connects the origin of the *left pulmonary artery* to the *aorta* and, in fetal life, allows most of the right ventricular blood to bypass the nonfunctioning lungs. After birth, and with the onset of respiration, its usefulness ends and it should normally close, at least functionally, within hours following birth. It is not known why, in some babies, the ductus arteriosus remains patent. It is a common cardiovascular anomaly in the rubella syndrome, which occurs in children whose mothers had German measles during the first 2 months of pregnancy. Patent ductus arteriosus is often associated with other cardiac anomalies and, in some (*e.g.*, aortic atresia), it is always present.

The *clinical features* of uncomplicated patent ductus arteriosus are characteristic in the majority of cases. Usually, the duct is rather small, and there are few or no symptoms in early childhood. Growth and development are normal. The heart is normal in size or may be enlarged slightly to moderately, depending upon the magnitude of the shunt across the ductus arteriosus. A thrill is often palpable over the left upper sternal border. Usually, it is systolic in time, but it may continue into diastole. There is a characteristic machinery- or fistulous-type murmur. It starts shortly after the first sound, increases in intensity, and decreases again after the end of systole. The characteristic features of the murmur are due to the fact that the aortic pressure is higher than the pulmonary-artery pressure during all phases of the cardiac cycle, since the pulmonary vascular resistance is considerably lower than that in the systemic vascular bed. The easy and rapid runoff of blood, during diastole, into the low-resistance pulmonary vascular bed results in a wide pulse pressure and explains the bounding peripheral pulses typically present in children with a patent ductus arteriosus.

Some infants with a very large ductus arteriosus may become symptomatic early in life or may even go into congestive heart failure. The symptomatology and physical findings resemble those seen in babies with large ventricular septal defects and massive left-to-right shunts.

The *roentgenographic findings* are similar to those in ventricular septal defect, but the aortic knob, instead of being small, is generally quite large. The *electrocardiogram* is normal in almost half of the cases; in the remainder, it shows left ventricular hypertrophy of the volume-overload type or, in a minority of cases, biventricular hypertrophy.

The *clinical* findings are generally so characteristic that *cardiac catheterization*

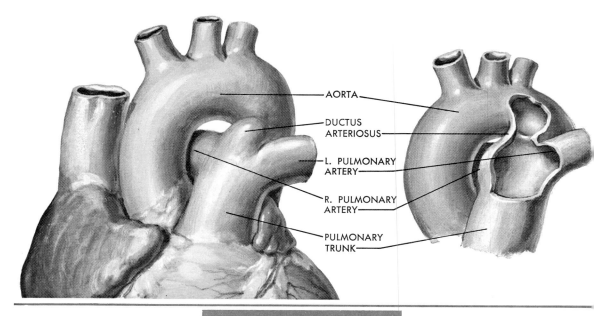

PATENT DUCTUS ARTERIOSUS

- AORTA
- DUCTUS ARTERIOSUS
- L. PULMONARY ARTERY
- R. PULMONARY ARTERY
- PULMONARY TRUNK

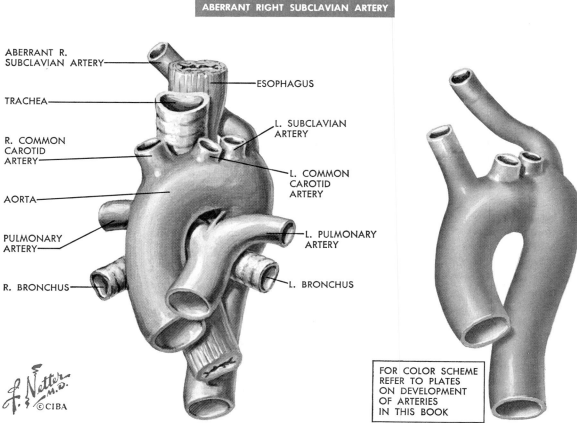

ABERRANT RIGHT SUBCLAVIAN ARTERY

- ABERRANT R. SUBCLAVIAN ARTERY
- TRACHEA
- R. COMMON CAROTID ARTERY
- AORTA
- PULMONARY ARTERY
- R. BRONCHUS
- ESOPHAGUS
- L. SUBCLAVIAN ARTERY
- L. COMMON CAROTID ARTERY
- L. PULMONARY ARTERY
- L. BRONCHUS

FOR COLOR SCHEME REFER TO PLATES ON DEVELOPMENT OF ARTERIES IN THIS BOOK

and *angiocardiographic* studies are not necessary. In cases of doubt, *aortograms* reveal the ductus arteriosus.

Treatment is simple and consists of *surgical* division of the patent ductus arteriosus. Where there is a left-to-right shunt initially, operation, as in all lesions, is contraindicated, once the patient has become cyanotic owing to a reversal of the shunt.

Aberrant Right Subclavian Artery

An *anomalous right subclavian artery*, originating from the descending *aortic arch* as a last branch and crossing behind the *esophagus* to the right arm, is very common both as an isolated anomaly and in association with other defects. It can be explained by postulating a disappearance of the right fourth aortic arch, which normally forms the most-proximal part of the right subclavian artery, and a persistence of the normally disappearing right dorsal aorta.

This anomaly can be detected *radiographically*, since it causes a posterior and oblique indentation of the barium-filled esophagus at the level of the fourth thoracic vertebra. It has been blamed for causing dysphagia (dysphagia lusoria) but only rarely does so. Usually, it is an incidental finding. The earlier notion that it may, at times, run between the *trachea* and the esophagus is almost certainly incorrect.

In an embryo of 7 to 8 mm C-R length, the first two pairs of *aortic arches* have disappeared, as such. The fifth pair, never well developed in man, has had only a fleeting existence. The remaining third, fourth, and sixth pairs of arches are well developed, originate from the truncoaortic sac, and encircle the developing esophagus and tracheobronchial tree to join the right and left dorsal aortas. All these aortic arches are normally retained, except for the distal portion of the right

(Continued on page 161)

ANOMALIES OF THE AORTIC-ARCH SYSTEM

(Continued from page 160)

sixth arch which has already disappeared in a 14-mm embryo. The establishment of a normal aortic-arch system involves the involution of three additional vessel segments (see pages 127 and 128).

The encirclement of the trachea and esophagus by the aortic-arch system in an early embryo does not constrict these structures, since the opening in the arterial ring is wide. With further development, however, there is relative shortening and widening of the arteries, and the ring becomes tighter. This will lead to compression of the esophagus and the trachea, unless the ring system is opened. To do this, it is only necessary for the distal portion of one of the dorsal aortas (in mammals, the right; in birds, the left) to disappear. If the distal right dorsal aorta persists as a major channel, a vascular ring can be prevented only if both the distal right sixth arch and the right dorsal aortic segment between the right fourth and sixth arches disappear. This simply results in an *anomalous right subclavian artery*, as shown in Plate 28. However, if only the right distal sixth arch vanishes, a *double aortic arch is formed*. If only the segment of dorsal aorta between the fourth and sixth arches is removed, the result will be a *right-side ductus of the posterior type*.

Double Aortic Arch

In cases of *double aortic arch*, the two arches may be equal in size but usually are not. Most commonly, the right-side arch is dominant, regardless of whether the *descending aorta* runs to the right or, more commonly, to the left of the spine. At times, the left arch is atretic. The *ductus (ligamentum) arteriosus*, in the majority of cases, is on the left side, but it may be on the right. Rarely, there is a bilateral ductus arteriosus. *Left* and *right common carotid* and subclavian arteries arise from their corresponding arches.

The *clinical symptoms* are those of obstruction of the trachea and esophagus, and their severity depends upon the tightness of the vascular ring. Symptoms generally are present in childhood, often in early infancy; occasionally, patients are asymptomatic, and the ring is discovered only accidentally. Wheezing, cough, inspiratory stridor, repeated respiratory infections, and aspiration pneumonia are common problems. Extension of the head and back tends to relieve respiratory difficulties, and infants often spontaneously assume such a position of hyperextension. Dysphagia varies in severity. It is often increased, or appears, when the child begins to take solid foods.

Roentgenographic examination, including an *esophagogram*, is of the utmost importance and demonstrates the ring's constriction of both the esophagus and the trachea.

Surgery is indicated in symptomatic patients and, at times, must be carried

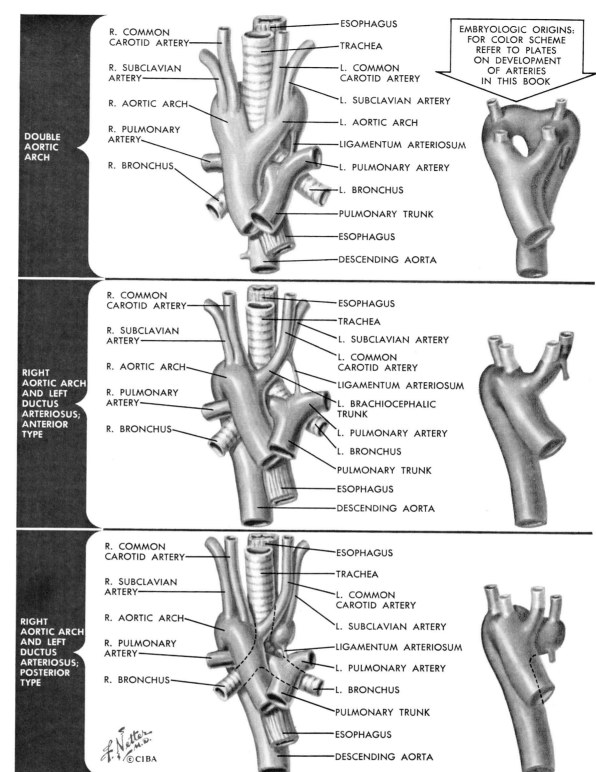

DOUBLE AORTIC ARCH — R. COMMON CAROTID ARTERY, R. SUBCLAVIAN ARTERY, R. AORTIC ARCH, R. PULMONARY ARTERY, R. BRONCHUS, ESOPHAGUS, TRACHEA, L. COMMON CAROTID ARTERY, L. SUBCLAVIAN ARTERY, L. AORTIC ARCH, LIGAMENTUM ARTERIOSUM, L. PULMONARY ARTERY, L. BRONCHUS, PULMONARY TRUNK, ESOPHAGUS, DESCENDING AORTA

EMBRYOLOGIC ORIGINS: FOR COLOR SCHEME REFER TO PLATES ON DEVELOPMENT OF ARTERIES IN THIS BOOK

RIGHT AORTIC ARCH AND LEFT DUCTUS ARTERIOSUS; ANTERIOR TYPE — R. COMMON CAROTID ARTERY, R. SUBCLAVIAN ARTERY, R. AORTIC ARCH, R. PULMONARY ARTERY, R. BRONCHUS, ESOPHAGUS, TRACHEA, L. SUBCLAVIAN ARTERY, L. COMMON CAROTID ARTERY, LIGAMENTUM ARTERIOSUM, L. BRACHIOCEPHALIC TRUNK, L. PULMONARY ARTERY, L. BRONCHUS, PULMONARY TRUNK, ESOPHAGUS, DESCENDING AORTA

RIGHT AORTIC ARCH AND LEFT DUCTUS ARTERIOSUS; POSTERIOR TYPE — R. COMMON CAROTID ARTERY, R. SUBCLAVIAN ARTERY, R. AORTIC ARCH, R. PULMONARY ARTERY, R. BRONCHUS, ESOPHAGUS, TRACHEA, L. COMMON CAROTID ARTERY, L. SUBCLAVIAN ARTERY, LIGAMENTUM ARTERIOSUM, L. PULMONARY ARTERY, L. BRONCHUS, PULMONARY TRUNK, ESOPHAGUS, DESCENDING AORTA

out as an emergency procedure. It consists of division of the smaller or atretic arch. If there is a ductus arteriosus or ligament on the same side, it also should be divided, or the patient will be left with a vascular ring of a different type, formed by the right arch, left ductus arteriosus, and pulmonary artery (see below).

Right Aortic Arch with Left-Side Contralateral Ductus Arteriosus

This condition may or may not cause symptoms. If the ductus originates from the bifurcation of the (here left-side) innominate artery, no ring is formed. However, if the ductus arteriosus arises *posteriorly* from a diverticulum (representing the left dorsal aorta) of the descending arch, a ring is formed by the *right arch, left ductus arteriosus*, and *pulmonary artery*.

The *symptoms* of this condition are similar to those

described above, but they generally appear later and tend to be less severe. Obviously, this type of anomaly can also occur in mirror-image fashion in cases with a left aortic arch.

Treatment is simple and consists of division of the ductus arteriosus or ligament.

Other variants of aortic-arch anomalies involving the third or fourth arches occur, but, as long as they do not form a constricting ring, they only occasionally cause symptoms and are of little clinical importance.

Anomalies of the aortic-arch system that mainly involve the sixth arches are rather uncommon. They are usually referred to as cases of absent left or right pulmonary artery, a terminology which is misleading.

It may be recalled that the embryonic pulmonary arteries proper arise as branches of the sixth arches and actually have made their appearance before the

(Continued on page 162)

ANOMALIES OF THE AORTIC-ARCH SYSTEM

(Continued from page 161)

ventral and dorsal primordia of the sixth arches have joined each other to complete these arches. In most cases of absent pulmonary artery, the derivatives of the (intrapulmonary) embryonic pulmonary arteries are present, even though they may have lost contact with the pulmonary trunk and receive their blood supply from a systemic arterial source. True and complete absence of a pulmonary artery and its terminal branches, with the lung supplied solely by anomalous systemic arteries arising from the aorta beyond the arch, is rare and will not be discussed here.

Cases of "absent" pulmonary artery fall into one of two categories: Either the distal pulmonary artery of the involved lung is continuous with a large artery originating from the ascending aorta, or it is supplied by a ductus arteriosus.

Pulmonary Artery Arising from Ascending Aorta

This anomaly may be of the *anterior* or *posterior type*. The pathogenesis of these two kinds is entirely different. As indicated in the plate, the *anterior-type* artery is made up of the left fourth arch, a segment of the dorsal aorta, the distal portion of the left sixth arch, and the left embryonic pulmonary artery. It is always contralateral to the aortic arch and can occur with either a right or a left aortic arch, and the subclavian artery contralateral to the aortic arch can be expected to arise anomalously from the descending aortic arch.

The *posterior-type* artery is made up of the proximal portion of the sixth arch and the embryonic pulmonary artery. Apparently, at the time of partitioning of the truncus and truncoaortic sac, it was left "stranded." It may be expected to be located always on the right side (in situs solitus individuals) with either a *right* or a *left aortic arch*, and the branching pattern of the aortic-arch vessels is normal, unless, of course, there is another independent anomaly of these vessels.

A pulmonary artery arising from the ascending aorta is generally large. The *clinical features* are similar to those seen in other conditions with anomalous communications at the arterial level, and they depend on the magnitude of the shunt. The *diagnosis* can best be established by *angiocardiography*.

Pulmonary Artery Arising from Ductus Arteriosus

If the proximal segment of one of the sixth arches disappears early, the corresponding embryonic pulmonary artery will be supplied, instead, by the *distal* sixth-arch segment, *i.e.,* the ductus arteriosus. Such a ductus arteriosus originates from the aortic arch if the arch is on the same side, or from the innominate artery if the aortic arch is on the opposite side. There is a tendency for the ductus arteriosus to close, and a large left-to-

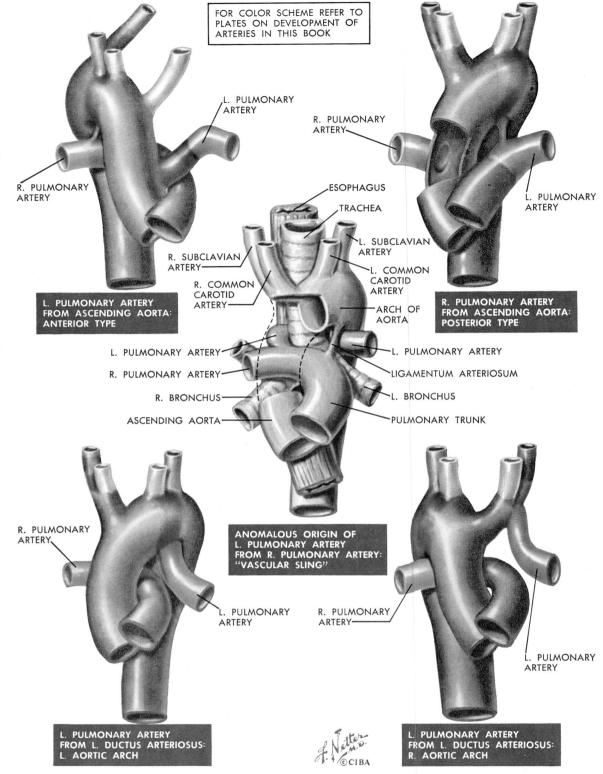

FOR COLOR SCHEME REFER TO PLATES ON DEVELOPMENT OF ARTERIES IN THIS BOOK

L. PULMONARY ARTERY

R. PULMONARY ARTERY

R. PULMONARY ARTERY

L. PULMONARY ARTERY

ESOPHAGUS

TRACHEA

R. SUBCLAVIAN ARTERY

L. SUBCLAVIAN ARTERY

R. COMMON CAROTID ARTERY

L. COMMON CAROTID ARTERY

L. PULMONARY ARTERY FROM ASCENDING AORTA: ANTERIOR TYPE

R. PULMONARY ARTERY FROM ASCENDING AORTA: POSTERIOR TYPE

ARCH OF AORTA

L. PULMONARY ARTERY

L. PULMONARY ARTERY

R. PULMONARY ARTERY

LIGAMENTUM ARTERIOSUM

R. BRONCHUS

L. BRONCHUS

ASCENDING AORTA

PULMONARY TRUNK

R. PULMONARY ARTERY

ANOMALOUS ORIGIN OF L. PULMONARY ARTERY FROM R. PULMONARY ARTERY: "VASCULAR SLING"

L. PULMONARY ARTERY

R. PULMONARY ARTERY

L. PULMONARY ARTERY

L. PULMONARY ARTERY FROM L. DUCTUS ARTERIOSUS: L. AORTIC ARCH

L. PULMONARY ARTERY FROM L. DUCTUS ARTERIOSUS: R. AORTIC ARCH

right shunt is therefore not present, as a rule. In many cases, this duct obliterates completely, and the involved lung then is supplied by bronchial-artery collaterals.

"Vascular Sling"

An *anomalous left pulmonary artery arising from the right pulmonary artery* is an interesting malformation. The vessel always comes off the posterior aspect of the right pulmonary artery at the level of the *right main bronchus* and carina, and runs between the trachea and the esophagus to the left lung. The ductus arteriosus is located normally on the left side. Other cardiovascular anomalies may be associated. In some cases, tracheobronchial anomalies, such as complete tracheal rings or a right upper-lobe bronchus arising independently from the trachea some distance above the carina (a "bronchus suis"), have been reported.

No dysphagia is present, but severe respiratory difficulties are usually manifest at a very early age. Inspiratory and expiratory stridor are pronounced, as a rule, and emphysema or atelectasis and pneumonitis of the right upper lobe — or even of the entire right lung — are usual.

On a lateral *chest roentgenogram,* an ovoid mass may be seen to separate the barium-filled esophagus and air-filled lower trachea. Though not pathognomonic, this finding should strongly suggest the presence of a *"vascular sling,"* as this anomaly has been called. A pulmonary-artery *angiogram* establishes the *diagnosis.*

Treatment is surgical and consists of detaching the anomalous vessel from the right pulmonary artery, followed by reimplantation into the main pulmonary artery. The *prognosis*, without treatment, is poor, the

(Continued on page 163)

Anomalies of the Aortic-Arch System

(Continued from page 162)

majority of infants succumbing within the first year of life.

Coarctation of the Aorta

This congenital narrowing of the descending aorta usually occurs in the vicinity of the ductus arteriosus, which may be patent. If the coarctation is located proximal to the ductus arteriosus, it is called *preductal;* if it is distal, it is termed *postductal. Preductal* coarctation is usually associated with other intracardiac anomalies, and the ductus arteriosus is often widely patent. It is the type most commonly seen in *infants. Postductal* coarctation is usually not associated with other intracardiac defects (except for aortic-valve anomalies, see below) and is the kind usually found in older children and *adults.* This has led to the older classification of coarctation of the aorta as infantile and adult types.

The coarctation may be mild but usually is quite tight or even atretic, and the distal aorta receives most of its blood by way of collaterals. These collaterals are generally extremely abundant, particularly in older children and adults. The main collateral routes are by way of branches of the *subclavian arteries (internal thoracic, transverse scapular,* transverse cervical) and the *intercostal arteries.* Other collateral routes are formed by cervical vessels at the thoracic inlet, the *vertebral* and the *anterior spinal arteries.* Aortic-valve anomalies are very common in coarctation of the aorta, occurring in about 80 percent or more of the cases. The reason for this curious association is not known.

The *clinical features,* in the majority of cases, are rather characteristic. Symptoms usually are absent in childhood, and growth and development are normal. As a rule, the *diagnosis* is arrived at indirectly and by accident, either because the femoral pulses are diminished or absent, a *chest roentgenogram* shows rib notching, or the patient is found to have hypertension. Some patients complain of coldness of the feet or of headaches. In older adults symptoms are due mainly to long-standing hypertension. Bacterial endocarditis (see page 181), generally of an anomalous aortic valve and rarely at the site of the coarctation, may occur at any age beyond early childhood. Rupture of the aorta and intracranial hemorrhage are most commonly seen in young adults. Some patients get into difficulty in infancy and develop severe congestive heart failure. Although very often there are associated cardiac defects which may be responsible for the early decompensation, this is by no means always the case. The most important findings are absent or greatly diminished femoral pulses, a pathognomonic sign in children and young adults, since other conditions causing obstruction of the lower aorta are so rare in these age groups. Hypertension in the

R. TRANSVERSE SCAPULAR ARTERY
R. TRANSVERSE CERVICAL ARTERY
R. THORACICOACROMIAL A.
R. LATERAL THORACIC A.
R. SUBSCAPULAR A.
R. CIRCUMFLEX SCAPULAR A.
VERTEBRAL ARTERIES
INFERIOR THYROID ARTERIES
L. COMMON CAROTID ARTERY
L. ASCENDING CERVICAL ARTERY
L. SUPERFICIAL CERVICAL ARTERY
L. COSTOCERVICAL TRUNK
L. TRANSVERSE SCAPULAR ARTERY
L. INTERNAL THORACIC (INT. MAMMARY) ARTERY
L. AXILLARY ARTERY
L. SUBCLAVIAN ARTERY
LIGAMENTUM ARTERIOSUM
ARTERIA ABERRANS
R. 4th INTERCOSTAL ARTERY
INTERNAL THORACIC (INT. MAMMARY) ARTERIES
COARCTATION OF THE AORTA
TO SUPERIOR AND INFERIOR EPIGASTRIC AND EXTERNAL ILIAC ARTERIES
L. INTERCOSTAL ARTERIES

(ADULT) POSTDUCTAL TYPE

(INFANT; 1 MONTH) PREDUCTAL TYPE

INTERCOSTAL ARTERY RETRACTED FROM RIB, DEMONSTRATING EROSION OF COSTAL GROOVE BY THE TORTUOUS VESSEL

proximal aortic bed usually is absent in young children, but it becomes increasingly frequent and severe with advancing age. Other findings are a systolic murmur and visible or palpable pulsations around the scapulae, in the axillae, and in the intercostal spaces.

Chest roentgenograms show a normal or somewhat enlarged heart (if no significant aortic-valve disease is present); notching of the ribs (in older children and adults) owing to *erosion of the ribs* by the *tortuous, dilated intercostal arteries;* and, often, a notch in the left border of the upper descending aortic shadow, indicating the site of the coarctation. An *esophagogram* may outline the opposite (also notched) border of the coarcted aortic segment. The *electrocardiogram,* in uncomplicated cases, is either normal or, more commonly, shows left ventricular hypertrophy. *Cardiac catheterization* is not essential. If information is desired concerning the status of the aortic valve, or

if other cardiac anomalies are suspected, cardiac catheterization is best postponed until after the coarctation has been corrected surgically.

Treatment is *surgical* and usually consists of resection of the coarcted segment and an end-to-end anastomosis of the aorta. Occasionally, if the coarcted segment is long, it is necessary to employ a synthetic-fiber graft to bridge the gap in the aorta, but its use should be avoided if at all possible. Surgery is carried out best in older children or young adults; in older adults, it may be hazardous, for technical reasons having to do with the quality of the aortic wall. When infants with coarctation of the aorta get into trouble early, they should be vigorously *treated medically* in the hope that surgery can be postponed for a few years. If the response to medical therapy is unsatisfactory, however, operation is indicated, even though the risk is high.

ENDOCARDIAL FIBROELASTOSIS AND GLYCOGEN STORAGE DISEASE

Endocardial Fibroelastosis

This is a distressingly common and serious cardiac disease of unknown etiology. Typically, it is a disease of early childhood, although it has occasionally been described in older children and even in young adults. Whether those few cases had the same disease is, however, not certain at present. Although the dilated as well as the contracted types have been distinguished, the former is by far the more common and important. The pathologic features are very characteristic. The left ventricle is hugely dilated and, sometimes, almost globular. The interior is coated by a shiny, white layer representing the tremendously thickened endocardium, and the trabeculae are coarse and relatively few in number. The mitral and aortic valves may be thickened, rather stiff, and (occasionally) incompetent. Endocardial fibroelastosis also occurs in association with severe cardiac malformations, such as aortic stenosis or atresia, congenital mitral stenosis, and coarctation of the aorta, and it is also seen—presumably as a secondary lesion—in various forms of acquired valvar disease. Its distribution, in these cases, is variable and spotty, however, and the clinical manifestations of endocardial fibroelastosis associated with other lesions are so different from the rather uniform picture seen in the isolated or "primary" form that the latter is generally treated as a separate entity, and it is the type which will be considered here.

The *clinical picture* is somewhat characteristic. The age of onset is generally between 2 and 7 months but sometimes earlier or later. Prior to onset, asymptomatic and perfectly healthy infants appear to get symptoms of a cold, followed by irritability, refusal to feed, tachypnea, dyspnea, fever, and cough. Many youngsters are *diagnosed* initially as having pneumonia, but, instead of improving with adequate treatment, they become progressively more sick or even die. Signs of cardiac failure, as evidenced by hepatomegaly, abdominal pain, generalized edema with puffy eyelids, and (often) the appearance of a systolic murmur, bring the realization that the problem is a more serious one. The heart is found to be greatly enlarged and there are a gallop rhythm and tachycardia.

Chest roentgenograms confirm the heart's size, with evidence of pulmonary venous congestion, with or without pneumonitis. The left upper lobe may be overinflated owing to compression of the left main bronchus. The *ECG* shows left axis deviation or, more commonly, a normal axis and, almost always, evidence of left ventricular hypertrophy with tall qR complexes and inverted T waves in the left precordial leads. Additional right ventricular hypertrophy may be present in

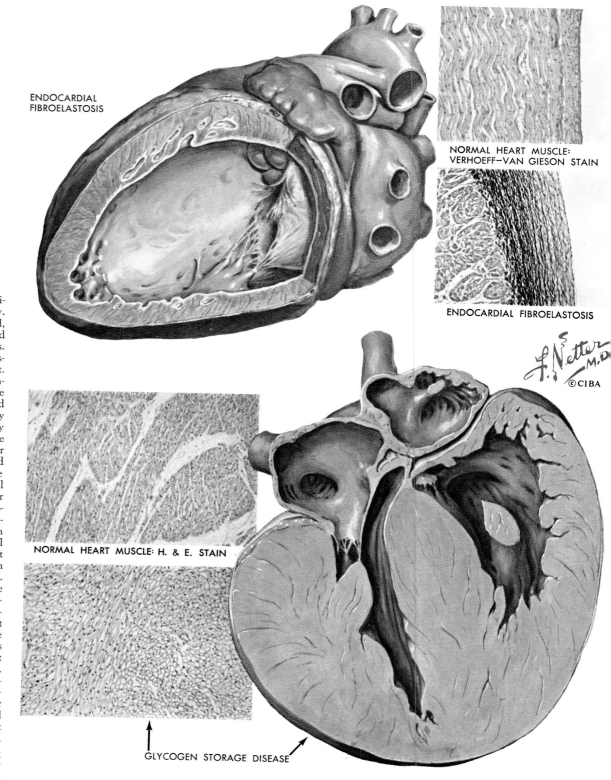

ENDOCARDIAL FIBROELASTOSIS

NORMAL HEART MUSCLE: VERHOEFF–VAN GIESON STAIN

ENDOCARDIAL FIBROELASTOSIS

NORMAL HEART MUSCLE: H. & E. STAIN

GLYCOGEN STORAGE DISEASE

infants with marked failure, but this disappears after successful anticongestive treatment. Arrhythmias and conduction disturbances are common. *Cardiac catheterization* and *angiocardiography* are usually not necessary, unless associated defects are suspected.

Treatment is medical. Digitalis therapy is often initially dramatically successful, with a good and rapid response. Sooner or later, however, within weeks or months, there is an exacerbation, and such recurrences respond less well to therapy. Almost all infants die within the first 2 years of life.

Glycogen Storage Disease

An excessive deposition of glycogen in the tissues characterizes this disease. It is due to a hereditary error in carbohydrate metabolism, is transmitted as an autosomal recessive gene, and occurs commonly in siblings. Several types are distinguished, and the enzyme defect of most of these is known. In the cardiac variety, first described

by Pompe, glycogen is deposited in abnormal amounts in all tissues but especially in the heart, which is enormously enlarged and globular, with tremendously thick and solid walls. Microscopically, large central vacuoles in the myocardial fibers, with a thin surrounding shell of cytoplasm, give the sections a peculiar lacelike appearance. Glycogen can be demonstrated with various histochemical staining technics.

Clinically, there are marked cardiomegaly and muscular weakness. Congestive heart failure appears early in infancy. There may be macroglossia, also owing to abnormal glycogen deposition in the tongue muscle (see CIBA COLLECTION, Vol. 4, page 246, for the metabolic aspects of glycogen storage).

Chest roentgenograms reveal marked cardiomegaly, and the *ECG* characteristically shows a short P-R interval, with or without the Wolff-Parkinson-White syndrome, and left ventricular hypertrophy.

The *prognosis* is very poor, and death usually occurs within the first year of life.

Section V

DISEASES—ACQUIRED

by
FRANK H. NETTER, M.D.

in collaboration with

ALDO R. CASTANEDA, M.D., Ph.D. and RICHARD L. VARCO, M.D.
Plates 26-31

J. N. P. DAVIES, M.D., Sc.D., F.C.Path.
Plates 42-46, 79

ARTHUR C. DeGRAFF, M.D.
Plates 91-93

THOMAS A. DOXIADIS, M.D.
Plate 80

JESSE E. EDWARDS, M.D.
Plates 3-14, 16-25

DONALD B. EFFLER, M.D.
Plates 69-75

LEONARD E. GLYNN, M.D., F.R.C.P., F.C.Path.
Plates 1-2

S. E. GOULD, M.D.
Plate 78

CHARLES A. HUFNAGEL, M.D.
Plates 32-34

DAVID KOFFLER, M.D. and HANS POPPER, M.D.
Plate 15

GEORGE KURLAND, M.D. and A. STONE FREEDBERG, M.D.
Plates 76-77

JAMES R. MALM, M.D.
Plates 35-36

AUBRE de L. MAYNARD, M.D., F.A.C.S.
Plates 89-90

LAWRENCE J. McCORMACK, M.D., M.S. (Path.)
Plates 49, 52-56, 61-63

HUBERT MEESSEN, Prof. Dr. Dr. h.c.
Plates 37-41, 82-83

EMIL A. NACLERIO, M.D., F.A.C.S., F.C.C.P., F.A.C.C.
Plates 84-88

IRVINE H. PAGE, M.D.
Plates 50-51, 58-60

ABEL LAZZARINI ROBERTSON, JR., M.D., Ph.D.
Plates 47-48

NORMAN E. SHUMWAY, M.D., Ph.D.
Plates 94-97

CH. STATHATOS, M.D.
Plate 81

RICHARD N. WESTCOTT, M.D., F.A.C.C.
Plates 64-68

PAUL DUDLEY WHITE, M.D.
Plate 57

RHEUMATIC FEVER;
SYDENHAM'S CHOREA

Rheumatic Fever

This condition can affect people of all ages except those in the first few years of life. It is characterized by a febrile onset, accompanied by a severe but temporary arthritis, and, often, by carditis in which all three cardiac layers may participate. Its etiologic relationship to *β-hemolytic streptococci* rests upon three main pieces of evidence:

1. Most cases have a history of an *acute streptococcal sore throat* some 2 to 3 weeks before the onset of arthritis.

2. The incidence of rheumatic fever, in any community, runs remarkably parallel to the incidence of streptococcal throat infections, and epidemics of streptococcal infection are invariably followed by epidemics of rheumatic fever, with a lag period, once again, of 2 to 3 weeks.

3. A high or rising titer of antibodies to streptococcal antigens may be taken as evidence of a recent streptococcal infection. If the response to a single antigen is studied, *e.g.*, the antistreptolysin-O titer, evidence of such a recent infection is found in about 70 percent of the cases. This figure rises progressively with the greater number of antibodies studied, and it reaches virtually 100 percent when a panel of four tests is employed.

The frequency with which rheumatic fever follows a streptococcal infection varies from 3 percent in epidemics to about 0.3 percent in sporadic infections. This discrepancy is largely due to the greater severity of epidemic types of infection, as revealed by clinical features and by the antibody titers induced. When streptococcal infections of comparable severity are studied, the incidence of subsequent rheumatic fever, even in sporadic cases, also reaches about 3 percent.

The lesions of this fever are not due to direct invasion by streptococci. When adequate precautions are taken against contamination, organisms cannot be isolated from the joints or the heart. The events connecting the primary infection to these lesions are still obscure. It is unlikely that circulating toxins, released from the organisms, are responsible, because then the clinical manifestations of rheumatic fever should coincide with the sore throat, in the same way as do the toxic symptoms of diphtheria. Furthermore, none of the many known streptococcal products produces comparable lesions in animals.

The relationship between streptococcal infection and rheumatic fever is therefore most widely regarded as an *immunologic* one, the lesions resulting from an *antigen-antibody reaction* in the affected tissues. This concept received strong support from the observation by Rich that lesions which resembled, at least superficially, those of rheumatic carditis could be produced in rabbits by the injection of massive doses of foreign serum.

It is difficult to conceive of a natural

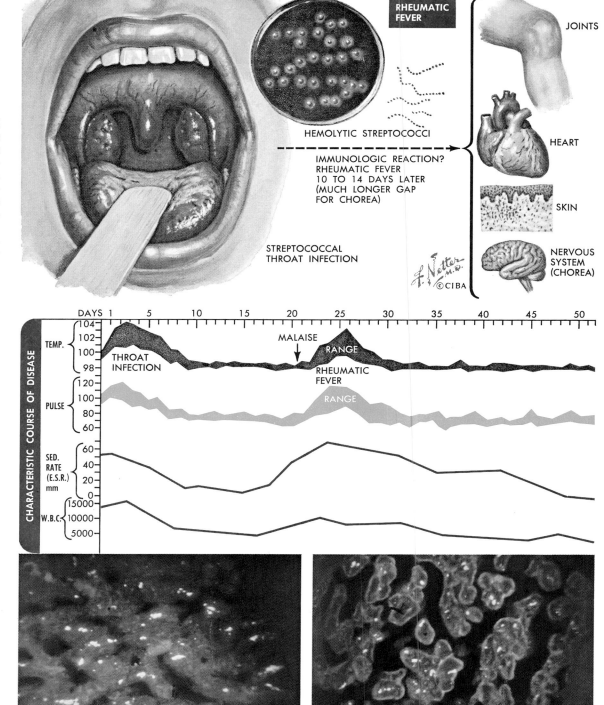

HEMOLYTIC STREPTOCOCCI

STREPTOCOCCAL THROAT INFECTION

IMMUNOLOGIC REACTION? RHEUMATIC FEVER 10 TO 14 DAYS LATER (MUCH LONGER GAP FOR CHOREA)

RHEUMATIC FEVER

JOINTS

HEART

SKIN

NERVOUS SYSTEM (CHOREA)

CHARACTERISTIC COURSE OF DISEASE

DAYS 1 · 5 · 10 · 15 · 20 · 25 · 30 · 35 · 40 · 45 · 50

TEMP. 104 102 100 98 — THROAT INFECTION — MALAISE — RANGE — RHEUMATIC FEVER

PULSE 120 100 80 60 — RANGE

SED. RATE (E.S.R.) mm 60 40 20 0

W.B.C. 15000 10000 5000

SECTION OF HUMAN HEART MUSCLE STAINED WITH PREIMMUNE SERUM OF RABBIT (X 200)

HUMAN HEART MUSCLE STAINED WITH ANTISERUM AGAINST TYPE-6 MATT GROUP-A STREPTOCOCCI (X 200). NOTE FLUORESCENCE OF SUBSARCOLEMMAL REGION OF MUSCLE FIBERS

situation in which a comparable massive exposure to antigen could occur in man. Therefore, it is more probable that any *immunological reaction* underlying the pathogenesis of rheumatic fever is of a more specific nature, directly involving one or more of the antigens native to the affected tissues. This concept is reinforced by Kaplan's finding that many strains of *β-hemolytic streptococci* contain, within their cell walls, an antigen which cross-reacts with an antigenic component of mammalian hearts, including the human. Furthermore, animals injected with such strains of streptococci produce antibodies which can be shown to react with the individual animal's cardiac antigens. Finally, similar antibodies have been found in a high proportion of patients with active rheumatic fever. Serious reservations remain, however. Despite the presence of firmly bound γ-globulin, presumably antibody, in the heart of many patients with rheumatic

fever, the correlation between circulating antibody and clinical severity is poor, and cardiac damage, in experimentally immunized animals, is unconvincing. Nevertheless, the closest resemblance to human rheumatic carditis obtained experimentally is that described by Murphy and Swift, in rabbits repeatedly infected by different types of *β-hemolytic streptococci*. Although the mechanism is still unclear, immunological cross-reactivity with myocardial and other antigens is, at present, the most probable answer.

The *clinical features* of an acute attack may range from the trivial to the fulminating — from easily overlooked pallor and fatigue to an exquisitely painful arthritis, with high fever, rash, and carditis sufficiently severe to lead to congestive heart failure. The *temperature* chart is characterized by a nonremittent type of *fever* with a *pulse rate raised* disproportionately.

(*Continued on page 167*)

RHEUMATIC FEVER;
SYDENHAM'S CHOREA
(Continued from page 166)

The *arthritis is migratory,* rarely lasting in any one joint for more than 1 or 2 days.

Swelling is slight and is accompanied by some flushing of the overlying skin. Large joints are more commonly affected than small ones, but these can become involved too, and the picture may then resemble rheumatoid arthritis.

Despite the many features common to rheumatic fever and rheumatoid arthritis (notably polyarthritis and subcutaneous nodules), there is no doubt that they are distinct nosologic entities. If there is difficulty in differentiation in the early stages, the difference in clinical evolution rapidly distinguishes them, and, even in the early stages, the *histology* of the synovium or of a biopsied *nodule* can be of help. The lesion is capsular rather than synovial, with areas of fibrinoid necrosis accompanied by focal infiltrations of histiocytes and lymphocytes.

The *joint lesions,* even when severe, are entirely reversible, and permanent damage does not result. This contrasts with the *cardiac lesions* which, even when the initial damage is mild, can occasionally progress to mitral stenosis and its sequelae.

Skin rashes, although relatively uncommon, can be characteristic, especially *erythema annulare,* a fleeting ring-shaped eruption, usually flat, and occurring typically on the trunk. Each lesion spreads centrifugally, leaving a slight staining in the center.

Another typical feature of the disease, seen especially in severe cases, consists of *subcutaneous nodules.* These are mainly confined to the tissues over bony prominences, where friction, combined with pressure, is apparently responsible for their development. They are most conspicuous when the illness has run some 2 to 3 weeks, although their impending development is often preceded by a more diffuse, boggy thickening. Histologically, a typical nodule shows an area of fibrinoid composed of parallel or interlacing bands sparsely infiltrated with histiocytes and fibroblasts. The adjacent tissue is edematous and contains groups of small vessels surrounded by similar cells. Fibrous tissue is inconspicuous.

Since permanent cardiac damage is closely correlated with persistent or recurrent activity of the disease, aids to the detection of such activity are important. The most helpful is the *erythrocyte sedimentation rate (E.S.R.),* which is almost never normal in the presence of active disease, except in patients with congestive heart failure. The converse, *i.e.,* a persistently raised E.S.R., does not, however, especially in girls, necessarily imply continued activity. For these reasons, estimations of C-reactive protein may more accurately reflect the state of the disease activity.

The greatest danger to the patient with a history of rheumatic fever is that of

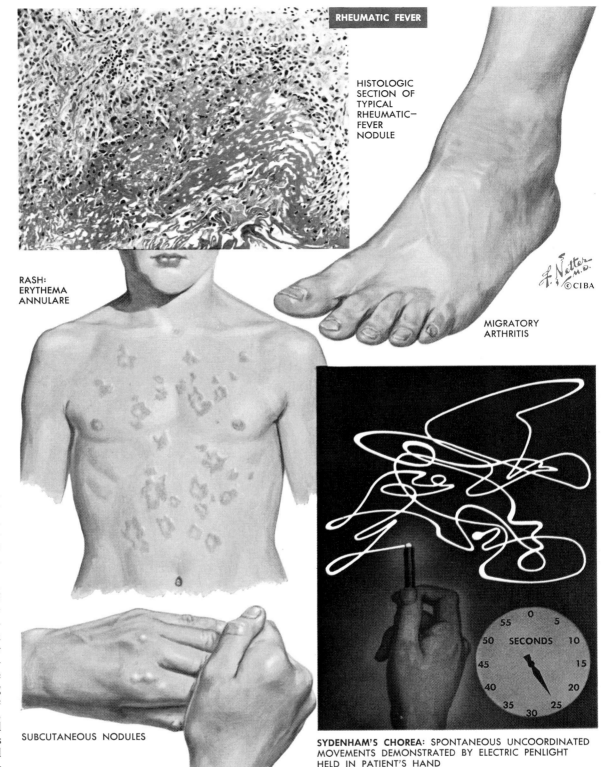

RHEUMATIC FEVER

HISTOLOGIC SECTION OF TYPICAL RHEUMATIC-FEVER NODULE

MIGRATORY ARTHRITIS

RASH: ERYTHEMA ANNULARE

SUBCUTANEOUS NODULES

SYDENHAM'S CHOREA: SPONTANEOUS UNCOORDINATED MOVEMENTS DEMONSTRATED BY ELECTRIC PENLIGHT HELD IN PATIENT'S HAND

incurring a fresh infection with *β-hemolytic streptococci,* as the chance of relapse is very much higher than after an initial attack. The undoubted success of chemoprophylaxis has confirmed both the importance of such reinfection in the development of a relapse and the role of the streptococci in rheumatic-fever pathogenesis.

Environmental and genetic factors have been studied widely in an attempt to account for the considerable geographic variation in the incidence of the disease. The most impressive data are those provided by Mills' map, showing the progressive decrease in mortality from rheumatic fever as one passes from the northern to the southern latitudes of the United States. Evidence of genetic factors, apart from the predominance in females, is less precise, but the increased incidence of nonsecretors of the blood-group substances in subjects with rheumatic fever points to

some genetic influence, although only a modest one. The dominant factor is undoubtedly environmental and related to the incidence and virulence of the local streptococci.

Sydenham's Chorea

The rheumatic nature of *Sydenham's chorea,* first recognized just over 100 years ago, is now established, by evidence similar to that invoked for rheumatic fever, as a poststreptococcal state. This is confirmed by the frequent subsequent development of rheumatic heart disease, in the absence of any clinical evidence of rheumatic fever. The outstanding *clinical features* are *ataxia, incoordination,* and *weakness,* accompanied by *spontaneous movements* which can be most clearly depicted by the *photographic record* of an *electric pencil torch held in the patient's hand.*

RHEUMATIC HEART DISEASE I

Rheumatic heart disease is a complication of recurrent upper-respiratory infection with group-A β-hemolytic streptococci. As streptococcal products are circulated from this source through the body, they engender a reaction in connective *tissues* which is called rheumatic inflammation. Sites of particular predilection are the heart, skin, and synovial membranes. In the latter two areas, inflammation usually heals by resolution, leaving no residual effects, but, in the heart, these recurrent respiratory infections may lead to severe deformities, usually of the valves.

For chronic rheumatic heart disease to occur, recurrent infections are required. Each attack of rheumatic inflammation goes through an active stage and is followed by healing. In the joints, active rheumatic involvement is characterized by migratory arthritis. In the skin, transitory subcutaneous nodules may appear. In the heart, each of the major anatomic components — the pericardium, the myocardium, the endocardium, and, particularly, the valves — may be involved.

Acute Pericarditis

Acute rheumatic pericarditis is characterized by the exudation of serum and fibrin, in varying amounts, into the pericardial cavity. Large effusions of fluid may cause *roentgenographic signs* of uniform cardiac enlargement and *physical signs* of pericardial effusion. Impairment of the inflow of blood to the heart, with the resultant increased systemic venous pressure, may be evidenced by distention of the cervical veins.

The fibrinous element of acute rheumatic pericarditis is manifested by particles of fibrin floating in the associated effusion and by the concentration of a fibrinous deposit on the visceral (epicardial) and parietal layers. The shaggy fibrin, evident when the two layers of the pericardium are separated, has given rise to the name "bread-and-butter" heart of rheumatic pericarditis. This gross feature is not specific, however, since it applies to any condition in which *fibrinous pericarditis* occurs.

Histologically, during the active stage of rheumatic pericarditis, one observes fibrin deposited upon the pericardial surfaces. Beneath this is a process of mobilization of capillaries and fibroblasts which gradually enter the fibrin as granulation tissue. The pericardium shows edema and a mild degree of leukocytic infiltration. Specific *Aschoff bodies,* which characterize acute rheumatic myocarditis, are not usually seen in the pericardium.

Acute Myocarditis

The specific *histologic lesion* of acute rheumatic carditis is usually restricted to the myocardium and takes the form of the *Aschoff body.* Aschoff bodies are reac-

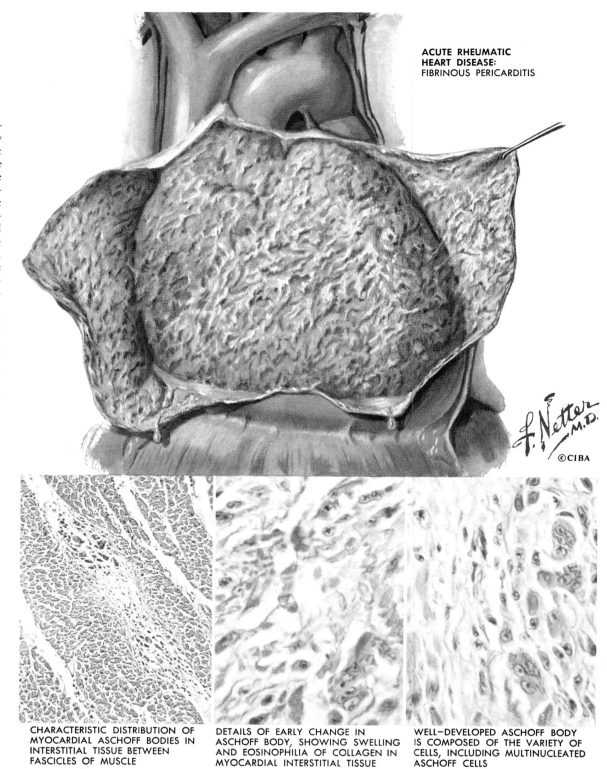

ACUTE RHEUMATIC HEART DISEASE: FIBRINOUS PERICARDITIS

f. Netter M.D.

©CIBA

CHARACTERISTIC DISTRIBUTION OF MYOCARDIAL ASCHOFF BODIES IN INTERSTITIAL TISSUE BETWEEN FASCICLES OF MUSCLE

DETAILS OF EARLY CHANGE IN ASCHOFF BODY, SHOWING SWELLING AND EOSINOPHILIA OF COLLAGEN IN MYOCARDIAL INTERSTITIAL TISSUE

WELL-DEVELOPED ASCHOFF BODY IS COMPOSED OF THE VARIETY OF CELLS, INCLUDING MULTINUCLEATED ASCHOFF CELLS

tive nodules within the connective tissue and therefore are predominantly found around blood vessels of the myocardium and in other bundles of connective tissue which separate *myocardial fascicles.* The primary lesion appears to be an alteration of *collagen* which shows a coagulationlike change with *eosinophilia,* a process commonly called fibrinoid necrosis. Secondary cellular reaction to the primary process in the collagen leads to the formation of the nodule. The involved cells include nonspecific phagocytes, myocardial histiocytes, and *multinucleated cells* (Aschoff giant cells). In the early Aschoff body, fibroblastic proliferation is not strongly evident, but, as the lesion becomes older, the phagocytic cells become less numerous and are replaced by fibroblastic cells. Toward the end of the activity of an Aschoff body, the nodule may be entirely fibrous and acellular in nature.

The characteristic scant loss of *muscle* in acute rheumatic carditis is paradoxical to the frequent occurrence of myocardial failure during this stage of the disease.

In subjects with *rheumatoid arthritis,* three types of cardiac disease may occur: The *first* comprises *all the changes* of rheumatic carditis, including typical valvular lesions. The *second* is the *rheumatoid granuloma,* which may involve the myocardium and/or the valves. It is characterized as a focal lesion with a central zone of caseouslike necrosis surrounded by radially oriented fibroblasts. It resembles the rheumatoid granuloma which occurs in subcutaneous tissue. The lesion does not usually contribute to cardiac failure. The *third* type is *amyloid infiltration* of the myocardium. It may be associated with cardiac failure and is part of systemic amyloidosis, a process that may complicate the course of disease in a patient with rheumatoid arthritis.

RHEUMATIC HEART DISEASE II

Acute Valvular Involvement

The gross changes which are exhibited in the cardiac valves, as a manifestation of acute *rheumatic* involvement, are highly characteristic. There is a strong tendency for the *mitral* and *aortic valves* to be involved, whereas the tricuspid valve is affected only occasionally and the pulmonary valve, classically, not at all. The primary change in the valve appears to be that of edema with minimal leukocytic infiltration. A secondary erosion of the *cusp along the line of closure* occurs as a complication of the trauma of closure of the edematous cusp. This is followed by a deposit of fibrin and platelets along the denuded area, accounting for the presence of a row of delicate, tan, translucent, regular, beadlike *vegetations* which tend to be confined to the line of closure. From the atrioventricular valves, the *vegetative material* may extend onto the chordae tendineae. Another characteristic feature of the gross changes in rheumatic endocarditis is the absence of destructive effects upon either the valvular tissue or the chordae tendineae, with little deformity of the valves at this stage.

Since *acute rheumatic endocarditis* is almost universally associated with acute rheumatic myocarditis, the gross effects of rheumatic myocarditis, in the form of ventricular dilatation, are frequently evident.

Mitral insufficiency may be present as a transient phenomenon during the acute stage of rheumatic carditis. The basis for this valvular disturbance is to be attributed primarily to the myocarditis and the associated ventricular dilatation rather than to intrinsic disease of the mitral valve. The involvement of the aortic valve by acute rheumatic endocarditis causes little functional change.

The existence of mitral insufficiency, during acute rheumatic carditis, may be associated with an area of regurgitant "jet lesions" on the posterior wall of the left atrium. Such lesions have been called MacCallum patches. In the past, such a lesion was thought to represent an area of specific predilection of the left atrium for rheumatic inflammation. The MacCallum patch is now considered a focus of response to regurgitation ("jet lesions") rather than a focus of primary rheumatic mural endocarditis.

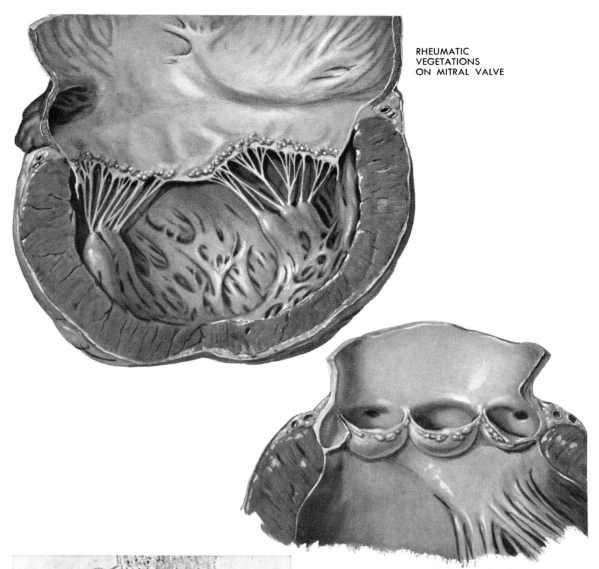

RHEUMATIC VEGETATIONS ON MITRAL VALVE

RHEUMATIC VEGETATIONS ON AORTIC VALVE

PHOTOMICROGRAPH OF MITRAL VALVE IN ACUTE RHEUMATIC ENDOCARDITIS. SWELLING ALONG LINE OF CLOSURE OF THE VALVE CUSP REPRESENTS HEALING OF VEGETATIVE MATERIAL, SOME OF WHICH STILL CAPS THE SUMMIT OF THE SWELLING

Acute rheumatic endocarditis occurring at a given time may represent either the first attack or one of several recurrent insults. The structural changes observed in a patient with acute rheumatic endocarditis will depend on whether the attack is the first event or is one of several recurrent episodes. Even in instances of a first attack, there may be evidence of a healing response to the inflammatory process. In such cases, there is little gross alteration, save for the presence of vegetations and the response to these.

The response to an initial attack has certain characteristics: In the cusp beneath the vegetation, various cells, including fibroblasts and macrophages, are mobilized in a palisade manner. Fibroblasts and capillaries grow into the vegetative material, replacing the fibrin. This sets the stage for the healed phase, when the sites of vegetative deposit are represented by fibrous nodules. In instances where the chordae tendineae also are involved by vegetative material, the process of *healing* leads to chordal thickening and, in some instances, to adhesions between the chordae tendineae.

If an attack is one of several recurrent episodes, the aforedescribed characteristic changes of acute rheumatic endocarditis are superimposed upon the residua of the healing of previous attacks. Under these circumstances, evidence of previous attacks includes such changes as shortening of the cusps, fibrous thickening along the line of closure, varying degrees of interadhesion between the chordae tendineae, shortening of the chordae, and vascularization of the cusps.

If valvular insufficiency has resulted from earlier attacks of acute rheumatic endocarditis, an enlargement of the chambers specific for the type of such insufficiency may be observed.

MITRAL VALVE: SOME FUSION OF CHORDAE TENDINEAE AND THICKENING OF CUSPS AT CONTACT AREAS; BLOOD VESSEL GROWING IN

AORTIC VALVE: FUSION OF RIGHT CUSP AND POSTERIOR CUSP, RESULTING IN A BICUSPID VALVE WHICH IS STILL COMPETENT

PHOTOMICROGRAPH OF INTERSTITIAL NODULE OF MYOCARDIUM REPRESENTING A HEALED ASCHOFF BODY

ADHESIVE PERICARDITIS WITH FOCAL CALCIFICATION

RHEUMATIC HEART DISEASE III

Residual Changes of Acute Rheumatic Carditis

Recurrent acute rheumatic carditis may lead to severe residual changes represented by stenosis or insufficiency of one or more valves; in some individuals, however, the rheumatic process leaves only minor damage. In some patients, each of the involved valves exhibits only minor changes, whereas in other subjects, one or two valves may show significant deformities. Also, minor residual changes of acute rheumatic carditis may be observed in the myocardium and pericardium, regardless of the specific damage to the valves.

In the *mitral valve*, minor residual changes are represented by fibrous *thickening* along the line of closure *of the cusps* at the sites of healed vegetations of acute rheumatic endocarditis. Minimal shortening of the free aspect of the cusp may occur, giving the impression of the insertion of *chordae tendineae* directly into the free edge of the cusp. Vascularization of the mitral valve is seen commonly as a sign of healed rheumatic involvement. Characteristically, the vascularization involves the anterior cusp. At its base, a *vessel* is seen to proceed toward the free aspect of the cusp, where it arborizes. Minor degrees of chordal shortening, thickening, and interadhesion may occur in competent valves. Also, minor degrees of fusion between the cusps, at their commissures, may be observed.

In the tricuspid valve, the minor residual effects bear a similarity to those which may occur in the mitral valve.

In the *aortic valve*, the minor residual changes include limited degrees of fibrous thickening along the line of closure, shortening of the *cusps,* and commissural *fusion*. Shortening of the cusps may be demonstrated by the fact that, in the conventional view of the opened aortic valve, a greater amount of the depth of the aortic sinuses can be observed than is revealed in the normal valve. Aortic-valve commissural fusion, of such a degree as to allow a near-normal function of that valve, is usually confined to one commissure. This results in one conjoined cusp which is about twice the width of

the second cusp. The latter is not adherent to its neighbors. An aortic valve so altered may be termed an *acquired bicuspid valve*. Although such a valve may be *competent* and also not stenotic, it fails to open with the freedom of a normal tricuspid aortic valve and is subject to the complication of slowly becoming calcified and stenotic.

Another potential complication of the minor residual effects of rheumatic disease in the valves is bacterial endocarditis, particularly of the mitral and the aortic valves.

In hearts with only minor residual valvular disease of rheumatic endocarditis, the *myocardium* is grossly normal and not hypertrophied, but small myocardial scars may exist. The latter are the residua of Aschoff bodies and are represented by avascular and acellular scars which tend to be located in perivascular positions. In many cases, the *healing of Aschoff bodies*

may be so complete that it is difficult to determine whether a strand of connective tissue in the myocardium is normal supporting tissue or a residual scar.

The healed effects of acute rheumatic pericarditis are rarely, if ever, responsible for significant disturbances of the circulation, regardless of the form that healing may take. Usually, acute rheumatic *pericarditis* heals by resolution, leaving a smooth-lined, nonadhesive pericardium. In other instances, the fibrinous exudate — either focally or diffusely — is replaced by fibrous *adhesions*. Even in those relatively uncommon instances where the entire pericardium is obliterated by fibrous adhesions, the adhesions are relatively thin and do not constitute a basis for cardiac constriction. In some instances of fibrous obliteration of the pericardial sac, *focal* plaques of *calcium* may be deposited in the adhesions, but, even in those, there appears to be no constrictive effect.

MITRAL STENOSIS, VIEWED FROM
BELOW AND LEFT: MINOR RHEUMATIC
INVOLVEMENT OF AORTIC VALVE

RHEUMATIC HEART
DISEASE IV

Mitral Stenosis:
Pathologic Anatomy

Mitral stenosis is the most common serious effect of recurrent *rheumatic fever*. Anatomically, it represents the culmination of recurrent attacks, leaving the *valve* highly deformed and obstructed. As the valvular vegetations of acute rheumatic fever heal, they cause not only fibrous *thickening* of the cusps but, more important, interadhesion between the cusps at the commissures and changes in the chordae tendineae. The healing of vegetations on the surfaces of the chordae is responsible for their fusion, with obliteration of the spaces between them. In the normal mitral valve, blood flows not only through that part of the orifice which lies between the papillary muscles but also through the spaces between the chordae, lateral to the papillary muscles. After interchordal adhesion, the secondary avenues for flow are obliterated.

An additional effect upon the chordae tendineae is that recurrent inflammation causes these strands to become shortened. This shortening is responsible for the cusps being held tautly in a downward position. The chordae related to each commissure exhibit a fanlike shape. The base of the fan is attached to the cusps, the apex to the papillary muscle. As the chordae become shortened and pull the cusps downward, they draw the base of the fan toward the apex. This tends to hold the cusps together and favors adhesion between the cusps at their commissures, as healing of the valvular vegetations occurs. The process of chordal shortening, with the resultant fixation of the cusps, is probably the major factor in restenosis after a commissurotomy has been performed.

In addition to the deformities already described, the *stenotic mitral valve* shows a typical deformity of its *anterior cusp*. This is characterized by a *convexity* directed toward the atrium. It is probable, in the absence of valvular calcification, that, during left ventricular diastole when the left atrial pressure exceeds the left ventricular pressure, the cusp at the site of this deformity buckles toward the ventricle. This buckling could be responsible for the "opening snap" which occurs at the beginning of diastole and which

THICKENED STENOTIC
MITRAL VALVE:
ANTERIOR CUSP HAS
TYPICAL CONVEXITY;
ENLARGED L. ATRIUM;
"JET LESION" ON L.
VENTRICULAR WALL

ENLARGEMENT OF R. VENTRICLE
WITH SOME THICKENING OF WALL
RESULTING FROM MITRAL STENOSIS;
PULMONARY ARTERY ENLARGED
AND THICKENED WITH SCATTERED
PLAQUES OF ATHEROMAS

is considered classic for mitral stenosis. During ventricular systole, the deformity buckles toward the atrium and impinges on the base of the posterior mitral cusp, to act as a flutter valve for the prevention of regurgitation through the valve.

The primary functional effect of mitral stenosis is obstruction at the valve.

The pressure rises in the left atrium, in the entire pulmonary vascular bed, and in the right ventricle. These functional changes result in secondary structural effects which aid in the *clinical diagnosis*. Included among these are *enlargement of the left atrium* and the main *pulmonary arteries,* and hypertrophy of the *right ventricle*.

The left atrial pressure exceeds the left ventricular end-diastolic pressure. This effect, coupled with the presence of a narrow mitral orifice, is responsible for the narrow, high-velocity stream of blood passing through the mitral orifice. At the sites where such streams strike the *left ventricular wall, "jet lesions"* may develop.

In cases with established mitral stenosis, functional studies indicate that there is a low cardiac output. This output is fixed. Therefore, the heart cannot respond, by an increase in output, to the need of the tissues for oxygen. With exercise and, in severe cases, even at rest, there is a greater-than-normal extraction of oxygen at the systemic capillary level. This results in the characteristic increased arteriovenous oxygen difference, in patients with mitral stenosis, as compared with the normal amount.

The low cardiac output of mitral stenosis is reflected in the size of the left ventricle and the aorta. The left ventricular cavity is smaller than normal, and the wall is thinner. The diameter of the aorta is narrower than normal.

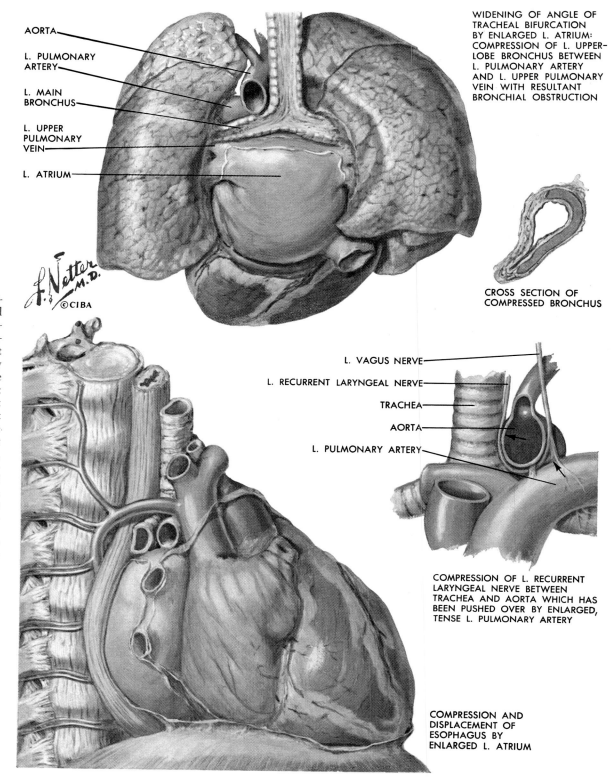

AORTA

L. PULMONARY ARTERY

L. MAIN BRONCHUS

L. UPPER PULMONARY VEIN

L. ATRIUM

WIDENING OF ANGLE OF TRACHEAL BIFURCATION BY ENLARGED L. ATRIUM: COMPRESSION OF L. UPPER-LOBE BRONCHUS BETWEEN L. PULMONARY ARTERY AND L. UPPER PULMONARY VEIN WITH RESULTANT BRONCHIAL OBSTRUCTION

CROSS SECTION OF COMPRESSED BRONCHUS

L. VAGUS NERVE

L. RECURRENT LARYNGEAL NERVE

TRACHEA

AORTA

L. PULMONARY ARTERY

COMPRESSION OF L. RECURRENT LARYNGEAL NERVE BETWEEN TRACHEA AND AORTA WHICH HAS BEEN PUSHED OVER BY ENLARGED, TENSE L. PULMONARY ARTERY

COMPRESSION AND DISPLACEMENT OF ESOPHAGUS BY ENLARGED L. ATRIUM

Rheumatic Heart Disease V

Mitral Stenosis: Secondary Anatomic Effect

The primary functional effect of mitral stenosis is obstruction at the mitral valve. This results in an elevation of pressure in the *left atrium,* in the entire pulmonary vascular system, and in the right ventricle, causing a number of secondary anatomic effects. Prominent among these are hypertrophy of the muscle in the left atrial wall and *enlargement* of the left atrial chamber. The wall of the right ventricle becomes hypertrophied, while the chamber may be of normal size or enlarged. If the latter effect is evident, it is probably a result of complicating congestive cardiac failure. Enlargement of the right ventricular chamber may, in turn, be responsible for dilatation of the tricuspid orifice and for secondary tricuspid insufficiency.

Dilatation of the major *pulmonary arteries* is another important secondary effect. The pulmonary hypertension, which brings about the latter effect, is also responsible for accentuating the second cardiac sound in the "pulmonary" area and for atherosclerosis of the major pulmonary arteries.

The left atrium is located inferior to the *tracheal bifurcation,* in such a position that its superior aspect is separated from the inferior aspects of the two major bronchi by only two structures. These are the tracheobronchial lymph nodes and the pericardium. The tracheal bifurcation arches over the left atrium. When the left atrium becomes dilated for any reason, as in mitral stenosis, the angle of the tracheal bifurcation increases. The latter effect results mainly from an upward displacement of the *left main bronchus,* whereas the right main bronchus is less affected. The close relationship between the *left upper pulmonary vein* and the left main bronchus may favor the upward displacement of the left main bronchus. The increased angulation (*widening of angle*) of the tracheal bifurcation may be identified in thoracic *roentgenograms,* and this serves as a parameter in identifying the *enlargement of the left atrium.*

Bronchial compression may also occur, being more evident in the left main bronchus than in the right. In extreme degrees of compression, the normally rounded lower aspect of the left main bronchus is represented by a sharp edge.

The impaired airway resulting from bronchial compression may cause recurrent pulmonary infection. This aspect of mitral stenosis may contribute to dyspnea, which is a common *symptom* among patients with this valvular disease.

Hoarseness, resulting from paralysis of the left vocal cord, may be observed in the occasional patient with mitral stenosis. This *sign* is to be taken as a complication of the associated pulmonary hypertension, since it is also observed in patients with other forms of cardiac disease in which pulmonary hypertension is involved. The paralysis of the left vocal cord is an ultimate effect of the enlargement of the major pulmonary arterial system. The aortic arch and the *left pulmonary artery* lie within a C-shaped angle formed by the left side of the *trachea* medially, the left main bronchus inferiorly, and the *left upper-lobe bronchus* laterally. Within this confined zone,

enlargement of the left pulmonary artery causes the aortic arch to be forced against the left side of the trachea. In this region, the *left recurrent laryngeal nerve* ascends after hooking around the lower aspect of the *aorta.* Compression of this nerve, as it runs between the trachea and the aortic arch, appears to be the explanation for the paralysis.

Enlargement of the left atrium is an important *sign* of mitral stenosis. This chamber may extend farther to the right than does the right atrium. Clinically, this is demonstrated by the yielding, in the *roentgenogram,* of two effects, namely, the *displacement of the esophagus* and the appearance of a "double" atrial shadow. As the left atrium lies closely applied to the esophagus, the enlarged left atrium frequently causes posterior displacement of the esophagus. In extreme cases, the esophagus may also be displaced laterally, usually toward the right.

RHEUMATIC HEART DISEASE VI

Mitral Stenosis: Secondary Pulmonary Effects

In *mitral stenosis*, obstruction at the diseased valve is reflected as an increase in pressure within the entire pulmonary vascular bed and *right ventricle*.

In the normal pulmonary vascular bed, there is a low-grade differential of pressure across the arteriolar level. The small, thin-walled *pulmonary arteries* and *arterioles* are incapable of exerting high levels of vasospasm. In mitral stenosis, on the contrary, these small arterial vessels exhibit medial *hypertrophy* and appear to be capable of displaying considerable degrees of vasospasm, which is associated with higher levels of differences in pressure between the pulmonary arterial and venous sides than those prevailing in the normal subject.

The pressure in the pulmonary capillary bed is determined by the factors of resistance to the flow of blood from the lungs (the stenotic mitral valve) and the amount of blood flowing into the bed. If the hydrostatic pressure within the capillary bed rises to certain levels, pulmonary edema may result. It is probable that the volume of flow into the capillary bed of the *lung* is determined by the degree of pulmonary arteriolar vasospasm. Pulmonary arteriolar vasoconstriction may be viewed as a protective phenomenon in mitral stenosis, guarding against flow to that degree at which pulmonary edema might develop.

Although the mechanism by which pulmonary arteriolar vasospasm is stimulated is unknown, it is conceivable that the pulmonary arteriolar bed exerts a constantly changing degree of vasoconstriction, depending upon pulmonary capillary pressure.

Pulmonary arteriolar vasospasm is significant under conditions of tachycardia. In the latter state, the diastolic period is shortened, and, in the presence of mitral stenosis, tachycardia is reflected in the retention of blood in the *left atrium* and in the *pulmonary venous* and capillary beds. Reduction of the flow of blood into the capillary bed tends to maintain the capillary pressure at a level lower than would be the case were no regulation present. Under conditions of tachycardia, the development of pulmonary edema may be ascribed to failure of the pulmonary arteriolar protective effect.

Among the structural changes in the pulmonary vascular bed is medial *thickening* of all classes of vessels, including the major arteries and veins. Intimal fibrous thickening may be apparent in

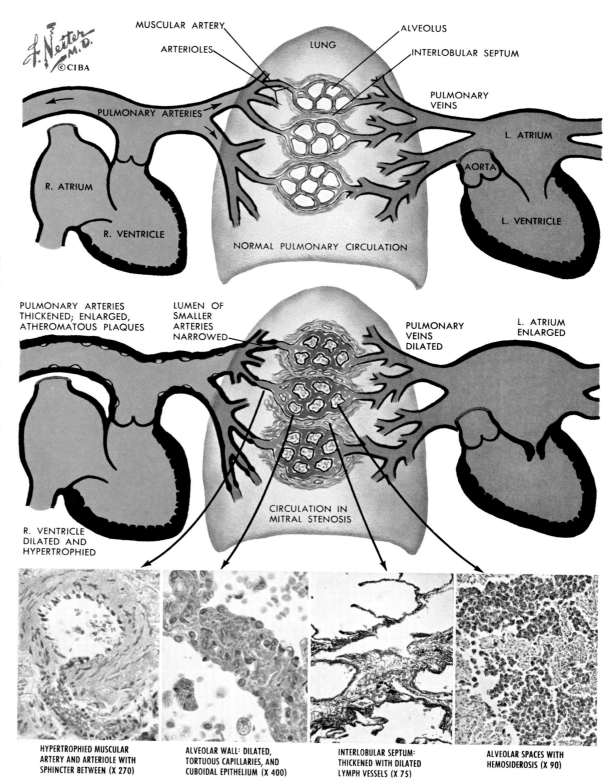

NORMAL PULMONARY CIRCULATION

CIRCULATION IN MITRAL STENOSIS

HYPERTROPHIED MUSCULAR ARTERY AND ARTERIOLE WITH SPHINCTER BETWEEN (X 270)

ALVEOLAR WALL: DILATED, TORTUOUS CAPILLARIES, AND CUBOIDAL EPITHELIUM (X 400)

INTERLOBULAR SEPTUM: THICKENED WITH DILATED LYMPH VESSELS (X 75)

ALVEOLAR SPACES WITH HEMOSIDEROSIS (X 90)

venules, arterioles, and small arteries. These changes are nonspecific and should not be compared with the characteristic *atherosclerosis* which may occur in the major pulmonary arteries. Intimal fibrous thickening of small arterial vessels is responsible for varying degrees of *luminal narrowing*. When severe changes are present, these are usually focal, many vessels being spared. This may relate to the phenomenon that pulmonary vascular disease, of the degree seen in mitral stenosis, does not preclude a fall in pulmonary arterial pressure if the mitral stenosis is relieved.

In addition to distention of the pulmonary *capillaries*, the parenchyma of the lung, in mitral stenosis, may show several significant alterations. These include *cuboidal* cells lining the *alveoli*, fibrosis of the *alveolar walls*, the organization of a fibrinous exudate in the alveolar spaces, the presence of occasional spicules of bone in the *alveolar spaces*, dilata-

tion of the pulmonary *lymphatics*, and *hemosiderosis*.

Dilatation of the pulmonary lymphatics is apparent in the visceral pleura and in the *interlobular septa*. The latter change probably contributes to the "straight lines" seen in the lower pulmonary lobes in *roentgenograms* of patients with mitral stenosis. It may represent evidence for the assumed phenomenon that, in mitral stenosis, some of the fluid of the blood in the lungs is diverted to the right side of the heart by way of the lymphatics.

Hemosiderosis is considered to be the result of recurrent hemorrhages from distended pulmonary alveolar capillaries. Characteristically, it is represented by the intraalveolar accumulation of macrophages laden with iron-containing pigment. Such accumulations are responsible for the stippled appearance of the lungs in the *roentgenogram*, and they are another *clinical sign* of mitral stenosis.

RHEUMATIC HEART DISEASE VII

Mitral Stenosis: Thromboembolic Complications

Thromboembolic complications are among the serious consequences of mitral stenosis. These stem from the common complication of *left atrial* thrombosis, of which a frequent secondary effect is systemic embolism. The susceptibility of the left atrium to develop thrombi in mitral stenosis is closely related to the fact that the left atrium may not empty completely with each cardiac cycle. In particular does this apply to the situation wherein atrial fibrillation is present. In this state, left atrial thrombosis and systemic embolism are significantly more common than they are in individuals with mitral stenosis and sinus rhythm.

Within the *left atrium,* there are two sites of predilection for thrombosis when mitral stenosis is present. These are the appendage of this chamber and the *posterior wall* of the chamber, beginning just above the posterior cusp of the *mitral valve.* Thrombosis of the *atrial appendage* (auricle) may be restricted to the territory of the appendage, or the *thrombus* may *extend* from the appendage into the main portion of the chamber. Under these circumstances, the thrombus may maintain its *attachment* to the wall of the main part of the left atrium and, in this way, be in a position for organization and firm attachment to the wall. More commonly, that part of the thrombus which protrudes from the atrial appendage, in a polypoid fashion, into the cavity has little opportunity for attachment to the atrial wall. This type of thrombus is particularly vulnerable to fragmentation, thus serving as a basis for embolism.

Thrombi originating against the posterior wall of the left atrium are less common than are those of the atrial appendage. The basis of the predilection for thrombosis against the posterior wall may be related to a local factor of injury, to this part of the left atrium, by a jetlike stream of blood striking the wall as an expression of a minor degree of associated mitral insufficiency.

There are examples of mitral stenosis in which the distribution of thrombi is so extensive as to result in descriptions of the left atrium as being *"filled"* with

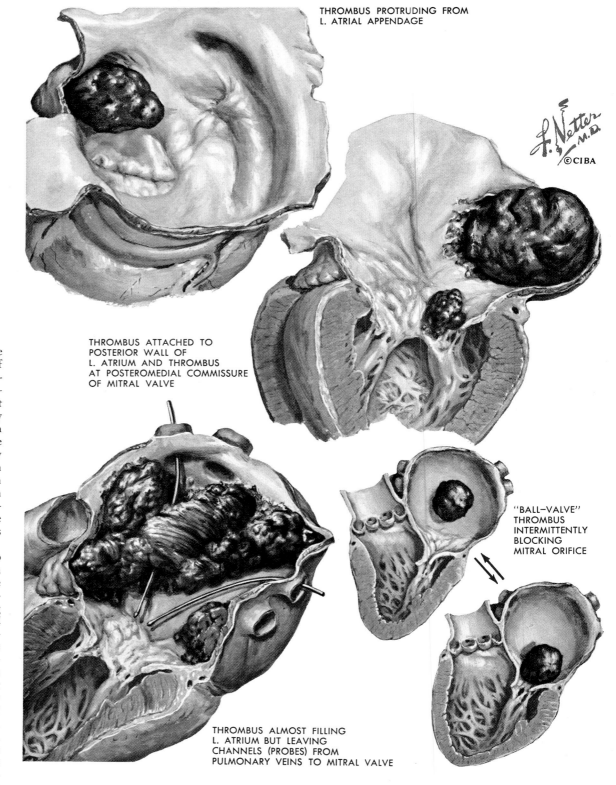

THROMBUS PROTRUDING FROM L. ATRIAL APPENDAGE

THROMBUS ATTACHED TO POSTERIOR WALL OF L. ATRIUM AND THROMBUS AT POSTEROMEDIAL COMMISSURE OF MITRAL VALVE

"BALL–VALVE" THROMBUS INTERMITTENTLY BLOCKING MITRAL ORIFICE

THROMBUS ALMOST FILLING L. ATRIUM BUT LEAVING CHANNELS (PROBES) FROM PULMONARY VEINS TO MITRAL VALVE

thrombi. Although such thrombi occupy considerable space within the left atrium, they do not literally fill the chamber, and, in fact, there is a characteristic distribution of the thrombotic material. As the flow from the *pulmonary veins* through the left atrium is maintained, the process of thrombosis spares those parts of the left atrial wall which are in relation to the streams of blood flowing from the pulmonary veins toward the mitral valve. Several factors are related to extensive thrombosis of the left atrium. These include (1) very severe degrees of mitral stenosis, (2) a tendency for the patient to be older than the average, (3) the likelihood of calcification of the left atrial wall, and (4) the presence of intractable congestive cardiac failure.

The factors concerning the severity of mitral stenosis and the increased age of the patient may, in turn, underlie the presence of alterations, in the left atrial wall, which predispose to extensive thrombosis. Such changes include fibrous endocardial thickening and calcification of the left atrial wall. In addition, in those patients whose *roentgenograms* exhibit signs of left atrial calcification, extensively distributed thrombi are likely to be harbored in the left atrium. The frequent presence of intractable congestive cardiac failure, among patients with extensive left atrial thrombosis, may be related to several interwoven factors, *e.g.,* the severity of the mitral stenosis and the tendency for the patient to be older than the average. The latter factor may be reflected as myocardial failure on the basis of a longer-than-average time during which the primary disease process has been present. Extensive thrombi occupy significant space in the left atrium and, in this way, represent an obstructive factor in addition to the primary process at the mitral valve.

(Continued on page 175)

RHEUMATIC HEART DISEASE VIII

Mitral Stenosis: Thromboembolic Complications

(Continued from page 174)

Another *site* for *thrombosis* leading to *embolism* is the mitral valve. Thrombosis of the mitral valve tends to involve one or both *commissural* areas (see page 174) in instances with valvular calcification. This relationship suggests that the basis for thrombosis of the mitral valve is a fracture of calcific valvular tissue, leaving exposed to the circulation the nonendothelialized altered valvular substance as a nucleus upon which thrombosis may occur. Thrombosis of the valve tends to increase the degree of the mitral stenosis.

A special form of *left atrial thrombosis* is that in which a thrombus has become detached from its site of origin (probably most often the atrial appendage) and remains as a loose body in the left atrium. As this mass moves about in the left atrium, it acquires a rounded or ovoid shape. It may engage the *mitral orifice* but, being too large to pass through the stenotic valve, the mass, acting as a *"ball valve"* (see page 174), occludes the circulation at this point. As a consequence, the patient loses consciousness and may die. Usually, however, the change in body position, incident to the loss of consciousness, may cause the mass to become dislodged from the mitral valve; if so, the circulation is reinstated and the patient regains consciousness. In a patient with mitral stenosis, the *clinical phenomenon* of recurrent fainting attacks should lead to a strong suspicion of the "ball-valve" phenomenon. A clinically similar state may be obtained in a patient with a primary myxoma of the left atrium.

Among patients with mitral stenosis, embolism may occur in either the pulmonary or the systemic vascular systems. Pulmonary embolism is generally a complication of cardiac failure, and the usual source of emboli is the venous system of the legs, even though thrombosis of the right atrial appendage may be associated.

Embolism of the systemic arterial system, when it occurs in mitral stenosis, is most often a complication of thrombosis within the left atrium, less commonly on the stenotic mitral valve. Any of the tissues or organs supplied by the systemic arterial system may be affected. The results of cerebral embolism may vary from one or several episodes of small *infarction,* in silent areas of the *brain,* through infarction of the *brain,* through infarction of the internal capsule and related structures (leading to a typical stroke),

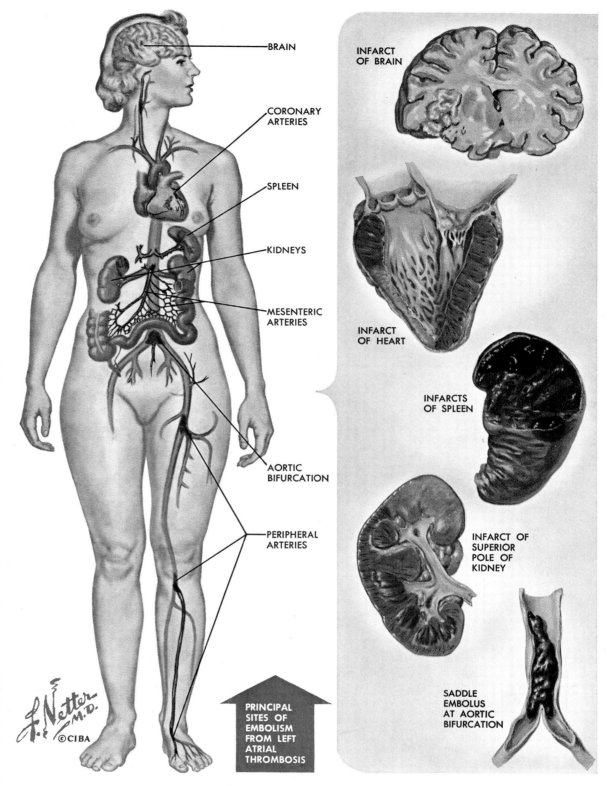

PRINCIPAL SITES OF EMBOLISM FROM LEFT ATRIAL THROMBOSIS

BRAIN

CORONARY ARTERIES

SPLEEN

KIDNEYS

MESENTERIC ARTERIES

AORTIC BIFURCATION

PERIPHERAL ARTERIES

INFARCT OF BRAIN

INFARCT OF HEART

INFARCTS OF SPLEEN

INFARCT OF SUPERIOR POLE OF KIDNEY

SADDLE EMBOLUS AT AORTIC BIFURCATION

or to infarction of most of a cerebral hemisphere. In instances of cerebral infarction, secondary hemorrhage may occur, making it difficult to distinguish between primary cerebral hemorrhage and infarction.

Depending upon the size of the vessel occluded, involvement of the *coronary arterial* system by embolism may lead to sudden death, to clinical evidence of typical *myocardial infarction,* or to silent infarction associated with nonspecific *electrocardiographic* manifestations.

Infarction of the spleen is common among patients with mitral stenosis. In some instances of splenic infarction the process is seemingly silent; in others, acute left upper abdominal pain may occur and may be associated with leukocytosis.

Embolism in the *kidneys,* with renal *infarction,* is also common. As with the spleen, some episodes may be associated with acute abdominal pain and may

be confused with conditions causing an "acute surgical abdomen." Under such circumstances, the frequent association of hematuria with renal infarction may be a helpful factor in the differential *diagnosis.*

Embolism in the arteries of the gastrointestinal tract is most likely to involve the superior *mesenteric artery,* whereas the celiac and the inferior mesenteric arteries are uncommon sites. Occlusion of the superior mesenteric artery leads to infarction of the entire small intestine (except the duodenum) and of the right half of the colon.

Embolism may occur in the branches of the extremities; but this is relatively uncommon, at least from the point of view of causing symptoms. More common is an embolism of the aorta. Characteristically, the embolus becomes impacted at the *aortic bifurcation,* a phenomenon often called *saddle embolism.*

RHEUMATIC HEART DISEASE IX

Mitral Insufficiency

In some hearts, the effects of recurrent rheumatic mitral endocarditis result in chordal shortening and *commissural fusion* — changes which make the valve stenotic but still competent. In other hearts, recurrent inflammation causes the *mitral valve* to be incompetent. The specific anatomic changes which result in mitral insufficiency include (1) intrinsic *shortening of the cusps,* (2) *commissural calcification,* and (3) *enlargement of the left atrium.* Characteristically, in instances of rheumatic mitral insufficiency, the *chordae tendineae* are relatively little affected. They may be somewhat thickened, but *shortening* is usually not present to any significant degree.

The feature of intrinsic *shortening of the mitral cusps* is more obvious in the *posterior* than in the anterior cusp. Evidence that the anterior cusp is shortened is the conversion of its free edge from a convex shape to a concave one. As a cusp becomes contracted, the tissue near its free end retracts, resulting in a pattern wherein some of the chordae tendineae attach directly to the free edge of the cusp. When intrinsic shortening of the cusps is responsible for mitral insufficiency, the basis for this functional disturbance is the inadequacy of tissue to guard the orifice.

It will be recalled that, in some instances of competent mitral stenosis (see page 171), there may be commissural calcification. In that condition, the involved commissures are held in a nearly closed position by the other changes responsible for mitral stenosis. In contrast, calcification in incompetent mitral valves involves commissures that are held in a nearly open position. In fact, the calcification is responsible for fixation of the cusps in such a position as to make them incapable of making contact, one with the other, in the area related to the calcified commissure. One or both commissures may be calcified. In the latter circumstance, the mitral valve is converted into a fixed structure which is open throughout the cardiac cycle.

Dilatation of the left atrium is a primary effect of mitral insufficiency, but, once established, left atrial enlargement may serve to increase the degree of incompetence of the valve. This applies when only one or neither commissure is *fused.* The aggravation of mitral insuf-

ficiency by left atrial enlargement depends primarily upon the anatomic phenomenon in which the left atrial wall and the mitral cusps may be considered as one continuous structure. When the left atrium dilates, its posterior wall extends backward and downward. This, in turn, causes the posterior mitral cusp to be pulled posteriorly and away from the anterior cusp, thereby accentuating the incompetence of the valve. In extreme cases, the posterior cusp may be displaced so much that it lies *over* the base of the *left ventricle.* In this position, the cusp being pulled posteriorly and downward by the left atrium is, at the same time, restricted from its other end by the attached chordae tendineae. This results in fixation of the posterior cusp as it lies *"hamstrung"* over the base of the left ventricle.

Mitral insufficiency is associated with enlargement of the left ventricular cavity and moderate hyper-

trophy of the left ventricular wall. Enlargement of the left atrium is constant, and the degree of enlargement is usually greater than that which occurs in mitral stenosis. Examples of "giant left atrium," in association with mitral valvular disease, are more apt to accompany mitral insufficiency than mitral stenosis.

Left atrial thrombosis may occur in mitral insufficiency, but this complication is distinctly less common than in mitral stenosis. The lesser tendency for left atrial thrombosis in mitral insufficiency is probably related to the constant turbulence of blood in this chamber, and there is less likelihood that blood will be retained in the left atrium in mitral insufficiency than in mitral stenosis.

The secondary effects upon the esophagus, tracheal bifurcation, right ventricle, and pulmonary vascular bed are like those described for mitral stenosis.

MITRAL INSUFFICIENCY: MITRAL VALVE VIEWED FROM BELOW; MARKED SHORTENING OF POSTERIOR CUSP, WITH ONLY SLIGHT COMMISSURAL FUSION, AND LITTLE FUSION AND SHORTENING OF CHORDAE TENDINEAE

MARKED ENLARGEMENT OF L. ATRIUM RESULTING FROM MITRAL INSUFFICIENCY

CALCIFIC PLATE AT ANTEROLATERAL COMMISSURE OF MITRAL VALVE, CONTRIBUTING TO INSUFFICIENCY

THICKENING AND SHORTENING OF MITRAL CUSPS WITH "HAMSTRINGING" OF POSTERIOR CUSP OVER THE MUSCULATURE OF L. VENTRICLE BY TRACTION OF ENLARGED L. ATRIUM

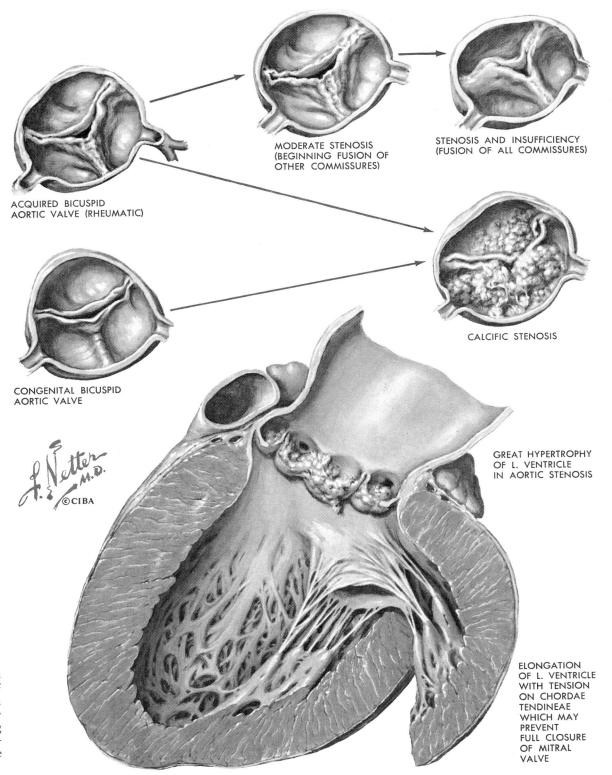

ACQUIRED BICUSPID
AORTIC VALVE (RHEUMATIC)

MODERATE STENOSIS
(BEGINNING FUSION OF
OTHER COMMISSURES)

STENOSIS AND INSUFFICIENCY
(FUSION OF ALL COMMISSURES)

CALCIFIC STENOSIS

CONGENITAL BICUSPID
AORTIC VALVE

GREAT HYPERTROPHY
OF L. VENTRICLE
IN AORTIC STENOSIS

ELONGATION
OF L. VENTRICLE
WITH TENSION
ON CHORDAE
TENDINEAE
WHICH MAY
PREVENT
FULL CLOSURE
OF MITRAL
VALVE

RHEUMATIC HEART DISEASE X

Aortic Stenosis

In the adult patient, obstruction at the *aortic valve* either may exist as a direct consequence of recurrent *rheumatic* endocarditis or may be a manifestation of the calcification of a *bicuspid* valve.

One may observe, in an aortic valve, various residua of rheumatic endocarditis which reduce, to some degree, the orifice of that valve. The simplest form of this type is characterized by *fusion of two of the cusps at one commissure*. The resultant pattern is that of an *acquired bicuspid aortic valve*. In this state, the orifice of the valve, though reduced, is usually sufficiently wide so as not to cause any recognizable obstruction to the egress of blood from the *left ventricle*. The next stage in severity is that in which the cusps are *fused at two of the commissures*. The restriction of motion of the cusps thus imparted by the adhesions may reduce the orifice sufficiently to cause significant aortic stenosis. The ultimate in restriction of motion is achieved in those cases where there is *fusion of adjacent cusps at each commissure*. Alteration of the valve in this manner is always associated with some degree of cusp shortening. The element of fixation of the cusps makes the valve severely *stenotic*, and the element of shortening is responsible for coexistent aortic *insufficiency* of a degree dependent upon the extent of shortening.

In the second way by which rheumatic endocarditis leads to aortic stenosis, the rheumatic endocarditis operates indirectly by first establishing an acquired bicuspid valve which, in turn, may become calcified. The resultant rigidity of the cusps makes the valve stenotic.

The most common type of aortic valvular stenosis is the *calcific* form. As indicated previously, this process may, in some cases, become established upon the acquired bicuspid valve; in others, however, it may represent a complication of a *congenital bicuspid valve*. From the examination of valves which have been involved in calcific aortic stenosis, it is readily apparent that such valves are almost invariably bicuspid in nature. The striking alterations in the valve make it difficult, however, to determine, for each case, whether the bicuspid state is acquired or congenital. As more experience is gained, it becomes increasingly evident that a congenital bicuspid valve is a common background for calcific aortic stenosis. Support for this concept comes not only from the intrinsic features of the valve but also from the fact that, in some cases of calcific aortic stenosis, a malformation known to be associated with a high incidence of congenital bicuspid valve, such as coarctation of the aorta, is also present.

In aged individuals, it is common that some calcification of the aortic cusps be present, and, in some of these, the changes may be sufficient to cause a murmur like that heard in true aortic stenosis, but the signs of left ventricular hypertrophy are usually absent. Such cases should not be considered examples of aortic stenosis.

Aortic stenosis is associated with elevation of the left ventricular systolic pressure to levels above the aortic systolic pressure. *Left ventricular hypertrophy* follows, giving a conical shape to the left ventricle, which extends beyond the border of the right ventricle.

In patients with aortic stenosis, coronary atherosclerosis may be present to the same extent seen in the general population. Areas of myocardial infarction are commonly observed in aortic stenosis. Usually, these lesions are small and occur both in patients with significant coronary atherosclerosis and in those with normal coronary arteries. Gross myocardial infarction associated with aortic stenosis is usually associated also with significant degrees of coronary arterial obstruction. As a rule, the latter process takes the form of atherosclerosis but, in an occasional case, coronary arterial narrowing results from embolism, the source of which is calcific material in the diseased aortic valve.

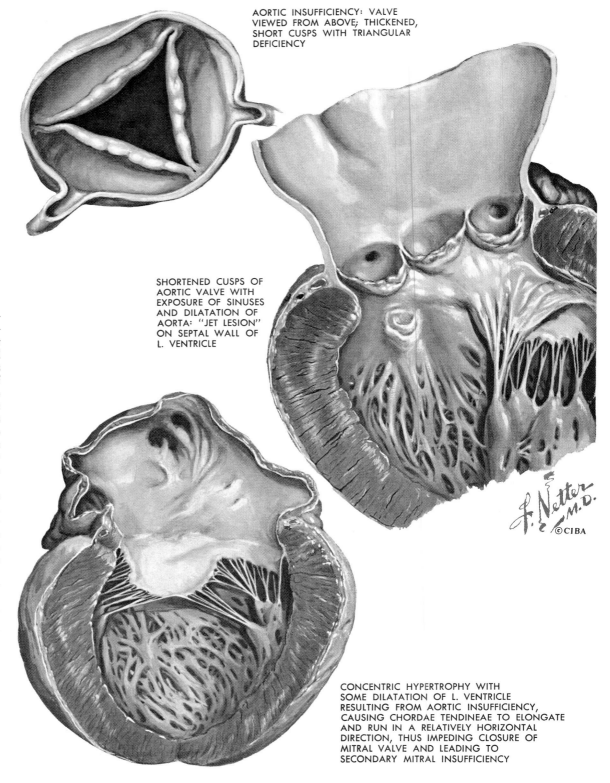

AORTIC INSUFFICIENCY: VALVE VIEWED FROM ABOVE; THICKENED, SHORT CUSPS WITH TRIANGULAR DEFICIENCY

SHORTENED CUSPS OF AORTIC VALVE WITH EXPOSURE OF SINUSES AND DILATATION OF AORTA: "JET LESION" ON SEPTAL WALL OF L. VENTRICLE

CONCENTRIC HYPERTROPHY WITH SOME DILATATION OF L. VENTRICLE RESULTING FROM AORTIC INSUFFICIENCY, CAUSING CHORDAE TENDINEAE TO ELONGATE AND RUN IN A RELATIVELY HORIZONTAL DIRECTION, THUS IMPEDING CLOSURE OF MITRAL VALVE AND LEADING TO SECONDARY MITRAL INSUFFICIENCY

RHEUMATIC HEART DISEASE XI

Aortic Insufficiency

If recurrent rheumatic endocarditis affects the aortic cusps but spares the commissures, isolated aortic insufficiency may result. This functional change is derived from *shortening* of the scarred *cusps*. As each cusp is shortened, there is a loss of some of the "extra length" of the cusp which, in the normal heart, makes the *valve* competent. If the deformation is sufficient, the cusps become too short to guard the aortic orifice. The incompetent orifice of the valve is then represented by a *triangular* opening bounded by the affected cusps.

Shortening of the cusps involves not only their width but also their length. Thus, when the *left ventricle* and the incompetent *aortic valve* are opened in the conventional pathologic dissection, more of the aortic *sinuses* is evident than is the case when the aortic valve is normal.

Secondary signs of aortic insufficiency include widening or *dilatation* of the ascending *aorta* and alterations in the left ventricle. Changes in the left ventricle include *hypertrophy* and the presence of regurgitant "jet lesions" on the wall of the subaortic region. The regurgitant "jet lesions" are responses to the trauma of the regurgitant stream striking the wall. These may be present on the *septal wall* of the outflow tract or on the ventricular aspect of the anterior mitral cusp. Characteristically, the fibrous tissue which constitutes the "jet lesion" is oriented in a cuspid pattern, the open parts of the cusps facing the source of the regurgitant stream. The presence of "jet lesions" in the subaortic area constitutes important anatomic evidence for aortic insufficiency, and their location may correspond to the site of origin of the diastolic murmur of aortic insufficiency.

The left ventricular hypertrophy of aortic insufficiency may be of extreme degree; among the heaviest hearts observed pathologically, aortic insufficiency is a common underlying problem. Along with thickening of the wall, there is enlargement (*dilatation*) of the cavity in both the lateral and the downward directions. The changes in the left ventricle may be responsible for the development of *secondary mitral insufficiency,* for the two following reasons:

1. In aortic insufficiency, as in aortic stenosis, while the left ventricle enlarges in a downward direction the papillary muscles may be moved downward as well. The resultant tension upon the *chordae tendineae* of the mitral valve may be responsible for undue restraint upon the mitral cusps, to such a degree that they cannot approximate each other adequately for *closure of the mitral valve* (see page 177). Mitral insufficiency results.

2. In aortic insufficiency, enlargement of the left ventricular cavity is responsible for the lateral displacement of the papillary muscles. This tends to change the axis of the papillary muscles and chordae tendineae from a near vertical position, with respect to the long axis of the left ventricle, to an axis which tends to be oriented toward the *horizontal* position. The change in direction of the pull of the papillary muscles may cause some inefficiency in the function of the papillary-muscle–chordal mechanism, with resultant mitral insufficiency.

The left ventricular hypertrophy accompanying aortic insufficiency or aortic stenosis may be looked upon as a basis for increased resistance to filling of the left ventricle. This manifestation is expressed functionally as an elevation of the left ventricular end-diastolic pressure. This change, in turn, may be considered as an obstruction to pulmonary venous flow, and, in this way, it is comparable to mitral stenosis. There is an elevation of the left atrial and pulmonary capillary pressures and pulmonary arterial pressures in the pulmonary vessels, and the parenchyma may simulate qualitatively that in mitral stenosis, although the degree of change is usually less in aortic valvular disease. The right ventricular hypertrophy accompanying aortic stenosis or aortic insufficiency may be derived in a manner similar to the right ventricular hypertrophy of mitral stenosis.

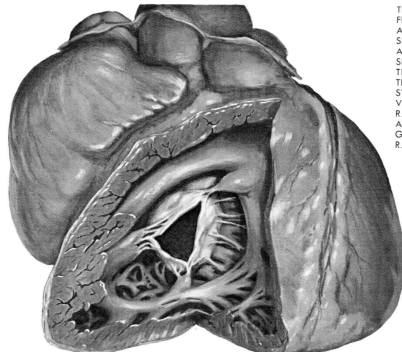

TRICUSPID VALVE VIEWED FROM BELOW: SOME FUSION AT EACH COMMISSURE, SHORTENING OF CUSPS, AND A LITTLE THICKENING AND SHORTENING OF CHORDAE TENDINEAE, LEAVING A TRIANGULAR ORIFICE OF A STENOTIC, INSUFFICIENT VALVE; HYPERTROPHY OF R. VENTRICLE DUE TO ASSOCIATED MITRAL DISEASE; GREAT ENLARGEMENT OF R. ATRIUM

RHEUMATIC HEART DISEASE XII

Tricuspid Stenosis and Insufficiency

Rheumatic deformity of the *tricuspid valve* is characterized principally by *fusion at each of the commissures* and *shortening of the cusps. Chordal changes* are usually minimal in degree. These changes are responsible both for a reduction in the caliber of the orifice and for incompetence of the valve. The usual coexistence of *stenosis* and *insufficiency* in the rheumatic tricuspid valve stands in contrast to the situation in the mitral valve. In the latter, the involvement is often manifested as stenosis *or* insufficiency. One characteristic effect of rheumatic tricuspid valvular disease is that the *right atrium* is *enlarged.* It is to be emphasized that chronic rheumatic involvement of the tricuspid valve is only rarely, if ever, an isolated phenomenon, since usually the *mitral valve* is also involved and, in some cases, the *aortic valve* as well.

In instances of mitral stenosis with evidence of tricuspid insufficiency, it remains to be determined whether the latter problem represents intrinsic involvement of the tricuspid valve or whether it is secondary to the mitral stenosis through right ventricular failure. There are certain features which favor secondary tricuspid insufficiency, in the patient with known mitral stenosis. Usually, congestive cardiac failure is evident. It has been indicated that in intrinsic rheumatic disease of the tricuspid valve, stenosis and insufficiency usually coexist, whereas in secondary tricuspid insufficiency stenosis is absent. Therefore, when, in the presence of tricuspid insufficiency, signs of tricuspid stenosis are lacking, one must view the tricuspid insufficiency as secondary rather than primary.

Multivalvular Disease

Involvement of more than one valve by deforming rheumatic disease generally consists of *disease* of the *mitral* and *aortic valves* while the tricuspid valve is essentially unaffected. The combination of aortic and mitral disease usually takes the form of predominant mitral stenosis and predominant aortic stenosis (of the fibrous type), with varying degrees of aortic insufficiency. Primary aortic insufficiency coupled with primary mitral

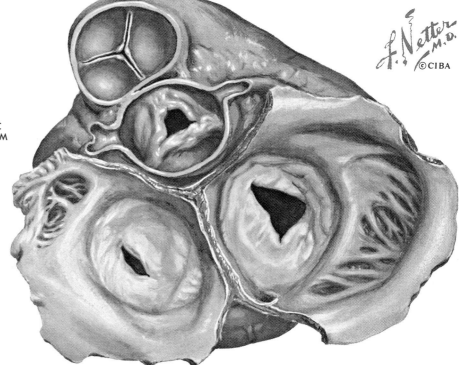

MULTIVALVULAR DISEASE VIEWED FROM ABOVE: AORTIC VALVE STENOTIC AND INCOMPETENT FROM FUSION OF ALL THREE COMMISSURES; MITRAL VALVE HAS ONLY A "SLITLIKE" STENOTIC ORIFICE, TRICUSPID VALVE A TRIANGULAR, FIXED, STENOTIC, AND INCOMPETENT ORIFICE; PULMONARY VALVE NORMAL

insufficiency, when each is of a severe degree, is rarely seen, possibly because of the tendency for the coexistence of the two to be a lethal combination.

When three valves are involved, the pulmonary valve is usually spared of major disease, but the tricuspid valve is affected. In trivalvular rheumatic disease, the lesions of the aortic and mitral valves are generally like those observed when only the left-side valves are affected. The tricuspid valve shows the characteristic features of intrinsic rheumatic disease, as described.

When multiple valves are involved, the effects upon the chambers vary both with the state of compensation of the heart and with the dominance of the disease in the various valves. Involvement of the tricuspid valve is universally associated with enlargement of the right atrial chamber. As a consequence of the mitral valvular disease, the *right ventricular*

wall is *hypertrophied.* When congestive cardiac failure is present, regardless of the state of the tricuspid valve, the *right ventricular chamber is enlarged.* In the compensated heart with mitral valvular disease and a normal tricuspid valve, the right ventricular chamber may be of normal size. The pulmonary trunk and the left atrium are enlarged as consequences of the mitral valvular disease.

In *multivalvular disease* in which the aortic valve also participates along with the mitral valve, the left ventricular wall is hypertrophied, but the degree of hypertrophy is considerably less than that observed in instances of isolated aortic valvular disease. The basis for this difference lies in the fact that the mitral valvular disease tends to be associated with a low cardiac output. As the cardiac output is lower than normal, the effects of aortic valvular disease — especially aortic stenosis — are minimized.

LUPUS ERYTHEMATOSUS

Systemic lupus erythematosus (SLE) is a disease which predominantly involves the vascular system. The major *clinical* and pathologic *features* of this disease reflect the site of vascular injury. Renal glomeruli, which are the vascular structures most susceptible to the injurious effects of the circulating agents, are frequently damaged during the course of SLE. In many patients a necrotizing vasculitis, affecting small and medium-sized blood vessels, is observed also. *Multiple visceral organs* may be affected, with *cardiac involvement* a prominent feature of this syndrome.

The cardiac lesions may be considered in relation to damage involving the valves and *mural endocardium,* blood vessels, and connective tissue of the myocardium and the pericardium. Most patients with SLE have *symptoms* attributable to involvement of the heart in the disease process. It is usually difficult to differentiate the primary signs, which reflect endocarditis and myocarditis, from the secondary symptoms resulting from fever, hypertension, anemia, and concurrent renal and pulmonary disease. *Pericarditis* is the most frequent and one of the earliest signs of SLE. *Endocarditis* may be associated with systolic or diastolic murmurs which have no distinguishing characteristics. The *vegetations* do not embolize. *Myocarditis* is exceedingly difficult to recognize, because the lesions are usually mild and do not lead to cardiac dilatation or failure.

Nonbacterial endocarditis, described by Libman and Sacks, was found originally in more than 50 to 60 percent of the hearts of the lupus erythematosus patients examined. The incidence of all cardiac lesions found at postmortem examination has changed radically since the institution of steroid therapy. The *mitral* and *tricuspid valves* are most frequently affected by single or mulberry-shaped excrescences, ranging in size from 1 to 4 millimicrons. They occur in a random fashion, both on and away from the line of closure on *both surfaces* of the valve. *Vegetations* also may be found on the *chordae tendineae,* the *papillary muscles,* and the *mural endocardium,* usually at the base of the ventricles. *Microscopically,* the excrescences have a superficial layer of partially hyalinized platelet and fibrin thrombi. Deeper layers may show evidence of *eosinophilic* collagen degeneration and *necrosis,* with a variable infiltrate of neutrophilic and mononuclear cells *(A).* Bacteria have not been demonstrated. In some instances, fibrous thickening of the valve, indicative of previous episodes of endocarditis, may be present. In the region of the valve ring,

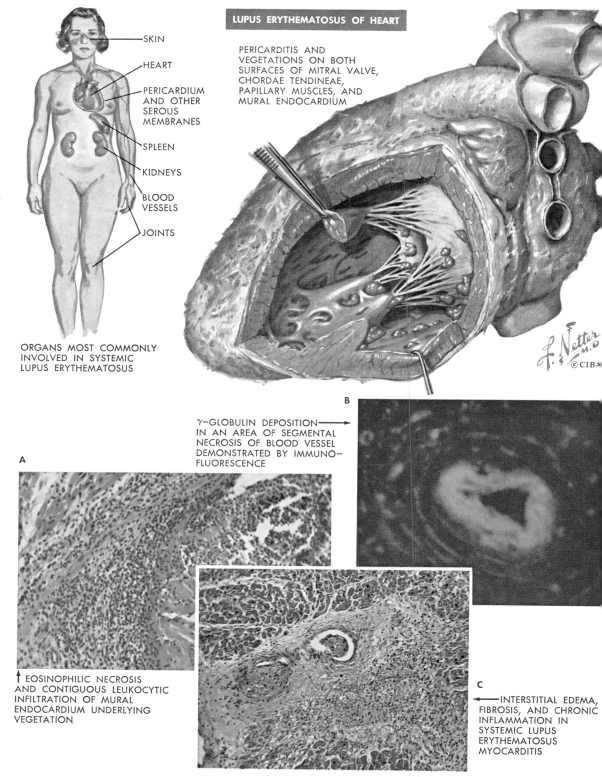

LUPUS ERYTHEMATOSUS OF HEART

ORGANS MOST COMMONLY INVOLVED IN SYSTEMIC LUPUS ERYTHEMATOSUS

SKIN
HEART
PERICARDIUM AND OTHER SEROUS MEMBRANES
SPLEEN
KIDNEYS
BLOOD VESSELS
JOINTS

PERICARDITIS AND VEGETATIONS ON BOTH SURFACES OF MITRAL VALVE, CHORDAE TENDINEAE, PAPILLARY MUSCLES, AND MURAL ENDOCARDIUM

A — ↑ EOSINOPHILIC NECROSIS AND CONTIGUOUS LEUKOCYTIC INFILTRATION OF MURAL ENDOCARDIUM UNDERLYING VEGETATION

B — γ-GLOBULIN DEPOSITION IN AN AREA OF SEGMENTAL NECROSIS OF BLOOD VESSEL DEMONSTRATED BY IMMUNO-FLUORESCENCE

C — INTERSTITIAL EDEMA, FIBROSIS, AND CHRONIC INFLAMMATION IN SYSTEMIC LUPUS ERYTHEMATOSUS MYOCARDITIS

the base of the valve and the valve-pocket proliferation of endothelial cells and myocytes may be prominent. Hematoxylin bodies may be found in the areas of endocardial inflammation.

Fibrinoid necrosis of the small and medium-sized arterioles may be associated with myocarditis. Endothelial proliferative and granular plugs of fibrin occlude the lumina of small vessels, showing *necrosis* of the wall. *Infiltrations* of neutrophils in the acute stage and mononuclear cells in the older lesions are prominent. Utilizing the *fluorescent*-antibody technic, deposits of γ-*globulin* and the C′$_3$ component of complement have been demonstrated in the acute vascular lesion *(B).* In the late stages of vessel involvement, endothelial proliferation, thickening, and partial occlusion may be found.

Foci of *myocardial inflammation,* associated with *interstitial edema* and eosinophilic degeneration of

collagen, may be prominent *(C).* Lymphocytes, plasma cells, and large histiocytic cells form the infiltrate. Hematoxylin bodies may be found in interstitial areas of *inflammation.* Degenerative changes in the myocardial fibers usually do not occur, and the myocarditis evident in SLE is usually not extensive, although areas of *fibrosis* may result.

Organizing fibrinous pericarditis, unassociated with uremia, is common, and fibrinoid necrosis of the pericardial connective tissue has also been observed. Serosanguineous effusions may accompany the pericarditis. Although fibrous adhesions may be seen, constrictive pericarditis does not occur.

The cardiac valvular lesions of SLE must be *differentiated* from those of rheumatic fever. Rheumatic vegetations occur on the atrial surface of the valve and have less tendency to undergo necrosis. The characteristic Aschoff nodule is absent in SLE.

BACTERIAL ENDOCARDITIS I

Portals of Entry and Predisposing Lesions

Bacterial endocarditis is a bacterial infection of the endocardium. Classically, the valves are involved primarily, but the mural endocardium of a cardiac chamber or the intima of a great vessel may also be subject to infection, yielding a clinical picture like that in classical valvular bacterial endocarditis.

In order for bacterial endocarditis to occur, two conditions must be satisfied: First, the offending organism must have a *portal of entry* into the *bloodstream,* in which bacteremia is established; second, a site susceptible to infection must be present. The latter may be identifiable as a lesion existing before infection, but, in instances of highly virulent bacteria, no predisposing lesion need be identifiable for infection to occur.

A portal of entry cannot always be recognized; when it can, the following are the important sites: The most common one is the mouth. The various *infectious lesions* associated with the *gums and teeth* may deliver *Streptococcus mitis (viridans)* to the bloodstream. The *male genital tract* is a source of another organism of relatively low virulence — *Streptococcus faecalis.* Its entry into the bloodstream usually follows some manipulation within the urethra, such as a prostatectomy. *Gonococcal urethritis* may be followed by bacteremia that may cause bacterial endocarditis. The *skin,* especially in infants with eczematous lesions, may permit entry of highly virulent staphylococci. From infection of the upper respiratory tract, *β-hemolytic streptococcus* is an occasional cause of bacterial endocarditis. *Pulmonary infections* are important sources of bacteremia, the organism commonly being the *pneumococcus.*

Just as a portal of entry is not recognized in all cases, so is a predisposing lesion not always identified. Particularly is the latter true if the infection is of the fulminating type. When a *predisposing lesion* is identified, it usually is of a type that will allow or cause trauma to a valvular or vascular lining. Fibrous thickening of freely movable cusps permits these structures to traumatize each other. A narrow stream of blood passing through a confined opening, with a considerable difference in pressure across the opening, is a basis for trauma. At the site of impact by such a stream, the lining of the vessel or endocardium involved is susceptible to infection.

The most common sites of bacterial endocarditis involve the *mitral* and/or the *aortic valve.* Predisposing lesions of the *mitral valve* are almost always *rheumatic* in nature. Classically, the degree of involvement of the valve by the rheumatic process is inadequate to cause significant hemodynamic changes, the patient often being unaware of any

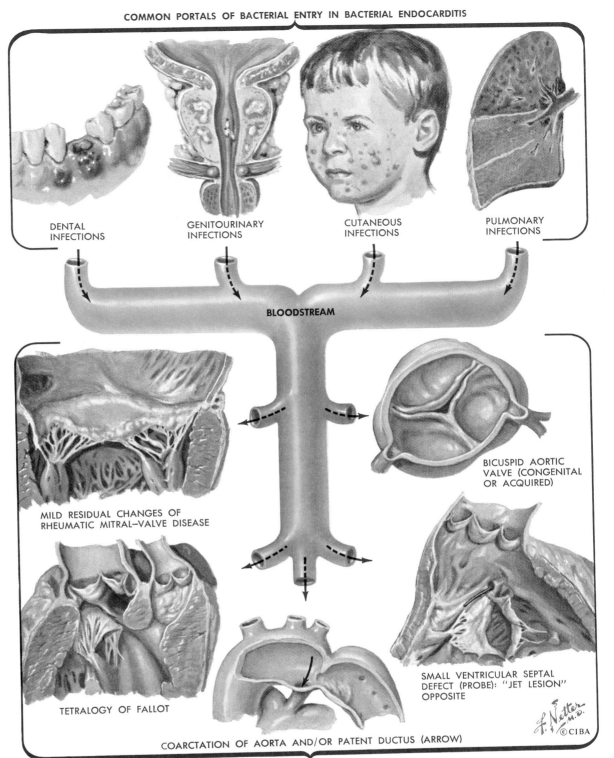

COMMON PORTALS OF BACTERIAL ENTRY IN BACTERIAL ENDOCARDITIS

DENTAL INFECTIONS   GENITOURINARY INFECTIONS   CUTANEOUS INFECTIONS   PULMONARY INFECTIONS

BLOODSTREAM

MILD RESIDUAL CHANGES OF RHEUMATIC MITRAL–VALVE DISEASE

BICUSPID AORTIC VALVE (CONGENITAL OR ACQUIRED)

TETRALOGY OF FALLOT

SMALL VENTRICULAR SEPTAL DEFECT (PROBE): "JET LESION" OPPOSITE

COARCTATION OF AORTA AND/OR PATENT DUCTUS (ARROW)

COMMON PREDISPOSING LESIONS

underlying cardiac disease. Characteristically, the changes are represented by mild fibrous thickening of the cusps along the line of closure. Chordal changes usually are minor, and commissural fusion, if present, is insignificant. Vascularization of the anterior mitral cusp is commonly present as a sign of antecedent rheumatic carditis. A valve affected as described displays free motion of its cusps, but denudation of endothelium may occur in relation to the areas of fibrous thickening. Such areas are susceptible if bacteria capable of causing infection are circulating in the bloodstream.

In the *aortic valve* a common anatomic background is the *bicuspid valve.*

In about half of the cases the bicuspid nature of the valve is of *congenital* origin, whereas in the remainder it is an *acquired* condition resulting from rheumatic endocarditis. In occasional instances of significant aortic stenosis, bacterial endocarditis may occur.

Bacterial endocarditis in the right side of the heart occurs under two circumstances. The first is that in which

a *highly virulent* organism, such as *staphylococcus, β-hemolytic streptococcus,* or *pneumococcus,* infects previously normal valves; the second, and more common, is that in which there is an underlying condition, which generally is congenital. Usually the malformation is responsible for forcing a stream of blood, at high pressure, through a narrow opening. Thus, the infundibulum of the right ventricle, in the *tetralogy of Fallot,* is susceptible, as is the tricuspid valve or the right ventricular wall ("*jet lesion*") in instances of *small ventricular septal defect.* In *patent ductus arteriosus* a similar condition exists, since that part of the pulmonary arterial wall opposite the ductus, struck by the stream of blood flowing through the ductus, is "fertile soil" for infection.

Peripheral blood vessels also may be subject to infection. These include the *aorta* (1) beyond a site of *coarctation,* (2) at an atheroma, or (3) within a saccular aneurysm, the latter usually of the abdominal segment of the vessel. In more-peripheral vessels, arteriovenous fistulas predispose to infection.

BACTERIAL ENDOCARDITIS II

Early Lesions

It is apparent, from the preceding plate, that valves and sites within blood vessels which become infected may exhibit preexisting lesions which make a susceptible area subject to trauma. The traumatic stimulus causes endothelial denudation, and, at the site of erosion, fibrin and *platelets* are *deposited*. Such deposits have a particular affinity for the arrest of circulating bacteria and for the nutrition of *organisms* caught in the adhesive material. Organisms meshed in fibrin and platelets multiply and invade the underlying tissue.

While a preexisting lesion's role in making an area susceptible to infection seems clear, the basis for the localization of infection, when no recognizable lesion is present, is less evident. It cannot easily be ascertained whether a preexisting lesion was present, in some cases, since it may be impossible to distinguish fibrous lesions either as being the result of bacterial endocarditis or as representing a preexisting lesion. Regardless of the presence or absence of a preexisting lesion, the early established lesion is similar. It is characterized by the features of bacterial attack, and later, as this process continues, by a reactive healing process coexisting with the first.

In the *early lesion,* bacteria invade the tissues while other events occur on the surface. Within the tissues are bacterial multiplication, *edema,* tissue destruction, and *leukocytic infiltration.* In later stages, granulation tissue, evidenced by proliferation of the capillaries and fibroblasts, may occur. At the same time, a *vegetation* forms on the surface of the infected area. The vegetation is characterized by deposits of varying amounts of platelets and fibrin and by proliferation of bacteria. The latter may be so extensive as to form colonies within and upon the surface of the vegetation. Fragmentation of vegetative material of this sort serves to maintain the bacteremia and to cause secondary occlusive effects in the peripheral circulation.

The most distinctive *gross feature* of the early lesion is the vegetation at the site of primary infection. Because of its basic content, the vegetation fundamentally appears tan, but, if erythrocytes become enmeshed in the fibrin, the vegetation may take on a purple color. An important gross characteristic of the vegetation is its friable nature. Considerable variation occurs in the gross appearance of these vegetations. In size, they range from barely visible flat plaques to verrucous masses.

Characteristically, the vegetations are deposited focally. Even in some early lesions, one or several vegetations may occur. Regardless of this detail, however,

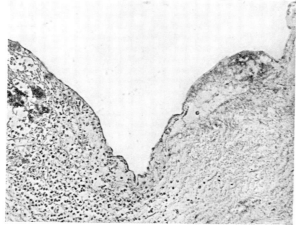

DEPOSIT OF PLATELETS AND ORGANISMS (STAINED DARK), EDEMA AND LEUKOCYTIC INFILTRATION IN VERY EARLY BACTERIAL ENDOCARDITIS OF AORTIC VALVE

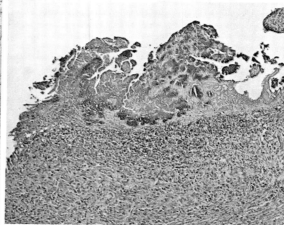

DEVELOPMENT OF VEGETATIONS CONTAINING CLUMPS OF BACTERIA ON TRICUSPID VALVE

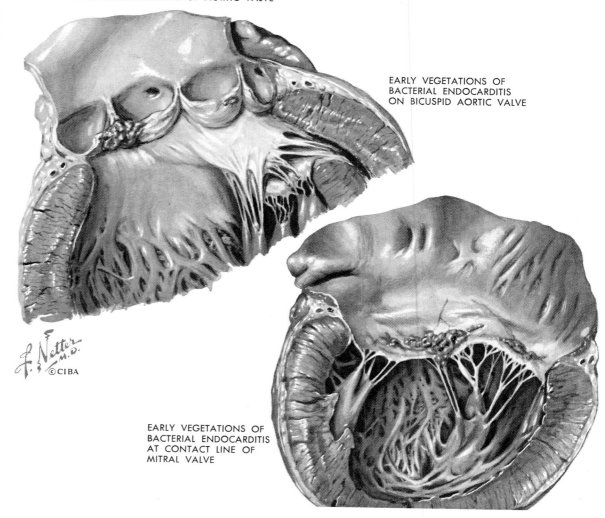

EARLY VEGETATIONS OF BACTERIAL ENDOCARDITIS ON BICUSPID AORTIC VALVE

EARLY VEGETATIONS OF BACTERIAL ENDOCARDITIS AT CONTACT LINE OF MITRAL VALVE

it is classic that the cusps are affected only in part.

In the *aortic valve,* which often is *bicuspid,* the *early vegetation* tends to involve either the fused commissure of an acquired bicuspid valve or the region related to the raphe of a congenital bicuspid valve.

In the *mitral valve,* vegetations are first deposited on the atrial surface, along the *contact line* of closure of the cusp.

Soon after the establishment of the primary site of infection, there may be evidence of secondary lesions on the same valve. These are derived from bacterial contamination of initially uninvolved segments of the valve that make contact with the site of primary infection. Secondary foci of infection so derived are called *contact* or *kissing* lesions. Once established, the secondary lesion appears similar to the primary one, so it is not always possible to determine which is the primary and which is the secondary site of infection.

In addition to contact lesions, an early lesion may show some tendency to spread, a feature exemplified by early extension of vegetations from the atrial surface of an atrioventricular valve onto its underlying chordae tendineae.

Grossly, the vegetations of bacterial endocarditis must be distinguished from other conditions which characteristically show vegetative deposits on the valves. These are active rheumatic endocarditis, endocardial lesions of lupus erythematosus, and marantic vegetations. The focal nature of the vegetations of bacterial endocarditis readily distinguishes them from the uniform small rheumatic vegetations. In the other two conditions, the focal nature of their vegetations makes gross distinction less simple. The general nature of the problem is an aid, but a specific *diagnosis* depends on the fact that bacteria are present only in the vegetations of bacterial endocarditis.

BACTERIAL ENDOCARDITIS III

Advanced Lesions

As *bacterial endocarditis becomes advanced*, it is truly a systemic disease with the potential of affecting each body organ. If the disease is not arrested in an early stage, heart changes become more advanced, leading to greater involvement of the valve primarily affected as well as to involvement of other valves. Spread from one valve to another may occur as a manifestation of forward infection, as when the *aortic valve* becomes secondarily involved to primary disease of the *mitral valve*. The reverse — a process which may be called regurgitant infection — may also happen.

Regurgitant infection depends upon the development of incompetence of the primarily involved valve. The incompetence may come about in one of several ways. The first, and more simple, is that bulky vegetations may prevent proper apposition of cusps, with resultant incompetence. More serious is the second phenomenon, characterized by *destruction* of valvular substance (and of *chordae tendineae*, in the case of the mitral valve), resulting in *perforation* and/or erosion of *cuspid tissue*. An additional route is simple *continuous spread* of the infection from one valve to another.

When the aortic valve is primarily involved, incompetence of the valve during the stage when the infection is active leads to infection of those sites against which regurgitant streams become impacted. This may cause either mural infection of the left ventricular-outflow tract or infection of components of the mitral valve.

As the anterior mitral cusp lies directly subjacent to the aortic valve, this cusp, in contrast to the posterior mitral cusp, is particularly vulnerable to secondary infection. Such a process is represented first by vegetations on the ventricular surface of this cusp. Destruction of tissue beneath such vegetations may lead either to focal weakness (with aneurysm formation in the cusp) or to perforation (with or without the intermediary stage of aneurysm formation). Perforation of a mitral cusp leads to mitral insufficiency, an additional cause for which is rupture of mitral chordae tendineae. If the regurgitant stream from the incompetent aortic valve is directed inferiorly, mitral chordae tendineae become sites of regurgitant infection. On the basis of anatomic orientation, chordae tendineae inserting into the anterior mitral cusp are more apt to be involved than those inserting into the posterior cusp, but the latter are not totally protected from this problem. Infected chordae tendineae may rupture, leading to inadequate support of a mitral cusp and to inevitable mitral insufficiency.

Direct spread from the aortic valve may involve structures other than the mitral valve. Extending inferiorly along the contact surface of the involved aortic cusps, the infection may attack the region

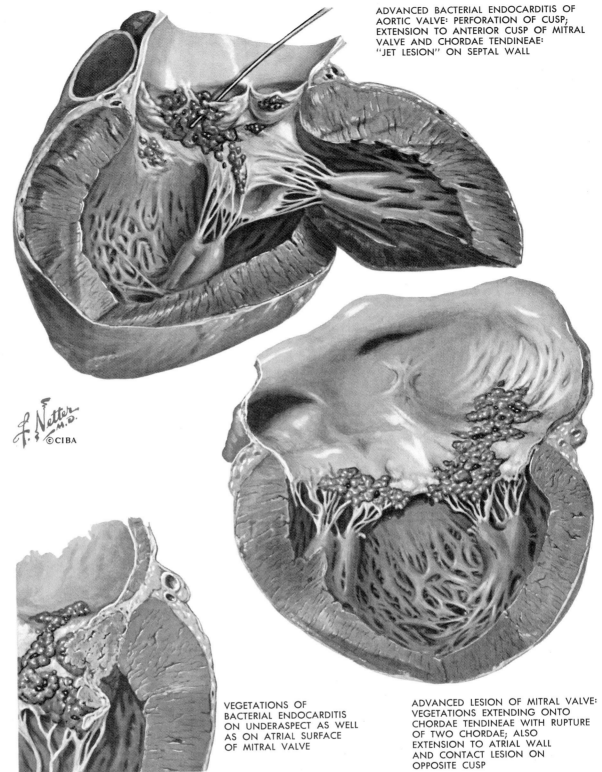

ADVANCED BACTERIAL ENDOCARDITIS OF AORTIC VALVE: PERFORATION OF CUSP; EXTENSION TO ANTERIOR CUSP OF MITRAL VALVE AND CHORDAE TENDINEAE: "JET LESION" ON SEPTAL WALL

VEGETATIONS OF BACTERIAL ENDOCARDITIS ON UNDERASPECT AS WELL AS ON ATRIAL SURFACE OF MITRAL VALVE

ADVANCED LESION OF MITRAL VALVE: VEGETATIONS EXTENDING ONTO CHORDAE TENDINEAE WITH RUPTURE OF TWO CHORDAE; ALSO EXTENSION TO ATRIAL WALL AND CONTACT LESION ON OPPOSITE CUSP

of the ventricular septum. From here, the destruction may cause an aneurysm of the ventricular septum, which, in turn, presents either into the right ventricle or the right atrium.

Extension of infection from an aortic cusp may advance into an aortic sinus, and this may cause an acquired type of aortic-sinus aneurysm. If the secondary infection involves the aortic valve above the level of the sinus and penetrates the aortic wall, it may lead to the rare complication of suppurative pericarditis.

When the mitral valve is primarily involved, regurgitation of blood through it may result in mural infection of the left atrium at those sites which are struck by regurgitant streams of infected blood.

Another advanced lesion involving the valves is infection of the posterior mitral cusp and the adjacent left ventricular mural endocardium in the angle

formed by these two structures. Although the infection characteristically starts on the contact aspect of the cusps, it rapidly extends through the full thickness of the cusp. In the case of the posterior mitral cusp, vegetations may then form on its *underaspect* or ventricular aspect. Organisms in this material may secondarily infect adjacent structures, including the left ventricular wall and the wedge of epicardium that extends to the nearby mitral ring.

Quite apart from the various types of intracardiac spread of infection which characterize advanced lesions, the destructive effects of the infection represent a common problem. Excavation of valvular tissue tends to cause loss of support and prolapse of valvular tissue. Perforations of cusps and *rupture* of chordae tendineae, on valves either primarily or secondarily involved, are additional important causes of valvular incompetence.

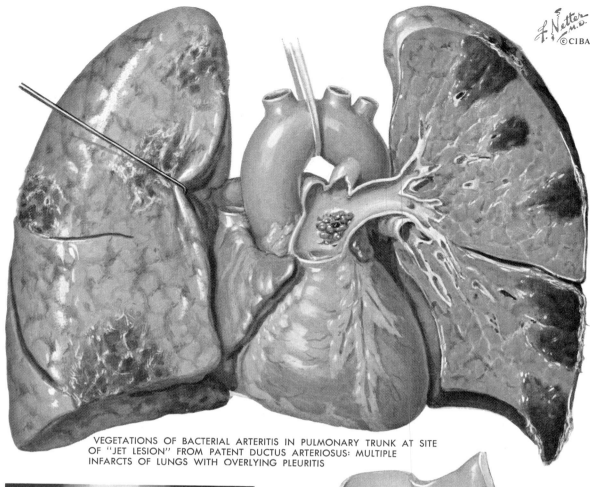

VEGETATIONS OF BACTERIAL ARTERITIS IN PULMONARY TRUNK AT SITE OF "JET LESION" FROM PATENT DUCTUS ARTERIOSUS: MULTIPLE INFARCTS OF LUNGS WITH OVERLYING PLEURITIS

BACTERIAL ENDOCARDITIS IV

Right-Side Involvement

Bacterial endocarditis involving the right side of the heart and/or pulmonary arterial system is far less common than is primary involvement of the left side.

Perhaps the most common kind of right-side bacterial endocarditis is that which complicates classical *patent ductus arteriosus*. In this form of patent ductus, aortic pressure is not fully transmitted into the pulmonary arteries, because of the relatively narrow state of the ductus. The stream of blood entering the pulmonary arterial system through the shunt strikes the pulmonary arterial wall opposite the ductus. Here, a *"jet lesion"* is set up, and this area will be predisposed to infection. While in the clinical state of "infected ductus arteriosus," the ductus itself may be involved, and, more often, the primary site of infection is in the *pulmonary trunk* or left pulmonary artery. The ductus itself may become secondarily involved.

A second anatomic situation leading to right-side bacterial endocarditis is ventricular septal defect. Here, as in patent ductus arteriosus, infection usually occurs when there is not full transmission of systemic arterial pressure through the defect. Thus, bacterial endocarditis is uncommon in cases of "large" ventricular septal defect — a condition in which right ventricular and pulmonary hypertension are present. On the contrary, the "small" ventricular septal defect — a state in which the right ventricular pressure is near normal — is particularly vulnerable to this infectious complication.

As in patent ductus arteriosus, the primary infection is at the site of impact of the shunted stream. Therefore, it tends to occur either on the anterior wall of the *right ventricle* or on the septal cusp of the tricuspid valve, since these structures lie opposite the defect. Infection of the edges of the defect occurs in some cases. When a left-side structure, such as the aortic valve, is involved, it usually follows infectious spread from the right-side structures through the defect.

Several types of congenital pulmonary stenosis, including the classical tetralogy of Fallot, isolated right ventricular infundibular stenosis, and pulmonary-valve stenosis, constitute the usual additional congenital conditions in which bacterial endocarditis may develop. In each, the right ventricular pressure is elevated, a feature which in-

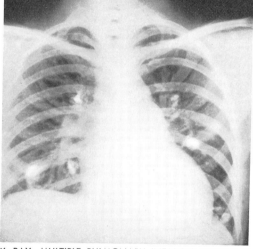

X-RAY: MULTIPLE PULMONARY INFARCTS RESULTING FROM PULMONARY ARTERITIS IN PATENT DUCTUS ARTERIOSUS

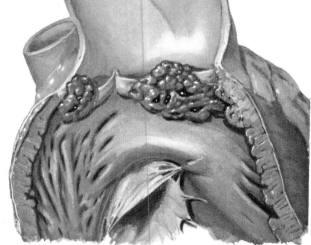

VEGETATIONS ON PULMONARY VALVE AND OUTFLOW TRACT OF RIGHT VENTRICLE

creases trauma to the tricuspid valve. In all these conditions, primary tricuspid bacterial endocarditis may occur. More commonly, however, when infection is present it involves that compartment beyond the obstructive lesion. In the tetralogy and in isolated infundibular stenosis, the right ventricular infundibulum is susceptible, and in pulmonary-valve stenosis the region of predilection for infection, in addition to the valve itself, is at the bifurcation of the pulmonary trunk — that area struck by the stream passing through the stenotic pulmonary valve.

The *gross appearance* of the lesions is essentially like that in left-side bacterial endocarditis. In the primary infection, vegetations vary considerably, from flat, hardly detectable aggregations to bulky masses. When a major pulmonary artery is infected, the destructive process may lead to formation of a mycotic aneurysm. In fact, more than half of the localized saccular aneurysms of major pulmonary arteries that have been described are of mycotic origin.

Whether right-side bacterial endocarditis starts in a

normal heart or in one with a congenital malformation, there is a *clinical picture* which differs, in many respects, from left-side endocarditis. Petechiae of the skin and mucous membranes and embolic phenomena in organs supplied by the systemic circulation are absent. The concentration of manifestations is in the lungs, as a result of embolism of vegetative material from the primary infection into many small branches of the pulmonary arteries. Classically, this causes widely distributed peripheral *infarcts of the lungs*. Commonly, a pleural reaction, characteristically fibrinous in nature, occurs over these lesions, leading to clinical evidence of pleurisy. When the organisms are virulent, the pulmonary infarcts suppurate, and the picture, both clinically and *roentgenographically*, is of widely distributed *pulmonary infiltrates*.

In protracted right-side bacterial endocarditis with pulmonary complications, heavy concentrations of organisms are fed through the pulmonary veins into the left side of the heart. This, in turn, may establish secondary foci of infection on either or both of the left-side cardiac valves.

BACTERIAL ENDOCARDITIS V

Cardiac Sequelae

Cardiac sequelae following *bacterial endocarditis* tend to fall into two groups: (1) those with residual changes that cause little functional disturbance of the valve and (2) those which are attended by a severe degree of anatomic change, usually manifested as valvular insufficiency.

Bacterial endocarditis, even though not recognized clinically, may heal. In some cases this may truly be spontaneous; in others, antibiotics administered for an undiagnosed condition may heal unsuspected bacterial endocarditis.

Healed lesions that have caused little functional disturbance are the end result of inflammation of the valve with surface deposit of vegetations. The site or sites of valvulitis are characterized by vascularization and varying degrees of fibrous *thickening*. The vegetation is replaced by fibrous tissue and by foci of calcification. One may observe focal thickenings on contact surfaces of cusps, representing not only the primary vegetation but also similar fibrous "kissing" lesions (see page 182).

Mural fibrous plaques in the left atrium or left ventricle may be observed as the residua of focal mural endocarditis which was present during the period of active infection.

Healed lesions which are responsible for valvular dysfunction commonly are characterized by the destruction of tissue. They take several forms, as follows:

Lesions of the *aortic valve*, responsible for hemodynamic disturbance resulting from bacterial endocarditis, may be characterized by (1) focal *erosion* leading to a serrated free edge of the involved *cusp or cusps*, (2) *perforation of the cusps*, and (3) destruction of that part of the cusp which attaches to the aortic wall, with resulting prolapse of the involved cusp. These lesions are responsible for aortic insufficiency and, in some cases, may be associated with mitral insufficiency. This form of aortic insufficiency causes secondary changes in the left ventricle—changes which are similar to those resulting from other etiologic types of aortic insufficiency. These changes include massive enlargement of the *left ventricular* cavity and an increase in its muscle mass. The *hypertrophy* often is severe, leading to cardiomegaly of a degree not exceeded by that caused by conditions other than aortic insufficiency.

"*Jet lesions*" resulting from the impact of the regurgitant stream may be observed either in the endocardium of the left ventricular-outflow tract or on the ventricular surface of the anterior mitral cusp.

Mitral insufficiency following bacterial

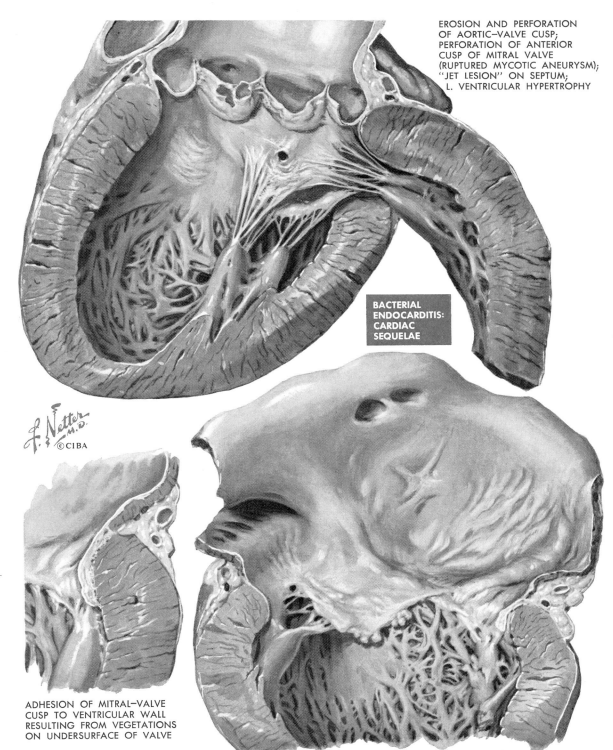

EROSION AND PERFORATION OF AORTIC–VALVE CUSP; PERFORATION OF ANTERIOR CUSP OF MITRAL VALVE (RUPTURED MYCOTIC ANEURYSM); "JET LESION" ON SEPTUM; L. VENTRICULAR HYPERTROPHY

BACTERIAL ENDOCARDITIS: CARDIAC SEQUELAE

ADHESION OF MITRAL–VALVE CUSP TO VENTRICULAR WALL RESULTING FROM VEGETATIONS ON UNDERSURFACE OF VALVE

THICKENING AND EROSION OF MITRAL VALVE WITH STUMPS OF RUPTURED CHORDAE TENDINEAE: ENLARGEMENT OF L. ATRIUM

endocarditis of the aortic valve may occur in one of several ways. When major left ventricular enlargement results from aortic insufficiency, there may be mechanical interference with the mitral-valve mechanism, causing valvular insufficiency.

In other instances, mitral insufficiency follows the destruction of mitral-valve elements or of mitral chordae tendineae, as a result of aortic regurgitation during the stages when the aortic-valve endocarditis was active.

It was shown earlier (see page 183) that active aortic-valve endocarditis could, by virtue of concomitant insufficiency, cause infection either of the mitral-valve anterior cusp or of mitral chordae tendineae. The end effects include mitral insufficiency from (1) perforation of the anterior mitral cusp or (2) rupture of chordae tendineae, with inadequate support of the cusps.

Primary mitral-valve endocarditis leading to mitral insufficiency may result from (1) destruction of cusp tissue, (2) *rupture of chordae tendineae*, or (3) *adhesion* of the posterior *mitral-valve cusp* to the left *ventricular wall*. The last process follows fibrous replacement of vegetations that, during the active stage of the disease, were deposited in the angle between the posterior mitral cusp and the left ventricular wall (see page 183). Because of this adhesion, the posterior mitral cusp ceases to function as a flap of valvular tissue.

When mitral insufficiency ensues from bacterial endocarditis, the usual secondary effects of mitral insufficiency are present. These include *left atrial enlargement* and right ventricular hypertrophy. Left ventricular hypertrophy is also present but to a lesser degree than that which results from aortic insufficiency.

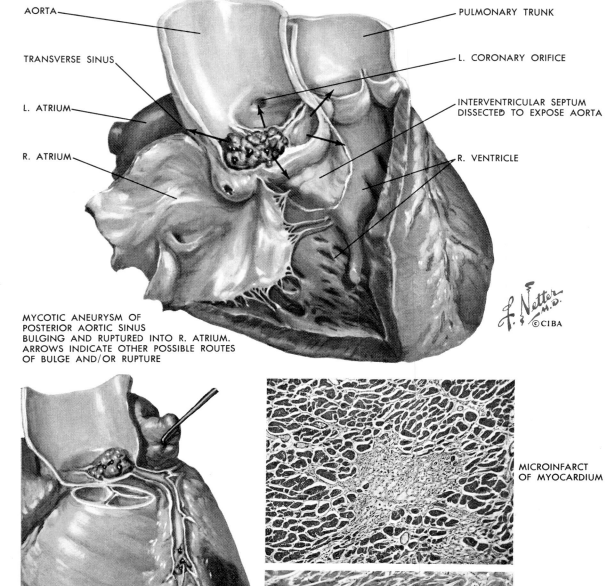

MYCOTIC ANEURYSM OF
POSTERIOR AORTIC SINUS
BULGING AND RUPTURED INTO R. ATRIUM.
ARROWS INDICATE OTHER POSSIBLE ROUTES
OF BULGE AND/OR RUPTURE

EMBOLUS FROM AORTIC-VALVE VEGETATIONS
OF BACTERIAL ENDOCARDITIS LODGED IN
CORONARY ARTERY RESULTING IN GROSS
MYOCARDIAL INFARCT

MICROINFARCT
OF MYOCARDIUM

MICROABSCESS
OF MYOCARDIUM

BACTERIAL ENDOCARDITIS VI

Mycotic Aneurysms and Emboli in the Heart

The manifestations of *bacterial endocarditis* range from localized valvular lesions to involvement of organs remote from the heart. Within this complex are secondary lesions at the origin of the *aorta* and a variety of embolic lesions within the *myocardium*.

Involvement of the aorta's origin may come from infection of either the mitral or the *aortic valve*, the latter being more common. Infection of the aortic origin from aortic-valve endocarditis may occur in one of three ways. The first is direct extension from the infected valve to the *aortic sinus* and the adjacent aortic wall. In the second mechanism, during systole an infected vegetation on an aortic cusp may make contact with the aortic wall, leading to bacterial deposit there. The third way is, in effect, embolic, as blood containing a high concentration of bacteria flows against the aortic wall.

Infection of the aortic origin starts in the intima and progresses through the underlying wall. Just as the infection is destructive to valves, so is it to the aorta. Weakness imparted to the aorta by this process may allow an aneurysm to form at the site of infection. Such aneurysms are usually called *mycotic aneurysms*, regardless of the specific organism characterizing the infection.

The ultimate effect of these mycotic aneurysms depends primarily on whether the aneurysm *ruptures*. Unruptured aneurysms are usually silent. Since the major portion of the aortic origin is intracardiac, aneurysms involving this part do not alter the contour of the cardiovascular shadow in *roentgenograms*. The only exception is an aneurysm involving the aorta near the *origin of the left coronary artery*. This part of the aorta lies against the epicardium, and an aneurysm here may create a shadow immediately superior to that of the left atrial appendage.

When a mycotic aneurysm of the aortic origin ruptures, the manifestations depend primarily on the site of the aneurysm. The upper illustration shows how diverse are the anatomic relations of the aortic origin and illustrates the several structures into which an aneurysm may, potentially, rupture. It should be recognized that mycotic aneurysms are derived from a destructive infectious process; thus, though certain basic anatomic rules obtain as to the potential for

rupture, variations do occur as expressions of fortuitous direction of the progression of the infection. Also, congenital aneurysms of the aortic sinuses (Valsalva), after rupturing into a cardiac chamber, may become infected, and it may be difficult to tell, from pathologic examination, whether a given aneurysm was primarily bland and secondarily infected or, conversely, primarily mycotic.

Mycotic aneurysms of the *posterior* (noncoronary) *aortic sinus* tend to present and rupture into the *right atrium*; rarely, into the *left atrium*. Since the right aortic sinus is closely related to the infundibulum of the *right ventricle*, an aneurysm involving this sinus usually leads to the right ventricle but rarely through the *ventricular septum* into the left ventricle. Because the left aortic sinus is related to the epicardium and to the *pulmonary trunk*, an aneurysm of this sinus has the potential either for leading to a suppurative pericarditis or for rupturing into the pulmonary trunk.

Embolism into the coronary arterial system is common in left-side bacterial endocarditis. Usually, this takes the

form of multiple small particles delivered into many intramyocardial ramifications of the coronary arteries. The consequences depend on the virulence of the organism involved in the valvular infection. In the more common situation, wherein the organism is of relatively low virulence, numerous small, seemingly bland, *microinfarcts* are seen in the *myocardium*. In the case of highly virulent organisms, such as β-hemolytic streptococci or staphylococci, the embolic process causes *microabscesses of the myocardium*.

Lodgment of an embolus in an epicardial branch of a *coronary artery* is a serious complication and may lead, shortly thereafter, to death from acute extensive myocardial ischemia. If the patient survives such an event, the effects may be apparent both in the involved artery and in the myocardium supplied by it. The latter may show typical *gross myocardial infarction*, while in the affected artery a mycotic aneurysm may result. A rare occurrence is the rupture of a coronary-artery mycotic aneurysm, leading to hemopericardium.

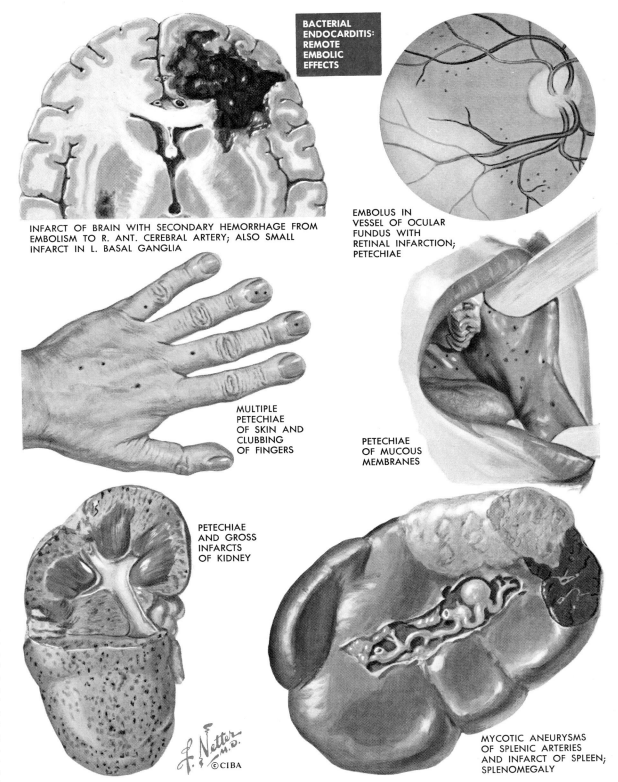

INFARCT OF BRAIN WITH SECONDARY HEMORRHAGE FROM EMBOLISM TO R. ANT. CEREBRAL ARTERY; ALSO SMALL INFARCT IN L. BASAL GANGLIA

BACTERIAL ENDOCARDITIS: REMOTE EMBOLIC EFFECTS

EMBOLUS IN VESSEL OF OCULAR FUNDUS WITH RETINAL INFARCTION; PETECHIAE

MULTIPLE PETECHIAE OF SKIN AND CLUBBING OF FINGERS

PETECHIAE OF MUCOUS MEMBRANES

PETECHIAE AND GROSS INFARCTS OF KIDNEY

MYCOTIC ANEURYSMS OF SPLENIC ARTERIES AND INFARCT OF SPLEEN; SPLENOMEGALY

BACTERIAL ENDOCARDITIS VII

Remote Embolic Effects

An important characteristic of *bacterial endocarditis* is its tendency for embolism; on this depend the many varied effects of the disease. Details of the embolic process depend on which side of the heart is involved. Concerning right-side bacterial endocarditis, it has been shown (see page 184) how the lungs become involved, usually dominating the *clinical picture*. In left-side bacterial endocarditis the potential *embolic effects* are more disseminated, since any organ or tissue supplied by the systemic arterial circulation may be affected. Important consequences are lesions of the *brain, myocardium,* or *kidney*. Involvement of *other body areas* may have significant sequelae representing important features leading to a clinical suspicion of the underlying disease.

Embolic lesions of the brain, as in the myocardium, are varied, depending fundamentally on the size of the obstructed artery or arteries and on the virulence of the organism. A dramatic effect results from obstruction of an element of the circle of Willis or one of its branches. Characteristically, the resulting lesion is an infarct. Initially a pale avascular lesion, the *cerebral infarct* may ultimately become *hemorrhagic*. It may be impossible to determine with certainty whether the hemorrhage is a primary lesion or one derived indirectly through infarction. Primary brain hemorrhages result from rupture of arteries infected from bacteria in an impacted embolus. Such hemorrhages may be single and massive or multiple and small.

More common than gross infarcts or hemorrhages of the brain are widespread microinfarcts. These may be silent or may cause variable signs or symptoms, often transient, including headache, focal paresis, aphasia, loss of memory, and confusion.

As highly virulent organisms may be responsible for multiple microabscesses in other organs, so may such lesions occur in the brain, causing the same types of cerebral disturbance as occur with disseminated microinfarcts.

Petechial lesions may form in any organ or tissue supplied by the systemic circulation. Whether these result from infection of small arterial vessels, with rupture, or from microinfarction, with secondary hemorrhage in the affected tissues, is debatable. In any event, the occurrence of *petechiae* is common and is of importance in alerting the

physician to the possibility of bacterial endocarditis. Areas in which petechiae may be readily observed are the *retina, skin,* and *mucous membranes;* when present, a *subungual* location also is common.

There may be *clubbing of the fingers* and toes, especially in those patients whose bacterial endocarditis has followed a protracted course.

The *kidney* may be affected either in its major arteries or in its parenchyma. The classical renal lesion is *focal embolic glomerulonephritis. Grossly, the picture* is that of the "flea-bitten" kidney, with widespread *petechiae* in the cortex. Histologically, the process is characterized by focal infarction of glomerular tufts and by glomerular and tubular hemorrhages. An uncommon parenchymal lesion is diffuse glomerulonephritis. Disseminated microabscesses generally occur if the infecting organism is highly virulent. Embolism to renal arteries is common, leading to infarction of portions of the renal substance, with attendant hematuria. That embolism may be episodic is evidenced by the fact that *renal infarcts* of various ages are

often encountered. Mycotic aneurysms of a renal artery or one of its smaller branches typify the involvement of major branches in this organ.

The *spleen* plays a prominent role in bacterial endocarditis. *Splenomegaly* is an important *clinical sign.* In addition, this organ may be the site of *mycotic aneurysm,* while *infarction,* as in the kidney, is common. The presence of splenic infarction may be marked by left upper-abdominal pain. Usually, the infarcts are relatively bland, but, in a rare instance, one may suppurate and rupture, leading to the formation of a subdiaphragmatic abscess.

Among other organs that may be involved is the gastrointestinal tract. The most common phenomenon is the occurrence of petechiae. Also, less often, intestinal infarction or the formation of mycotic aneurysms of mesenteric arteries may result from embolism of gross vegetative particles.

In the extremities mycotic aneurysms, with or without surrounding cellulitis or abscess formation, are observed in an occasional case.

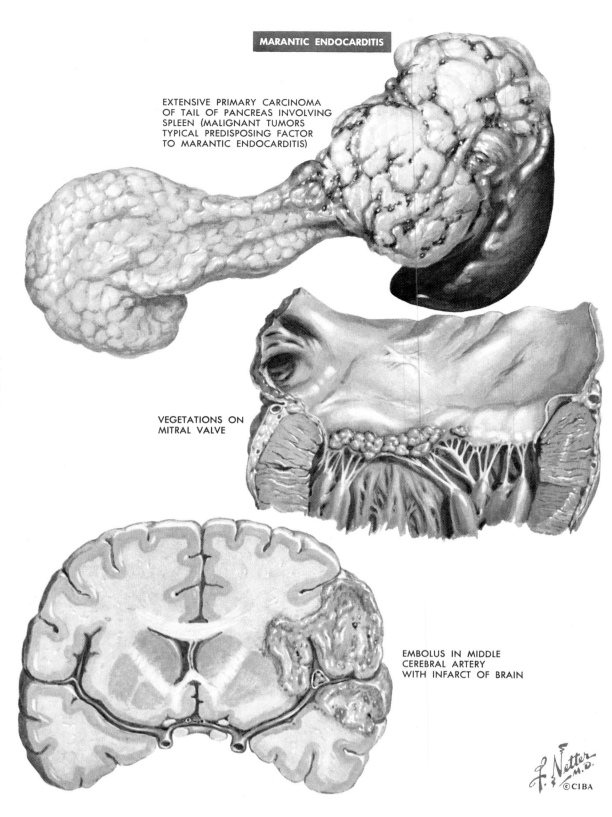

MARANTIC ENDOCARDITIS

EXTENSIVE PRIMARY CARCINOMA
OF TAIL OF PANCREAS INVOLVING
SPLEEN (MALIGNANT TUMORS
TYPICAL PREDISPOSING FACTOR
TO MARANTIC ENDOCARDITIS)

VEGETATIONS ON
MITRAL VALVE

EMBOLUS IN MIDDLE
CEREBRAL ARTERY
WITH INFARCT OF BRAIN

Marantic Endocarditis

Among the various forms of so-called verrucous or vegetative endocarditis is *marantic endocarditis*. Sharing a feature with rheumatic endocarditis and the endocarditis of lupus erythematosus, marantic endocarditis is a nonbacterial form. The name "marantic" has the same derivation as the word "marasmus" and was originally applied as a condition seen in wasting diseases. Although this feature still holds true, marantic endocarditis may also be seen in individuals who do not exhibit wasting, for any reason, but who harbor *malignant tumors*. One of the *clinically important features* of marantic endocarditis revolves about the latter point. In some patients the complication of marantic endocarditis, in the form of embolism to systemic arteries, may represent the primary evidence of a malignant tumor when specific manifestations have not yet become apparent. Particularly is this observed when the tumor is relatively occult, as when *primary in the body or tail of the pancreas.*

Marantic vegetations may occur on any valve but do so most commonly on the left-side valves, and it is not rare to find both the *mitral* and *aortic valves* involved simultaneously.

The *gross appearance* of marantic vegetations is that of friable, brown-to-gray material attached focally to the contact surface of the valve cusps. As the vegetations are focal in distribution and of varying size, they do not resemble the fine, regularly deposited vegetations of acute rheumatic endocarditis. On the other hand, marantic vegetations may be confused grossly with those of either bacterial endocarditis or lupus erythematosus. There are, however, other distinguishing features.

In contrast to bacterial endocarditis, marantic vegetations are not associated with destructive lesions of the valve cusps or chordae tendineae. Moreover, marantic vegetations are sterile, failing to contain bacteria as determined by histologic examination.

In lupus erythematosus the vegetations are deposited not only on the contact surface of the valve cusps, as in the case of marantic vegetations, but also on the mural endocardium of the chambers. Also, vegetations may be present in the angle between the posterior mitral cusp and the left ventricular wall. Histologically, lupus endocarditis, as characterized by nonbacterial inflammation of the valve cusp, is a process in which a heavy leukocytic infiltration is present. The valve cusp beneath a marantic vegetation, on the contrary, shows little, if any, leukocytic infiltration.

Some controversy exists as to whether marantic endocarditis is, in fact, a disease of the cusp or merely one in which vegetative material is deposited on a normal cusp. The exhaustive study by Allen provided evidence that the primary process is in the substance of the cusp. In essence, this shows focal swelling of collagen and secondary microrupture of the overlying portion of the cusp. Upon such areas, products derived from the blood, platelets, and fibrin are deposited, constituting marantic vegetations.

Marantic vegetations do not cause significant deformity of the valve. Their only serious potential is that of embolism. Since most of these vegetations occur on valves in the left side of the heart, embolism may involve any organ except the lung. Depending on the sites of lodgment of marantic vegetations, the results of *embolism* include *infarction* of the *brain, kidney, spleen,* etc.

While embolism from marantic vegetations is recognized as a cause of systemic arterial occlusion in patients with malignant tumors, other causes should be mentioned. Uncommonly, in such a patient, metastases may be deposited in the left side of the heart. Either the mural endocardium or the valves may be involved, the latter lesions requiring histologic examination for distinction from marantic vegetations. When metastases are present in the left side of the heart, systemic embolism may result from fragmentation of neoplastic nodules or of thrombotic material that may be deposited on intracavitary foci of secondary tumors.

Among patients with malignant tumors, systemic venous thrombosis is more common than marantic endocarditis. The primary effect of venous thrombosis is pulmonary embolism, a situation which yields pathologic and clinical features unlike those of marantic vegetations. In an unusual situation of pulmonary embolism, however, paradoxical embolism to the left side of the heart may occur (usually through a patent foramen ovale). Paradoxical embolism, in turn, may lead to systemic arterial occlusion and infarction of organs. In this regard, systemic venous thrombosis and marantic endocarditis may exhibit features in common.

CYSTIC MEDIAL NECROSIS OF THE AORTA

Cystic medial necrosis of the *aorta* is yet another cause of aortic insufficiency. In some patients the aortic valve may be competent, while other manifestations, such as mitral insufficiency or dissecting aneurysm of the aorta, may appear.

Cystic medial necrosis is seen in elastic arteries and is characterized histologically by deposits within the media of amorphous basophilic accumulations. Essentially, these are microcysts, and they account for the name of the condition. Initially tiny isolated lesions, these microcysts tend to coalesce and, in extreme cases, replace broad areas of the elements of the media. While the microcysts are small, the elastic laminae of the aorta may be intact. In the presence of coalesced microcysts, a number of elastic laminae in a given area are interrupted, and such fibers then recoil. The histologic effect is that multiple areas of the media are devoid of elastic fibers. The overall *gross effect* of this process is an increase in the diameter of the aorta in the involved segments.

In the aorta the greatest effect of cystic medial necrosis is evident from the root of the vessel distally to include the entire ascending aorta and varying extents of the arch.

Among patients with significant cystic medial necrosis of the aorta, variation occurs as to body habitus. In some, this is normal, and the dilatation of the aorta is called *idiopathic dilatation of the aorta*. Others exhibit distinct characteristics of body habitus and other effects which, collectively, are called arachnodactyly or *Marfan's syndrome*. Such subjects, characteristically, are unusually tall and have correspondingly long bones of the arms, legs, feet, and hands. The arm span exceeds the total body height. These patients also have a high-arched palate, dislocation of the optic lenses, and a tendency toward emphysema. Biochemical abnormality may be detected by high values of hydroxyproline in the urine.

Patients with extensive cystic medial necrosis of the aorta, including those with arachnodactyly, have a strong tendency to cardiovascular disease. Though certain congenital malformations of the heart have been identified, these are not common, and this association may be fortuitous. Lesions involving the aorta, the *aortic valve*, the atrioventricular valves, and the pulmonary trunk appear to have a direct association with cystic medial necrosis.

The aortic-valve effect is among the common manifestations and results in aortic-

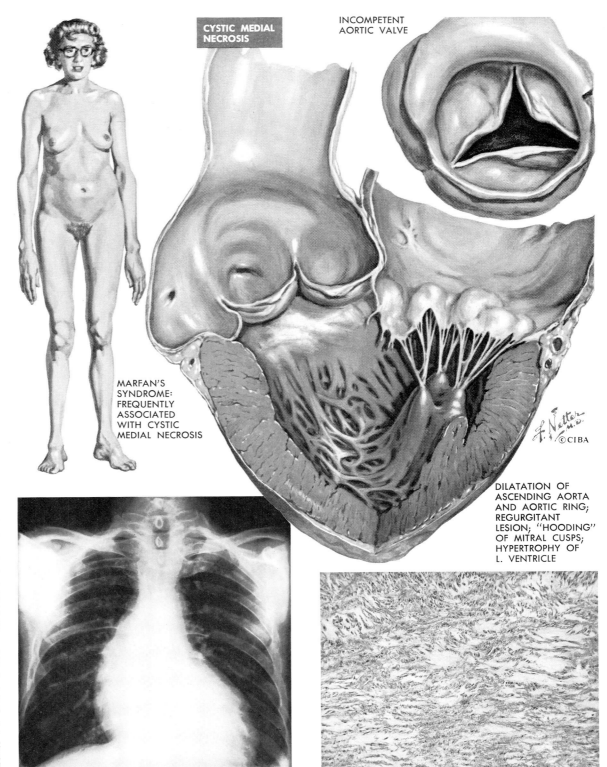

CYSTIC MEDIAL NECROSIS

INCOMPETENT AORTIC VALVE

MARFAN'S SYNDROME: FREQUENTLY ASSOCIATED WITH CYSTIC MEDIAL NECROSIS

DILATATION OF ASCENDING AORTA AND AORTIC RING; REGURGITANT LESION; "HOODING" OF MITRAL CUSPS; HYPERTROPHY OF L. VENTRICLE

DILATION OF ASCENDING AORTA

CYSTIC MEDIAL NECROSIS OF AORTA

valve insufficiency. This abnormality in function may be brought about in several ways. The simplest is *extensive dilatation of the aortic root,* including each sinus. This process may be the sole cause of *aortic-valve incompetence.* Some patients show extreme enlargement with *prolapse of the aortic cusps,* a change which compounds the effect of aortic dilatation in causing *aortic insufficiency.*

The aorta which harbors significant degrees of cystic medial necrosis has a decided tendency to rupture. This complication may take several forms. The first is that of simple hemorrhage, resulting in either exsanguination or cardiac tamponade from hemopericardium. The second effect is a classical dissecting aneurysm with several possible complications. The third effect pertains to the situation in which the tear does not extend through the entire wall of the aorta and results in a localized aneurysm. If such an aneurysm is present in the ascending aorta, it may distort the aortic valve sufficiently to either initiate aortic insufficiency or compound its degree, if already present.

The *ascending aorta dilated* by cystic medial necrosis, whether or not a localized aneurysm is present, may cause some alteration in the shape of the cardiovascular shadow in thoracic *roentgenograms,* but it is significant that, since the aortic origin is within the cardiac shadow, major degrees of aortic dilatation may go undetected.

In the atrioventricular valves of patients with cystic medial necrosis of the aorta, there may be changes indicating the weakness of connective tissues. Characteristically, the valvular substance between the insertion of the chordae tendineae has a tendency to balloon up toward the atrium, and there may also be elongation of the chordae. These changes may account for insufficiency of either atrioventricular valve, although the *mitral valve* is more commonly affected than is the tricuspid valve. In the pulmonary arterial system, cystic medial necrosis is manifested as dilatation of the involved vessels, and it is suggested that idiopathic dilatation of the pulmonary trunk may be a manifestation of cystic medial necrosis in this vessel.

SYPHILITIC HEART DISEASE

Syphilis of the aorta is a classic cause of aortic-valve insufficiency. In rheumatic heart disease or bacterial endocarditis, changes in the valve cusps represent the primary causes of valvular incompetence. In syphilis, in contrast, aortic insufficiency results primarily from changes in the aortic wall rather than in the cusps. Moreover, syphilitic heart disease has another manifestation; this relates to coronary-artery obstruction. In addition to the secondary changes within the heart, syphilis of the aorta exerts direct effects, such as atherosclerosis, aneurysm, and rupture, upon the aorta.

The primary affected site is the *media of the thoracic aorta* which shows many microscopic foci where tissue has been lost and replaced by delicate *stellate scars*. Lymphocytes and plasma cells may be present in the scars. In addition, alterations may occur within the adventitial and intimal layers. The adventitia shows fibrous thickening and lymphocytic and plasma-cell infiltration. Also, the vasa vasorum may show nonspecific fibrous proliferation of the intima, with corresponding degrees of narrowing of the lumen. This change has led investigators to wonder whether the medial change of syphilis is an effect of direct infection of the media or a result of faulty nutrition, secondary to the alterations in the vasa vasorum.

Certain *gross characteristics* are displayed by the aorta, which is the end organ in syphilitic disease. *Clinical identification* of these features provides circumstantial evidence for a syphilitic background in the patient with aortic insufficiency.

The combination of two features of this disease, namely, (1) widening of the affected portion of the aorta, and (2) localization to the thoracic portion of the vessel, results in a characteristic appearance of the syphilitic aorta. Beginning at the *root of the aorta* and extending for a variable distance along the *thoracic portion,* the vessel is *widened.* In the classic example, widening extends to the level of the diaphragm where, by virtue of lack of dilatation of the abdominal portion, the descending aorta assumes a funnel shape as it becomes continuous with the abdominal segment.

Grossly, another feature is usually apparent; there is a strong tendency for the involved portion to show *diffuse atherosclerosis.* This lesion may display focal calcification and may be ulcerated. *Calcification* in the secondary atherosclerotic lesion of the thoracic aorta, *involving the ascending aorta,* may be observed in clinical *roentgenograms.* This process, together with evidence of dilatation of

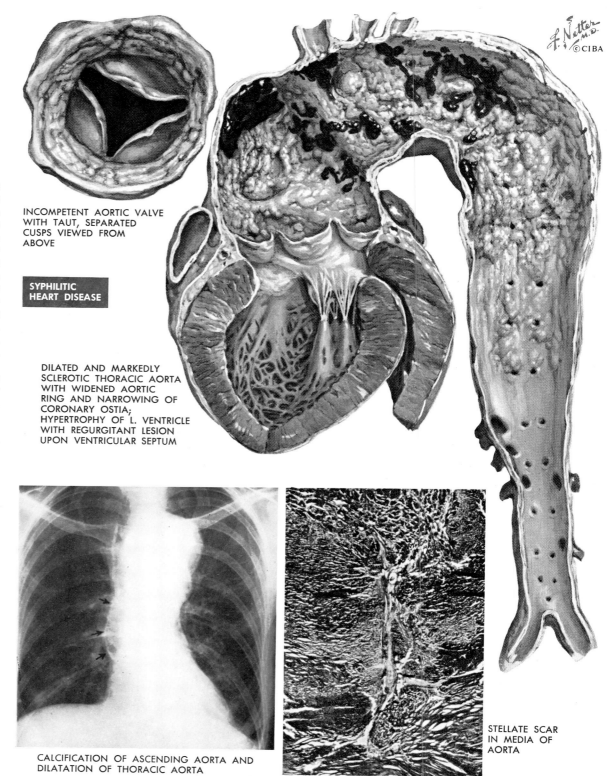

INCOMPETENT AORTIC VALVE WITH TAUT, SEPARATED CUSPS VIEWED FROM ABOVE

SYPHILITIC HEART DISEASE

DILATED AND MARKEDLY SCLEROTIC THORACIC AORTA WITH WIDENED AORTIC RING AND NARROWING OF CORONARY OSTIA; HYPERTROPHY OF L. VENTRICLE WITH REGURGITANT LESION UPON VENTRICULAR SEPTUM

CALCIFICATION OF ASCENDING AORTA AND DILATATION OF THORACIC AORTA

STELLATE SCAR IN MEDIA OF AORTA

the ascending aorta, presents very strong—though not absolutely specific—evidence of syphilitic aortitis.

The complicating process of atherosclerosis may result in one of the classic features of this disease — a *narrowing of the coronary arterial ostia.* The same process in the aorta may also compromise the lumina of the branches arising from the arch.

In addition to the effects of secondary atherosclerosis, the syphilitic aorta may show complications of the medial disease beyond simple uniform dilatation. These include formation of saccular aneurysms in any segment of the thoracic aorta, except in the wall of the aortic sinuses. The latter segment appears to be spared of any significant effect. Rupture of the thoracic aorta, either into a serous cavity or into an adjacent vessel, such as the superior vena cava or the pulmonary artery, may be a complication of either a saccular aneurysm or a simple dilatation.

In the specific area of the ascending aorta, the process of widening may be responsible for aortic insufficiency. As the aorta widens, each *aortic-valve cusp* may be pulled away from its neighbor at the commissure, resulting in the classical feature of so-called *commissural separation.* More important, as it relates to complicating aortic insufficiency, the widening of the aorta causes undue *tension* on the individual cusps. These become bowed, and the length of the cusps, relative to the size of the aortic orifice, shortens. A triangular deficiency in the aortic valve appears, and aortic insufficiency ensues. Once the valve becomes incompetent, secondary fibrotic changes may occur in the free extremities of the cusps. The *aortic-valve incompetence* causes *left ventricular hypertrophy.* Also, at the site of impact of the regurgitant stream, the outflow tract of the left ventricle may show regurgitant *"jet lesions."*

SURGERY FOR ACQUIRED HEART DISEASE (VALVAR REPLACEMENT)

Effective surgery for acquired heart disease probably began about 1897 when Rehn first successfully sutured a wound of the heart. Operations for acquired valvar disease were initiated with Cutler's pioneering effort (1920), which converted mitral stenosis into mitral insufficiency by using a valvulotome inserted transventricularly. Souttar had an early success (1925) with a transatrial *mitral commissurotomy* for mitral stenosis. Contributions by Bailey and Harken to closed mitral operations aided in the meteoric development and popularization of cardiac surgery during recent decades. The symptomatic improvement achieved by closed mitral commissurotomy was not duplicated by attempts at closed operations on the aortic valve; premonitions of such limitations were aroused by Tuffier's incomplete result in a case of aortic stenosis which he attempted to relieve by invaginating the aortic wall (to open the valvar chink).

A true breakthrough in curative efforts was achieved when the technics of cardiopulmonary bypass (see page 193) were introduced in 1954. Then, for the first time, direct surgical approach to all cardiac valves became feasible. These benefits and advantages are so demonstrably sound that, although closed mitral commissurotomy still is suitable in some cases, open-heart technics are preferable for the correction of valvar pathology in the majority of patients.

With the introduction of direct-vision procedures, it was hoped that restoration of valvar function could be accomplished with the natural valvar structures. Hence, for both calcific aortic and mitral stenoses, debridement and mobilization of fixed valve cusps were attempted. Unfortunately, success was usually incomplete and transient. Somewhat better results have been obtained following plication of a dilated insufficient valvar annulus of the type present in some cases of mitral or tricuspid insufficiency. Also, plication of valve cusps, in the management of certain kinds of ruptured chordae tendineae, has functioned acceptably. The overall immediate and long-term accomplishments of operations for acquired valve disease were substantially amplified by the introduction and (shortly thereafter) ready availability of prosthetic devices which permitted total valvar replacement. To be realistic, however, it must be emphasized that none of the presently available prosthetic valves achieves the physiological and mechanical features

DIGITAL MITRAL COMMISSUROTOMY BY MEANS OF FINGER INTRODUCED VIA LEFT ATRIAL APPENDAGE WITH EXTERNAL COUNTERPRESSURE

TUBBS DILATOR INTRODUCED THROUGH LEFT VENTRICULOTOMY, GUARDED BY OPPOSED MATTRESS SUTURES, AND GUIDED INTO MITRAL ORIFICE BY FINGER

DILATOR TIP CLOSED

DILATOR TIP OPENED

of a normal human valve. Certainly, improvements in valve design leading to superior flow characteristics, the development of prosthetic materials which arouse less adverse reactions in soft tissues or blood, and the elimination of mechanical breakdown are critical goals to be strived for in the near future.

The caged ball valve of Starr and Edwards was used in the accompanying illustrations describing the insertion of prostheses in the aortic, mitral, and tricuspid areas.

Mitral Valve

Acquired Mitral Stenosis. Acquired calcific mitral stenosis is the most common valvar lesion resulting from rheumatic fever. Pure mitral stenosis accounts for about two thirds of functional mitral-valve disease. It is four times more common in women than in men.

A history of rheumatic fever is obtainable in over 50 percent of the cases.

Valve-orifice narrowing, to a clinically significant degree (usually less than 1 sq cm), occurs at least 2 years after the acute attack of rheumatic fever. Once that state has been reached, the left atrial pressure is elevated and the pulmonary-artery pressure rises passively to maintain a pressure difference in the pulmonary arteries and veins. The work of the *right ventricle* is thereby increased so that, in certain far-advanced cases, right heart failure and secondary tricuspid insufficiency develop. More frequently encountered complications created by mitral stenosis are atrial fibrillation, hemoptysis, bacterial endocarditis, and embolization from thrombi developing in the left atrium.

SURGICAL INDICATIONS. Patients in class II and class III (New York Heart Association classification)

(Continued on page 192)

SURGERY FOR ACQUIRED
HEART DISEASE
(VALVAR REPLACEMENT)

(Continued from page 191)

are appropriate candidates for surgical relief of mitral stenosis. Those in class IV, although operable, clearly have a higher operative risk. Closed mitral commissurotomy is still indicated for patients with pure mitral stenosis who reveal minimal amounts of or no calcium at fluoroscopy. Coexisting heart failure should surely be treated, whenever possible, until compensation has been achieved. However, a few patients with severe right heart failure, acute pulmonary edema, or severe hemoptysis may fail to respond to all forms of medical management. These may require an emergency mitral valvotomy. Rheumatic activity and bacterial endocarditis are relative temporal contraindications for surgery. On the other hand, neither pregnancy nor advancing years represents an absolute contraindication.

Closed Mitral Commissurotomy. The patient is positioned for a left *anterolateral thoracotomy.* The chest is entered through the bed of the resected fifth rib. The *pericardium* is incised posterior and parallel to the left phrenic nerve, extending the *incision* from the left pulmonary artery to the apex of the *left ventricle.* A purse-string suture of heavy nonabsorbable material is placed at the base of the *left atrial appendage,* and both ends are left long; these are threaded through a Rumel tourniquet. Prior to the application of a noncrushing clamp at the base of the appendage in the area immediately distal to the purse-string suture, the appendage is palpated. If no clot can be felt, the clamp is applied, and the appendage is incised and thoroughly flushed. Next, the interior is carefully inspected for retained clots. Trabeculae within this chamber are divided for ready access of the right index *finger.* Now the clamp is loosened, and hemostatic control is secured by the Rumel tourniquet snugged about the operator's digit.

The *mitral valve* is first gingerly palpated to determine the line and the extent of *fusion* of the valve cusps and to estimate the *orifice's size,* the degree of insufficiency, and the extent of calcification. While *finger fracturing* of the anterior commissure is accomplished, *counterpressure* is applied *externally* over the *atrioventricular groove* to *avoid injury* to the left circumflex coronary artery. An adequate opening of the anterolateral commissure should always be sought. Fracture of the posterior medial commissure is often less satisfactory. If a wide opening cannot be obtained by simple finger fracture, then recourse regularly

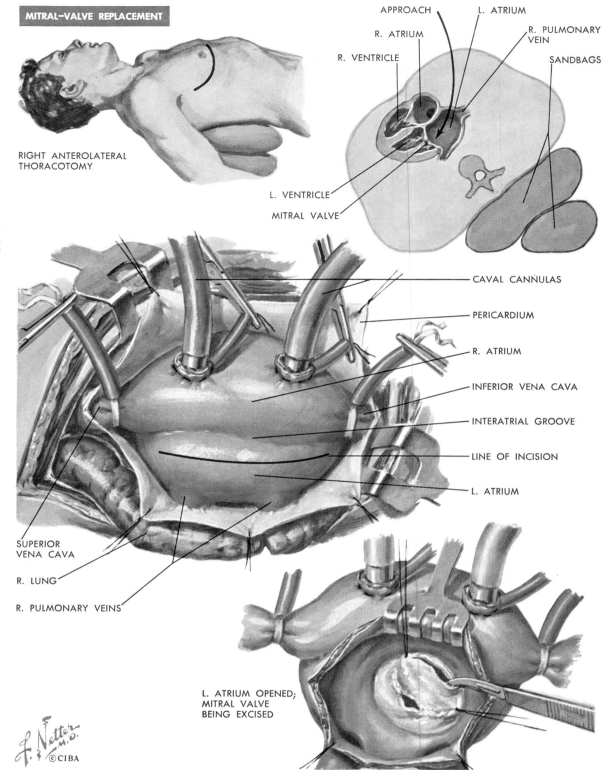

MITRAL-VALVE REPLACEMENT

RIGHT ANTEROLATERAL
THORACOTOMY

APPROACH
L. ATRIUM
R. ATRIUM
R. PULMONARY VEIN
R. VENTRICLE
SANDBAGS
L. VENTRICLE
MITRAL VALVE

CAVAL CANNULAS
PERICARDIUM
R. ATRIUM
INFERIOR VENA CAVA
INTERATRIAL GROOVE
LINE OF INCISION
L. ATRIUM

SUPERIOR VENA CAVA
R. LUNG
R. PULMONARY VEINS

L. ATRIUM OPENED;
MITRAL VALVE
BEING EXCISED

should be made to the use of an expandable metal *dilator* (Logan-Tubbs). *Rarely* will a *valvotomy knife* be necessary. For the introduction of the dilator, an avascular area on the anterior surface near the apex of the left ventricle is selected, and two *mattress sutures* of nonabsorbable material are placed there. A small stab wound between these stitches permits the dilator to be inserted bloodlessly into the *left ventricle.* It is then advanced into the *mitral-valve orifice* with *guidance from the fingertip* protruding through the mitral valve. Care must be exercised, while maneuvering this instrument, to prevent tearing or rupture of either chordae tendineae or papillary muscles. Then, with the dilator precisely in place, the blades of the instrument are *opened slowly* to a preset extent, in an effort to tear the valve edges apart along the line of their fusion. It is *critical* that one should not attempt to open each valve to the maximum expand-

able width of the dilator. Allowance should always be made for the individual patient's valvar anatomy. When heavy calcium deposits are present, the valve may have a tendency to split unevenly; in that case, excessive dilatation can split through the annulus and lead to severe mitral insufficiency. The presence of calcium also creates additional hazards from *embolization,* since flecks readily break loose, during valvar manipulations, and are difficult to control.

After the valve has been opened as much as possible, the instrument is removed, and the *ventriculotomy* is carefully closed by tying the previously placed mattress sutures. Then the atrial base is closed with the purse-string suture. Redundant tissue should be excised and the cut edge oversewn with a nonabsorbable suture. Interrupted stitches to close the pericardial sac should be so spaced as to allow for drainage of any

(Continued on page 193)

SURGERY FOR ACQUIRED HEART DISEASE (VALVAR REPLACEMENT)

(Continued from page 192)

fluid subsequently accumulating therein.

When a hitherto unrecognized thrombus or atrial tumor is encountered during mitral commissurotomy, the procedure should be converted to an open-heart operation, using a pump oxygenator. If this is unavailable, the operation should be terminated, if consistent with the state of the patient's cardiac condition; in general, delay until a more propitious opportunity, when proper equipment is available, will usually be in the patient's best interest. If the necessary equipment is at hand, however, cannulation of the left common femoral artery is first carried out. Then, a large-bore catheter is positioned in either the *right atrium* or the right ventricular-outflow tract. Partial extracorporeal bypass can now be safely established. After some decompression of the right heart with this technic, it is possible to cross-clamp the main pulmonary artery, thus creating total cardiopulmonary bypass. The heart can now be electrically fibrillated prior to opening the *left atrium*. The exposure thereby provided is quite satisfactory for almost all necessary surgical manipulations within the left atrial chamber and on the mitral valve.

Mitral-Valve Operations Under Direct Vision. Whenever an operation is indicated, direct-vision mitral-valve surgery is the method of choice for managing significant mitral insufficiency, either alone or in combination with mitral stenosis. Bypass is also the best technic if the mitral valve is heavily calcified or when the mitral-valve disease coexists with aortic or tricuspid valvar problems. Also, bypass should be utilized primarily in most instances of a history of peripheral embolization. Certain patients in class II, and virtually all in classes III and IV (New York Heart Association), are candidates. Those in class II and class III are, of course, safer risks. Preferably, all patients will come to operation restored to cardiac compensation by an adequate period of treatment with digitalis and diuretics (if required), and without potassium depletion. However, in isolated instances of class-IV patients, mitral-valve replacement may represent the sole remaining resource, and therefore the operation must be undertaken, despite residual cardiac failure.

Prosthetic-valve replacement is nearly always necessary in severely calcific mitral stenosis. This is true also for most cases of acquired mitral insufficiency. An exceptional instance of ruptured papillary muscles or chordae tendineae can be real-

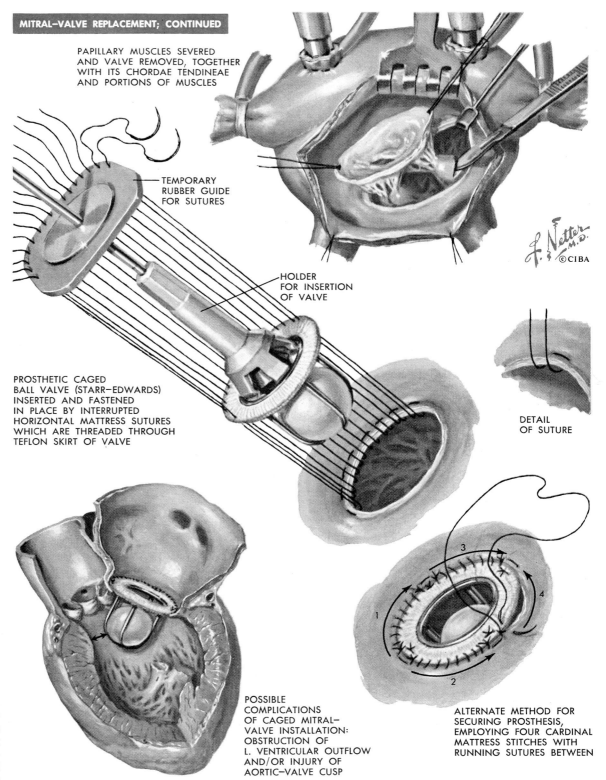

MITRAL-VALVE REPLACEMENT; CONTINUED

PAPILLARY MUSCLES SEVERED AND VALVE REMOVED, TOGETHER WITH ITS CHORDAE TENDINEAE AND PORTIONS OF MUSCLES

TEMPORARY RUBBER GUIDE FOR SUTURES

HOLDER FOR INSERTION OF VALVE

PROSTHETIC CAGED BALL VALVE (STARR-EDWARDS) INSERTED AND FASTENED IN PLACE BY INTERRUPTED HORIZONTAL MATTRESS SUTURES WHICH ARE THREADED THROUGH TEFLON SKIRT OF VALVE

DETAIL OF SUTURE

POSSIBLE COMPLICATIONS OF CAGED MITRAL-VALVE INSTALLATION: OBSTRUCTION OF L. VENTRICULAR OUTFLOW AND/OR INJURY OF AORTIC-VALVE CUSP

ALTERNATE METHOD FOR SECURING PROSTHESIS, EMPLOYING FOUR CARDINAL MATTRESS STITCHES WITH RUNNING SUTURES BETWEEN

istically corrected by suture approximation of the cusps. Pericardial-patch closure of a perforated valve cusp, secondary to bacterial endocarditis, does not require prosthetic replacement. Plication of the mitral annulus, in order to reduce the size of the valve's orifice and to improve the approximation of the cusps, has been practically discontinued by the authors, because of unsatisfactory long-term results.

TECHNIC OF TOTAL CARDIOPULMONARY BYPASS. The authors' patients are currently operated upon with the use of a roller-pump console and the DeWall-Bentley disposable bubble oxygenator with a built-in heat exchanger. This oxygenator is primed with 5 percent dextrose in water (16 cc/kg body weight) and 100 to 400 cc of 25 percent mannitol. Heparinized (70 mg/500 cc) fresh blood is added in a quantity sufficient to obtain a total priming volume of about 20 cc/kg body weight. Prior to the institution

of bypass, the patient receives heparin intravenously in the amount of 2 mg/kg body weight. During bypass flow, the rates may vary between 40 and 100 ml/minute/kg body weight. The rate is determined by the quantity of venous return and the temperature of the patient at the time. Moderate hypothermia (30 to 33° C) is utilized in many cases.

Mitral-Valve Replacement. For isolated elective mitral-valve replacement, a *right anterolateral thoracotomy,* with subperiosteal excision of the fifth rib, provides excellent exposure (see page 192). *Cannulas* are placed within the *superior* and *inferior venae cavae,* via incisions in the right atrium, and are maintained there with purse-string sutures. The femoral artery is used for arterial return flow via another catheter. Ventricular fibrillation is induced electrically, before the *left atrium* is opened, to prevent air embo-

(Continued on page 194)

Surgery for Acquired Heart Disease
(Valvar Replacement)

(Continued from page 193)

lization. A longitudinal (vertical) left atriotomy allows adequate visualization of this chamber and the mitral-valve area, particularly after the *right atrium* has been retracted. If there is a need for prosthetic replacement, *excision of the mitral valve* (including the *chordae tendineae* and *papillary muscles*) is customarily carried out. Appropriately positioned *interrupted horizontal mattress sutures* of 2-o Tefdek®, placed securely in the valve's rim, are then *threaded through the Teflon® skirt of the ball-valve prosthesis.* To maintain order and allow proper spacing, these stitches are passed through a *temporary rubber flange* which is attached to the valve holder.

Some cases of mitral insufficiency and/or mitral stenosis can be dealt with also by a somewhat less tedious *alternative method.* In these instances, *four cardinal mattress sutures* are placed at 12, 3, 6, and 9 o'clock. After tying down one, *running stitches* are continued *between* the Teflon® skirt and the valvar remnant, moving in a clockwise fashion, and interrupted only at each of the fixed points until the prosthesis has been firmly sutured in place. During closure of the left atriotomy, the heart is rewarmed. It is d-c (direct-current) defibrillated, unless this occurs spontaneously.

Aortic Valve

Rheumatic endocarditis may be responsible for as much as two thirds of the cases of aortic stenosis and/or insufficiency. When aortic stenosis becomes *clinically* serious, the valve cusps are often fused, thickened, distorted, and heavy with calcific deposits. These changes increase the total work of the heart with each beat. Consequently, progressive left ventricular hypertrophy and failure, including arrhythmias, ensue. The chamber's size is usually small, and left ventricular compliance is poor. On the other hand, in cases of aortic reflux, left ventricular diastolic filling is enhanced by the volume of the leak. The chamber volume is often greater than normal, and the heart has a tendency to dilate. Failure is slower in onset, but nonetheless inevitable, if the regurgitant factor is large.

Prosthetic *aortic-valve replacement* has steadily assumed an ever-more-significant role in the management of patients with aortic stenosis or insufficiency, in whom clinical manifestations of cardiac decompensation, syncope, and/or angina regu-

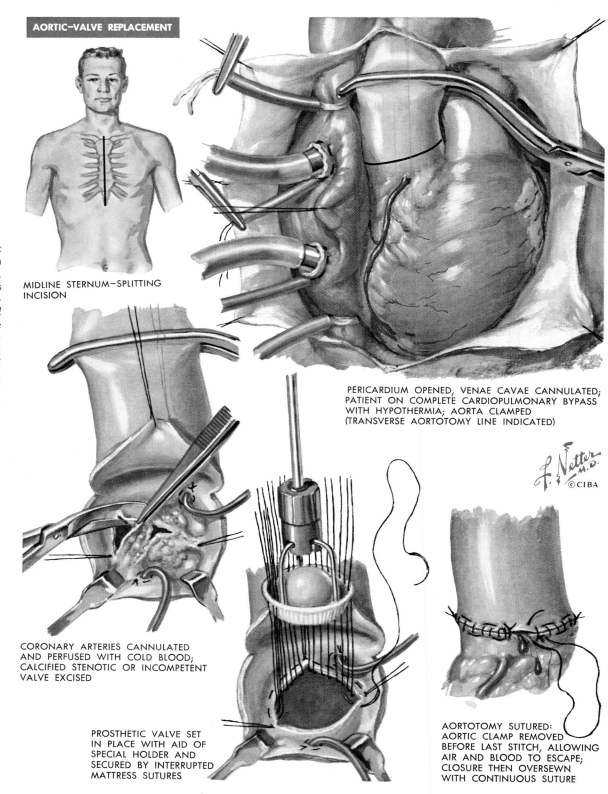

AORTIC-VALVE REPLACEMENT

MIDLINE STERNUM–SPLITTING INCISION

PERICARDIUM OPENED, VENAE CAVAE CANNULATED; PATIENT ON COMPLETE CARDIOPULMONARY BYPASS WITH HYPOTHERMIA; AORTA CLAMPED (TRANSVERSE AORTOTOMY LINE INDICATED)

CORONARY ARTERIES CANNULATED AND PERFUSED WITH COLD BLOOD; CALCIFIED STENOTIC OR INCOMPETENT VALVE EXCISED

PROSTHETIC VALVE SET IN PLACE WITH AID OF SPECIAL HOLDER AND SECURED BY INTERRUPTED MATTRESS SUTURES

AORTOTOMY SUTURED: AORTIC CLAMP REMOVED BEFORE LAST STITCH, ALLOWING AIR AND BLOOD TO ESCAPE; CLOSURE THEN OVERSEWN WITH CONTINUOUS SUTURE

larly affect their life activities. This role prevails because patients with hemodynamic evidence of a serious compromise of cardiac function (particularly those with significantly elevated left ventricular end-diastolic pressure) are unlikely to be benefited long by procedures other than aortic-valve replacement. The authors definitely prefer to have all potential candidates for aortic-valve replacement undergo *cardiac catheterization* (including right- and left-heart catheterization) and *cardioangiography,* in order to evaluate more precisely their hemodynamic functional state. Furthermore, these data are essential if postoperative accomplishments are to be studied meaningfully.

Aortic-Valve Replacement. The aorta is exposed through a *midline sternotomy.* The *pericardium is opened* longitudinally, and standard *cannulations* are made of the *venae cavae* (through the right atrium) and of the

femoral artery. After beginning *total cardiopulmonary bypass, hypothermic perfusion* is employed to carry the esophageal temperature to 33° C. Now the aorta is cross-clamped proximal to the innominate branch. Then, through a low *transverse aortotomy,* the valve is widely exposed. The *left and right coronary arteries are cannulated* and *perfused* (during valve placement), employing an independent pump for each ostium. The authors strive not to exceed 80 mm Hg pressure within the coronary-perfusion system. With the situation now in hand, the *diseased valve cusps* are carefully *excised,* and calcium is removed from the valve's annulus or even from the left ventricular-outflow tract, preserving a small valvar remnant on the wall. Into this remnant, *interrupted and inverted mattress sutures* of 2-o Tefdek® are placed. Each is threaded symmetrically through the *Teflon® skirt* of

(Continued on page 195)

SURGERY FOR ACQUIRED HEART DISEASE (VALVAR REPLACEMENT)

(Continued from page 194)

the *ball-valve prosthesis* prior to tying the latter into position. *Particular care* must be exercised to *assure* that the *upper rim* of the valvar prosthesis *lies well below the coronary ostia*. This is done best by proper placement of each stitch. No attempt is made to induce fibrillation during this procedure. Cardiac action may cease at times, whenever the cardiac temperature is low. However, once the heart has been rewarmed, spontaneous defibrillation may occur.

A secure *aortotomy closure* can be obtained by a *running horizontal mattress suture* which is subsequently *reinforced* with an over-and-over *continuous suture*. *Before* completing the central portion of this suture line, the *aortic clamp is temporarily released to force out residual air.* After that, final closure is secured. Decannulations are deferred until a hemodynamically acceptable total body perfusion has been achieved by the beating heart. Temporary partial bypass may serve to smooth this transition.

Aortic-Valvular Insufficiency. This can result not only from intrinsic aortic-valve disease but also from lesions of the ascending aorta. Syphilitic aortic disease, dissecting aneurysms, weakness of the aortic media in Marfan's syndrome, or idiopathic dilatation of the aorta, senile dilatation of the aorta, and traumatic and nonspecific inflammatory disease of the aorta may lead to aortic insufficiency either by dilatation of the aortic annulus and/or because of structural fatigue of the tissue supporting the aortic cusps.

Aortic-valve insufficiency, associated with idiopathic *cystic medial necrosis* producing *aneurysmal dilatation* of the ascending aorta, occurs with sufficient frequency to warrant discussion. In this disease entity, the *aortic valve* is usually tricuspid and contains no calcifications. Aortic insufficiency is secondary to dilatation of the annulus, thereby increasing the area of the valvar orifice. The cusps are thinned out, and, at times, the free edges of the valve cusps are rolled. The ascending aortic wall proper is dilated and thinned, and microscopically small accumulations of basophilic material are found within the aortic media. This material is composed mainly of acid mucopolysaccharides. In addition, there are disruption and fragmentation of the elastic fibers. At times, early dissecting aneurysms with limited extravasations within the media are observed.

These patients may exhibit classical *signs and symptoms* of aortic insufficiency

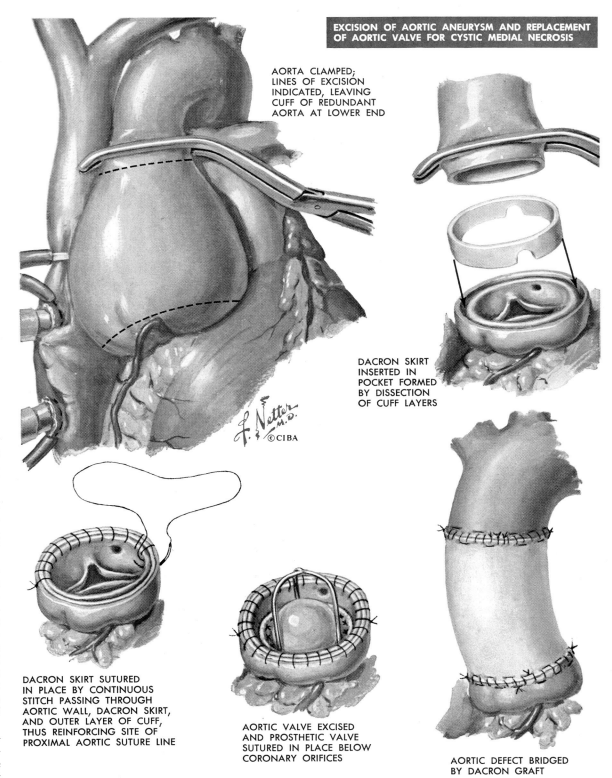

EXCISION OF AORTIC ANEURYSM AND REPLACEMENT OF AORTIC VALVE FOR CYSTIC MEDIAL NECROSIS

AORTA CLAMPED; LINES OF EXCISION INDICATED, LEAVING CUFF OF REDUNDANT AORTA AT LOWER END

DACRON SKIRT INSERTED IN POCKET FORMED BY DISSECTION OF CUFF LAYERS

DACRON SKIRT SUTURED IN PLACE BY CONTINUOUS STITCH PASSING THROUGH AORTIC WALL, DACRON SKIRT, AND OUTER LAYER OF CUFF, THUS REINFORCING SITE OF PROXIMAL AORTIC SUTURE LINE

AORTIC VALVE EXCISED AND PROSTHETIC VALVE SUTURED IN PLACE BELOW CORONARY ORIFICES

AORTIC DEFECT BRIDGED BY DACRON GRAFT

and cardiac disability of class III or class IV. Simple anteroposterior and lateral *roentgenograms* show marked dilatation of the ascending aorta. Left-heart *catheterization* and *angiocardiography* usually confirm the evidence for the *diagnosis* of massive aortic insufficiency in the presence of a widely dilated ascending aorta.

SURGICAL TECHNIC. After clinical, roentgenologic, and hemodynamic evaluation, surgical correction of this lesion includes (1) prosthetic valvar replacement, (2) resection of the ascending aortic aneurysm, and (3) replacement with a prosthetic graft. Through a *midline sternotomy*, the patient is placed on *full cardiopulmonary bypass*, and moderate systemic *hypothermia* is induced. The *aorta is cross-clamped* distal to its point of dilatation — usually immediately proximal to the takeoff of the innominate artery. The proximal line of resection is about 1 cm above the

level of the coronary arterial takeoffs. The *aneurysm is completely excised,* and then the *coronary arteries are cannulated and perfused continuously* throughout the procedure. Not uncommonly, hematomatous dissection within the *proximal aortic cuff* is encountered. To obliterate this resultant cleft and, particularly, to ensure a firmer base for suturing the graft to the diseased and thinned aortic wall, a *Dacron® skirt* is fashioned and *positioned within* the split residual aortic root. This Dacron® cylinder is *sutured in place by continuous stitches, passing successively through the inner aortic wall, the Dacron® skirt, and the outer aortic layer.* This procedure *reinforces* the proximal aorta. Once this has been accomplished, the *aortic valve is resected* and *replaced by a prosthesis.* It is our belief that prosthetic valvar replacement is necessary, since these secondarily deformed aortic valves are not suitable

(Continued on page 196)

SURGERY FOR ACQUIRED HEART DISEASE (VALVAR REPLACEMENT)

(Continued from page 195)

for enduring reconstructive procedures.

Subsequently, the *aortic defect is bridged by a crimped Dacron® graft*. The posterior row of the proximal suture line is completed first, followed by the entire distal suture line. The proximal anastomosis is then continued and almost completed before the coronary cannulas are removed. The heart usually requires defibrillation with d-c countershock, and the patient is kept on partial bypass until adequate cardiac function resumes.

Multiple Valve Replacement. Significant involvement of more than one cardiac valve is more complicated to evaluate quantitatively and to handle surgically. Aortic- and mitral-valve disease is the most common combination, and it requires particularly careful study. The wisest decision, in the more complex cases, is based on the physical findings, the left- and right-heart-*catheterization studies,* and the analysis of the *angiocardiographic* findings. These data can usually be relied upon to provide appropriate qualitative and quantitative estimations of the overall state of valvar disease.

Decisions involving the tricuspid valve are less precisely based on derivable data. In general, however, when serious organic involvement of the tricuspid valve is present, prosthetic replacement will be required. Functional tricuspid insufficiency (most commonly occurring in mitral stenosis), on the other hand, will usually improve after correction of the primary problem. To intervene or not, therefore, may create a dilemma which can be only partially resolved by experience. Patients who, despite prolonged bed rest and intense medical treatment for multivalve-induced cardiac failure, show little or no improvement in the signs and symptoms of tricuspid-valve disease, usually turn out to require prosthetic tricuspid-valve replacement. The same need holds true for patients who, in the presence of normal or nearly normal pulmonary-artery pressure (at catheterization), have significant tricuspid insufficiency. Finally, an additional opportunity is provided, at operation, for evaluating the tricuspid-valve function, both by inserting a finger into the right atrium, while the heart is beating, and by direct inspection within the atrium after instituting a cardiopulmonary bypass. In general, if the tricuspid valve has seemed to be organically involved, it has proved wiser to replace it.

SURGICAL TECHNIC. A *midline sternotomy incision* is used for *multiple valve*

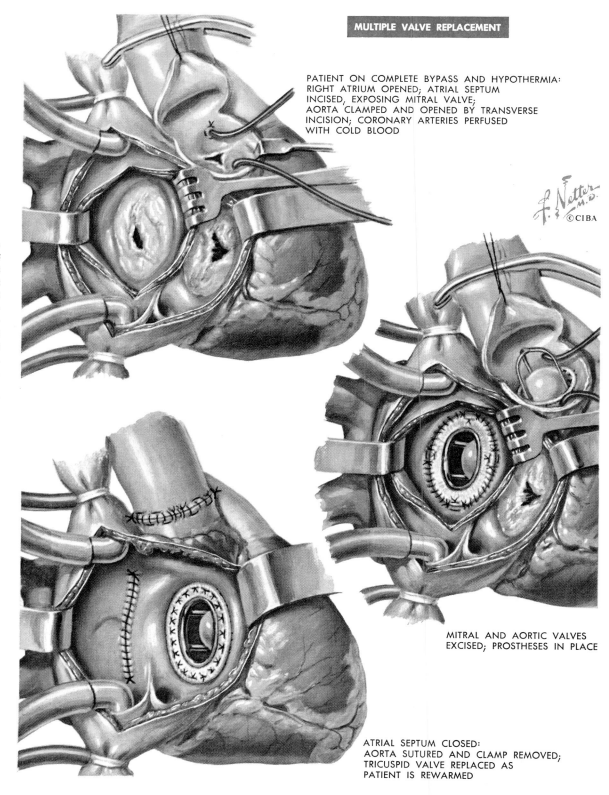

PATIENT ON COMPLETE BYPASS AND HYPOTHERMIA: RIGHT ATRIUM OPENED; ATRIAL SEPTUM INCISED, EXPOSING MITRAL VALVE; AORTA CLAMPED AND OPENED BY TRANSVERSE INCISION; CORONARY ARTERIES PERFUSED WITH COLD BLOOD

MITRAL AND AORTIC VALVES EXCISED; PROSTHESES IN PLACE

ATRIAL SEPTUM CLOSED: AORTA SUTURED AND CLAMP REMOVED; TRICUSPID VALVE REPLACED AS PATIENT IS REWARMED

replacements which include the aortic valve. In these cases, as previously outlined, the patient is placed on *complete cardiopulmonary bypass, and moderate systemic hypothermia* is achieved. First, the *ascending aorta is cross-clamped*. Then, via a low-lying *transverse aortotomy*, both *coronary arteries are cannulated,* and *perfusion* of the myocardium is maintained. The *aortic valve* is now *resected*. If only aortic- and mitral-valve replacement (double valve insertion) is planned, the heart is arrested electrically at this point, and the left atrium is opened anteriorly to the right pulmonary veins. However, if tricuspid-valve replacement is contemplated also (triple valve insertion), the *right atrium* is opened widely and the left atrium is then entered via an *incision* into the *atrial septum*. This approach provides excellent *exposure of the mitral valve,* unless the patient has extensive adhesions between the peri- and epicardium. After excision

of the mitral valve, the prosthesis is inserted according to either of the two previously described technics. Subsequently, the aortic-valve prosthesis is positioned. With both in place, the *atrial septum* and the *aortotomy are properly closed,* care being taken to evacuate all air from the left side of the heart.

After the aortic clamp has been removed, hypothermia is discontinued. *During the period required for rewarming, the tricuspid valve is resected and replaced.* This prosthesis is seated and anchored into the annulus by either of the two previously described technics for the mitral area. Since the tricuspid valve is easily accessible, and because calcification is only rarely encountered in this valve, its replacement is readily accomplished. The right atriotomy is then closed, and the heart is defibrillated with d-c countershock. Partial bypass is maintained until adequate cardiac action has been resumed.

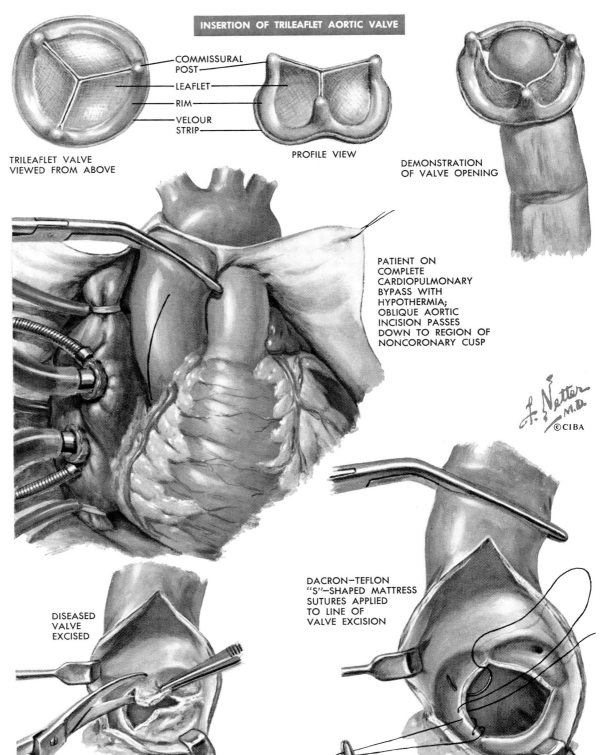

INSERTION OF TRILEAFLET AORTIC VALVE

COMMISSURAL POST
LEAFLET
RIM
VELOUR STRIP

TRILEAFLET VALVE
VIEWED FROM ABOVE

PROFILE VIEW

DEMONSTRATION
OF VALVE OPENING

PATIENT ON
COMPLETE
CARDIOPULMONARY
BYPASS WITH
HYPOTHERMIA;
OBLIQUE AORTIC
INCISION PASSES
DOWN TO REGION OF
NONCORONARY CUSP

DISEASED
VALVE
EXCISED

DACRON–TEFLON
"S"–SHAPED MATTRESS
SUTURES APPLIED
TO LINE OF
VALVE EXCISION

INSERTION OF TRILEAFLET AORTIC VALVE

The basic concept of an artificial valvular mechanism which would function permanently and reliably in the human body was first introduced in 1952. Since that time, many variations of the original ball valve have been evolved. The free-floating discoid was a later type, which was first used clinically in 1962. Though all these variations have produced progressively better results, they also have had an inherent problem, common to all: The central space was occupied by the occlusive portion of the valve mechanism. All such valves (1) produced an alteration in the direction of blood flow, (2) introduced a resistance imposed by the ball or disc in this area of high pressure and high-velocity flow, and (3) depended upon a marginal or restricted space being available at the periphery of the occlusive part of the mechanism in the plane of maximum travel.

Presented here is a new kind of aortic-valve prosthesis which provides a full central flow pattern similar to that of the normal natural valvular mechanism. This has been termed the unitized *trileaflet valve*. It embodies the principle of self-suspended flexible leaflets (cusps) and

has certain features which have not been used previously in prosthetic valves. The leaflets are made of polypropylene covered with silicone rubber. Polypropylene is extremely resistant to flexion fatigue, and no other currently available plastic material approaches it in flex life. The three leaflets are suspended from the base and lie within the aortic sinuses, without attachment to the aortic wall at their commissures. This makes closure independent of changes in the aortic diameter and configuration, since these may vary widely from individual to individual and under different physiologic conditions. The leaflets are very pliable, and the valve has an extremely low opening pressure.

The proximal orifice of the valve is equal to the size of the ventricular-outflow tract. Its *profile* is sufficiently low to permit the entire valve to lie within

the sinuses of Valsalva. The base of the valve follows a scalloped contour, which duplicates the configuration of the normal aortic-cusp attachments to the aortic root. Because of this design of the base, which provides a new cushion, the need for a cuff is essentially eliminated. A small area of *Dacron*® velour is provided for the ingrowth of tissue along the line of suture attachment. All other areas of the base are composed of Hepacone®, which inhibits the clotting of blood. Thus, for the first time, there is available a valve which requires only the secure attachment of its base to the *aortic annulus*; once this has been achieved, the *opening and closure of the valve* are ensured. *Nine to twelve sutures* are required for *fixation* of the valve. Its very light weight and its low

(Continued on page 198)

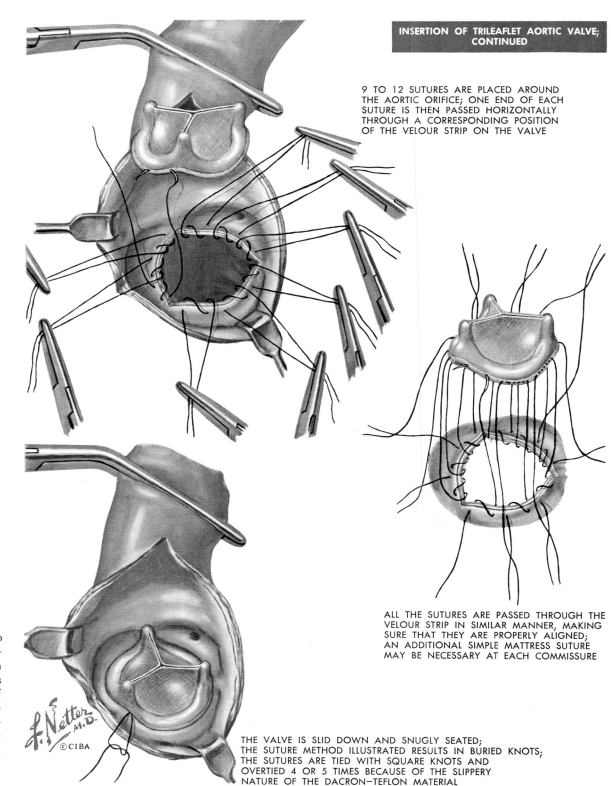

9 TO 12 SUTURES ARE PLACED AROUND THE AORTIC ORIFICE; ONE END OF EACH SUTURE IS THEN PASSED HORIZONTALLY THROUGH A CORRESPONDING POSITION OF THE VELOUR STRIP ON THE VALVE

ALL THE SUTURES ARE PASSED THROUGH THE VELOUR STRIP IN SIMILAR MANNER, MAKING SURE THAT THEY ARE PROPERLY ALIGNED; AN ADDITIONAL SIMPLE MATTRESS SUTURE MAY BE NECESSARY AT EACH COMMISSURE

THE VALVE IS SLID DOWN AND SNUGLY SEATED; THE SUTURE METHOD ILLUSTRATED RESULTS IN BURIED KNOTS; THE SUTURES ARE TIED WITH SQUARE KNOTS AND OVERTIED 4 OR 5 TIMES BECAUSE OF THE SLIPPERY NATURE OF THE DACRON—TEFLON MATERIAL

INSERTION OF TRILEAFLET AORTIC VALVE

(Continued from page 197)

resistance to blood flow permit fixation to be achieved with minimal technical difficulty. The problem of an accumulation of clots, and subsequent embolism, has been a serious one in previous types of valvular prostheses. In an effort to minimize those factors tending toward thrombosis, several *methods for burying the fixation sutures* between the valve and the aortic wall have been developed. The method which the author and his associates currently use is as follows:

Three sutures are required in *each* of the three portions of the aortic annulus. The first of these begins below the superior portion of the *commissure* at the level where the leaflets begin to diverge from each other. It passes through the aortic annulus, first from below upward, and the same suture is then passed in a similar fashion, from below upward, 5 to 6 mm toward the lower portion of the aortic-leaflet insertion. The second suture occupies the inferior central area, and the third corresponds, on the ascending limb, to the first. When all nine sutures have been placed, they are inspected to be sure that they closely approximate each other and that no gaps remain between them.

If the leaflet insertions diverge widely, an *additional simple mattress suture* may be required through one or more of the commissural zones, just above the highest portion of the preceding sutures. After all sutures have been *properly placed, one limb of each* of the double-ended sutures is *passed through the velour cuff* in the *corresponding position* of the *valve base.* This suture does not penetrate any of the surfaces of the valve that contact the bloodstream but occupies only a position which will be buried between the ingrowth section of the valve and the aortic wall. Each suture is placed through the *corresponding position* of the prosthesis, in rotation. Then, using the thumb and three fingers of the right hand, the valve is *gently set in snug* contact with the aortic annulus. The sutures are *tightened to ensure an accurate*

approximation of the annulus and the valve base. The three leaflets are pushed aside gently to view the interior of the ventricle, and it is important that no loops of loose suture be visible. The sutures are then tied in rotation, each with a *square knot* followed by a surgeon's knot. The suture is then cut close to the knot, which is pushed gently downward into the groove between the valve and the aortic annulus, where it disappears.

Valve sizes must be selected in relationship to the aortic root. Because of the very wide valve orifice and the low resistance to flow, care should be taken not to attempt the insertion of a valve too large in size, since even the smaller trileaflet valves provide an orifice which approaches normal. Accurate sizing is obviously desirable and makes insertion simple and rapid.

FREE-FLOATING DISCOID VALVE FOR MITRAL AND TRICUSPID REPLACEMENT

The replacement of mitral and tricuspid *valves* has posed a particularly difficult problem because of several factors: (1) low pressure in the atrium and the resultant tendency toward thrombus formation with systemic embolization; (2) overgrowth of tissue on the metallic or plastic parts, which results in valvular dysfunction, necrosis of tissue, and embolization; (3) inertia of the valvular mechanism; (4) occlusion of a portion of the mechanism, with regurgitation prior to complete closure and dislodgment of the sewing ring produced by the large mass striking the areas of suture; (5) incomplete ventricular filling due to the large size of the occluding portion of the mechanism, thus requiring the use of a valve of small orifice size; and (6) obstruction to the left ventricular-outflow tract because of the angulation of any mechanism with a long travel.

The free-floating *discoid valve* was evolved, between 1960 and 1962, primarily for the atrioventricular position. Since then, it has been modified to its present form and its use, during the last year, has uniformly produced essentially normal hemodynamics and excellent clinical results, without embolization.

The valve mechanism is made entirely of polypropylene and consists of a free disc in an open cage. It does not impinge upon the ventricular septum or obstruct the left ventricular-outflow tract. The extremely light weight of the polypropylene disc allows for a very rapid response with minimal *pressure* variations. Closure of the valve is complete upon the initiation of systole. The sewing ring has a core of Hepacone® (see page 198), and the entire valve seat and base are covered with Dacron® velour. Thus, the entire base of the valve mechanism is covered by a controlled thickness of material that will support tissue ingrowth.

The total coverage of the base prevents pannus formation and thrombus formation from interfering with valve function. The replacement of mitral and tricuspid valves has not resulted in embolism, in any case, during a period of 8 months. Valve malfunction and peribasilar insufficiency have not occurred.

A buried-suture technic is used to implant this mechanism, thus eliminating the hazardous protrusion of sutures into the atrial lumen. Two methods have been devised. The first and simplest of these requires twelve to fourteen *sutures* of the type illustrated, leaving the *cuff of the valve* on the auricular surface. The sutures are tied so that they lie beneath the cuff. When the individual ends are cut, no suture is visible from the auricular surface. The obstructing *balloon* is

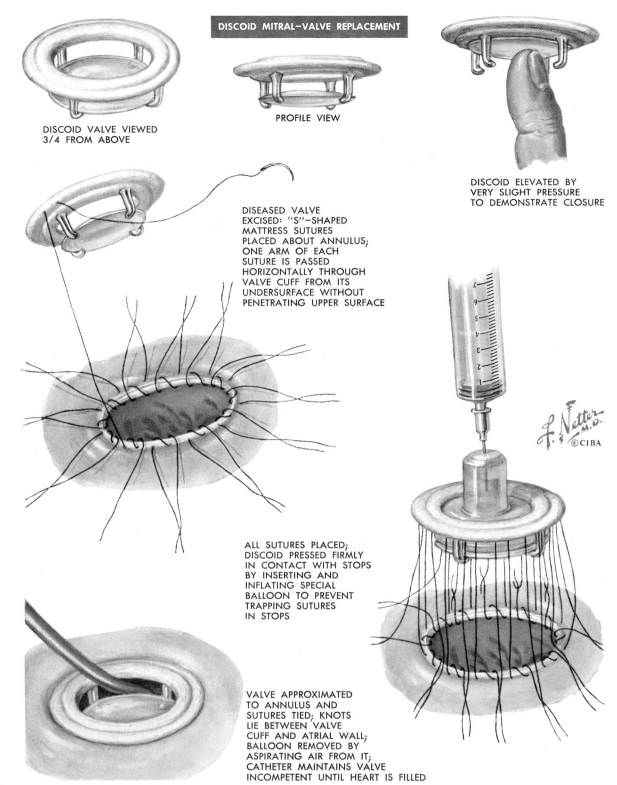

DISCOID MITRAL–VALVE REPLACEMENT

DISCOID VALVE VIEWED 3/4 FROM ABOVE

PROFILE VIEW

DISCOID ELEVATED BY VERY SLIGHT PRESSURE TO DEMONSTRATE CLOSURE

DISEASED VALVE EXCISED: "S"–SHAPED MATTRESS SUTURES PLACED ABOUT ANNULUS; ONE ARM OF EACH SUTURE IS PASSED HORIZONTALLY THROUGH VALVE CUFF FROM ITS UNDERSURFACE WITHOUT PENETRATING UPPER SURFACE

ALL SUTURES PLACED; DISCOID PRESSED FIRMLY IN CONTACT WITH STOPS BY INSERTING AND INFLATING SPECIAL BALLOON TO PREVENT TRAPPING SUTURES IN STOPS

VALVE APPROXIMATED TO ANNULUS AND SUTURES TIED; KNOTS LIE BETWEEN VALVE CUFF AND ATRIAL WALL; BALLOON REMOVED BY ASPIRATING AIR FROM IT; CATHETER MAINTAINS VALVE INCOMPETENT UNTIL HEART IS FILLED

then removed by *aspirating the air* from within it. Also available are closed-cage modifications of the valve, which do not require the use of a balloon to prevent catching of the sutures.

An *alternative method* employs the ventricular placement of the prosthesis. When this technic is used, a *mattress suture* is passed through the annulus, from above and downward. One or both arms of this suture are then placed through the upper surface of the valve cuff. With this procedure the valve is brought upward from the ventricular side into contact with the valve remnant and the annulus. As each knot is tied, it lies between the valve remnant and the cuff of the valve.

Although both methods have been very satisfactory, the latter is particularly useful when an extremely dilated annulus is present. In such instances, the presence of the valve cuff below the mitral annulus tends to force the cuff into contact with the tissues of the annulus to prevent peribasilar insufficiency.

The advantages of the free-floating discoid may be summarized as follows: (1) complete coverage of the base by ingrowth of tissue; (2) prevention of excessive clot buildup, prior to the ingrowth of tissue, by the use of a Hepacone® core; (3) an extremely low *profile*; (4) a short travel of the occlusive member of the valve; (5) extremely light weight of the entire prosthesis; (6) great durability of the discoid, eliminating the problems of wear; (7) absence of outflow-tract obstruction; (8) extreme sensitivity and rapidity of response to pressure changes; (9) minimal tendency to disruption of the suture line, because of the small mass of the moving part and the short distance over which it travels; and (10) the minimal volume occupied by the valve mechanism within the ventricular cavity.

AORTIC-VALVE HOMOGRAFT

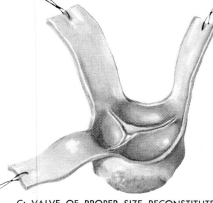

A: HOMOGRAFTS ARE STERILIZED BY RADIATION; STORED FROZEN IN SEALED DOUBLE–PLASTIC ENVELOPES AND CATALOGUED BY SIZE; QUARTZ BEAD WHICH TURNS BROWN ON RADIATION IS STERILIZATION CONTROL

C: VALVE OF PROPER SIZE RECONSTITUTED IN WARM SALINE, TRIMMED AND SHAPED

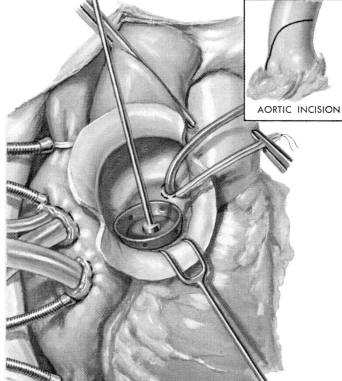

AORTIC INCISION

B: UNDER COMPLETE CARDIOPULMONARY BYPASS AND HYPOTHERMIA, AORTA OPENED BY CURVED INCISION PASSING DOWN TO NONCORONARY CUSP; DISEASED VALVE EXCISED AND ORIFICE SIZE DETERMINED BY CALIBRATED MEASURING CUP

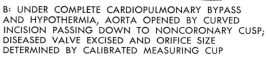

D: FIRST LINE OF SUTURES BEGUN BY A STITCH WELL DOWN IN AORTIC ROOT BENEATH LEFT CORONARY ORIFICE AND PASSING OUTWARD THROUGH LOWER EDGE OF HOMOGRAFT

Aortic-valve replacement, utilizing *homograft* or heterograft valves, has been evaluated clinically during the past 4 years. The advantages of these nonviable tissue grafts are the absence of late peripheral arterial emboli and the elimination of postoperative long-term anticoagulation therapy.

The technic of harvesting, preparing, sterilizing, and storing these homograft valves has an influence on their structure and function. Laboratory tests have shown that the freeze-irradiation method of *sterilization* and *storage* of the aortic-valve homografts causes the least change in their gross morphology and tensile strength. The principal feature of this technic is irradiation of the graft in the *frozen* state to bactericidal energy levels of 2 to 2.2 megarads in a short-time exposure of 5 to 6 seconds.

The first insert (*A*) shows the *packaged* sterilized valve available from the valve bank. Note the discolored *quartz bead* used as an indicator of the degree of irradiation exposure. The aortic valves are obtained unsterile from autopsy speci-

mens less than 12 hours following death. All valves are *trimmed* of fat and cardiac muscle to reduce the bulk of muscle that may become interposed between the graft and the host. Careful dissection of the aortic root is required to preserve the aortic sinuses. The internal diameter of the valve is measured and recorded prior to packaging and freezing the graft to −50° C.

A graft is selected *equal* in size to the internal diameter of the patient's *aortic root* following *excision of the diseased aortic valve* (*B*). The 2- to 3-mm wall thickness of the graft ensures a replacement that is somewhat greater in diameter than the aortic-root implant site. The valve selected is *reconstituted in warm saline* solution under sterile conditions (*C*). Excess muscle and mitral-valve tissue are trimmed from the homograft valve, leaving a 2-mm rim below the

sinuses of Valsalva. Portions of the homograft aortic wall are excised into the sinuses to accommodate the host's coronary-artery orifices. The struts of the aortic wall remaining on the homograft valve will be utilized later, during implantation, to provide added support for the cusp commissures.

Access to the aortic root is gained through an *oblique aortotomy extended into the noncoronary cusp.* Continuous perfusion of both coronary arteries is employed during the period of total *cardiopulmonary bypass.* While the valve is being prepared, the *lower suture line* for valve implantation is placed (*D*). A series of *interrupted sutures* is placed in the left ventricular-outflow tract (*E*). Interrupted sutures are placed sufficiently deep in the aortic root to include

(*Continued on page 201*)

E: LOWER LINE OF INTERRUPTED SUTURES IS CONTINUED COMPLETELY AROUND GRAFT; WHEN HOMOGRAFT IS SETTLED INTO POSITION, KNOTS WILL BE BURIED BETWEEN GRAFT AND AORTIC WALL

AORTIC-VALVE HOMOGRAFT

(*Continued from page 200*)

F: UPPER MARGIN AND STRUTS OF HOMOGRAFT ARE SUTURED TO AORTIC WALL BY DOUBLE–NEEDLE CONTINUOUS SUTURES; MATTRESS STITCHES THROUGH AORTIC WALL (REINFORCED WITH TEFLON PLEDGETS INSIDE AND OUT) SECURE STRUTS, AND EXCESS OF STRUTS IS EXCISED (BROKEN LINES); ENDS OF CONTINUOUS SUTURES PASS THROUGH AORTIC WALL AND ARE TIED TO MATTRESS–SUTURE ENDS

G: PHANTOM VIEW OF HOMOGRAFT IN PLACE

the mitral cusp and junction of the ventricular septum and aortic root. The graft is positioned so that the mitral-valve remnant lies below the left coronary orifice to reduce bulk and to ensure placement well *below the lumen of the coronary artery.* Sutures are then passed *through the base of the homograft* from inside out, thus placing the suture line *between the host aorta and the graft.* A second suture line is required to attach the graft *aortic-wall struts* to the host aorta. Interrupted or continuous sutures are used, with completion of the insertion at the *upper end* of each valve commissure by reinforced *mattress sutures* placed through the host aortic wall (*F*).

The technic of valve implantation is more precise and time-consuming than that required for the artificial prosthesis. Correct positioning and suturing of these grafts are essential for proper valve function postoperatively. The operative mortality and clinical results following aortic-homograft-valve replacement compare favorably with those reported after insertion of the ball-valve prosthesis. The

absence of late peripheral arterial emboli and of the need for postoperative anticoagulation therapy are the strongest arguments for the use of the homografts. A significant incidence of postoperative aortic diastolic murmurs has been reported, being 20 percent in our series. In only 1 case, however, did this prove to be of hemodynamic significance. The double-suture-line technic has prevented suture-line disruption and has reduced suture-line leakage.

A satisfactory size relationship must exist between the host aortic root and the homograft, and the homograft valve selected must be large enough in diameter to remain sufficient when the aortic ring is distended by systemic pressure. In our series, allowance was made for this change (*B*) by calibrating all homografts by their internal diameter. The graft size selected is

based on the internal diameter of the aortic root of the recipient; hence, the wall thickness of the graft, namely 2 to 3 mm, represents the excess area available when the aortic root dilates. Tailoring of the aortic root was not required in our series, but it has been helpful in reducing the diameter of large aortic bases to accommodate the homograft.

The clinical follow-up (for 2 years postoperatively in this series) suggests that the aortic-homograft valve functions satisfactorily, with no evidence of breakdown or restenosis. No late peripheral arterial emboli were noted, and no postoperative anticoagulation was required. Although changes in the design of artificial prostheses will ultimately solve the thromboembolism problem, at present the aortic homograft remains far superior in this regard.

AMYLOIDOSIS

Among cardiomyopathies caused by disturbances of protein metabolism, amyloidosis should be mentioned first. Amyloid infiltration of the heart may occur under four circumstances: (1) as part of primary systemic amyloidosis, (2) as part of amyloidosis complicating multiple myeloma, (3) as part of secondary systemic amyloidosis, and (4) as a localized phenomenon in the aged. Rare *primary systemic amyloidosis,* often called atypical amyloidosis or paramyloidosis, can involve the heart only. Amyloid may be deposited also in the lungs, skin, thyroid gland, intestinal tract, and arterial walls throughout the body. In primary systemic amyloidosis, the liver, spleen, and kidneys are usually (but not universally) found without amyloid deposits. In 99 cases of primary amyloidosis, 92 showed severe involvement of the heart. Generally, the etiology of primary systemic amyloidosis of the heart is not known.

The clinician should entertain the *diagnosis* of amyloidosis of the heart when chronic, intractable heart failure develops in a patient 50 or more years of age, particularly if the heart failure remains unexplained, even in the presence of the usual symptoms and signs. The heart is enlarged in almost every case, but hypertension is absent. The excursions of the heart are slow, and noncharacteristic murmurs may be heard. Murmurs typical of valvular disease can be detected only if the valves are affected by depositions of amyloid. The *electrocardiogram* indicates a *low voltage.* Disturbances of the atrioventricular conduction may be caused by amyloidosis of the bundle of His and of the bundle branches. The Congo-red absorption test is rarely positive in amyloidosis of the heart; however, biopsies of the skin, the rectal mucosa, or the myocardium may help to establish the diagnosis.

Grossly, one may detect plaquelike or, more commonly, tiny nodular deposits of gray-yellow amyloid in the endocardium, particularly in the left atrium. The myocardium shows a markedly increased consistency, and its cut surface exhibits a peculiar pale-tan and waxy appearance. The epicardial fat tissue may also be affected by gray and gelatinous pearllike deposits of amyloid. The heart weighs 500 gm or more.

Microscopically, the homogeneous deposits of amyloid are translucent and refract the light strongly. Sections of myocardium stained with Congo red exhibit a network of homogeneous bands surrounding the bundles of myocardial fibers and separating these. The myocardial fibers are compressed and often are atrophied to very flat fibers with pinlike nuclei. The interstices are diffusely widened but not infiltrated by inflammatory cells. The pseudomyocardial hypertrophy explains the insufficiency of both chambers of the heart. Rarely, as a result of obstruction of a coronary artery by nodular deposits of amyloid, infarction or disseminated necroses of the myocardium

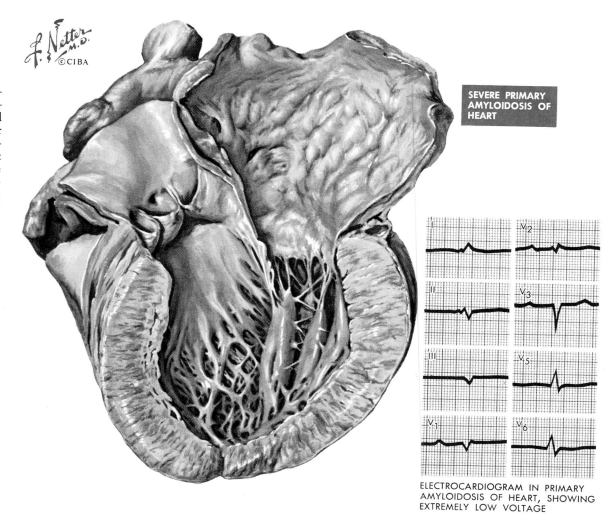

SEVERE PRIMARY AMYLOIDOSIS OF HEART

ELECTROCARDIOGRAM IN PRIMARY AMYLOIDOSIS OF HEART, SHOWING EXTREMELY LOW VOLTAGE

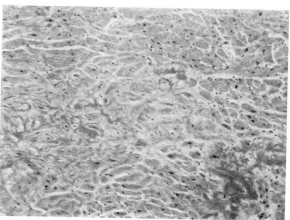

FOCAL DEPOSITION OF AMYLOID AROUND MUSCLE CELLS OF HEART WITH DEAD MYOCARDIAL FIBERS

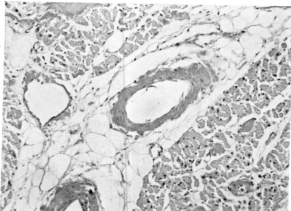

PERIVASCULAR AMYLOID DEPOSITS IN MYOCARDIUM (X 40)

may occur. When amyloidosis complicates multiple myeloma (20 percent of the cases), the distribution of amyloidosis is like that in primary systemic amyloidosis. Cardiac involvement is common.

Secondary typical or systemic amyloidosis occurs in diseases with chronic suppuration and severe tissue necrosis. Chronic tuberculosis of the lungs or other organs is the most frequent cause. Other primary underlying diseases may be bronchiectasis, empyema of the pleural cavities, chronic osteomyelitis, and tumors, as well as leprosy, syphilis, or echinococcosis. The incidence of secondary amyloidosis has decreased, during the last 20 years, as a result of antibiotic therapy. In systemic amyloidosis, the liver, spleen, and kidneys are affected predominantly, but in one third of these cases the heart also may be involved. The depositions of amyloid are much less extensive than in primary systemic amyloidosis of the heart, and they

demonstrate a different pattern. Amyloid is usually deposited in the media of the arteries and veins and in the capillaries between the endothelial cells and the basement membrane. The lumina of the capillaries remain patent, as in the arteries and veins, and thus the complications are not so serious as in primary systemic amyloidosis of the heart.

Deposits of amyloid may be found in the blood vessels and in relation to myocardial fibers of the *myocardium* of old people without special underlying diseases. The incidence of presenile or senile amyloidosis (which also may involve the brain) is low in patients under 60 years of age. However, the heart can be affected in 25 percent of all patients over 80 years of age.

Electron *microscopic* studies of homogeneous amyloid demonstrate delicate fibers which are thought to be responsible for the effect of birefringence.

SEPTIC MYOCARDITIS

HEART SERIALLY SECTIONED
REVEALING MULTIPLE INTRAMURAL
AND SUBEPICARDIAL ABSCESSES
WITH PERICARDITIS

SEPTIC MYOCARDITIS

ABSCESS IN HEART MUSCLE: CENTRAL MASS OF BACTERIA
SURROUNDED BY LEUKOCYTES, DESTROYED MUSCLE,
AND DILATED BLOOD VESSELS

MASTOIDITIS

TONSILLITIS,
SEPTIC SORE THROAT

CARBUNCLE

CARDIAC CATHETERIZATION

STAPHYLOCOCCAL
ENTERITIS

OMPHALITIS

APPENDICITIS

PERITONITIS

SEPTIC ENDOMETRITIS

SURGICAL—WOUND INFECTION

HAND INFECTION

OSTEOMYELITIS

MAJOR FOCI OF ORIGIN

Septic or suppurative *myocarditis,* which can lead to myocardial abscesses and other complications, has been encountered only rarely since the introduction of antibiotics, but it has not disappeared completely because of the development of antibiotic-resistant strains of bacteria. The number of known *major foci* permitting the spread of infection via septicemia (which precedes suppurative myocarditis) increases with the use of new diagnostic and therapeutic methods, *e.g.,* the use of indwelling intravascular catheters.

The most common causative organisms in suppurative myocarditis are strains of Staphylococcus, Pseudomonas, Proteus, Aerobacter-Klebsiella, and (rarely) Pneumococcus. Newborns, nursing mothers, and patients who have had preceding viral infections are predisposed, as are diabetics and those with severe burns. In some cases the process is associated with, or is a complication of, bacterial endocarditis; in other instances the valves are not affected.

The first *nonspecific signs* indicative of myocarditis in septicemia are fever, leukocytosis, and shock. Circumscribed areas of necrotic and damaged myocardium may lead to changes in the *electrocardio-*gram. Murmurs can be heard only in those patients in whom endocarditis or pericarditis has developed.

Frequently, in acute *pyemia,* no macroscopic changes are visible in the heart, because the rapid course of the septicemia does not allow the tissues to react against the spreading bacteria. *Clinically, signs of sepsis are predominant.*

Important for the specific *diagnosis* and *treatment* of septic myocarditis is the culturing of the strains taken from the myocardium. Dense colonies of bacteria, within the *dilated capillaries and veins,* comprise the earliest detectable finding in *microscopic* sections of the myocardium. In later stages these are *small abscesses,* showing abundant bacteria *in their centers,* with a circular wall of numerous polymorphonuclear *leukocytes.* The surrounding myocardial fibers can reveal a homogeneous cytoplasm whose nuclei are not stained or are pyknotic. The entire focus is surrounded by a hemorrhagic marginal zone.

Myocardial abscesses are often visible as small yellow points or stripes, measuring 1 or 2 mm, beneath the thin endocardium of the right ventricle. The irregular and bizarre formation of the abscesses is usually determined by the anatomical course of the muscle bundles. Subendocardially located abscesses can perforate into the ventricular lumen and cause bacterial endocarditis. Subepicardial abscesses can involve the pericardium also. Frequently, the focus can be detected easily, *e.g.,* after perforation into the pericardial sac, but, in a few instances, it may be impossible to find. Therefore, primary hematogenous spread cannot always be ruled out with certainty.

DIPHTHERITIC AND VIRAL MYOCARDITIS

Microorganisms (viruses, rickettsiae, bacteria, and protozoa) or the toxins thereof can produce myocarditis. The morphological findings alone do not permit the elucidation of the etiology of myocarditis. Focal or diffuse myocarditis may develop without clinical manifestations. Therefore, in order to ascertain the *diagnosis* of myocarditis, all clinical information and the results of the bacteriological and the virological examinations should be evaluated together.

Diphtheritic Myocarditis

In *diphtheria* of the upper respiratory tract, or as a consequence of wound diphtheria, myocarditis is caused by the powerful exotoxins of the Corynebacterium diphtheriae (Klebs-Löffler bacillus). This kind of toxic myocarditis occurred quite frequently before the introduction of active immunization, and, even today, small epidemics may occur.

In acute diphtheria the heart is flabby, and the myocardial fibers have a boiled appearance. Both ventricles are *dilated,* and small *mural thrombi* may be found between the trabeculae. The left ventricle, and particularly the apex, may be filled with large ball thrombi. Decreasing blood pressure, arrhythmias, and complete heart block may precede acute heart failure.

Microscopically, in cases of acute *diphtheritic myocarditis,* the myocardial fibers are swollen and demonstrate a dustlike fatty degeneration. The interstices are edematous. In subacute cases the myocardial fibers show granular or hyaline necrosis. Polymorphonuclear leukocytes and mobilized histiocytes are distributed throughout the interstitial connective tissues.

The *secondary inflammatory reactions* are frequently arranged focally but also may be diffuse. In the surrounding areas of *toxic necrosis,* circulatory disturbances also may develop, leading to further necrosis. The *protracted shock* finally affects the coronary blood supply in such a manner that additional disseminated *hypoxic necrosis* occurs. After several weeks the necrotic myocardial fibers will be organized and replaced by fine reticular fibrosis. The extent of such diffuse fibrosis can often be determined only by quantitative methods, measuring the components of connective tissue and myocardial fibers. Fibrosis, and even scarring, can be so severe that death occurs as a consequence of chronic heart failure.

Viral Myocarditis

The incidence of *viral myocarditis* has increased during recent years. Known

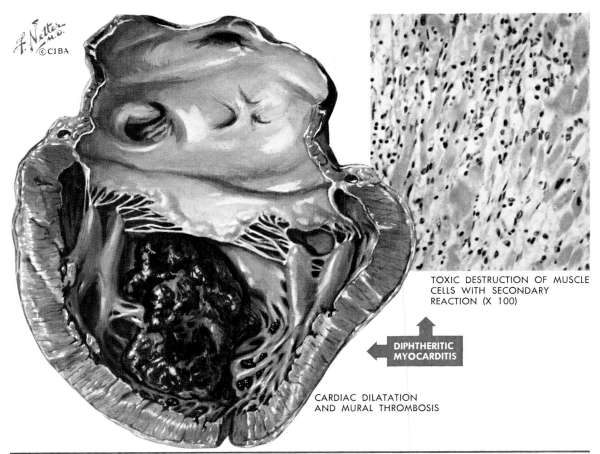

TOXIC DESTRUCTION OF MUSCLE CELLS WITH SECONDARY REACTION (X 100)

DIPHTHERITIC MYOCARDITIS

CARDIAC DILATATION AND MURAL THROMBOSIS

VIRAL MYOCARDITIS

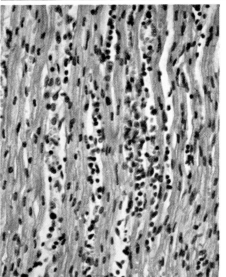

COXSACKIE GROUP–B VIRUS INFECTION: DIFFUSE AND PATCHY INTERSTITIAL EDEMA; CELLULAR INFILTRATION WITH ONLY MODERATE MUSCLE–FIBER DESTRUCTION (X 100)

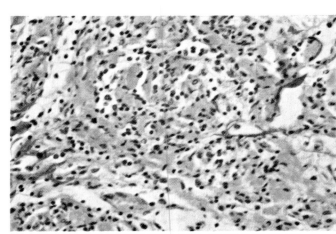

DIFFUSE CELLULAR INFILTRATION OF BUNDLE OF HIS AND RIGHT AND LEFT BUNDLE BRANCHES (X 100)

causative organisms of viral myocarditis in man are the *Coxsackie group-B viruses,* some cardiotropic strains of poliovirus, and, occasionally, certain types of influenzal virus. The etiology can be ascertained only if virological examinations are successful. Epidemiological studies are able merely to give hints about the possible organism. Newborns, infants, children, and adolescents are predisposed.

Myocarditis can be preceded by meningitis, encephalitis, pleurisy, and pericarditis, as well as by gastrointestinal symptoms. After 3 to 10 days, fever, tachycardia, cyanosis, and, finally, signs of cardiac failure may develop. The *electrocardiogram* reveals severe changes suggestive of *damaged myocardium* or *alterations of the conduction system.* X-ray examination demonstrates enlargement of the heart.

Except for dilatation of both ventricles of the heart, the myocardium appears *macroscopically* unchanged.

Several tissue blocks should be sampled for *microscopic* examination, because viral myocarditis affects the myocardium *focally,* and large areas of the heart may be spared. The histologic findings also depend largely on the stage of the inflammatory process. The first stage of the invasion by the virus into the myocardial fiber can be studied only under experimental conditions. During the following stage (disturbances of cell metabolism), a few or several *myocardial fibers* may undergo *necrosis.* In the third stage, *interstitial* accumulations of lymphocytes, plasma cells, and histiocytes are the predominant features. These third-stage changes are observed most frequently in sections of the myocardium and the conduction system, at necropsy. The *diffuse* interstitial fibrosis of the fourth stage does not differ from the fibrosis caused by toxic myocarditis. The extensive scarring may cause chronic congestive heart failure.

MYOCARDITIS IN
SARCOIDOSIS AND
SCLERODERMA

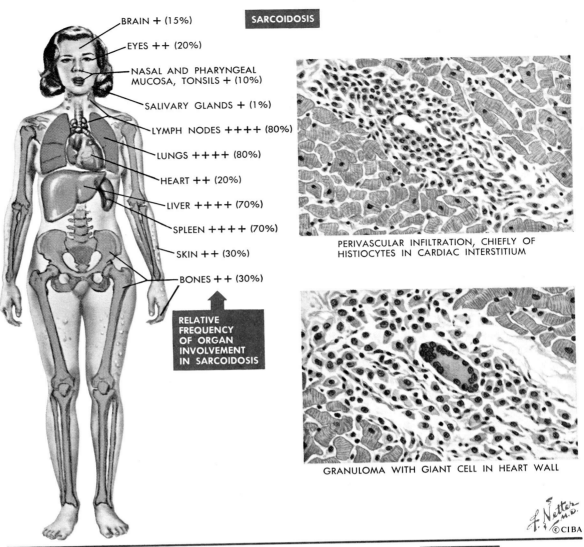

SARCOIDOSIS

- BRAIN + (15%)
- EYES ++ (20%)
- NASAL AND PHARYNGEAL MUCOSA, TONSILS + (10%)
- SALIVARY GLANDS + (1%)
- LYMPH NODES ++++ (80%)
- LUNGS ++++ (80%)
- HEART ++ (20%)
- LIVER ++++ (70%)
- SPLEEN ++++ (70%)
- SKIN ++ (30%)
- BONES ++ (30%)

RELATIVE FREQUENCY OF ORGAN INVOLVEMENT IN SARCOIDOSIS

PERIVASCULAR INFILTRATION, CHIEFLY OF HISTIOCYTES IN CARDIAC INTERSTITIUM

GRANULOMA WITH GIANT CELL IN HEART WALL

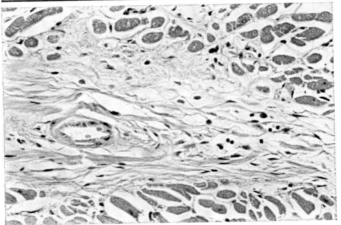

SCLERODERMA

EXTENSIVE FIBROSIS BETWEEN AND AROUND CARDIAC MUSCLE FIBERS AND IN ARTERIAL WALL WITH ONLY MODERATE LYMPHOCYTIC AND HISTIOCYTIC INFILTRATION

Sarcoidosis

Among the interstitial myocarditides, *sarcoidosis* (Besnier-Boeck-Schaumann disease) is second in incidence to rheumatic myocarditis. In sarcoidosis the *lungs, liver, spleen,* and *lymph nodes* are involved much *more frequently* and more extensively than is the *heart*. However, the heart may be affected in 20 *percent* of all cases, and, in 6 percent, death may result from myocarditis. Sarcoidosis of the lungs leads to pulmonary hypertension and, consequently, to right heart failure and cor pulmonale without myocarditic changes.

Myocarditic *granulomas* are found particularly in the *wall of the left ventricle,* but they may be present also in other portions of the heart. Some of the granulomas measure up to 4 mm in diameter and are recognizable grossly. Granulomas of the right atrium may cause arrhythmias and sinus tachycardia. Granulomas involving the bundle of His can lead to abnormalities in atrioventricular conduction, including complete A-V block. Therefore, death may occur during Morgagni-Adams-Stokes seizures.

At the beginning, the myocarditic foci are composed of *perivascular accumulations of histiocytes*. Later, granulomas develop and demonstrate a few Langhans *giant cells*. Finally, granulomas may be replaced by hyaline scars. The recurrent course of the disease may result in diffuse fibrosis of the myocardium. However, the granulomatous lesions are nonspecific. Similar changes can occur in tuberculosis, brucellosis, and tularemia. Therefore, the *histological* findings can be interpreted only within the entire picture of the disease.

The *etiology* of sarcoidosis is unknown. Some authors believe that the disease is caused by a single specific agent, *e.g.,* a virus, a fungus, or an unidentified acid-fast bacillus. Other investigators regard the condition as a response to a variety of agents, *e.g.,* pine pollen and mycobacterium tuberculosis. Sarcoidosis shows a special predilection for Negroes. Why more than one case of sarcoidosis can be observed in families or in siblings is still undetermined.

Scleroderma

An *interstitial myocarditis* can also occur in *scleroderma*. The focal myocardial lesions consist mainly of *lymphocytes* and *histiocytes*. In later stages, perivascular interstitial *fibrosis* progresses, and *scarring* extends *diffusely* throughout the myocardium. Similar changes are seen in systemic lupus erythematosus and in dermatomyositis. Therefore, the *diagnosis* can be made only after a review of all clinical data.

The *etiology* of scleroderma is unknown. Initially, the disease is characterized by edema and erythema of the skin. This phase is followed by hardening and atrophy of the skin. In addition to involvement of the heart, other internal organs, such as the lungs, the kidneys, and the alimentary tract, are frequently affected.

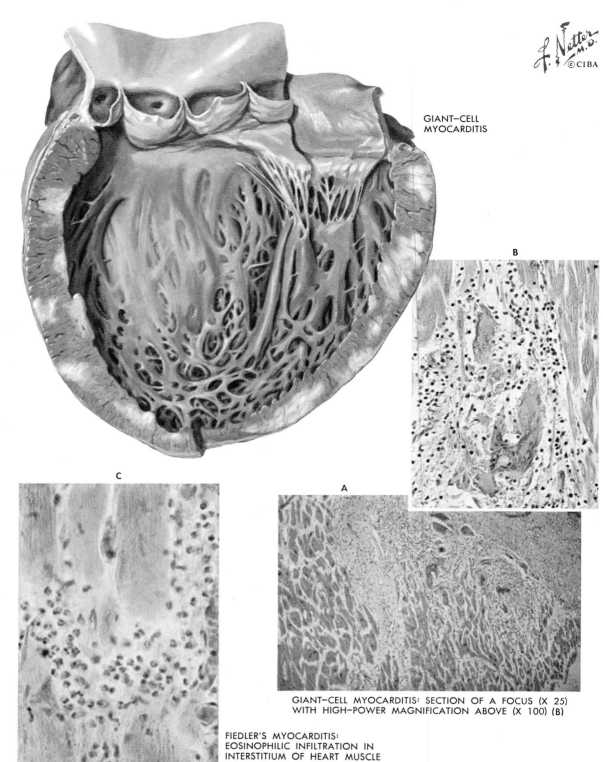

GIANT-CELL
MYOCARDITIS

IDIOPATHIC MYOCARDITIS

GIANT-CELL MYOCARDITIS: SECTION OF A FOCUS (X 25)
WITH HIGH-POWER MAGNIFICATION ABOVE (X 100) (B)

FIEDLER'S MYOCARDITIS:
EOSINOPHILIC INFILTRATION IN
INTERSTITIUM OF HEART MUSCLE
WITH DILATED BLOOD VESSELS; ONLY
SPOTTY DESTRUCTION OF MUSCLE FIBERS

Giant-Cell Myocarditis

Among the isolated myocarditides of unknown origin (also called *primary idiopathic myocarditis*), *granulomatous myocarditis with giant cells* should be distinguished.

In granulomatous myocarditis the enlarged heart shows dilatation of both ventricles and atria, and usually weighs 500 gm or more. The cut surface of the myocardium has a patchy, gray, and dim appearance. The focal lesions are not surrounded by hemorrhagic marginal zones. The coronary arteries are delicate. The typical *gross findings* often facilitate the *diagnosis*.

Microscopically, the focal granulomatous lesions are composed of dense infiltrates of lymphocytes, plasma cells, and histiocytes, together with giant cells of the Langhans type. As remnants of myocardial fibers, giant cells with numerous nuclei may also be present. Other areas of the myocardium show fibrosis.

Because some cases of *giant-cell myocarditis* also reveal granulomas in other organs, some investigators have regarded the condition as being related to sarcoidosis. However, as long as the *etiology* of granulomatous myocarditis with giant cells is not clarified, final classification will remain unresolved.

The *diagnosis* of giant-cell myocarditis often can be made only at autopsy. Clini-

cal examination will reveal an enlargement of the heart, with passive congestion of the lungs and abdominal organs. Usually, the body temperature is not elevated, but, in a few cases, it may reach septic levels. The *electrocardiogram* shows abnormalities suggestive of *myocardial damage* or of disturbances of the conduction system. A diagnosis of giant-cell myocarditis is justified only if other causes of cardiac failure (rheumatic heart disease, idiopathic hypertrophy of the heart, amyloidosis, etc.) can be excluded.

Fiedler's Myocarditis

Isolated *eosinophilic myocarditis (Fiedler)* reveals *necroses of myocardial fibers* associated with dense *interstitial infiltrates of eosinophilic leukocytes*, as

well as a few lymphocytes and plasma cells. Parietal thromboses may develop over foci located directly beneath the endocardium. These thrombi may be as extensively spread out as in cases of parietal fibroplastic endocarditis (Löffler, see page 208). In some instances of eosinophilic myocarditis, vascular lesions can occur also, as in the course of pericarditis.

Idiopathic myocarditis usually takes a rapid and fatal course, and, for this reason, it often is called pernicious myocarditis.

Some authors assume that idiopathic myocarditis is viral in origin. On the other hand, certain morphological features suggest that allergic reactions may play an important role. Regardless of these two theories, however, the etiology and pathogenesis are, as yet, not known.

ENDOMYOCARDIAL FIBROSIS

Endomyocardial fibrosis is common in many tropical countries, but typical cases are seen also in temperate regions. The pathologic lesion is a scar replacement of the endocardium and subjacent myocardium; this is strictly confined to the inflow-tract areas of the ventricles, and a raised, firm, *hard ridge marks the junction of the inflow and outflow tracts,* best seen in the *left ventricle.* The part of the endocardium which is not scarred may show a mild opacification from elastomyofibrosis. Lesions may be focally distributed in the inflow tract, and the areas of preference are the apex and the site behind the *posterior cusp* of the A-V valve, the cusp becoming *adherent* to the *mural endocardium.* In more severe cases the posterior cusp is lost in a mass of fibrous tissue extending from atrium to apex and partway up the septal and anterior walls, engulfing the *papillary muscle* and rendering the A-V valve completely incompetent. The A-V valves themselves exhibit no specific lesions, and the semilunar valves are entirely unaffected.

On the right side the ventricular configuration results in the process filling the ventricular cavity with a mass of thrombus and organizing *fibrous tissue* so that the cavity is *obliterated.* This can be recognized *externally* by a severe *recession of the right apex* or, less commonly, a recession higher up on the ventricular wall. The effective cavity is reduced to a shallow saucer, and fibrous tissue extends high up toward the pulmonary valve, but the endocardium immediately below the valve is normal or opacified by elastomyofibrosis. The *right atrium may be enormously dilated,* like a rubber balloon.

In both ventricles the endocardium may be covered by *thrombi* which, rarely, may detach and produce a massive embolus. Usually, it is extremely firmly attached and does not loosen, so that infarctions are quite uncommon. Beneath the thickened endocardium there are small blood lagoons — dilated thebesian veins — and, from these and the endocardial scar tissue, tongues of fibrous tissue extend into the inner third or half of the myocardium but never involve its full thickness. The major coronary vessels are normal; no changes are seen in the minor vessels save for an occasional small focus of inflammatory cells and, in late stages when fibrosis is severe, an obliterative arteritis. Severe *calcification* may develop in the valve or mural endocardium, important *radiologically** as indicating that the constriction is endocardial, not pericardial, though sometimes there is a large pericardial effusion. No constant extracardiac lesions are seen except for those

*The X-ray picture is reproduced through the courtesy of Dr. P. Hutton of Makerere College, Kampala, Uganda, and the Wellcome Museum of Medical Science.

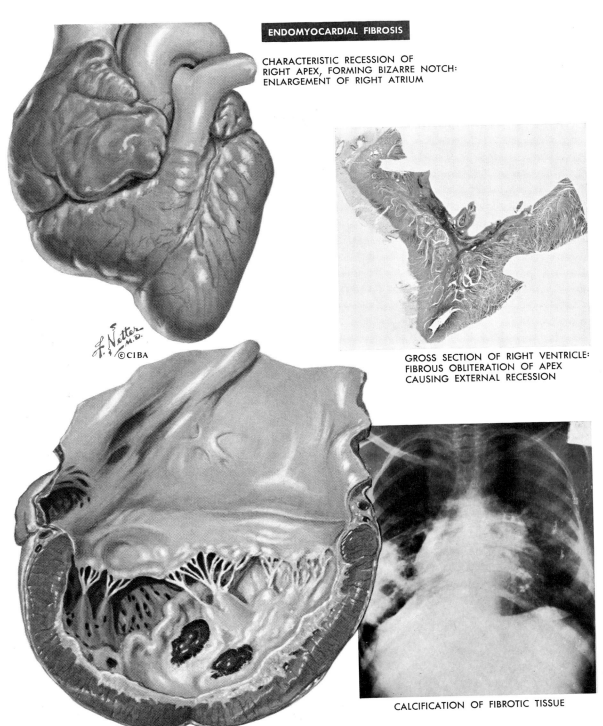

ENDOMYOCARDIAL FIBROSIS

CHARACTERISTIC RECESSION OF RIGHT APEX, FORMING BIZARRE NOTCH: ENLARGEMENT OF RIGHT ATRIUM

GROSS SECTION OF RIGHT VENTRICLE: FIBROUS OBLITERATION OF APEX CAUSING EXTERNAL RECESSION

CALCIFICATION OF FIBROTIC TISSUE

DENSE COLLAGEN LAYER LINING L. VENTRICLE, INVOLVING POSTERIOR PAPILLARY MUSCLE AND CHORDAE TENDINEAE, DEMARCATED BY A RIDGE, SPARING OUTFLOW TRACT; POSTERIOR MITRAL CUSP ADHERENT TO WALL; MURAL THROMBI

of congestion. The heart weight may be increased but is often reduced, and, despite the voluminous atria, the ventricles often are small and shrunken.

The cause of the disease is unknown, and the early lesions have not yet been identified. Most cases are seen only when endocardial scarring is advanced. The disease may be biventricular, and the *clinical manifestations* may change from time to time, depending on which ventricle is bearing the brunt of the disease. If the left ventricle alone is affected, the disease runs a rapid course, with very severe pulmonary hypertension developing. If the right side alone is involved, the progress of the disease is much slower. The patients have a very high central venous pressure and may show exophthalmos. They have no peripheral edema but a severe and extremely tense ascites, the ascitic fluid having a very high protein content. The liver is exceptionally large. The high venous pressure apparently substitutes for the incapacitated right ventricle.

In some cases, differentiation from constrictive pericarditis may be extremely difficult, but *diagnosis* of endomyocardial fibrosis has been much facilitated by *angiocardiography.* Whichever ventricle is affected, there is severe damage to the posterior A-V valve cusp, with resulting mitral and tricuspid incompetence and, in rare cases, stenosis. There is some evidence that the early lesion may be a pyrexial form of carditis followed, after a relatively short period, by evidence of progressive cardiac damage. Whatever the cause, the pathogenesis of the disease is destruction of the endocardium and underlying myocardium of the ventricular-inflow tracts, with the formation of scar tissue. Elastic tissue in the affected areas is almost entirely lost, and elastosis is uncommonly seen, save at the edges of the scar tissue. No significant diagnostic blood changes have been found.

LÖFFLER'S DISEASE

MULTIPLE EMBOLIC INFARCTS (LUNG, BRAIN, SPLEEN, KIDNEY) AND DIFFUSE ARTERIOLITIS

BRAIN

HEART ENLARGED

LIVER ENLARGED

ASCITES

EDEMA

LEUKOCYTOSIS, EOSINOPHILIA

LÖFFLER'S DISEASE

Löffler's disease is an uncommon but distinctive form of disease in which the heart is the organ mainly affected by an *eosinophilic arteritis,* probably of an allergic type. In recorded series, males predominate, and the disease occurs between 7 and 65 years of age.

At autopsy the changes of congestive cardiac failure are seen, usually with considerable effusion into the serous cavities. *Infarcts,* fresh or of some standing, are often found in the *brain, kidneys,* and other organs. The *heart* may be of normal size but is usually *enlarged,* either generally or on one side only, most commonly the left side. In acute cases, little change may be observed, save for marked pallor of the *endocardium* and *subjacent myocardium,* but microscopy shows swelling and necrosis of the endothelial cells, an *eosinophilic infiltration* of both the endocardium and the thebesian veins, focal necrosis of myocardial fibers with an eosinophilic infiltration, and an eosinophilic arteritis of the small coronary arteries with an occasional focus of fibrinoid necrosis. A similar eosinophilic arteritis will be found in the small arteries of the *brain, kidneys, lungs,* and *striated muscle,* but the main coronary arteries are not involved.

More advanced cases will show extensive lesions. The *endocardium* is *thickened* and *scarred,* gray-white in color, and covered with *mural thrombi,* both atrial and ventricular, in varying stages of organization and attachment. Scar tissue may cover the *papillary muscle* and shorten and thicken the *chordae tendineae,* thus distorting the A-V valve which itself usually exhibits valvulitis with vegetations. The *semilunar valves* may also show these lesions. The myocardium will have areas of necrosis, sometimes with frank hemorrhage, and organization and scarring, the lesions often involving the full thickness of the ventricular myocardium. Between the myocardium and the thickened endocardium, small blood lagoons may be detected in dilated thebesian veins. In the necrotic and fibrosing areas of the myocardium, a great eosinophilic infiltration usually is present. The cells are abundant also in the thickened endocardium. The original endocardium is largely destroyed, being replaced by scar tissue with some elastosis. In more chronic cases, tissue eosinophilia may diminish or disappear, the arteries show only an obliterative arteritis, and severe endomyocardial scarring is found, usually

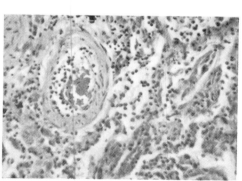

GREATLY ENLARGED HEART: EXTENSIVE FIBROSIS OF ENDOCARDIUM AND SUBENDOCARDIAL MYOCARDIUM WITH EXTENSION THROUGH ENTIRE THICKNESS OF HEART WALL AND INVOLVEMENT OF PAPILLARY MUSCLES, CHORDAE TENDINEAE, AND VALVE CUSPS; MURAL THROMBI

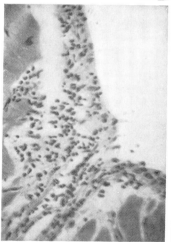

ACUTE EOSINOPHILIC AND NEUTROPHILIC INFILTRATION OF SUBENDOCARDIUM

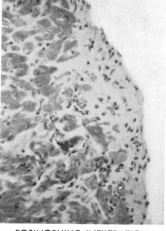

EOSINOPHILIC INFILTRATION AND EARLY MYOCARDIAL DAMAGE

ACUTE EOSINOPHILIC ENDARTERITIS IN LUNG; SIMILAR LESIONS OCCUR IN SMALL VESSELS OF BRAIN, KIDNEY, AND OTHER ORGANS

maximal at the apex and spreading thence to involve both the inflow- and outflow-tract endocardium.

The basic arteritis may cause the initial manifestations to be cerebral, abdominal, or renal, or to commence with arthralgias, muscle pains, and, in some cases, polyneuritis. The *symptoms* may come on acutely, with a fulminant course, or slowly, with a progressive evolution. A particular group is comprised of those in whom the disease develops after several years of attacks of respiratory disease with bronchospasm. Cardiac decompensation develops, often with major embolic accidents. Pyrexia is common. *Radiology* may demonstrate cardiac enlargement, and evidence of myocardial necrosis, especially of the subendocardial myocardium, may be found by *electrocardiography.* Mitral insufficiency may develop. Most important in *diagnosis* is an absolute *high eosinophil count* in the blood; figures of up to 130,000 per cubic

millimeter have been recorded. The eosinophilia may not be marked or even present at the onset, and it frequently diminishes and may disappear terminally or in the chronic stages when the disease may closely mimic all the signs and symptoms of a constrictive pericarditis.

No specific cause of Löffler's disease is known. It is of worldwide distribution. The important points in its distinction are blood and tissue eosinophilia (in the endocardium and myocardium particularly), eosinophilic arteritis, endocardial scarring which may involve the inflow or outflow tracts, valvulitis, and involvement of the whole thickness of the ventricular myocardium.

The microscopic slides are reproduced through the courtesy of Horst W. Weber, M.D., Professor of Pathology, University of Stellenbosch, South Africa.

BECKER'S DISEASE

Becker's disease, common in all races in South Africa but occurring in other areas also, appears to be a specific type of heart disease, the basic lesion being a form of *verrucous angiitis* which particularly affects the *subendocardial* blood vessels. The lesions found at autopsy reflect the acuteness or chronicity of the disease. At whatever stage death occurs, severe lesions of *congestive cardiac failure,* with large *effusions* in the serous cavities, are found, as well as *multiple infarctions.* The latter are present in the *lungs* in all cases and, commonly, also in the *brain, spleen, kidneys,* and other organs. The *heart* is greatly *dilated* and usually considerably increased in weight. *Mural thrombi* are always present in the *ventricles,* sometimes small, sometimes covering two thirds of the mural endocardium and interfering mechanically with the A-V valve function. The heart valves show no specific lesions, and the main coronary arteries are normal. In acute cases the endocardium not covered by thrombus is neither thickened nor opaque, though a fine surface deposition of fibrin may be seen. Small dark spots may be visible; these are small *hemorrhagic polyps* on the *endocardial surface.* In acute cases, pallor of the myocardium under the mural thrombi is seen, and, in the later stages, small areas of granulation tissue and streaks of fibrous tissue are visible in the inner third of the myocardium. In more chronic cases, irregular plaques of fibroelastotic endocardial thickening are found, scattered irregularly over the inflow and outflow tracts though most evident at the apex. The hearts often have a stiff rubbery feel and a curious *tan* or *yellowish color.*

Microscopically, progressive changes are recognizable. In the acute stage the *endocardium* is thickened with a serous and mucinous *edema,* and it may be acellular or infiltrated with inflammatory cells, wholly polymorphonuclear or mixed in type. Fibrin is diffusely or focally deposited on the endocardial surface, and, where damage is severe, the thrombus accretes. The focal fibrin deposits may form polyps, and hemorrhage into these may produce the black spots. The organization of the deposited fibrin and elastic-tissue proliferation leads to the fibroelastotic plaques of the late stages. A verrucous angiitis of the subendocardial vessels commences with ectatic dilatation and deposits of fibrin on the walls. These may develop into narrow-stalked polyps, which break loose and produce microembolic lesions, or they may be organized into a fibrinofibrous cushion, rich in capillary tissue, to one side of the vessel or, occasionally, occluding it. Similar changes

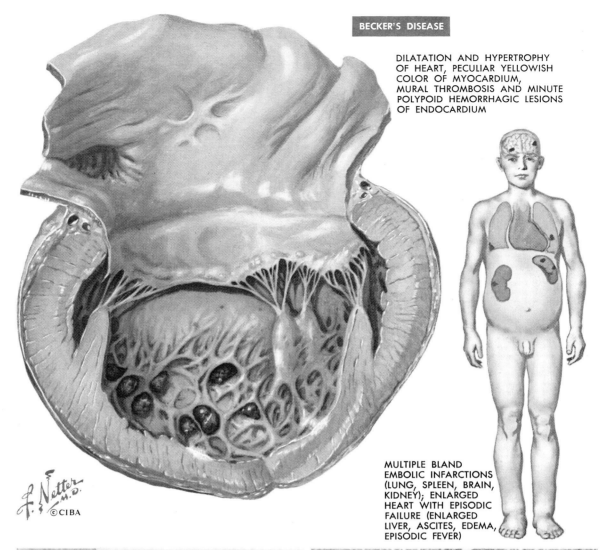

BECKER'S DISEASE

DILATATION AND HYPERTROPHY OF HEART, PECULIAR YELLOWISH COLOR OF MYOCARDIUM, MURAL THROMBOSIS AND MINUTE POLYPOID HEMORRHAGIC LESIONS OF ENDOCARDIUM

MULTIPLE BLAND EMBOLIC INFARCTIONS (LUNG, SPLEEN, BRAIN, KIDNEY); ENLARGED HEART WITH EPISODIC FAILURE (ENLARGED LIVER, ASCITES, EDEMA, EPISODIC FEVER)

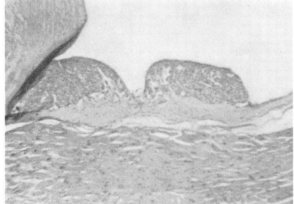

VERRUCOUS LESIONS ON THICKENED, EDEMATOUS ENDOCARDIUM

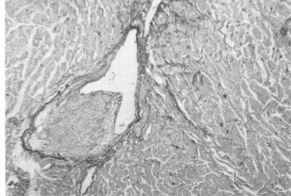

HYALINIZED POLYPOID PROTRUSION INTO LUMEN OF SUBENDOCARDIAL VEIN

are found in pulmonary blood vessels. In the acute stages the myofibers show little change, and what is seen — loss of striation, nuclear hyperchromatism, and fragmentation — appears to be anoxic. Interstitial edema may be marked, and the changes are confined to the inner third of the myocardium. In the chronic stages, some interstitial fibrosis may develop. Small perivascular inflammatory-cell infiltrates are sometimes seen, but, for the most part, there is little myocardial inflammatory-cell infiltration.

The cause of this disease is unknown. It may develop acutely, with very severe congestive cardiac failure, and the serous effusions are commonly out of proportion to the severity of the cardiac failure. Abdominal pain from acute *liver congestion* may be intense. There is often a fever with a neutrophil polymorphonuclear leukocytosis but no eosinophilia with tachycardia or cardiomegaly, *radiology* revealing only

an *enlarged and flaccid heart. Electrocardiographic* changes are not distinctive, and low-voltage patterns are usual. *Embolic accidents,* large or small, are common. The patient may progress to death in cardiac failure, unresponsive to all treatment, or may recover completely. After a variable interval there will be a relapse, which may result in death or in recovery. The *episodes* may be repeated over many months, the intervals of improvement becoming progressively shorter, the periods of congestive failure progressively more protracted. Treatment at all stages is disappointing, as the disease is refractory to all therapy. Ultimately, death occurs, often rapidly, in a final episode of heart failure.

Pathologically, the cardiac lesions can be recognized by the enlargement and stiffness of the heart, the fibroelastotic patches, and the distinctive verrucous angiitis of the subendocardial blood vessels.

BERIBERI

The term "beriberi" should be confined to the lesions which result from a dietary deficiency of thiamine. Cardiovascular beriberi is seen as a fulminant disease of small breast-fed infants, reflecting severe thiamine deficiency in the mothers. It has a seasonal incidence, as does adult cardiovascular beriberi, in regions where the disease is due to a deficient diet of a simple staple such as husked rice. Small epidemics may occur in prisons, camps, and fishing boats. It is sometimes seen as an acute disease in alcoholics who consume a very restricted diet. The crucial feature of all these types is that they *respond to adequate thiamine* very quickly, save in the most severe of terminal cases. The response is rapid and dramatic.

The circulation rate in cardiovascular beriberi is extremely *rapid,* the pulse is bounding, and the *blood pressure is raised;* "pistol-shot" sounds are heard over the extremities, the hands and feet are warm despite peripheral *edema* of rapid onset, and *ascites,* possibly with a polyneuritis, may occur. The heart has to increase its work load considerably to meet the demand of this hyperkinetic circulation, and the rapid return of blood to the heart leads to disproportionate *right-side dilatation and hypertrophy.* It seems that the basic change is in the peripheral circulation, with a great opening up of arteriovenous anastomoses, especially in striated muscles. The initial effect of thiamine seems to be on the peripheral circulation; the work load on the heart is abruptly diminished, and rapid alteration in heart size and rate results. These changes are so rapid that thiamine administration can be used as a *therapeutic test* for cardiovascular beriberi. If the patient should die, it is from the sudden failure of the heart to meet the sustained call for *high output.* The terminal failure may be sudden, with severe *pulmonary edema.*

It has been impossible thus far to define specific changes due to thiamine deficiency in the hearts of human cases of cardiovascular beriberi. The hearts will invariably exhibit a degree of right-side dilatation and hypertrophy, but the microscopic findings may show only myofiber hypertrophy, with enlargement and hyperchromatism of the nuclei, which are cigar-shaped or blunt-ended. Watery *vacuolation* of the *myofibers* and *interstitial edema* have often been recorded, as have fatty infiltration and varying degrees of

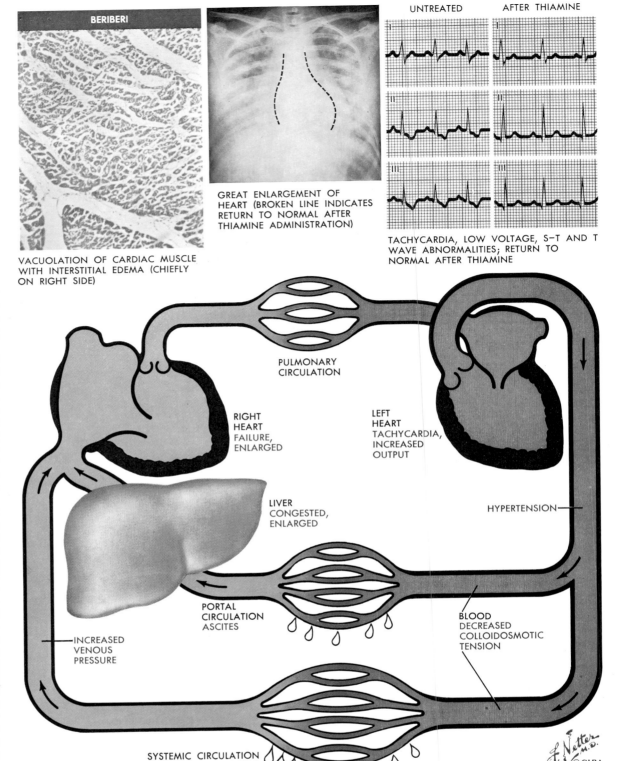

VACUOLATION OF CARDIAC MUSCLE WITH INTERSTITIAL EDEMA (CHIEFLY ON RIGHT SIDE)

GREAT ENLARGEMENT OF HEART (BROKEN LINE INDICATES RETURN TO NORMAL AFTER THIAMINE ADMINISTRATION)

UNTREATED   AFTER THIAMINE

TACHYCARDIA, LOW VOLTAGE, S–T AND T WAVE ABNORMALITIES; RETURN TO NORMAL AFTER THIAMINE

PULMONARY CIRCULATION

RIGHT HEART FAILURE, ENLARGED

LEFT HEART TACHYCARDIA, INCREASED OUTPUT

LIVER CONGESTED, ENLARGED

HYPERTENSION

INCREASED VENOUS PRESSURE

PORTAL CIRCULATION ASCITES

BLOOD DECREASED COLLOIDOSMOTIC TENSION

SYSTEMIC CIRCULATION EDEMA

myocardial fibrosis. These changes seem to reflect the general nutritional status of the patient rather than being specific lesions of thiamine deprivation. They do not resemble the lesions found in experimental animals on thiamine deficiency. The latter die suddenly, with focal patchy necrosis of muscle cells with an inflammatory infiltrate. Lesions of this type are not recorded in humans. The lesions seen in animals are similar to those induced by extreme potassium deficiency, but a combination of thiamine and potassium deficiency does not produce the lesions.

In Western countries a high-output type of cardiovascular disease is sometimes seen in alcoholics. This may respond completely to thiamine administration. Some patients in this state, to whom thiamine is given, may have their status changed from high-output failure to low-output failure, in all probability the result of an alcoholic cardiomyopathy.

Nutritional deficiencies in humans are only very rarely due to some single essential dietary lack. While thiamine deficiency may occur in otherwise-well-nourished individuals, most of those affected will be on diets that usually are low in protein and fat but high in carbohydrates. Thus, they suffer from multiple deficiencies. Since the administration of thiamine is so highly effective in cardiovascular beriberi, it should be given in appropriate dosage, by an effective route, as quickly as possible. If improvement does not follow, or if only some of the cardiovascular modifications are altered, it would be well to regard the remaining cardiovascular lesions as being due to some cause other than thiamine deficiency. In the light of current views on the metabolic derangements in thiamine deficiency (see CIBA COLLECTION, Vol. 4, pages 252 and 253), it seems unlikely that a state of chronic beriberi heart disease could exist.

CARDIAC MYOPATHIES

In any cardiac clinic an occasional patient is seen who exhibits evidence of cardiac disease, almost invariably with a *greatly enlarged heart* but with no evidence of valvular disorder, coronary-artery disease, or hypertension. Clues to the possible cause and nature of the disease may be found in the family history, by a history of a past episode of infections, or by the evidence of accompanying endocrine disturbance, a generalized vasculitis, or some form of systemic disease. Hemochromatosis, amyloidosis, glycogen storage disease, and disorders of the nervous system have to be excluded, and evidence of some persisting or past episode of bacterial, viral, or protozoan-induced disease evaluated. Eventually, there remains a group in whom the cause of the cardiomegaly is still obscure. These will include some women in the later stages of pregnancy or in the postpartal state. In numerous parts of the world, this group of patients with "idiopathic cardiomegaly" is a sizable one. With many of these there is a suspicion of malnutrition and perhaps a history of alcoholism — often difficult to elicit in detail — which leads to a consideration of thiamine deficiency, but administration of the vitamin often produces no improvement. Some patients may recover spontaneously, apparently fully and permanently, only to relapse later; in some, the disease may progress rapidly and relentlessly, or a slow deterioration may set in. Physicians should be alert to epidemics of cardiomyopathies. Several of these have been described, particularly in beer drinkers. There is reason to believe that, in many, alcohol is a most important factor, and this may be so in special groups (*e.g.,* palm-wine drinkers), but similar conditions also affect those who do not take alcohol.

Radiologic examination is usually not helpful other than in demonstrating a grossly enlarged heart which ordinarily continues to increase in size. *Electrocardiography* confirms the comparative weakness and poverty of the heart's action. As a rule, only symptomatic relief can be given, and the clinician finally is hopeful that autopsy will reveal the cause of the condition. Unhappily, it too often happens that, if the cause was not uncovered in life, it cannot be satisfactorily established at autopsy. Evidence of congestive failure is found with an enlarged heart, the enlargement being compounded of varying degrees of *hypertrophy* and *dilatation*. Some degree of coronary arteriosclerosis may be found, especially in communities where this condition is common, but this is usually not sufficient to explain the lesions, and, very

GREATLY ENLARGED HEART

GREATLY DILATED AND MODERATELY HYPERTROPHIED HEART: LITTLE OR NO FIBROSIS OF ENDOCARDIUM; MURAL THROMBI IN L. VENTRICLE AND L. AURICLE

DIFFUSE FOCI OR IRREGULAR FIBROSIS, REPLACING CARDIAC MUSCLE FIBERS

INFILTRATION OF CARDIAC MUSCLE WITH LYMPHOCYTES AND MONOCYTES; EDEMA AND OCCASIONAL GIANT CELL

VACUOLATION OF MYOCARDIAL FIBERS AND INTERSTITIAL EDEMA SIMILAR TO THAT SEEN IN BERIBERI

often, the coronary vessels are normal or widely patent. The myocardium is often soft and flabby, or it may be stiffer than normal. It may exhibit pallor, and there may be evidence of some *myocardial fibrosis.* The *endocardium* may be normal, or may be covered in part by *mural thrombi,* or it may be patchily thickened and opaque.

The histologic changes may be equally indeterminate, and some cases may show nothing beyond hypertrophy of myocardial fibers, with enlarged hyperchromatic blunt-ended or cigar-shaped nuclei. There may be watery *vacuolation* of *myofibers* with, perhaps, some accumulation of lipid droplets. The myofibers may be separated by *interstitial edema. Diffuse fibrosis* or *focal scars* may be present. There may be cellular infiltration of varying degrees of intensity; the cell types vary, but commonly there is an *infiltrate* of *lymphocytes and monocytes* and, *occasionally, a giant*

cell. Histochemical studies may show a great diminution in oxidative enzymes.

Study of the endocardial lesions, especially areas of endocardial thickening, may help in understanding some of the pathogenetic mechanisms involved. Thus, a considerable degree of endocardial smooth-muscle hypertrophy indicates a past stage of acute cardiac dilatation. From the pathological aspect, study of many carefully oriented blocks and exact mapping of lesions, as well as careful correlation with any extracardiac lesions that may be found, are the steps to better understanding of these hearts, and, ultimately, to a knowledge of the causes of these presumed metabolic cardiomyopathies. In these cases, however, nothing can equal in importance the most detailed and meticulous clinical history taking, as well as the most careful probing into the patient's background and the circumstances surrounding the onset of the disease.

STRUCTURE OF CORONARY ARTERIES

In man, the *coronary arteries* are susceptible to atherosclerosis as well as to its complications, particularly intravascular thrombosis, often resulting in myocardial infarction. Atherosclerosis is a form of arteriosclerosis characterized by initial involvement of the inner layer of the arterial wall or intima; the intimal localization of early atheromas helps to differentiate this form from other types of arteriosclerosis, such as Mönckeberg's medial sclerosis or periarteritis nodosa, that primarily involve the muscular or adventitial layers.

Recent histochemical, organ-culture, and electron microscopic studies have brought out further evidence of the complexity of the arterial wall. As shown, a medium-sized muscular artery, such as a main coronary vessel, consists of a series of concentric tubes or coaxial coats of differentiated cellular and extracellular components in three layers: tunica intima or *intima,* tunica *media* or *muscular,* and tunica *adventitia.* In the intima the innermost cell layer in direct contact with the bloodstream consists of a sheet of polygonal *endothelial* cells, usually less than 1 micron thick, except at the site of the cell nucleus, and elongated in a direction parallel to the vessel's axis. Many of these endothelial cells have pinocytotic vesicles of "caveolas" in their cytoplasm, abundant mitochondria, well-developed granular endoplasmic *reticulum,* and Golgi complex. The areas of contact between endothelial cells, under the electron microscope, vary from simple mutual contact of the cell membranes to well-defined intercellular bridges or *desmosomes,* corresponding to the so-called intercellular cement lines described in earlier light microscopic studies. A distinct *basement membrane* separates these endothelial cells from the subendothelial space, which varies in thickness not only because of the size of the artery under study but according to the age of the subject. In fetal life and shortly after birth, the endothelium in the coronary arteries lies in *direct contact* with the *internal elastic membrane* or *lamina,* without the *subendothelial space* that appears by the end of the first decade of life. In adulthood the intima consists of a matrix of ground substance containing small amounts of acid mucopolysaccharides and elastic and *collagen* fibers separating scattered intimal cells or *intimacytes.*

Because of morphological and cytochemical difficulties in classifying intimacytes, their response to in vitro incorporation of serum lipids has been used to identify them. Some intimacytes or *atherophils* incorporate lipid rapidly and show ultrastructural characteristics of modified smooth-muscle cells, with typical bundles of myofilaments in their cytoplasm, pinocytotic vesicles, and portions of limiting basement membrane on the cell surface. On the other hand, other cells, *fibrophils,* are spindle-shaped, have fingerlike cytoplasmic projections, an

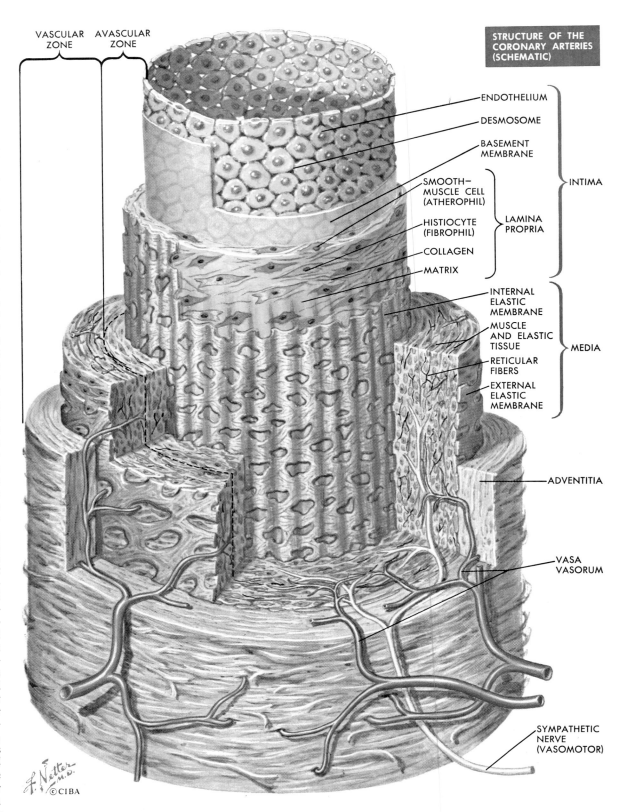

VASCULAR ZONE — AVASCULAR ZONE

STRUCTURE OF THE CORONARY ARTERIES (SCHEMATIC)

ENDOTHELIUM
DESMOSOME
BASEMENT MEMBRANE
INTIMA
SMOOTH-MUSCLE CELL (ATHEROPHIL)
HISTIOCYTE (FIBROPHIL)
LAMINA PROPRIA
COLLAGEN
MATRIX
INTERNAL ELASTIC MEMBRANE
MUSCLE AND ELASTIC TISSUE
MEDIA
RETICULAR FIBERS
EXTERNAL ELASTIC MEMBRANE
ADVENTITIA
VASA VASORUM
SYMPATHETIC NERVE (VASOMOTOR)

absence of basement membrane, and few pinocytotic vesicles. Occasionally, large mononuclear ovoid cells appear. These contain cytoplasmic inclusions with "single-unit" acid phosphatase positive granules or lysosomes, resembling macrophages. Separating the *lamina propria* from the underlying *smooth-muscle cells* of the media is usually a well-developed *internal elastic membrane* consisting of a tenacious *matrix* containing fibrils approximately 500 angstroms in diameter and with abundant fenestrations. This internal elastic membrane or lamina is usually wavy in cross sections, and the fenestrations are oval or rounded openings extending across its surface.

The underlying tunica media is characterized by concentric layers of *smooth-muscle cells* measuring from 10 to 25 microns in length, oriented transversely to the main axis of the artery.

Individual smooth-muscle cells are surrounded by

a network of collagenous and elastic fibers, which continue without transition into both the internal and external elastic membranes. The *external elastic membrane* separates the media from the adventitia and is characterized by the presence of loosely packed collagen and elastic fibers. Small blood vessels or *vasa vasorum* as well as both *sympathetic* and *parasympathetic nerve fibers* from the autonomic nervous system are also found.

These morphologic and functional characteristics of the coronary arteries are modified early in the presence of the intimal changes characteristic of *atherosclerosis* (see page 213).

The most important *clinical difference* between coronary and aortic atherosclerosis is the high incidence of acute thrombosis in coronary vessels, resulting, through infarction, in irreversible damage to the underlying myocardium.

HYPOTHESIS ON PATHOGENESIS OF HUMAN ATHEROSCLEROSIS

Some of the histological and functional characteristics of the intimal lining of the arteries, particularly the presence of different cell types in a ground-substance matrix and the absence of a direct blood supply (see page 212), help one to understand the histogenesis of spontaneous atheromas, often initiated, in man, shortly after birth.

The well-developed atherosclerotic plaque, resulting from the interplay of inflammatory and reparative processes, is a complex lesion, containing *extracellular deposits of calcium salts,* blood components, cholesterol crystals, and acid *mucopolysaccharides.* The initial changes, however, seem to occur at the cellular level; electron microscopy has shown that they are often accompanied by an abnormal intracellular storage of *lipids,* particularly cholesterol esters, fatty acids, and *lipoprotein* complexes. These findings have strengthened the thesis that lipid infiltration from the bloodstream may be a significant factor in the growth of the atheromatous plaque. Furthermore, since lipids may be recognized by cytochemical technics, they have been used as helpful indicators of abnormal cell behavior, independent of their role in the etiology of atheroma.

Because of the severity and frequent occurrence of atherosclerosis, the use of short-term organ-culture technics for the isolation of human arterial intimal cells or *intimacytes* has been applied to the identification of susceptible cell populations, based on their response to incorporation of homologous-serum lipids in vitro. Intimacytes from arteries, with and without histological evidence of atherosclerosis, have shown, respectively, two different types of cells or *atherophils* — one which is *genetically highly susceptible* to intracellular *lipid accumulation,* the other *genetically resistant.*

Based on these findings, the following hypothesis is advanced: Susceptible atherophils, in the presence of increased perfusion rates of plasma lipoproteins due to local hemodynamic changes, hypertension, elevated serum lipids, or changes in the permeability of the endothelial surface (trauma, *fibrin deposition, platelet aggregation*), will be transformed into lipid-laden atherocytes. The secondary release of intracellular lipids from these cells will induce surrounding atherophils to incorporate them, creating a self-feeding process with cytological changes that increase metabolic requirements, including *oxygen*-consumption rates, which, if not met, result in increased permeability

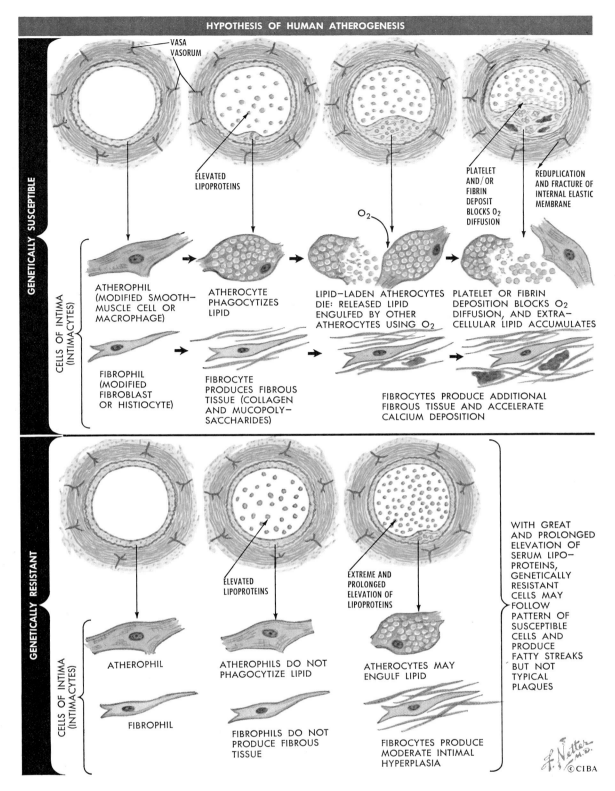

of the cell membrane to lipids. These events set up a vicious circle that favors further expansion of focal atherosclerotic changes. The latter include the laying down of collagen fibers by *fibrophils* that are then transformed into *fibrocytes* surrounded by acid mucopolysaccharide deposits; this eventually results in a characteristic intimal hyperplasia, following ground-substance changes. These histological lesions are self-perpetuating, resulting in the replacement of intimacytes by an acellular area of arterial intima that stimulates further surface involvement of the vascular wall in this interplay between deposition, inflammatory response, and scarring, ending with the eventual production of a *typical* atherosclerotic *plaque.*

In contrast, genetically resistant atherophils, even in the presence of *elevated serum-lipid levels,* do not respond (or respond in only a limited fashion) to an increased perfusion of plasma lipids. If some athero-

cytes appear, they are few in number, and only superficial *fatty streaks* are developed, resulting in minimal intimal elevations with few fibrophils and the absence of a well-organized plaque. This type of cytological response seems also less susceptible to the clinical complications of atherosclerosis (particularly thrombosis or rupture) owing to the limited involvement of the vascular wall.

This concept of the pathogenesis of human atherosclerosis emphasizes the clinical significance of identifying, at the earliest possible time, those individuals whose arteries are susceptible to atheroma, in an effort to modify or prevent those environmental conditions, for the cells of the arterial intima, which favor the acceleration of atherogenesis. This hypothesis also stresses the importance of local factors in the localization of the lesions, suggesting possible therapeutic approaches for their arrest or inhibition.

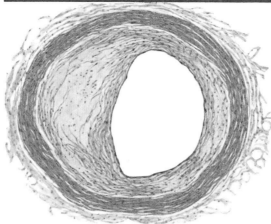

MODERATE ATHEROSCLEROTIC NARROWING OF LUMEN

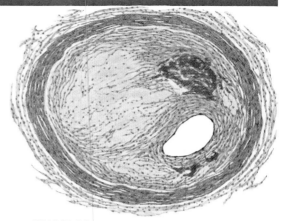

ALMOST COMPLETE OCCLUSION BY INTIMAL
ATHEROSCLEROSIS WITH CALCIUM DEPOSITION

PATHOLOGIC CHANGES IN CORONARY-ARTERY DISEASE

Disregarding the various theories concerning the etiology and pathogenesis of *atherosclerosis* (and directly, *coronary*-artery disease), the alterations produced by this greatest destroyer of modern Western man are awesome, presenting a panorama of structural changes that defies the determination of an orderly sequence of events. As a consequence, there has been much speculation concerning the various stages visible within the coronary artery. The earliest recognizable atheromatous change seems to be the accumulation of aggregates of lipid-laden macrophages in the intima (see page 213). The appearance of this lesion is similar to that seen in many of the experimentally produced vascular lesions. Another apparently early phenomenon, difficult to correlate and possibly not related, is a subintimal deposit of collagen that often is primitive and, hence, rich in acid mucopolysaccharides. Lesions of this type shadow atherosclerosis wherever it occurs and, as previously described, can involve the peripheral arteries of the body. The relationship of this vascular lesion to the kind seen in Oriental races has not been elucidated, but this disorder does occur in that racial group also. A further complication of this lesion is the deposition of fibrin either on or within its superficial layers. As a consequence, the complicating theories of zonal layers of thrombosis have crept into speculations concerning etiology and pathogenesis. Problems arise in relating this collagenosis to atherosclerosis.

As more lipid accumulates, an atheromatous plaque, which contains many constituents, is formed. This plaque may involve only a segmental portion of the artery or can involve its entire circumference. (One can only admire the choice of the French term in calling this grumous material "putty.") When the macrophages die, their contained lipid is released and serves as an irritant. Fibrin is accumulated, as are other blood constituents, and the final reaction is a stimulation of *calcium deposition* and the proliferation of fibroblasts. How some of these lesions thicken is a matter of debate, but many stenotic lesions appear to accumulate more surface material by the deposition of superficial layers of thrombosis. That this lesion, even though extensive, can regress is demonstrated, in part, in individuals with cirrhosis of the liver and in those who have died of starvation.

Even a segmental *atheroma* can cause atrophy of the underlying arterial wall, and the concentric type seems to be associated with major destruction of the interna elastica and portions of the media. Such changes appear secondary to interference with the nutrients permeating the intima. Careful observation of these various stages of the atheroma strongly leads to the belief that an inability to clear hemic constituents, which have permeated the media, is a major feature in the lesion's development. That such a permeation is a most dynamic affair

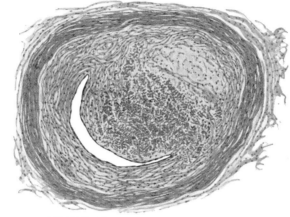

HEMORRHAGE INTO ATHEROMA, LEAVING
ONLY A SLITLIKE LUMEN

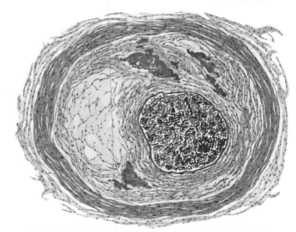

COMPLETE OCCLUSION BY THROMBUS IN LUMEN
GREATLY NARROWED BY ATHEROMA

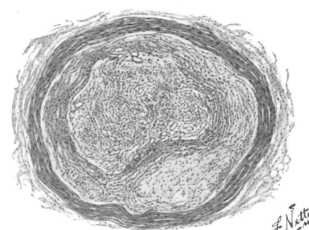

ORGANIZATION OF THROMBUS

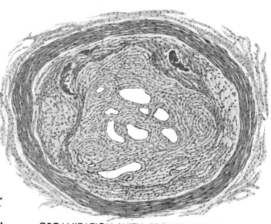

ORGANIZATION WITH RECANALIZATION
MAY OCCUR

can be demonstrated easily by perfusing isolated segments of living canine arteries and observing the quantity of lipid found in the vasa vasorum of the adventitia.

It is difficult to realize that, when the atheroma reaches the stage described above, it is still dynamic and still can undergo many changes. It can be dislodged from its moorings and thereby serve as an embolus, or pieces of it may break off and embolize. The occurrence of *hemorrhage* into such a lesion has been described, and it still is debatable whether blood is dissecting into the plaque from the surface or by hemorrhage from the vasa vasorum; both routes probably contribute. As can be predicted, thrombosis is a complication that *may completely occlude* the artery. If this occurs and the individual survives, *organization* of the fibrin clot progresses, with small new vessels *recanalizing* the organized area. However, the ability of these small vessels to supply any appreciable volume of blood beyond the area of blockade is doubtful, and this doubt is still further fortified by their appearance in arteriography. It also would seem possible that, on occa-

sion, a thrombus could completely disappear.

In addition to atheromatous and thrombotic blockade of the coronary arteries, emboli of all types can lodge within an otherwise-normal coronary artery. Such emboli can consist of bits of thrombi, valvular calcification, bits of tumor, and even, on occasion, small foreign bodies. Various kinds of inflammatory aortitis can involve the vessels; syphilis of the aortic wall can occlude the ostia, and surgeons can inadvertently disturb the blood flow. All these events can result in severe myocardial difficulties.

The atheroma, however, is the main disorder, but it would probably not be significant if it were not for its distribution. In the case of the coronary arteries, there is usually diffuse involvement by the time anatomic studies are done, and the involvement seems to be predominantly in the "free" portions of the arteries, prior to their branches entering the cardiac muscle. Those closest to the aorta are the plaques usually seen and exclaimed over, since, logically, they would seem to be the ones most likely to interfere with cardiac circulation.

CRITICAL AREAS OF ATHEROSCLEROSIS

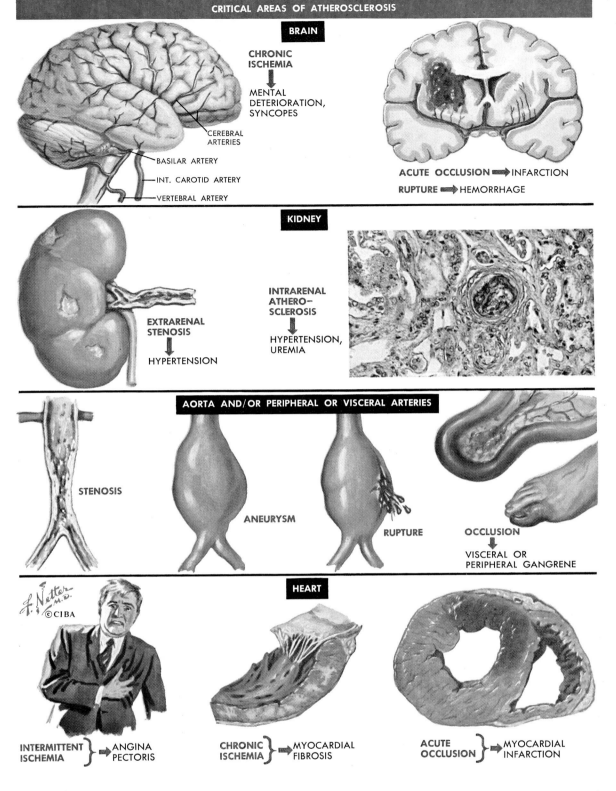

CRITICAL AREAS OF ATHEROSCLEROSIS

BRAIN

CHRONIC ISCHEMIA → MENTAL DETERIORATION, SYNCOPES

CEREBRAL ARTERIES

BASILAR ARTERY

INT. CAROTID ARTERY

VERTEBRAL ARTERY

ACUTE OCCLUSION → INFARCTION

RUPTURE → HEMORRHAGE

KIDNEY

EXTRARENAL STENOSIS → HYPERTENSION

INTRARENAL ATHERO-SCLEROSIS → HYPERTENSION, UREMIA

AORTA AND/OR PERIPHERAL OR VISCERAL ARTERIES

STENOSIS

ANEURYSM

RUPTURE

OCCLUSION → VISCERAL OR PERIPHERAL GANGRENE

HEART

INTERMITTENT ISCHEMIA → ANGINA PECTORIS

CHRONIC ISCHEMIA → MYOCARDIAL FIBROSIS

ACUTE OCCLUSION → MYOCARDIAL INFARCTION

For reasons not altogether clear, vascular disease, and hypertensive vascular disease in particular, suffers from comminution into special areas. This has resulted, often, in the failure to recognize that all are part of the *same general process*. For example, the recent federal law initiating the regional program for heart disease, cancer, *and* stroke illustrates the fact that the legislators did not wholly associate stroke with heart disease, and neither term clearly delineated the concept that both were, in reality, mostly vascular disease. This dichotomy has also resulted in a curious subdivision of specialists into neurologists who care for

strokes; cardiologists, the *heart;* and nephrologists, the *kidney.* Ultimately, there must be those with an overview of the whole circulation.

The *cerebral* circulation is particularly vulnerable in hypertensives. Stroke is the major cause of death. Hypertensive vascular disease is usually a combination of the specific arteriolar lesions resulting from the *hypertension* and *atherosclerosis.* The latter disease clearly seems to be accelerated by elevated blood pressure. *Infarction* of the *brain* is more common than *bleeding.* Bleeding seems to be chiefly the result of *rupture* of microaneurysms of the small arteries.

The coronary vessels are the ones next most vulnerable. *Angina pectoris* and *myocardial infarction* are the common results of the accelerated atherosclerosis. This fact heavily underscores the need for the

concurrent treatment of both the hypertension and the atherogenesis. Many persons have their blood pressure return to normal levels, only to die of the results of atherosclerosis.

The results of the increased rate of atherogenesis are to be seen in the *large vessels* besides the coronary arteries. Thus, *aneurysms* of the *aorta* and *renal arteries* are frequent, leading to dissection and ultimate *rupture.* Reducing blood pressure seems to have a clearly beneficial action on these lesions.

It needs to be stressed that about half of the problem of arterial hypertension is the problem of atherogenesis or atheropoiesis. Treatment should encompass both. Currently, much of the treatment of atherosclerosis is corrective. This is necessary, but prevention is the more important aspect.

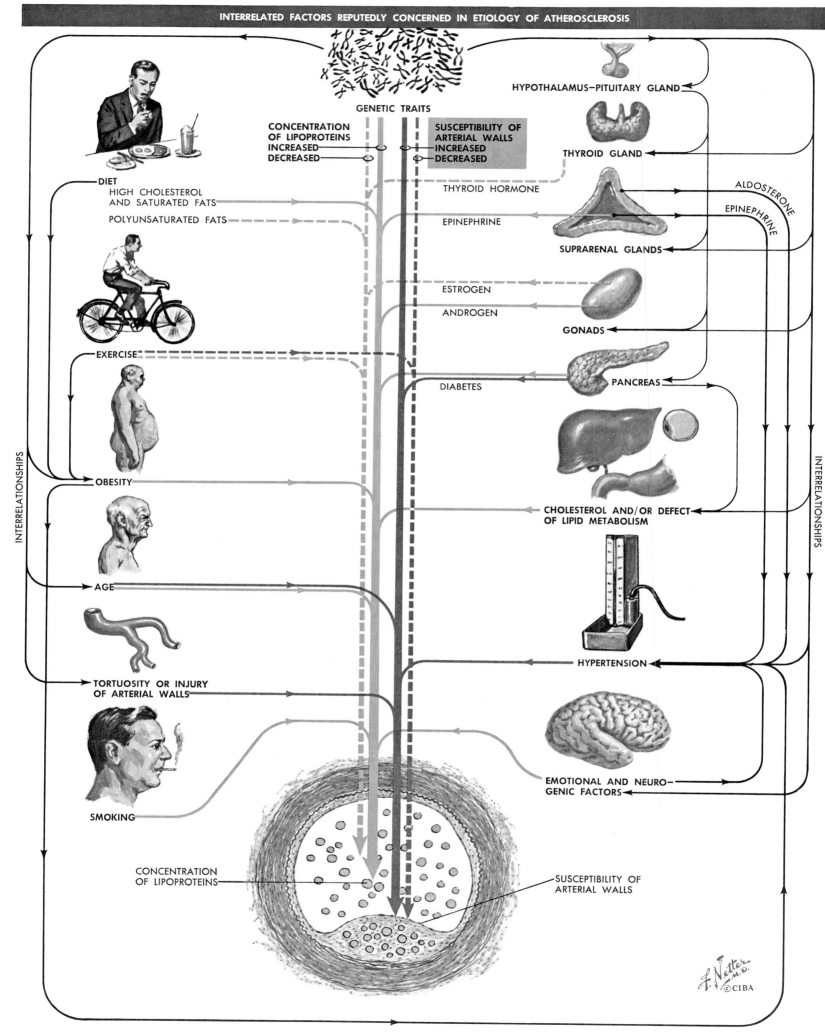

INTERRELATED FACTORS REPUTEDLY CONCERNED IN ETIOLOGY OF ATHEROSCLEROSIS

GENETIC TRAITS

CONCENTRATION OF LIPOPROTEINS INCREASED DECREASED

SUSCEPTIBILITY OF ARTERIAL WALLS INCREASED DECREASED

HYPOTHALAMUS–PITUITARY GLAND

THYROID GLAND

THYROID HORMONE

ALDOSTERONE

EPINEPHRINE

SUPRARENAL GLANDS

ESTROGEN

ANDROGEN

GONADS

DIABETES

PANCREAS

DIET
HIGH CHOLESTEROL AND SATURATED FATS
POLYUNSATURATED FATS

EXERCISE

OBESITY

CHOLESTEROL AND/OR DEFECT OF LIPID METABOLISM

AGE

TORTUOSITY OR INJURY OF ARTERIAL WALLS

HYPERTENSION

EMOTIONAL AND NEURO-GENIC FACTORS

SMOKING

INTERRELATIONSHIPS

INTERRELATIONSHIPS

CONCENTRATION OF LIPOPROTEINS

SUSCEPTIBILITY OF ARTERIAL WALLS

F. Netter
©CIBA

FACTORS IN ETIOLOGY OF ATHEROSCLEROSIS

In terms of mortality, certainly the most important single problem facing the more highly developed countries is *atherosclerosis* of the cardiac and cerebral blood vessels. In the past 2 decades it has become increasingly evident that there is no single cause of atherosclerosis (see also CIBA COLLECTION, Vol. 4, pages 212 and 213), and this is why Page, years ago, labeled it a "multifaceted disease" and a "disease of regulation." Atherosclerosis seems to reflect the culmination of many *factors* acting over a lifetime, and it usually becomes clinically manifest only when complications, such as thrombosis or aneurysm, occur.

All students of the subject are agreed that it has a strong *hereditary* background. So far, no one has been able to alter this aspect. The environment also may have an important contribution to make, but specific factors in it have not been positively identified. The hardness of the water is said by some to be correlated with the incidence of atherogenesis, but, as yet, there is no general acceptance of this thesis.

Recently, *cigarette smoking* has been found to be closely correlated with the incidence of coronary atherosclerosis and, as a result, cigarettes are being widely, if not altogether successfully, interdicted. Lack of *exercise* is also believed to be one of the deficiencies associated with myocardial infarction and coronary atherosclerosis. Some believe that the function of exercise is to improve collateral circulation and to increase the efficiency of oxygenation of the myocardium. It is being widely recommended for victims of an infarction.

Excessive saturated fat in the diet is still another factor believed to be involved importantly in atherogenesis. Countries in which the fat content of the diet approaches 40 percent of the total calories have an inordinately high incidence of coronary heart disease. The high-fat diets are believed to achieve their deleterious effects by increasing the levels of the blood lipids. Some consider that the *cholesterol* content of the blood is the most important constituent, while others stress *triglycerides*. Probably both are concerned through mediation of the *lipoproteins*, which act as the primary transport mechanism for lipids in the blood. Cholesterol is a convenient clinical measure of certain types of lipoproteins. Strong evidence suggests that *unsaturated fatty acids* with two or more double bonds aid in reducing cholesterol blood levels when their relationship to saturated fatty acids is increased. These are the bases for the current thinking regarding dietary control of atherogenesis.

Currently there are two mainstreams of thought about atherogenesis: (1) that it is chiefly due to infiltration of the blood vessel by fat from the bloodstream, and (2) that it is due to laying down of fibrin and/or platelet aggregates on the surface endothelium, followed by overgrowth of the latter to form a plaque; lipid infiltration is then a secondary phenomenon. Doubtless, both are correct and both simplistic.

The first hypothesis has led to an enormous increase in the study of the metabolism of cholesterol and other lipids that are found associated in atherosclerotic lesions. It has also led to a frantic search for drugs that lower blood lipids, because of the repetitive demonstration of the close association between cholesterol levels and the incidence of heart attacks. Currently d-thyroxine, nicotinic acid, Atromid-S®, and *estrogen* are under the most intensive study. Estrogens were introduced largely because it had been found that women, before the menopause, were about one fourth as susceptible to myocardial infarction as men.

The second hypothesis also has many adherents. Attempts have been made to associate the "stickiness" of the platelets to their aggregation as well as to injury of the blood-vessel endothelium. The conversion of fibrinogen to insoluble fibrin is also important in providing a matrix for surface thrombi. Capillary hemorrhage within the blood-vessel wall is usually considered to be secondary to the primary facets of atherogenesis, but any hemorrhage large enough to reduce the lumen of a coronary artery is potentially dangerous.

The endocrine glands have been closely associated with atherogenesis through a variety of mechanisms. The *pituitary gland* seems to exert some effect indirectly, through its regulatory arteries, on other endocrine glands. Reduced *thyroid* secretion is believed to accelerate atherogenesis. There has been no specific implication of the *suprarenal* corticoids but the *catecholamines* have been widely suspected. One view is that their effects are chiefly on the oxygenation of the myocardium, while others suggest that they mediate the effects of *emotional* strain and tobacco. There is clearly no unanimity on the mechanism of their participation. The influence of "femaleness" and the estrogen has already been mentioned. "Maleness" and the *androgen* may accentuate atherogenesis, but the proof for this effect is less convincing. The *pancreas* has been associated with atherogenesis because of the part it plays in *diabetes* and carbohydrate metabolism. One of the major complications of this disease is atherosclerosis; it appears earlier and is more severe than in healthy persons.

Obesity may or may not be associated with endocrine disturbance, but it is associated, to some degree, with increased atherogenesis, although probably not as importantly as it formerly was supposed.

The clinical effects of atherosclerosis are often determined by secondary factors. The *anatomy of the blood supply* to an organ may be critical, especially in the *pattern of the coronary vessels*. A strategically located atherosclerotic plaque may do far more damage than extensive, diffuse atherosclerosis. The formation of a clot, either on the surface of a plaque or by rupture of an atheromatous ulcer, may be the first clinical evidence of the presence of atherosclerosis. The effects of the latter have even been seen by the appearance of cholesterol crystals in the vessels of the eyegrounds.

Much emphasis has been given recently to identifying what is known as the "coronary profile." These are persons believed to be highly susceptible to coronary atherosclerosis and myocardial infarction. They are characterized by being male, short, stocky and muscular, and excessively aggressive, smoking large numbers of cigarettes, being obese, taking little exercise, being under *emotional pressure,* and having elevated blood cholesterol and triglyceride levels and, often, abnormal glucose tolerance. Friedman and Byers place more emphasis on the psychological responsiveness as a means of characterizing the people. While the "coronary profile" is a useful clinical generality, it often is inexact in its predictions.

In summary, it is now clear that atherosclerosis results from intimal and medial cellular defects that depend on the cellular *genetic* makeup interacting over long periods of time with exogenous and endogenous environmental factors. This is why it has been called a "multifaceted disease of regulation."

ARTERIOSCLEROTIC HEART DISEASE

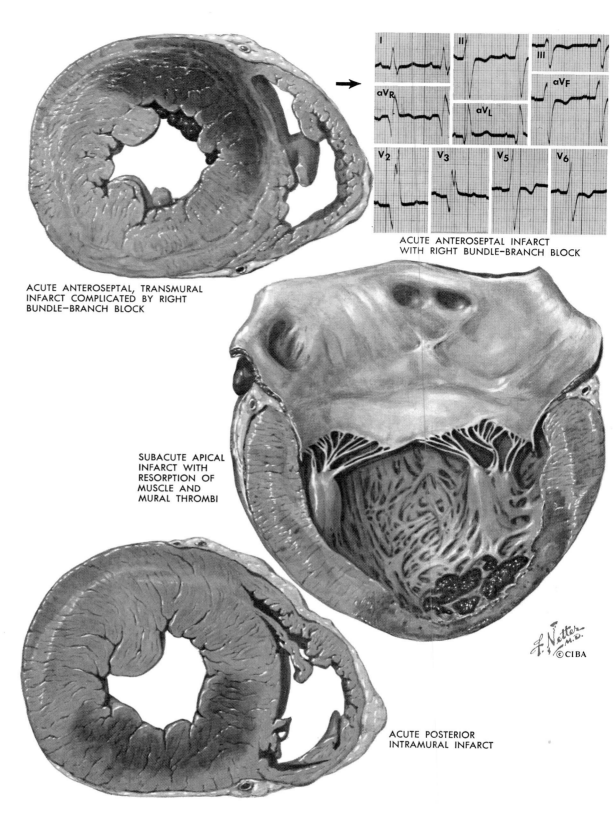

ACUTE ANTEROSEPTAL, TRANSMURAL
INFARCT COMPLICATED BY RIGHT
BUNDLE—BRANCH BLOCK

ACUTE ANTEROSEPTAL INFARCT
WITH RIGHT BUNDLE-BRANCH BLOCK

SUBACUTE APICAL
INFARCT WITH
RESORPTION OF
MUSCLE AND
MURAL THROMBI

ACUTE POSTERIOR
INTRAMURAL INFARCT

Myocardial infarction is the other side of the coin in the problem of coronary-artery disease and, again, it exhibits an extensive panorama of changes. Death of the cardiac muscle may occur as a zonal variety or as multiple foci scattered diffusely throughout the heart. The latter can be found following suboptimal perfusion of the heart, utilizing a pump oxygenator, wherein all the minute necrotic foci are of the same age. More commonly, however, the multiple minute foci can be found as destroyed zones of varying ages. In the acute phases these

microinfarcts may be extremely difficult to see and may be recognizable only microscopically as areas showing variable myofibril destruction and replacement by collagen. Chronically, these small foci may be minute white patches salted throughout the myocardium.

A larger myocardial infarct shows a variety of change that, in part, is dependent on the duration of the patient's survival following the episode of infarction. The earliest changes are associated with the resulting paralysis of vessel walls, engorgement of the capillaries, and migration of polymorphonuclear leukocytes. Some autolytic changes then occur, and the dead muscle fibers can be recognized as showing

a loss of striations and an increase in eosinophilia, fragmentation, and the gradual disappearance of nuclei. The dead muscle, by this time, has become an irritant, and a larger number of polymorphonuclear leukocytes appear. Finally, the subsequent activities of repair include macrophage infiltration and replacement fibrosis. If the *infarct* is minute, such a sequence is of relatively short duration, but, if it is large, remnants of necrotic muscle may be found several years later. It appears that such dead tissue has been effectively sealed away from the physiologic activities.

The infarct may be named according to the area

(Continued on page 219)

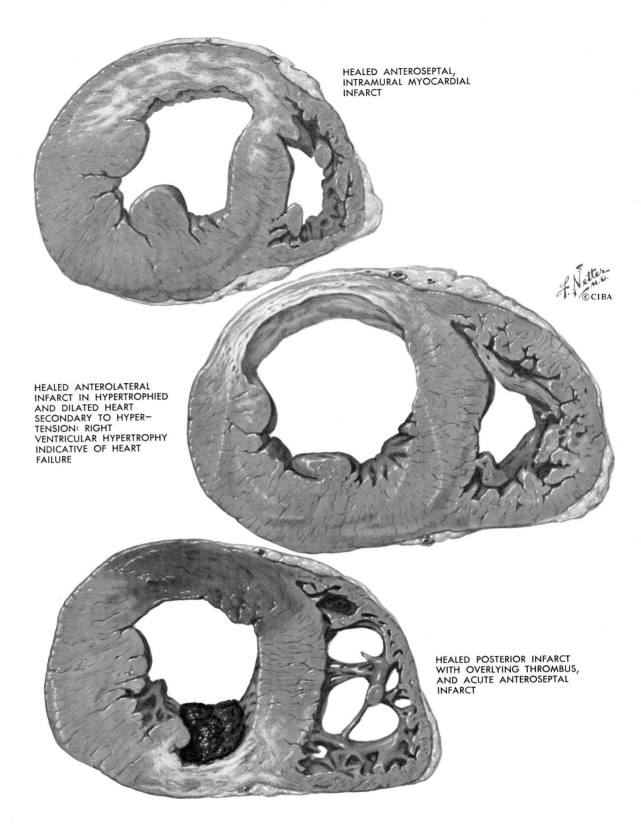

HEALED ANTEROSEPTAL,
INTRAMURAL MYOCARDIAL
INFARCT

HEALED ANTEROLATERAL
INFARCT IN HYPERTROPHIED
AND DILATED HEART
SECONDARY TO HYPER-
TENSION: RIGHT
VENTRICULAR HYPERTROPHY
INDICATIVE OF HEART
FAILURE

HEALED POSTERIOR INFARCT
WITH OVERLYING THROMBUS,
AND ACUTE ANTEROSEPTAL
INFARCT

ARTERIOSCLEROTIC HEART DISEASE

(*Continued from page 218*)

of the heart involved. Most of the posterior infarcts affect areas of the septum as well, and many of the anterior ones involve anterior portions of the septal wall, hence the terms *anteroseptal* and *posteroseptal*. In addition, a *lateral infarct* is found, occasionally, in a small percentage of the cases. The above-described sequence of events — muscle death, removal, and repair — may or may not result in thinning of the myocardium.

It is the author's opinion that myocardial infarction, at necropsy, appears to be different in various parts of the country: The farmers in southern Minnesota have a type of myocardial infarction different from those found in steelworkers of Cleveland.

Myocardial infarction may also be classified according to the thickness of the ventricular wall involved. If all layers of the ventricular wall are affected, the term *transmural* is used, and this type of lesion is associated, most commonly, with complete occlusion of the coronary artery. In about 90 percent of these lesions, complete occlusion is demonstrated, as contrasted with a lesser incidence in the other type known as *subendocardial*. In this latter type, a thin zone of muscle is spared between the endocardium and the zone of infarction. The infarcted muscle apparently

is the deep bulbospiral bundle area. It is easy to see how *mural thrombosis* may be a more common accompaniment of transmural myocardial infarction, but both of these lesions can show endocardial sclerosis, with much elastic-tissue deposition in the chronic phase.

One of the difficult enigmas, among many in the problem of coronary-artery disease, is the lack of many correlations between this disease and myocardial infarction, in an individual who has died. Although the appearance of a lesion in the anterior descending coronary artery or the main left coronary artery is a common finding in sudden death and,

(*Continued on page 220*)

ARTERIOSCLEROTIC HEART DISEASE

(Continued from page 219)

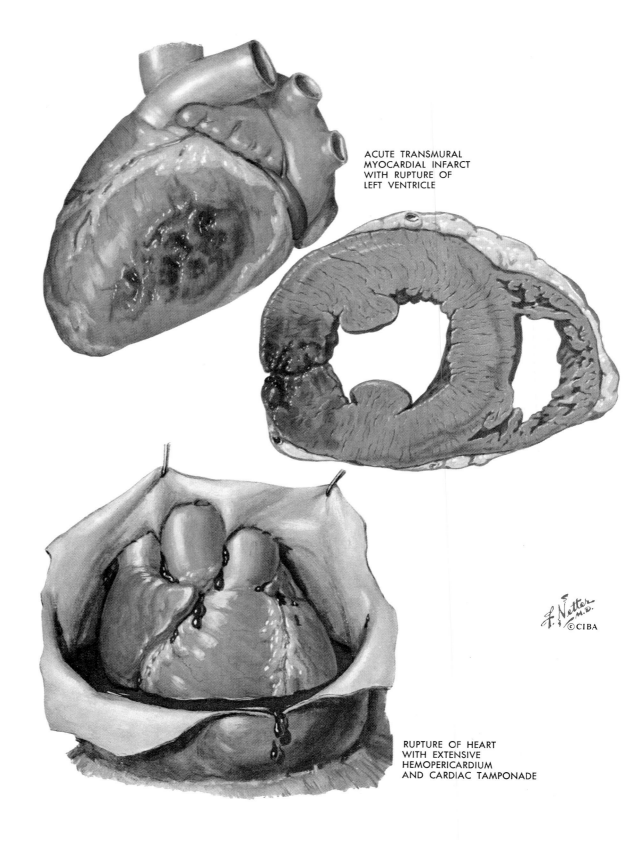

ACUTE TRANSMURAL
MYOCARDIAL INFARCT
WITH RUPTURE OF
LEFT VENTRICLE

RUPTURE OF HEART
WITH EXTENSIVE
HEMOPERICARDIUM
AND CARDIAC TAMPONADE

on occasion, may be the only lesion discovered, we do not know the status of the underlying cardiac muscle, since morphologic myocardial infarction cannot be demonstrated. In approximately 25 percent of the examples of myocardial infarction encountered at autopsy — either acute or chronic but, especially, chronic — no history can be elicited as to when such a disorder occurred. In hearts with acute myocardial infarctions, only about half show complete occlusion of the coronary artery, although the remainder exhibit a significant to marked

narrowing. In addition, an appreciable number of people, in whom the immediate cause of death was believed to be coronary-artery disease, have no demonstrable recent acute myocardial infarction.

These unknown quantities then leave one with a sense of frustration and a query as to whether, for all people with myocardial infarction, some sort of sensing equipment should be developed that might stimulate the heart in case it stopped beating. If the cause of death, in some of these individuals, is thalamic, hypothalamic, or conductive, they might be saved by such a device.

Exercise may be extremely valuable in all these situations, as recent studies seem to indicate that,

although the incidence of myocardial infarction is not lessened, the severity of the disease is less in those individuals who have maintained a tonic circulatory system.

In only a portion of the deaths can acute damage to areas of the conduction system, such as hemorrhage or infarction, be demonstrated. However, other complications are common. The immediate results of the changes in the circulatory status and constituents of the blood apparently can produce all types of thrombotic activity. These lead to a deposition of fibrin at numerous sites, including the coronary arteries, with a further extension of the myocardial

(Continued on page 221)

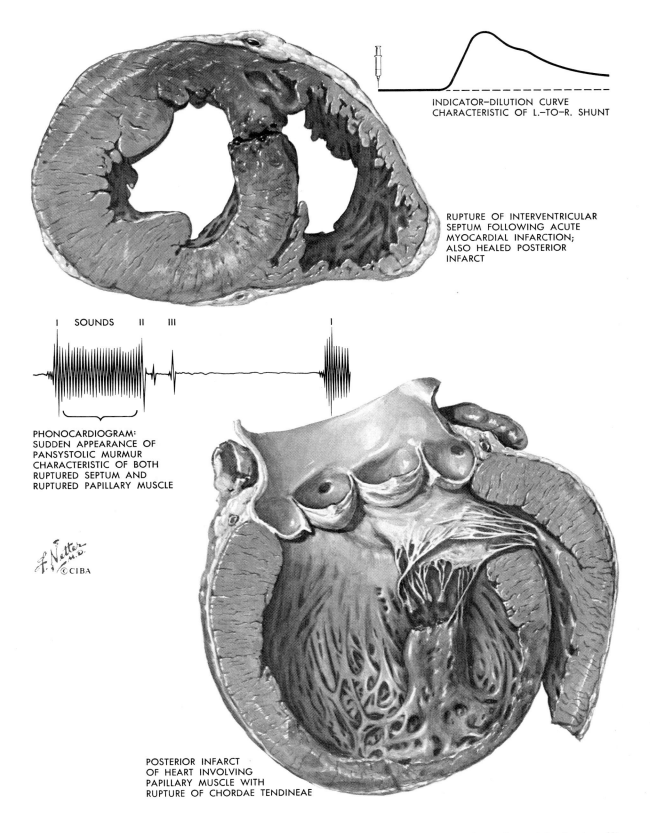

INDICATOR—DILUTION CURVE
CHARACTERISTIC OF L.-TO-R. SHUNT

RUPTURE OF INTERVENTRICULAR
SEPTUM FOLLOWING ACUTE
MYOCARDIAL INFARCTION;
ALSO HEALED POSTERIOR
INFARCT

SOUNDS II III

PHONOCARDIOGRAM:
SUDDEN APPEARANCE OF
PANSYSTOLIC MURMUR
CHARACTERISTIC OF BOTH
RUPTURED SEPTUM AND
RUPTURED PAPILLARY MUSCLE

POSTERIOR INFARCT
OF HEART INVOLVING
PAPILLARY MUSCLE WITH
RUPTURE OF CHORDAE TENDINEAE

ARTERIOSCLEROTIC HEART DISEASE

(Continued from page 220)

infarction. Mural thrombi form on the endocardium, in the auricles (much more commonly on the left than on the right), and possibly, at all sites where previous atheromas had existed. As a consequence, cerebral anoxia can occur not only as a result of the slowed circulation but also because of superimposed thrombosis during the early stages of the disease. Thrombosis also occurs in the systemic veins.

Unfortunately, embolism is a natural sequela of thrombosis, and systemic embolization occurs in an appreciable number of those individuals with thrombi in the left side of the heart. Cerebral embolism is the most damaging and the most severe, but saddle embolism of the aorta is also an extremely difficult situation, as is an embolization in an extremity. Smaller emboli may produce focal, splenic, and renal infarction. Mesenteric embolism, although not so common, may occur, and this is a medical disaster. Unfortunately, mural thrombi persist for a long period of time, and systemic embolization may occur at various periods following apparent recovery from the acute infarct. Pulmonary embolism is also common.

The hypoxic heart, like the hypertensive heart in failure, can dilate, with resultant valvular insufficiency and subsequent regurgitation. In the chronically failing hypertensive heart, jet lesions may occur on the endocardium, but they usually are not so common in the cardiac failure associated with coronary-artery disease. The collagenous tissue that forms valvular rings must be highly dependent upon oxygen to maintain its integrity, and, when oxygen is not supplied, these fibers will stretch, destroying valve competency.

Rupture of the heart is another necropsy finding that is subject to considerable variation. The incidence of cardiac rupture ranges from 1 to 10 per-

(Continued on page 222)

ARTERIOSCLEROTIC HEART DISEASE

(Continued from page 221)

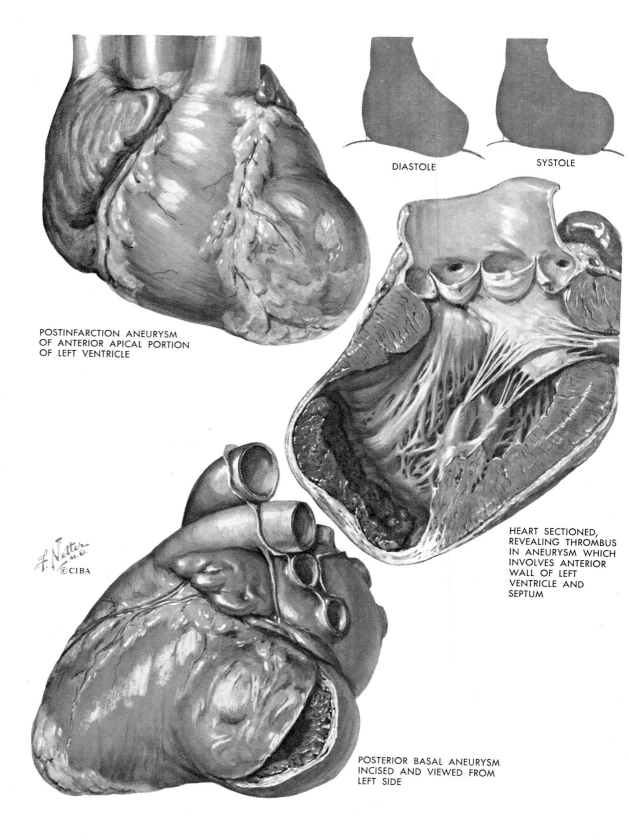

POSTINFARCTION ANEURYSM
OF ANTERIOR APICAL PORTION
OF LEFT VENTRICLE

DIASTOLE

SYSTOLE

HEART SECTIONED,
REVEALING THROMBUS
IN ANEURYSM WHICH
INVOLVES ANTERIOR
WALL OF LEFT
VENTRICLE AND
SEPTUM

POSTERIOR BASAL ANEURYSM
INCISED AND VIEWED FROM
LEFT SIDE

cent, in those deaths from acute myocardial infarction studied, and may be related to the amount of physical activity in the early phases of myocardial infarction. For some unknown reason, the area of rupture often shows the peculiar morphologic change of a large increase in polymorphonuclear leukocytes and at a much later time than such cellular elements are usually encountered. (Ruptures of the heart usually occur in the first week.) The possibility that an increased number of proteolytic enzymes may be available for myocardial lysis has

been implicated as an important cause of the rupture.

In addition to free rupture of the heart into the pericardial cavity and the resulting *cardiac tamponade, rupture of the interventricular septum* can occur on occasion. Rarely, *papillary muscles rupture,* and, for some unknown reason, the *posterior* muscle is more likely to do so than the anterior.

Anterior and apical aneurysm, as a chronic complication, has been alluded to clinically, and it too has some interesting pathologic problems. Mural thrombi are commonly found within, and, as a consequence, the patient is continually exposed to the problem of embolism. There is no good reason why the papillary muscles should not be incorporated within

the lesion, but such a lack seems to be the usual circumstance.

Finally, and unfortunately, it can be said of coronary-artery disease that it is never over. In addition to all the complications of embolism, cardiac aneurysm, sudden death, and rupture of the heart, there is the problem of reinfarction. In an appreciable number of hearts, there can be demonstrated not only the zone of an old infarct but also areas of a new one. The new infarct may be adjacent to the old, or it can occur in an entirely different area of the distribution of other coronary arteries. The ultimate is the finding of an *old* posterior, an *old* anterior, and a *new* lateral zone of infarction.

ANGINA PECTORIS

Angina pectoris, which literally means "strangling of the chest," has been recognized as a serious symptom ever since William Heberden first described it in 1768. His description has never been excelled, even though he did not connect it with disease of the coronary arteries, an association discovered later by Jenner. The one other most-vital discovery concerned with coronary arterial disease was that by Herrick who, in 1912, described the clinical condition of acute coronary thrombosis, the pain of which is like that of angina pectoris except that it lasts for hours instead of a few minutes, is often much more severe, is not usually brought on by effort or emotion, and is *not* relieved by nitroglycerin, which practically always subdues the pain of angina pectoris within 1 or 2 minutes.

Angina pectoris varies somewhat from patient to patient, but an average description of the *symptoms* includes a feeling of a heavy weight, oppression, or a choking sensation under the middle of the breastbone, and *pain,* extending a few inches to both sides of the *chest* and sometimes to the *arms* (especially the *left*), almost never to the back, and rarely to the neck and jaws. It resembles the discomfort that occurs in any muscle under a tourniquet. It is produced, as a rule, by *effort* or emotion, especially in the *cold* or when hurried or excited, and, particularly, *after meals* or *smoking*. It rarely lasts more than 2 or 3 minutes and may be *relieved quickly* by dissolving a nitroglycerin tablet under the tongue. (It is often prevented in the same way.) It must be differentiated from other symptoms, particularly from spasm of the esophagus or upper end of the stomach (cardiospasm) which is not induced by effort, and also from gallbladder pain, arthritis or bursitis in the left shoulder, neuritis, and the heart pain of nervous exhaustion or neurocirculatory asthenia.

Angina pectoris is *caused* by the aching of the ischemic myocardium. Ischemia of the heart muscle results from a decrease in the flow of blood from the coronary arteries due to the "rusting process" of the inner lining of the arteries (atherosclerosis).

The close relationship between angina pectoris and the pain of coronary thrombosis is well known. Fundamentally, they are due to the same disease process, but the prolongation of the pain when blood is clotting in the arteries — that is, coronary thrombosis — is caused by the protracted blockage of the blood supply. During that time, some heart muscle may perish, being replaced by a scar — a *myocardial infarct* — which takes several weeks to become solid.

The *prognosis* of angina pectoris varies greatly. Many patients who are sensible and reasonably careful, especially of their diet

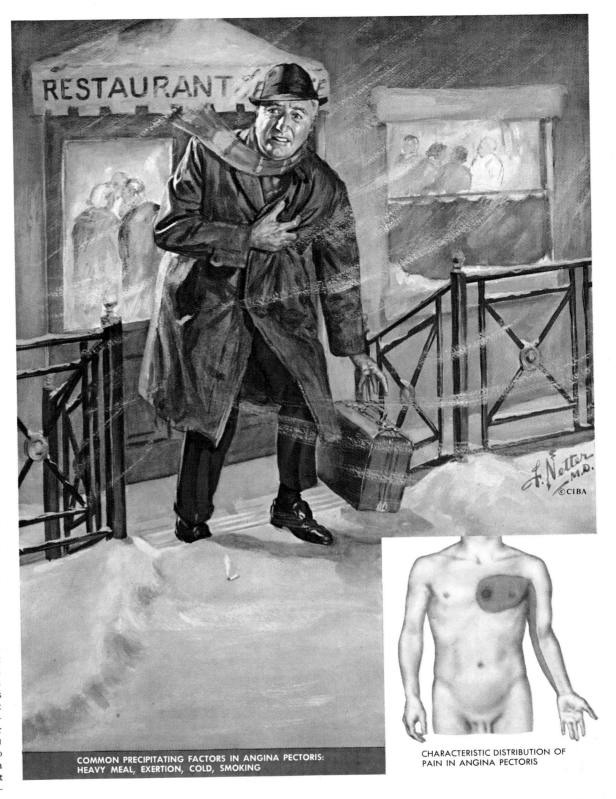

COMMON PRECIPITATING FACTORS IN ANGINA PECTORIS: HEAVY MEAL, EXERTION, COLD, SMOKING

CHARACTERISTIC DISTRIBUTION OF PAIN IN ANGINA PECTORIS

and weight, can continue to carry on their program of living, avoiding unnecessary stress. In the course of time (months or years), they may slowly get rid of their angina pectoris through the natural development of an adequate collateral circulation in their coronary arterial tree. If attacks come very frequently and occur at night, waking a patient from sleep (angina decubitus), the problem is more serious, and the individual should be advised to get more rest. Angina decubitus is always an important symptom, threatening life whenever it occurs, although this may happen hundreds of times. It probably kills by ventricular fibrillation. It is possible, by electrical means, to abolish such fibrillation and restore a normal heartbeat; many individuals who have been intensively watched, with suitable facilities at hand, have thus had their lives saved.

The *treatment* of angina pectoris is chiefly *medical* (see page 103), although *surgical* measures are now being proposed and tried, in an attempt to bring more blood to the heart muscle (see page 236) or to clear the coronary arteries of their obstructions. Rest and the avoidance of extra effort or emotional stress are essential, but mild exercise (walking) is helpful. The use of medicines, particularly nitrites, to dilate the vessels of the body and relieve the heart of some of its load as well as to flush out the heart muscle, is a routine measure. When coronary thrombosis threatens or prevails, more complete rest is necessary, and it is now generally customary to use anticoagulants also, at least for some months.

Most important of all is the *prevention* of the underlying disease which causes angina pectoris, and measures of this sort are now being studied with intensity. Such prevention, as far as our present knowledge is concerned, consists (especially in candidates for the disease, as shown by family history and a high serum cholesterol) of the avoidance of obesity, the establishment of a sensible diet low in animal fat, routine vigorous exercise in the absence of heart disease, and no smoking. These measures deserve first priority in any program, and they should start in early youth.

INTERDEPENDENT AND INTERACTING FACTORS IN BLOOD-PRESSURE REGULATION

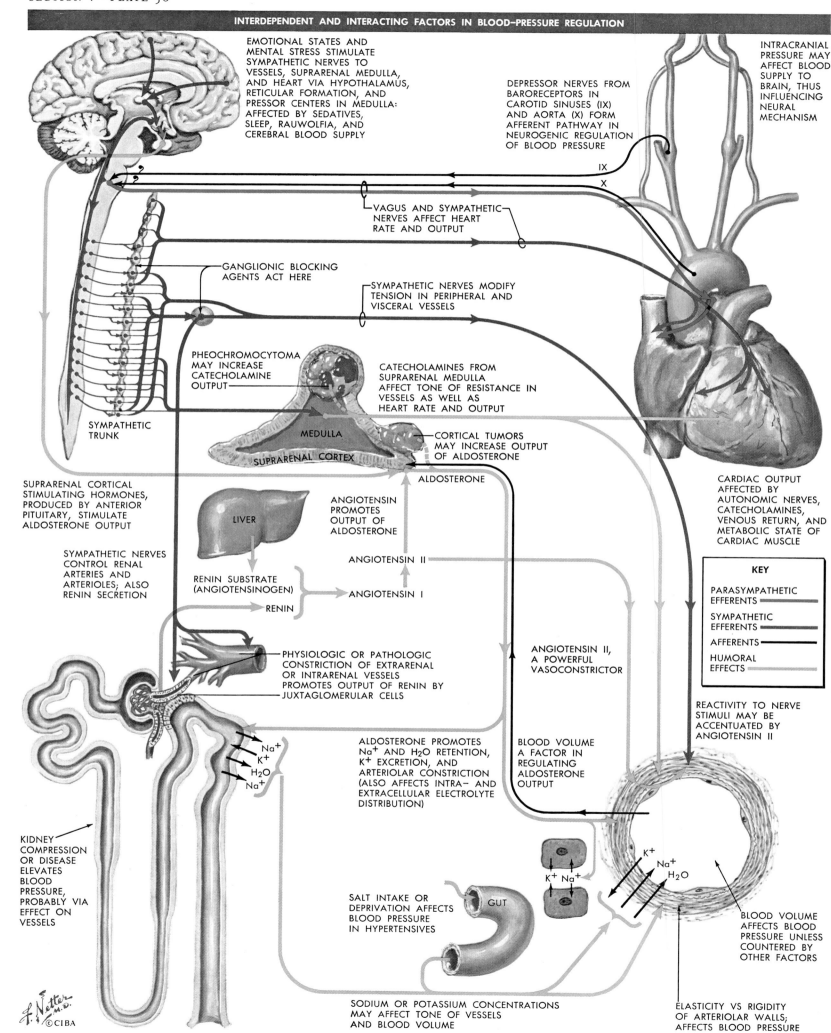

EMOTIONAL STATES AND MENTAL STRESS STIMULATE SYMPATHETIC NERVES TO VESSELS, SUPRARENAL MEDULLA, AND HEART VIA HYPOTHALAMUS, RETICULAR FORMATION, AND PRESSOR CENTERS IN MEDULLA: AFFECTED BY SEDATIVES, SLEEP, RAUWOLFIA, AND CEREBRAL BLOOD SUPPLY

DEPRESSOR NERVES FROM BARORECEPTORS IN CAROTID SINUSES (IX) AND AORTA (X) FORM AFFERENT PATHWAY IN NEUROGENIC REGULATION OF BLOOD PRESSURE

INTRACRANIAL PRESSURE MAY AFFECT BLOOD SUPPLY TO BRAIN, THUS INFLUENCING NEURAL MECHANISM

IX

X

VAGUS AND SYMPATHETIC NERVES AFFECT HEART RATE AND OUTPUT

GANGLIONIC BLOCKING AGENTS ACT HERE

SYMPATHETIC NERVES MODIFY TENSION IN PERIPHERAL AND VISCERAL VESSELS

PHEOCHROMOCYTOMA MAY INCREASE CATECHOLAMINE OUTPUT

CATECHOLAMINES FROM SUPRARENAL MEDULLA AFFECT TONE OF RESISTANCE IN VESSELS AS WELL AS HEART RATE AND OUTPUT

SYMPATHETIC TRUNK

MEDULLA

SUPRARENAL CORTEX

CORTICAL TUMORS MAY INCREASE OUTPUT OF ALDOSTERONE

ALDOSTERONE

CARDIAC OUTPUT AFFECTED BY AUTONOMIC NERVES, CATECHOLAMINES, VENOUS RETURN, AND METABOLIC STATE OF CARDIAC MUSCLE

SUPRARENAL CORTICAL STIMULATING HORMONES, PRODUCED BY ANTERIOR PITUITARY, STIMULATE ALDOSTERONE OUTPUT

LIVER

ANGIOTENSIN PROMOTES OUTPUT OF ALDOSTERONE

ANGIOTENSIN II

SYMPATHETIC NERVES CONTROL RENAL ARTERIES AND ARTERIOLES; ALSO RENIN SECRETION

RENIN SUBSTRATE (ANGIOTENSINOGEN)

ANGIOTENSIN I

RENIN

KEY

PARASYMPATHETIC EFFERENTS

SYMPATHETIC EFFERENTS

AFFERENTS

HUMORAL EFFECTS

ANGIOTENSIN II, A POWERFUL VASOCONSTRICTOR

PHYSIOLOGIC OR PATHOLOGIC CONSTRICTION OF EXTRARENAL OR INTRARENAL VESSELS PROMOTES OUTPUT OF RENIN BY JUXTAGLOMERULAR CELLS

REACTIVITY TO NERVE STIMULI MAY BE ACCENTUATED BY ANGIOTENSIN II

Na^+
K^+
H_2O
Na^+

ALDOSTERONE PROMOTES Na^+ AND H_2O RETENTION, K^+ EXCRETION, AND ARTERIOLAR CONSTRICTION (ALSO AFFECTS INTRA- AND EXTRACELLULAR ELECTROLYTE DISTRIBUTION)

BLOOD VOLUME A FACTOR IN REGULATING ALDOSTERONE OUTPUT

KIDNEY COMPRESSION OR DISEASE ELEVATES BLOOD PRESSURE, PROBABLY VIA EFFECT ON VESSELS

K^+
Na^+

K^+
Na^+
H_2O

SALT INTAKE OR DEPRIVATION AFFECTS BLOOD PRESSURE IN HYPERTENSIVES

GUT

BLOOD VOLUME AFFECTS BLOOD PRESSURE UNLESS COUNTERED BY OTHER FACTORS

SODIUM OR POTASSIUM CONCENTRATIONS MAY AFFECT TONE OF VESSELS AND BLOOD VOLUME

ELASTICITY VS RIGIDITY OF ARTERIOLAR WALLS; AFFECTS BLOOD PRESSURE

Hypertension — A Disease of Regulation

Arterial blood pressure is only one of the functions that serves the purpose of perfusing tissues. Because organs require different amounts of blood at different times, blood must be withdrawn from one part of the body and transferred to the part in need, in the right amount and at the right time. This is a hemodynamic problem of great complexity. To solve it, the body has many regulatory devices, all working in concert. It is the interrelated and equilibrated system which has been called "the mosaic theory" of hypertension.

To understand the many factors which control arterial blood pressure, it is necessary to grasp the physiology and biochemistry of these multiple mechanisms. This is not merely an academic exercise but applies to diagnosis, treatment, and prognosis. The varied facets of this regulatory mechanism may be divided into four groups: (1) the renal, (2) the endocrine, (3) the neural, and (4) the cardiovascular factors. These divisions are wholly artificial since, in life, they are all interdependent and maintain themselves in equilibrium. Several of these regulatory mechanisms are of the feedback type, which means there are mechanisms that sense the need for blood and those for the delivery of it in an orderly way, so as not to deprive an essential organ, such as the brain, of blood because of the demand of other less essential tissues.

Chemical Mechanisms

Renal Factors. An enzyme, *renin,* is contained in the *juxtaglomerular cells* surrounding the afferent arterioles in the *kidneys*. Its secretion is under the influence of *mean arteriolar pressure, sodium content* of the tubular fluid, and the *neural innervation* of the juxtaglomerular cells. Released into the bloodstream, it splits *renin substrate (angiotensinogen)* to produce *angiotensin I,* which, in turn, is split by converting enzymes to *angiotensin II,* a polypeptide containing 8 amino acids. Angiotensin II is the most powerful known pressor substance, has a powerful regulating influence on the secretion of *aldosterone,* and is actively involved in the genesis of renovascular hypertension.

Angiotensin has become the focal point of the proposed mechanisms responsible for renal hypertension. It is believed that *obstructive lesions* of the renal artery cause hypertension by the large release of renin, with formation of angiotensin. If only for this reason, several methods have been proposed recently for clinical use in determining the blood levels of angiotensin and renin. So far, none of them has proved simple in application.

Angiotensin has a complex pharmacological action. It is not certain whether the small, almost immeasurable, amounts present in normal blood have any important action. The notion is growing that they participate normally in the *regulation of salt excretion by the kidneys*. It appears that when its level rises to easily detectable amounts, overt arterial *hypertension* occurs. There are many effects of angiotensin which have not been adequately studied but which suggest that it acts in concert with other humoral agents in the control of tissue perfusion. As an example, one may cite the action of minute amounts of angiotensin injected into the blood supply of the suprarenal gland, causing the large secretion of catecholamines. Instead of the trivial rise in blood pressure to be expected from so small an amount of angiotensin, a preternaturally large one occurs. While efforts have been made to find an antagonist to angiotensin similar to those blocking the action of norepinephrine, they have not been successful.

The kidney also has other methods of regulating blood pressure. One of them is by control of *salt and water* metabolism. It has long been known that low-salt diets reduce blood pressure, and this is one of the reasons for the use of diuretics in the treatment of hypertension. Salt causes the *retention of water,* and the increase in water raises the *blood volume* which, in turn, *increases blood pressure*. This phenomenon is seen clearly, especially when both kidneys are removed from a patient preparatory to renal transplantation. As salt and water are retained, blood volume rises, as does arterial pressure. If the salt is dialysed away, pressure usually returns to normal. There are probably other ways through which·salt elicits hypertension, as illustrated by especially bred salt-sensitive rats.

There is growing evidence that substances of a phospholipid nature, capable of regulating the function of the enzyme renin, also are contained in the kidneys, but their participation in the mechanisms of hypertension has not been proved.

Several experimental models of renal hypertension have been developed. The two most commonly used are the adjustable clamp on the renal artery, and the fibrous capsule resulting from the application of cellophane to the renal parenchyma. Much of the knowledge of the mechanism of human hypertension has come from the study of these experimental counterparts.

Human renal hypertension has multiple causes, some of which are correctable by surgery or drugs. The detection of obstructive lesions in the renal arteries by renal angiography has greatly aided the surgeon in their removal, and this has resulted in a reasonably high cure rate. Treatment of pyelonephritis may also result in lowering the blood pressure, provided the parenchyma of the kidneys is not too badly scarred.

Endocrine Factors. Tumors of the *suprarenal medulla* produce paroxysmal types of hypertension, and those of the *cortex* a more moderate but sustained hypertension. These are illustrated by pheochromocytoma and primary aldosteronism. Since *angiotensin* has a strong *controlling influence on aldosterone secretion* and the latter strongly retains salt, it is believed that this retention of salt and water is one of the important mechanisms of hypertension. Another possible mechanism is the stimulation by angiotensin of the release of catecholamines from the suprarenal medulla.

Recently, there has been much discussion as to whether many patients with a diagnosis of essential hypertension do not, in fact, have primary aldosteronism, many of them being normokalemic. Decreased tolerance to carbohydrate is believed to be one of the characteristics. The finding of *suprarenal cortical* adenomas has also been used as evidence to bolster this notion. However, most students of the subject categorize this as a rare syndrome, seldom involved in patients diagnosed as having essential hypertension.

Aldosterone antagonists have found limited usefulness in the treatment of not only hypertension of suprarenal origin but also early essential hypertension. When the patient is losing large amounts of *potassium* as a part of secondary hyperaldosteronism, such antagonists are especially helpful.

Other Mechanisms

Neural Factors. The neural network regulating blood pressure is vast and complicated. A *mental component,* characterized chiefly by *emotions of hostility,* may play some part in the mechanisms of hypertension. The *sympathetic nervous system,* and to a much lesser degree the parasympathetic, actively participates in vascular regulation. Probably the most powerful *regulatory device* is the *carotid-sinus baroreceptor*. The central integrating areas for vasomotor control are widely scattered in the brain but occur especially in the midbrain and medulla. The efferent pathways end on the blood vessels, heart, suprarenal medulla, and juxtaglomerular cells.

The neural component exhibits the phenomenon of negative feedback and baroreceptor resetting. When arterial pressure rises in the carotid sinus, the vasomotor activity, especially of the medulla oblongata, is inhibited, and peripheral resistance falls, and vice versa. Normal average blood-pressure levels are thus maintained. But if the elevation in arterial pressure is persistent, resetting of the barostat occurs, and now the carotid-sinus regulatory mechanism tries to maintain the elevated pressure. In short, inhibition does not occur until the preternaturally high pressure has been further exceeded. The normal level has now been reset upward. This is one reason, among several, why it is necessary to maintain blood pressure *persistently* at lower levels, with drugs, to have treatment be maximally effective. The same sort of resetting phenomenon appears to exist in the control of renin release by the kidneys.

Cardiovascular Factors. Arteries and *arterioles* have an inherent *tone* which responds with change to the needs of tissue; it is autoregulatory. Besides this, the anatomy of the blood vessels is so tailored to the particular needs of an organ as to aid in the regulation of its blood supply. Lastly, the responsiveness of blood vessels to a great variety of stimuli may change; for example, under some circumstances the blood vessels may constrict about ten times as powerfully in response to the same stimulus. This phenomenon has been called "cardiovascular reactivity." One of the results of hypertension is the increase in the rate of development of atherosclerosis.

Blood vessels exhibit what is called "autoregulation" which is just what the name indicates — the ability to adjust their caliber to the needs of the tissue with a changing blood pressure. Thus, kidneys need not become ischemic when arterial pressure falls. The mechanism of autoregulation is not known, although it has been extensively studied. It is a powerful regulatory force that seems to be inherent in the function of the smooth muscle of blood vessels, although this, admittedly, is no true explanation of the phenomenon.

CAUSES OF SECONDARY HYPERTENSION POSSIBLY AMENABLE TO SURGERY

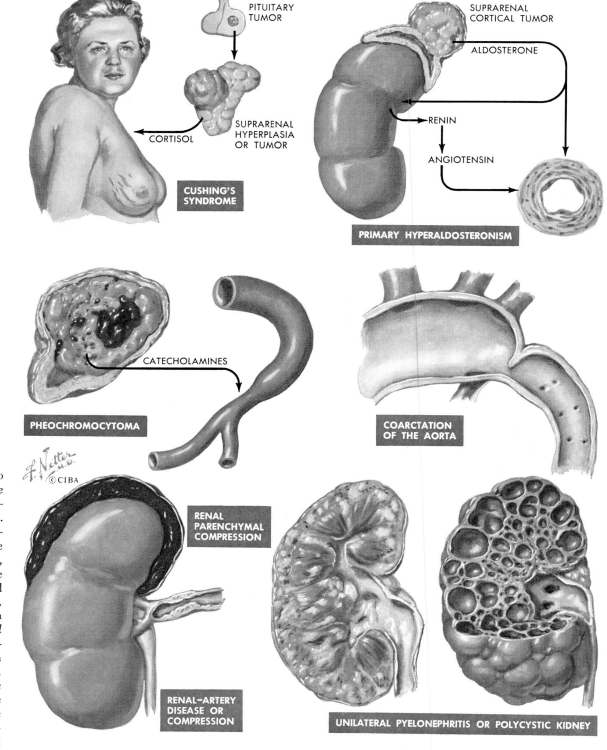

CAUSES OF SECONDARY HYPERTENSION WHICH MAY BE AMENABLE TO SURGERY

PITUITARY TUMOR

SUPRARENAL HYPERPLASIA OR TUMOR

CORTISOL

CUSHING'S SYNDROME

SUPRARENAL CORTICAL TUMOR

ALDOSTERONE

RENIN

ANGIOTENSIN

PRIMARY HYPERALDOSTERONISM

CATECHOLAMINES

PHEOCHROMOCYTOMA

COARCTATION OF THE AORTA

RENAL PARENCHYMAL COMPRESSION

RENAL–ARTERY DISEASE OR COMPRESSION

UNILATERAL PYELONEPHRITIS OR POLYCYSTIC KIDNEY

Certainly, *hypertension secondary to obstruction to the flow of blood to the kidneys* is the most common form of arterial hypertension correctable by surgery. The recognition of this form of renovascular hypertension is chiefly by the use of radiography, with which the vessels, both large and small, are visualized. The most common obstruction is produced by arteriosclerosis. To elicit hypertension, there must be a substantial reduction in mean blood pressure within the *renal artery*. Surgical correction of such stenosis has been notably successful and often has restored blood pressure to normal. Much less common is *compression of the renal parenchyma* by a connective-tissue hull or by blood clots pressing on the parenchyma. Such lesions have been followed by malignant hypertension, and their correction by cure. Because of this success, even though rare, these conditions should not be overlooked.

Primary aldosteronism is now a well-recognized cause of what is usually very moderate arterial hypertension. The hypertension is abolished when the *tumor of the suprarenal cortex* is surgically removed. Since *aldosterone* secretion is importantly determined by *angiotensin* from the kidneys, increased amounts of aldosterone may be secreted in hypertension of primary renal origin. This may be one reason why low-salt diets and aldosterone antagonists are often valuable in the treatment of renovascular hypertension.

Pyelonephritis, especially in its ad-

vanced stages, is a relatively common cause of arterial hypertension. Often it occurs *unilaterally,* thus providing an opportunity for surgical treatment by nephrectomy. Since pyelonephritis is commonly bilateral, it is important that nephrectomy not be performed in such patients unless there are indications other than the treatment of the hypertension. *Polycystic disease of the kidneys* may also be associated with hypertension, especially when the kidneys have become scarred, and pressure on the parenchyma is occurring. Draining of the cysts is rarely helpful.

Pheochromocytoma is not common, but, when it occurs, this tumor of the suprarenal medulla usually produces dramatic clinical signs and symptoms. There are several well-known provocative diagnostic tests. Surgical removal of the tumor usually, but not always,

results in the maintenance of normal blood pressure. Occasionally, the blood pressure does not return to normal, because there are other, very small, undetected tumors not removed, or other causes for the hypertension.

Correction of *coarctation of the aorta* is usually followed by cure of the hypertension, both proximal and distal to the obstruction. This operation was one of the first to be performed in the now-burgeoning field of cardiac surgery.

A rare form of hypertension is that associated with *Cushing's syndrome*. It is believed to be chiefly of suprarenal origin, although Cushing himself thought of it as primarily of *pituitary* origin. Removal of the *pituitary tumors* is believed to be useful, although the evidence is not substantial.

EYEGROUNDS IN HYPERTENSION

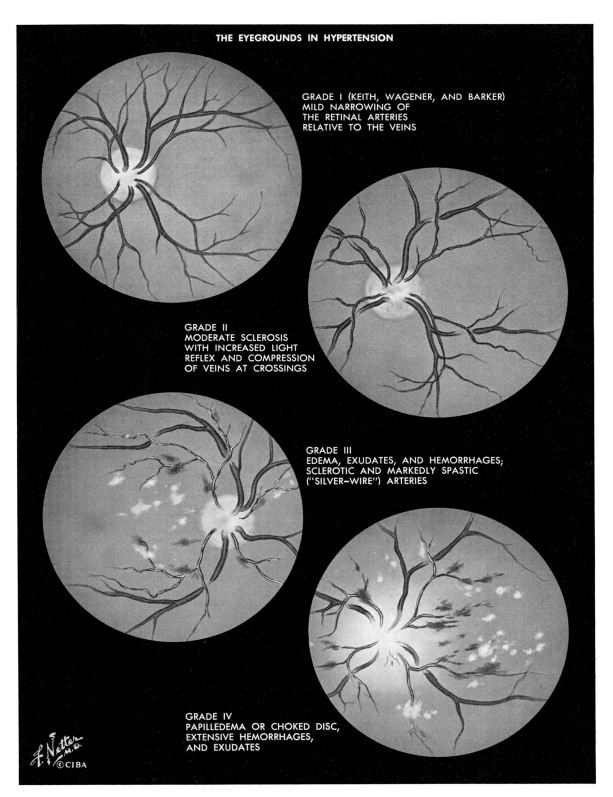

THE EYEGROUNDS IN HYPERTENSION

GRADE I (KEITH, WAGENER, AND BARKER)
MILD NARROWING OF
THE RETINAL ARTERIES
RELATIVE TO THE VEINS

GRADE II
MODERATE SCLEROSIS
WITH INCREASED LIGHT
REFLEX AND COMPRESSION
OF VEINS AT CROSSINGS

GRADE III
EDEMA, EXUDATES, AND HEMORRHAGES;
SCLEROTIC AND MARKEDLY SPASTIC
("SILVER-WIRE") ARTERIES

GRADE IV
PAPILLEDEMA OR CHOKED DISC,
EXTENSIVE HEMORRHAGES,
AND EXUDATES

Direct observation of *eyegrounds* is of the greatest importance in following the course of hypertensive vascular disease. It is the only part of the body where *arterioles* may be seen, and it is the arterioles which constitute the greatest locus of resistance to blood flow.

Various schemes are used for the *grading of eyegrounds,* but the most commonly used, over the longest period, has been that of Keith, Wagener, and Barker, as follows:

Grade I. Retinal changes consist of *mild narrowing* or *mild sclerosis* of the *arterioles.* It is compatible with good health for many years. The blood pressure is not excessively high, and it falls during rest.

Grade II. The changes in the retinal vessels are *more marked* than in grade I, but retinitis is not present. The disease is more progressive and the blood pressure is higher and more sustained, but the general health is good, and cardiac and renal function are satisfactory.

Grade III. Angiospastic retinitis, together with *definite sclerotic changes* in

the arterioles, occurs, but edema of the disc is not always present. The hypertension is high and sustained. Although cardiac and renal function may be adequate, sometimes there are alterations, as indicated by dyspnea on exertion, changes in the electrocardiogram, and nocturia. Nervousness, headache, vertigo, and visual disturbances may occur. Proteinuria and hematuria may be present.

Grade IV. The important retinal alteration is *edema of the discs.* There is also *marked* spastic and organic narrowing of the arterioles with *diffuse retinitis.* Characteristic *symptoms* are nervousness, asthenia, loss of weight, headache, visual disturbances, dyspnea on exertion, and nocturia. Proteinuria, cylindruria, and red blood cells are usually present. The prognosis is serious.

It is important for the physician to become thoroughly familiar with the appearance of the retinal blood vessels *during the varied stages of hypertension.* For this reason, it is best that he examine the eyegrounds repeatedly himself, rather than rely on a consultant. The left eye often may have more extensive changes in it than the right. The normal cupping of the nerve head should be carefully noted so that, when *papilledema* occurs, it will not be overlooked. Papilledema may occur in the presence of normal or only slightly elevated spinal-fluid pressure. The *hemorrhages* of hypertension should be differentiated from those of diabetes. *Exudates* may be fresh or mature.

Under *proper treatment,* the severe changes characterizing malignant hypertension may be *reversed.*

OCCLUSIVE DISEASE OF MAIN RENAL ARTERY

The recognition of a naturally occurring renovascular hypertension in man, that closely parallels Goldblatt's experiments with constriction of the renal artery, has progressed rapidly during the last decade. Such a cause as stenosis of a renal artery is eagerly sought, for many patients with this condition can, by surgery, be returned to a normotensive state. Undoubtedly, the erroneous designation of an ischemic kidney as an example of pyelonephritis (either by the original observer or, secondarily, by an expert interpreter of an earlier literary effort) contributed to a long period when hypertension due to *renal-artery disease* was thought, by most students of the disorder, not to exist. This misapprehension prevailed, in the face of evidence to the contrary, until the late 1930s.

The early studies of Howard and of Poutasse did much to stimulate the search for another anatomic cause of hypertension. The development of *aortography* (and, subsequently, selective renal *angiography*) was probably the greatest single achievement in diagnosing disease of the main renal artery. Not only have experts in this field been able to demonstrate constricting lesions in general, but further refinements have allowed the recognition of exact types of renal-artery disease, in the vast majority of cases, by distinguishing similar lesions that differ from one another clinically, anatomically, and symptomatically.

Atherosclerosis

Atherosclerosis is the most common cause of occlusive arterial disease in general and of renal-artery stenosis in particular. Although this variety of renal-artery disease predominates in older men, it also is found in women. It usually involves the origin and first portion of the renal artery, although, occasionally, plaques may be found more distally in a *renal-artery branch*. Arteriographically, the lesion commonly appears eccentric and is a *plaque* that involves merely a portion of the circumference of the artery. The lesion, in addition to its eccentric form, also dominantly involves the intima. For these reasons, endarterectomy can be performed, as a decreased plane may be developed between the diseased portion and the remainder of the arterial wall. (This is not true in other types of renal-artery disease.) At times, the lesions may be completely *concentric*, even involving most of the *media* in addition to destroying the *intima*.

Besides hypertension and damage to the kidney, two other complications may be found: As in general atherosclerosis, *thrombosis* may be superimposed upon the lesion. Also, a most unusual morphologic problem — a *dissecting aneurysm* — may be encountered. Blood striking an endothelial-lined channel in an abnormal manner, as must

SEVERE CONCENTRIC ATHEROSCLEROSIS OF RENAL ARTERY WITH LIPID DEPOSITION AND CALCIFICATION, COMPLICATED BY THROMBOSIS (COMPOSITE, X 12)

TRANSLUMBAR AORTOGRAM AND RENAL ARTERIOGRAM, REVEALING ATHEROSCLEROTIC AND THROMBOTIC OCCLUSION OF R. RENAL ARTERY

SELECTIVE ARTERIOGRAM DEMONSTRATING ASYMMETRICAL NARROWING OF PROXIMAL L. RENAL ARTERY BY ATHEROSCLEROTIC PLAQUE

INTIMAL FIBROPLASIA IN RENAL ARTERY CLOSE TO AORTA IN AN INFANT (VERHOEFF—VAN GIESON STAIN, X 55)

ANEURYSMAL LESIONS OF R. RENAL ARTERY

INTIMAL FIBROPLASIA IN BRANCH OF RENAL ARTERY:
L=LUMEN OF ARTERY
A=CAVITY OF DISSECTING ANEURYSM
(VERHOEFF—VAN GIESON STAIN, X 18)

occur distal to these plaques, results in breaks in the intima, with channels of blood dissecting into the arterial wall. Much of the time, these channels dissect merely for short distances, forming what might, more logically, be called an intramural hematoma. At other times, they dissect for appreciably greater distances along the renal artery. However, the pressure gradient distal to the plaque appears to be so much less that sufficient force is not exerted for dissection into the main aorta. It seems that, as soon as blood passes beneath the occluding zone, distal pressure lessens, and no more dissection occurs.

Fibrotic Lesions

The second general group of renal arterial lesions may be classified as fibrotic (nonatheromatous). A general term applied to all these fibromuscular hyperplasias has been sufficient in some instances, but a variety of clinically and pathologically distinctive lesions also may be encountered, and, since no etiologies have been ascer-

tained for any of these, a descriptive nomenclature has been developed that is based primarily on the location of the arterial damage.

Intimal Fibroplasia. This disease affects the main renal artery or its branches and is found, most commonly, in young males, although it may occur in both sexes and all age groups. When not complicated by dissection, the lesion produces a fusiform narrowing of the renal artery. This lesion may not be limited to a renal artery and has been described in many locations; its morphology is very similar to that of endarteritis obliterans of the smaller arteries. Even in children, other main arteries have been involved. *Microscopically,* most commonly a diffuse circumferential thickening of the media is seen, but, on occasion, it seems as though a thin layer of collagen has been applied to an underlying *elastica interna* that has been thrown into marked folds. In addition, those affected arteries found in the young show marked alterations of the internal elastic membrane (usually, reduplication).

(Continued on page 229)

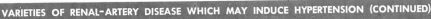

OCCLUSIVE DISEASE OF MAIN RENAL ARTERY

(Continued from page 228)

Medial Fibroplasia with Aneurysms. This renal-artery disorder was originally interpreted, roentgenographically, as fibromuscular hyperplasia. Characteristically, the *roentgenogram* resembles a *"string of beads,"* with dilated irregularities of the artery; this beading appears larger than the diameter of the origin of the artery, which is usually spared. The disease is primarily a disorder of women and, unfortunately, is commonly bilateral. It does not, exclusively, affect the renal artery but has been reported in other locations.

The morphology is most unusual. When opened longitudinally, the afflicted artery appears similar to the diverticulosis of the colon (in miniature). Small outpouchings can be seen, distorting the arterial wall. A most bizarre *microscopic* picture is found, with *varying thicknesses of the arterial wall,* ranging from fibrous accumulations superimposed on intact internal elastic membrane, to areas where the external elastic membrane is the only portion left. The recognizable remaining media shows, in many areas, a marked loss of muscle and an increase in collagen. It is suspected that this increased collagen saves the vessel from longitudinal dissection by tethering segments of the artery to the external elastic membrane.

Subadventitial Fibroplasia. This lesion usually afflicts young women. It is, on occasion, bilateral; in the only reported series, 25 percent of the patients had such involvement. Again, it frequently is a disease of the right renal artery. The disorder usually affects variable lengths of the renal artery beyond its origin but rarely involves its main branches, either primarily or by extension. *Microscopically,* the lesion appears to be a unique involvement of the renal artery, consisting of a *dense, circumferential collar of collagen* external to and, at times, partially or completely replacing varying segments of the *media.* A considerable amount of the *adventitial* elastic tissue still remains, as well as what seems to be much of the external elastic lamellae, hence the origin of the term *subadventitial fibroplasia.* The collagen is remarkably dense and, with special stains, appears to be completely mature, in contrast to some of the changes seen in intimal fibroplasia; this difference is best shown by any of the technics for demonstrating acid mucopolysaccharides. In longitudinal sections the collagen appears to vary in thickness. Consequently, *renal arteriograms* show an irregularity in the outline of the arterial lumen. In contrast to medial fibroplasia with aneurysms, the diameter of the vascular irregularity is less than the diameter of the uninvolved proximal segment of renal artery. Here again, dissecting hematoma does not occur, and secondary thrombosis is a distinct rarity.

Fibromuscular Hyperplasia. In the restricted sense this is, at least in part, another fibrotic

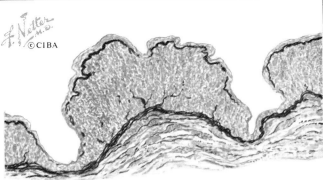

LONGITUDINAL SECTION OF RENAL ARTERY WITH MEDIAL FIBROPLASIA: GREAT VARIATION IN THICKNESS OF ARTERIAL WALL, CHIEFLY OF MEDIA, WITH ANEURYSMAL EVAGINATION (VERHOEFF—VAN GIESON STAIN, X 20)

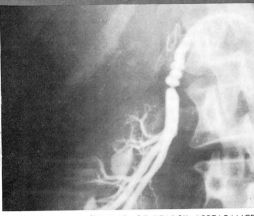

CHARACTERISTIC "STRING OF BEADS" APPEARANCE OF RENAL ARTERIOGRAM: ALTERNATE STENOSES AND ANEURYSMAL DILATATIONS

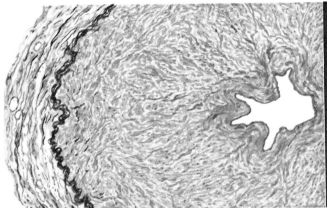

FIBROMUSCULAR HYPERPLASIA: MEDIAL THICKENING CONSISTING OF FIBROUS AND MUSCULAR TISSUE; INTERNAL ELASTIC MEMBRANE NOT PRESENT (VERHOEFF—VAN GIESON STAIN, X 100)

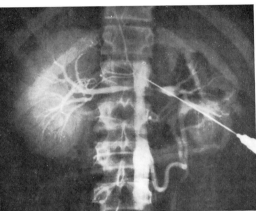

ARTERIOGRAM SHOWING STENOSES AT ORIGINS OF BOTH RENAL ARTERIES WITH POSTSTENOTIC DILATATION OF THE LEFT VESSEL

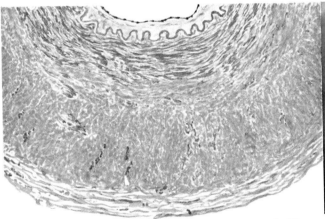

SUBADVENTITIAL FIBROPLASIA: A CONCENTRIC RING OF DENSE COLLAGEN IS PRESENT BETWEEN MEDIA AND ADVENTITIA (MASSON TRICHROME STAIN, X 80)

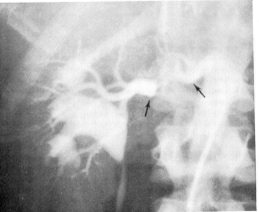

EXTENSIVE VARIED STENOSIS OF RIGHT RENAL ARTERY IN SUBADVENTITIAL FIBROPLASIA REVEALED BY ARTERIOGRAM

stenosing lesion of the main renal artery. It is the rarest of all fibrotic renal arterial problems and, as such, is difficult to analyze statistically. Once again, there seems to be a difference between the lesions in young children and those in adults. In the young, the lesion appears to consist predominantly of *muscle,* although the concentric lesion can be a uniform mixture. Rarely is it bilateral. In older individuals it seems to involve men and is complicated by distal dissecting hematomas. The *arteriographic* picture, in the young, is very similar to that of intimal fibroplasia, with a smooth, uniform *stenosis;* in older men, any narrowing is obscured by dye filling the *aneurysmal* dilatation. In addition, children apparently show some abnormality of the aorta, as it appears to be irregularly stenosed. This coarctation extends from above the origin of the renal arteries to, or nearly to, the aortic bifurcation.

Other Hypertensinogenic Changes

In addition to the rather characteristic lesions described,

other hypertensinogenic changes afflict the main renal arterial vasculature. *Primary dissecting aneurysms* can occur, causing partial to complete occlusion of the renal artery, as well as hypertension. The underlying etiology is obscure, but, apparently, a discontinuity in the internal elastic membrane can allow the intramural dissection of blood. Such lesions have been found even in children. The relationship between this lesion and the so-called aneurysm of the renal artery has not been completely clarified, but the same lack of elastic-tissue continuity might be responsible for either condition. The presence of a dissection may depend upon whether the forces can pass longitudinally in the vessel or must remain contained within a pouch and form an aneurysm. *Periarterial fibroplasia* has been seen as a part of *retroperitoneal fibrosis,* and it can be responsible for hypertension. Large *perinephric hematomas* apparently can also interfere with the main renal vasculature and, possibly, the small vasculature, to produce a remedial type of elevated blood pressure.

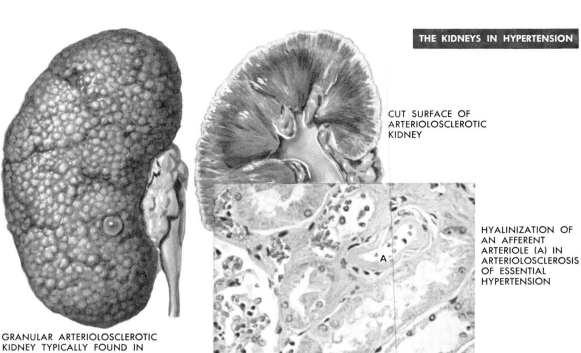

CUT SURFACE OF ARTERIOLOSCLEROTIC KIDNEY

HYALINIZATION OF AN AFFERENT ARTERIOLE (A) IN ARTERIOLOSCLEROSIS OF ESSENTIAL HYPERTENSION

GRANULAR ARTERIOLOSCLEROTIC KIDNEY TYPICALLY FOUND IN ESSENTIAL HYPERTENSION

KIDNEYS IN HYPERTENSION

CHARACTERISTIC "ONIONSKIN" LAMINATION AND DETERIORATION OF A RENAL ARTERIOLE IN MALIGNANT PHASE OF ESSENTIAL HYPERTENSION

KIDNEY IN MALIGNANT PHASE OF ESSENTIAL HYPERTENSION: NUMEROUS VARIEGATED HEMORRHAGES

NECROSIS OF A GLOMERULUS (G) AND OF AN AFFERENT ARTERIOLE (A) IN MALIGNANT HYPERTENSION

It should be clearly understood that there are no lesions of the renal vasculature (either large or small vessels) which guarantee the development of hypertension, nor are there any lesions within the kidney which assure that the patient has an elevated blood pressure. There is much interrelation between renal disease and hypertension, but some other mechanism must also be operative; e.g., angiograms to demonstrate aortic disease will also, at times, show renal-artery disease, but the patients have no hypertension. One is best served by remembering that there is no all-inclusive relationship among vascular disease, renal disease, and elevated blood pressure.

Certain facts must be elaborated whenever one examines the problem of a change in the kidney and hypertension. Whether the kidney has been "protected" from an elevation in blood pressure can be a major determining factor in morphologic alterations within the structure. The "protected" kidney (i.e., one that has been partially or completely removed from systemic circulation by alterations in the main renal-artery flow) may show no changes at all but usually displays a wide variety of differences occurring as a result of the decrease in renal blood flow. Study of the "protected" kidney, using only the alkaline phosphatase stain, may show a loss of this enzyme when the morphology is, otherwise, apparently normal. However, the fully developed "protected" kidney shows marked tubular atrophy, with a loss of all identifying characteristics as to specialized cell type; the tubules are lined by a thin, undifferentiated epithelium, with individual cells showing a sparse amount of cytoplasm. As a result of this parenchymal loss, the glomeruli appear crowded, lying much closer to each other, though their structure seems unaltered. Since this is common, even in total occlusion of the main renal artery, collateral circulation from the capsular branches, extending deep into the renal parenchyma, must be responsible for the lack of infarction. Zones of old infarction are rare; those seen are, most commonly, in association with lesions involving branches of the main renal artery. It is unusual to find any alteration in the vasculature of this type of kidney.

There is, however, an important variation that is found in association with atherosclerosis. It is necessary to recognize this, lest one inadvertently misinterpret the changes present in a biopsy of such a kidney. It must be remembered that atherosclerosis is a dynamic disorder, and an occlusive plaque may develop in a main renal artery after the kidney has

(Continued on page 231)

experienced some vascular changes. The presence of this prior change does not negate the possibility that removal of the plaque will correct the hypertension. It is then possible to have considerable changes in the vessels in the renal parenchyma of a kidney that has been partially or completely blocked from the main circulation. The vessels in this kidney can show *arteriosclerosis* of the smaller arteries and arterioles, and obliterating fibrotic and atherosclerotic changes in the medium-sized and large arteries, without these findings being of any great significance.

The changes in the kidney (or kidneys, in *essential hypertension*) exposed to the full force of hypertension depend, in part, on the duration of the disease. Many renal biopsies, done at the time of such operations as sympathectomy, have shown no significant morphologic alterations in the renal vasculature. The first change may be a thickening of the musculature of the small arteriole, but its interpretation is open to some question. *Hyaline arteriolosclerosis* is common in chronic hypertension with, at first, only hyaline masses being present in arteriolar walls, but later, and in severe cases, the arteriolosclerosis can become thick and circumferential. The constituency of this peculiar waxy material is complex, and one cannot help but believe that it represents merely some type of conglomeration of the constituents of blood that have focally leaked through the vessel wall. There has always been a question as to how significant this lesion is in producing alterations of a major character in renal dynamics.

A more important lesion may be the one found with great frequency in the larger arteries of the renal parenchyma. A good term has not been developed for this lesion, but possibly the old one of "endarteritis obliterans" is sufficient. The disorder consists of a marked intimal thickening in the arcuate, interlobar, and interlobular arteries. The thickening consists predominantly of collagen, but slight atheromatous changes can also be seen. This lesion is not limited to the kidney but can, on occasion, be seen in any small artery. Its importance in the kidney seems related to a loss of renal parenchyma, since careful search will reveal that these lesions are most likely responsible for much of the *granular* scarring and the larger wedge-shaped scars so common in the kidney in hypertension. A physiologic "circus maneuver" may develop because of this vascular change. It can be postulated that hypertension causes the intimal thickening, and, as a result, hypoxia of the kidney occurs. This, in turn, stimulates a vasopressor mechanism to elaborate substances responsible for either the maintenance of blood pressure or its further increase. Under these circumstances, it may well be that these fibrotic changes in the medium-sized and small arteries are the most important ones, as far as alterations in renal physiology in hypertension are concerned. Although these changes are extensive in the kidney in essential hypertension, they are sufficiently patchy to allow adequately functioning renal parenchyma to remain. As a consequence, renal failure is not the common cause of death in essential hypertension.

In contrast, the renal lesions in *malignant hypertension* are so extensive that renal failure has been one of the common causes of death in untreated cases. All areas of the renal arterial tree are involved. The arteriole shows a wide variety of lesions. Its walls may become necrotic, with fibrin being deposited and forming minute thrombi. For this change, the terms "necrosis" and "thrombonecrosis" have been used. In addition, a most peculiar *lamellar* hyperplasia, which appears to be alternating collagen and elastic tissue, can be seen. This is the characteristic *"laminated onion"* of malignant nephrosclerosis which must not be confused with the subintimal changes that can occur in any of the medium-sized or small arteries in any variety of hypertension. Both of these lesions can be responsible for changes in the *glomerulus,* with either partial or complete *necrosis* of the tuft. Whenever this extensive damage occurs, *hemorrhage* in either the glomerulus or the arteriolar wall can result. As a consequence, a wide variety of cellular elements can be found in the urine.

In addition to the arteriolar changes, extensive alterations can also occur in the arteries. The extreme pressures will drive blood constituents into and beyond the arterial walls, with large pools of fibrin and necrotic muscle being formed. Here again, interference with the blood flow can occur by thrombosis superimposing on these lesions. Under these circumstances there may be small areas of infarction that eventually atrophy. Other evidence of material being driven into the arterial and arteriolar walls is the presence of *lipid* accumulations (microatheromas) within these structures. This finding serves as additional proof that atherosclerosis is basically a filtration disease. The arteries also show the same type of intimal fibroplasia as that seen in essential hypertension. In some patients it may not have had time to develop, but, in others, the arteries will show such major occlusive change, especially if life is prolonged by extensive antihypertensive therapy. The intimal fibroplasia, under these circumstances, has been demonstrated to be of such severity that the hypertension and renal failure, in some of these patients, recurs. In this particular situation only atrophy of the kidneys is found at necropsy. The intimal changes in the medium-sized and small arteries, at that time, have apparently exerted a "protective effect."

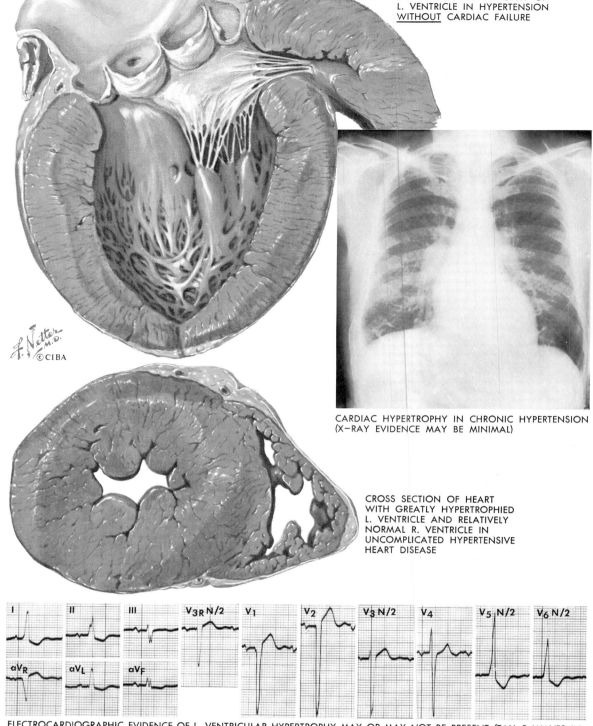

CONCENTRIC HYPERTROPHY OF
L. VENTRICLE IN HYPERTENSION
<u>WITHOUT</u> CARDIAC FAILURE

CARDIAC HYPERTROPHY IN CHRONIC HYPERTENSION
(X–RAY EVIDENCE MAY BE MINIMAL)

CROSS SECTION OF HEART
WITH GREATLY HYPERTROPHIED
L. VENTRICLE AND RELATIVELY
NORMAL R. VENTRICLE IN
UNCOMPLICATED HYPERTENSIVE
HEART DISEASE

ELECTROCARDIOGRAPHIC EVIDENCE OF L. VENTRICULAR HYPERTROPHY MAY OR MAY NOT BE PRESENT (TALL R WAVES IN V_4, V_5, & V_6; DEEP S WAVES IN V_{3R}, V_1, V_2, III, AND aV_R; DEPRESSED S–T AND INVERTED T IN V_5, V_6, I, II, aV_L, AND aV_F)

HEART DISEASE IN HYPERTENSION

Although the heart often is affected adversely in patients who have various forms of elevated blood pressure, the detectable changes in the heart correlate poorly with the degree and duration of hypertension in any individual patient. Whereas from 60 to 75 percent of the patients with hypertension die with a cardiac complication, the timing, incidence, and severity of the heart disease are quite variable.

Numerous investigators, in the past, have demonstrated that the elevation of blood pressure, in hypertensive patients, is due to an increased peripheral resistance to blood flow in the presence of well-preserved stroke volume and cardiac output. It is, therefore, an attractive theory that the resulting increase in the work of the heart causes *concentric hypertrophy of the left ventricular* myocardium. Thickening of the wall of the heart ensues, over a variable period of time, and serves as a compensatory mechanism maintaining the normal cardiac output against the increased peripheral resistance that, in turn, results from arteriolar constriction due to a variety of causes and mechanisms, depending on the etiology of the hypertension (see page 224).

During this phase of concentric left ventricular hypertrophy, a high index of suspicion is necessary in order to make a *diagnosis* of *hypertensive heart disease.* The clinician may detect some increased forcefulness of the point of maximum impulse over the left precordium, together with an increased intensity of the aortic component of the second heart sound, and an increased palpable pulsation of the great vessels at the base of the neck.

There may be some *roentgenographic* evidence of left ventricular enlargement, especially in the left anterior-oblique projection, where a rounded posterior left ventricular border may be seen

to overlap the anterior margin of the vertebral column.

One of the *earliest* and most reliable *signs* of left ventricular hypertrophy, at this stage, may occur in the *electrocardiogram,* which will show left axis deviation, an *increased amplitude of the R wave* in leads I, V_5, and V_6, as well as of the S wave in leads III, V_2, and V_3. (The electrocardiographic changes depicted are indicative of *more advanced* left ventricular hypertrophy.) It has recently been demonstrated that electrocardiographic signs of left atrial enlargement are also often present even before an increase in the diameter of the left ventricle can be measured, and these frequently correlate with the presence of a fourth heart sound or atrial gallop. These abnormalities may disappear if effective lowering of the systemic blood pressure can be accomplished.

During this phase of compensated hypertensive heart disease, the patient may have no particular cardiac *symptoms,* except for some fatigability and a sensation of increased forcefulness of the heartbeat, particularly with excitement or exercise. Measurements of circulation time, blood volume, and venous pressure will be normal, as will the cardiac output, whether measured by dye-dilution or catheterization technics.

The incidence of coronary atherosclerosis is moderately increased in patients with hypertensive heart disease, and it is for this reason that angina pectoris, coronary insufficiency, and myocardial infarction appear more commonly than in the normal population. Theoretically, this situation prevails because the left ventricular myocardium tends to outgrow its own blood supply, which is also intrinsically compromised because of the apparently traumatic effects of higher blood pressure on the coronary arterial walls themselves.

(Continued on page 233)

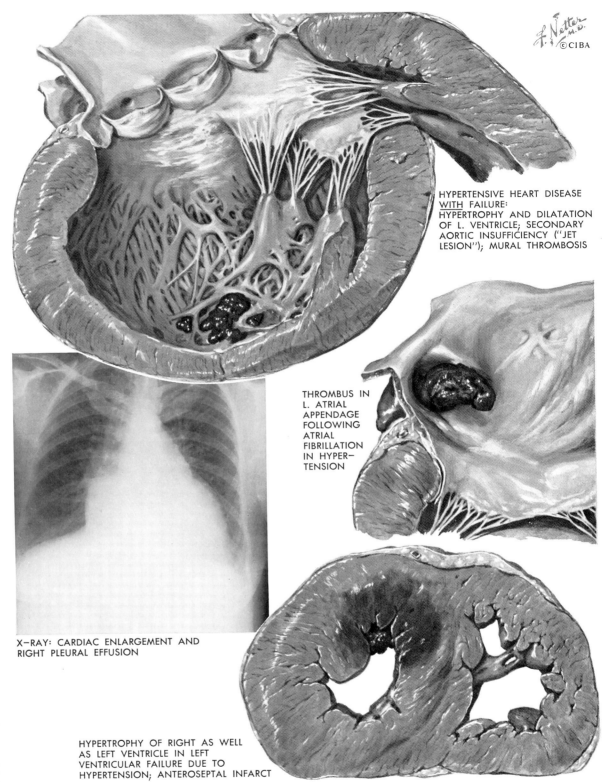

HYPERTENSIVE HEART DISEASE WITH FAILURE: HYPERTROPHY AND DILATATION OF L. VENTRICLE; SECONDARY AORTIC INSUFFICIENCY ("JET LESION"); MURAL THROMBOSIS

THROMBUS IN L. ATRIAL APPENDAGE FOLLOWING ATRIAL FIBRILLATION IN HYPERTENSION

X-RAY: CARDIAC ENLARGEMENT AND RIGHT PLEURAL EFFUSION

HYPERTROPHY OF RIGHT AS WELL AS LEFT VENTRICLE IN LEFT VENTRICULAR FAILURE DUE TO HYPERTENSION; ANTEROSEPTAL INFARCT

HEART DISEASE IN HYPERTENSION

(Continued from page 232)

At some point in the progression of hypertensive heart disease, which cannot be accurately forecast either from the severity or from the duration of the hypertensive history, the compensatory mechanism of concentric hypertrophy is no longer sufficient. Evidence of cardiac decompensation and congestive heart *failure* supervenes, but this state is usually ushered in by the appearance of coronary atherosclerosis, the malignant phase of hypertension, or the retention of sodium and water because of the frequently associated changes in renal function.

The first stage in the development of congestive failure is the elevation of end-diastolic pressure in the *left ventricle,* which, subsequently, begins to show *dilatation* in addition to the previously mentioned hypertrophy. Progressive *cardiac enlargement* then develops, and dilatation of the mitral annulus may result in functional mitral regurgitation and a characteristic pansystolic blowing murmur at the cardiac apex. A ventricular-gallop sound, pulsus alternans, or increased intensity of the pulmonic component of the second heart sound may all be detected at the bedside. *Atrial fibrillation* may occur in about 25 percent of the patients, depending on the duration and degree of associated coronary atherosclerosis.

At this stage the patient usually has definite symptoms of pulmonary congestion, with exertional dyspnea, orthopnea, and paroxysms of unprovoked nocturnal dyspnea. Frank pulmonary edema occasionally may be precipitated, requiring emergency treatment with oxygen administration, rapid digitalization, vigorous diuretic therapy, and control of systemic hypertension.

The subsequent course of hypertensive heart disease depends largely on the inci-

dence and severity of the associated coronary atherosclerosis, the control of blood-pressure levels, and the incidence of renal insufficiency. Provided the patient survives for an adequate period, pulmonary-artery pressure rises because of pulmonary vascular changes similar to those found in rheumatic mitral stenosis. *Hypertrophy* of the *right ventricle* and sometimes right ventricular failure may follow, in which dependent edema and hepatic congestion cause more of the symptoms than does the left ventricular failure per se.

Additional complications of hypertensive heart disease include the appearance of peripheral *emboli,* particularly in those patients who have myocardial infarction, and especially in the presence of chronic atrial fibrillation. If renal insufficiency and azotemia develop, fibrinous pericarditis occasionally is seen (with characteristic friction sounds heard over

the precordium) and electrocardiographic changes. If there is consequent difficulty in controlling the electrolyte balance, considerable care must be exercised in the use of diuretic or hypotensive drugs as well as digitalis preparations.

The *treatment* of hypertensive heart disease, especially in the so-called decompensated stage, has improved considerably in the last few years, because of the more effective hypotensive agents and the more sensitive diuretic drugs currently available. Weight reduction, control of complicating factors such as diabetes mellitus, maintenance of adequate nutrition, and proper balance of physical activity are all important features of the program for the hypertensive cardiac patient, and the prognosis remains relatively satisfactory unless myocardial infarction, cerebral vascular disease, the malignant phase of hypertension, or renal failure aggravate the overall problem.

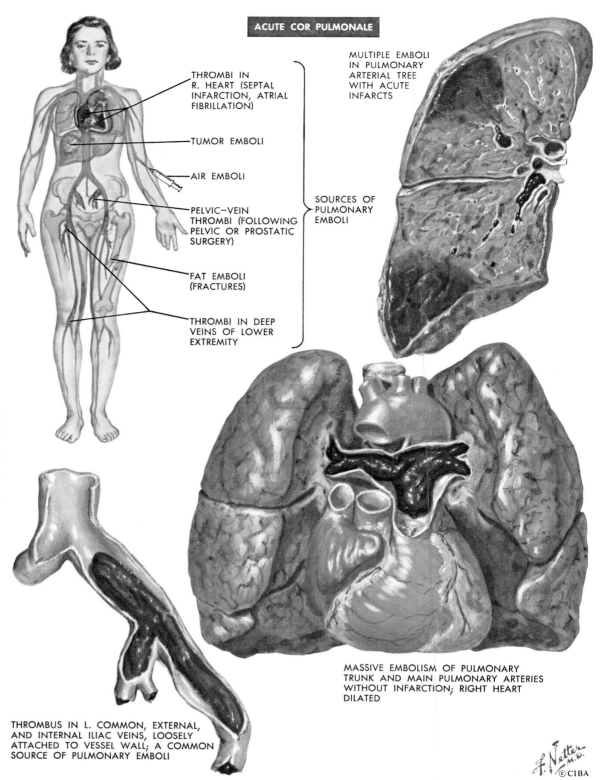

ACUTE COR PULMONALE

THROMBI IN
R. HEART (SEPTAL
INFARCTION, ATRIAL
FIBRILLATION)

TUMOR EMBOLI

AIR EMBOLI

PELVIC–VEIN
THROMBI (FOLLOWING
PELVIC OR PROSTATIC
SURGERY)

FAT EMBOLI
(FRACTURES)

THROMBI IN DEEP
VEINS OF LOWER
EXTREMITY

MULTIPLE EMBOLI
IN PULMONARY
ARTERIAL TREE
WITH ACUTE
INFARCTS

SOURCES OF
PULMONARY
EMBOLI

MASSIVE EMBOLISM OF PULMONARY
TRUNK AND MAIN PULMONARY ARTERIES
WITHOUT INFARCTION; RIGHT HEART
DILATED

THROMBUS IN L. COMMON, EXTERNAL,
AND INTERNAL ILIAC VEINS, LOOSELY
ATTACHED TO VESSEL WALL; A COMMON
SOURCE OF PULMONARY EMBOLI

ACUTE COR PULMONALE

In the field of cardiovascular disease, the interdependence of the heart and lungs, as a unit, is nowhere more apparent than in *cor pulmonale*—heart disease caused by hypertension in the pulmonary circulation—which, in turn, results from an abnormal resistance to blood flow and to perfusion of the lungs by the right ventricular output.

Acute cor pulmonale most often results from *pulmonary embolism* due to a clot dislodged somewhere in the *venous system* or to a mural thrombus in the right side of the heart. The embolus may arise in an area of thrombophlebitis, in which case there may be some prior warning, but, more often, silent phlebothrombosis occurs in the large *veins of the legs* or of the *pelvis,* the ensuing clinical syndrome being determined chiefly by the size and number of the pulmonary arteries obstructed.

Pulmonary emboli are related to other forms of heart disease in that they may precipitate or aggravate existing congestive heart failure or produce a clinical picture simulating acute myocardial infarction. There is a predisposition to embolism in persons confined to bed, especially when they have heart failure, malignant disease, or polycythemia; when they are obese or of advanced age, particularly if varicose veins are present; or when they recently have undergone *pelvic or prostatic surgery*. Pulmonary emboli occasionally arise in the right side of the heart from mural thrombosis superimposed on a *transseptal infarction,* or when there are long-standing right-side heart failure and *atrial fibrillation*.

Pulmonary emboli occasionally may consist of *tumor* fragments from a carcinomatous invasion of the large abdominal veins, or there may be *fat emboli* initiated by soft-tissue trauma. Amniotic-fluid emboli after delivery and, occasionally, *air bubbles* accidentally introduced into the veins during certain types of *surgical procedures* may cause obstruction either

to the *pulmonary arteries* or to the right ventricle itself.

Although it is well known that a 50 percent reduction of the cross-sectional area of the pulmonary circulation (as after pneumonectomy) results in no elevation of resting pulmonary-artery pressure, pronounced pulmonary hypertension may occur after pulmonary embolism; this can later be shown to have obstructed only a small proportion of the *pulmonary arterial tree*. Therefore, considerable controversy has developed over the years (based on animal experimental evidence and clinical observation) as to the relative contribution of pulmonary vasoconstriction and of vascular obstruction to the demonstrated rise in pulmonary-artery pressure. However, it has been shown, in more recent human studies, that the administration of 100 percent oxygen or of acetylcholine, to a patient with acute pulmonary embolism, results in a signifi-

cant lowering of pulmonary-artery pressure, thus indicating the presence of a significant reflex vasoconstrictive factor.

There is general agreement that, in embolization of the lungs, because of the increased resistance to pulmonary blood flow there is a significant decrease in cardiac output, with an associated fall in systemic blood pressure. In addition, pulmonary-artery pressure rises, and there are consequent effects on right ventricular function. Many of the *clinical features* of a large pulmonary embolism result from myocardial ischemia due to the resulting fall in coronary blood flow, which may be further aggravated by reflex coronary constriction mediated via the vagus nerves. If significant elevation of right ventricular pressure occurs, theoretically there may also be impairment of the thebesian venous drainage.

(Continued on page 235)

Acute Cor Pulmonale

(Continued from page 234)

Another clinical aspect results from associated bronchospasm, which may be due to the release of serotonin from platelets in the vicinity of or, perhaps, in the clot itself. Both experimental animal data and human observations confirm the appearance of hyperventilation, tachypnea, diminished lung compliance, a rise in airway resistance, reduced arterial oxygen content caused by venous admixture, and a decreased alveolar-arterial pCO_2 difference, presumably owing to underperfused but still-ventilated segments of the lung.

The typical picture of *massive pulmonary embolism* is characterized by the sudden onset of dyspnea, tachycardia, substernal pain, a dramatic sense of impending doom, and systemic hypotension. Clinical evidence of right ventricular strain and failure may develop rapidly and should be suspected when increasing prominence of the pulmonic component of sound II (S II) is detected phonocardiographically, together with a ventricular gallop along the right sternal border and a distention of the cervical veins. The failure of these symptoms and signs to respond to the administration of vasopressor drugs, oxygen, and digitalis suggests a poor prognosis.

At this point, an *electrocardiogram* is perhaps the simplest and most useful diagnostic aid available. The typical pattern includes a prominent S wave, with a depressed S-T segment in lead I and perhaps lead II, and a deep Q and a late inversion of T in lead III. There usually are prominent precordial P waves, a movement of the transition zone to the left, and an inversion of precordial T waves of variable degree and distribution.

Occasionally, in this setting, the decision must be made quickly as to whether a surgical embolectomy is indicated in a critically ill patient, who possibly might recover spontaneously. The prompt availability of cardiopulmonary-bypass facilities, a qualified surgeon, and selective pulmonary angiography must all be considered, since there are only a few reports of successful pulmonary embolectomy.

Pulmonary embolism of less massive proportions may be associated with dyspnea, hyperventilation, cyanosis, restlessness, chest pain of a pleuritic nature, and (sometimes) syncope. Evidence of right ventricular strain, as mentioned above, may develop, to be followed later by hemoptysis, fever, roentgenographic evidence of pulmonary consolidation, pleural friction rub, and jaundice. In this setting there usually is time for laboratory determinations to be made, and a rise in serum lactic dehydrogenase, accompanied by a normal serum glutamic oxalacetic transaminase, with subsequent increase in the serum bilirubin, provides confirmatory evidence.

Most patients, who have normal hearts and lungs before pulmonary embolism occurs, show a striking ability to reabsorb emboli, so that subsequent study of right-side heart pressures, even with pulmonary angiography and respiratory-function tests, shows no significant abnormality. However, such recovery depends on the prevention and avoidance of recurrent thromboembolism and sometimes requires ligation of the inferior vena cava and the use of anticoagulants.

In the acute stage of pulmonary embolism, heparin is recommended both as an anticoagulant and as an antiserotonin factor in the reduction of bronchospasm with its attendant respiratory disturbance. Prompt digitalization usually is indicated if there is evidence of right ventricular failure. Symptomatic relief with meperidine hydrochloride and the use of atropine, papaverine, and pressor agents must be considered according to the details and indications of the individual problem.

Although recurrent, small, pulmonary emboli may often go unrecognized, the alert clinician should have a high index of suspicion if he encounters unexplained fever, transient increases in pulse rate and respiration, the complaint of chronic fatigue, and (especially) the unexplained appearance of right ventricular hypertrophy without evidence of intrinsic pulmonary disease (see page 237). This clinical syndrome may be avoided largely by early ambulation of postoperative patients, wide application of elastic stockings to bedridden patients, and recognition of the problem, especially in persons with malignant disease, congestive heart failure, polycythemia, varices of the lower extremities, recent pelvic trauma, or splenectomy.

Chronic Cor Pulmonale

Although chronic pulmonary hypertension occurs in disorders of the left side of the heart, such as left ventricular failure and mitral stenosis, or left-to-right shunts in congenital cardiac lesions, the term *cor pulmonale* is usually applied to heart disease caused by intrinsic disorders of the lungs and pulmonary circulation.

Whereas the normal pulmonary circuit is characterized by low pressure, low resistance, and a capacious and distensible vascular bed, notable changes in these features may occur in a variety of pulmonary disorders in which either some anatomic restriction of the pulmonary parenchyma and vascular structures occurs, or vasoconstriction in the arterial tree results from an associated disturbance in pulmonary function. Studies of lung function, in the various diseases that cause hypertension of the lesser circulation, may show alteration of ventilation (as in chronic obstructive lung disease), or there may be, primarily, a disturbance in the ventilation-perfusion relationships, or a reduction of diffusing capacity, as in alveolar-capillary block syndromes. The apparent common denominator of these various functional disturbances is hypoxia, affecting either the pulmonary-capillary and venous blood, or the alveolar gas itself. It has been shown, in a number of ways, that hypoxia is capable of producing vasoconstriction of the pulmonary bed, thus contributing to an increase in pulmonary vascular resistance.

Clinically, there are four general categories of pulmonary diseases that result in cor pulmonale:

1. *Chronic obstructive lung disease* causes from 85 to 90 percent of cor pulmonale as it is seen in most parts of the world today. This category includes cases of chronic bronchial asthma, in which there is widespread intermittent narrowing of the airways, and obstructive *emphysema,* in which there are loss of elasticity, increase of residual volume, decrease of lung compliance, and, particularly, reduction in the number and size of the alveolar capillaries. Some degree of chronic bronchitis is usually present, and, in fact, the British diagnosis of "chronic bronchitis-emphysema" scarcely attempts to separate the two entities. Disturbances occur in many facets of overall pulmonary function, but the chief disorder is that of ventilatory insufficiency, and the principal symptom is dyspnea.

2. *Pulmonary fibrosis* of various types, sometimes associated secondarily with emphysema, also comprises a large group of pulmonary disorders that commonly lead to hypertension and cor pulmonale. *Tuberculosis,* bronchiectasis, and other pulmonary infections have been associated with cor pulmonale less frequently in recent years, probably because of the widespread use of antibiotics and antimicrobial agents. Pulmonary hypertension may result from some of the pneumoconioses owing to inhalation of foreign substances (particularly *silicon,* bauxite, diatomaceous earth, and beryllium) possibly only in patients who are hyperreactive to these agents.

Sarcoidosis, scleroderma, and fibrosing interstitial pneumonitis (Hamman-Rich syndrome) may likewise result in severe reduction of the pulmonary vascular bed, with alteration of the alveolar capillary membrane and impairment of oxygen diffusion as well as impairment of lung compliance and some distortion of ventilation-perfusion relationships. In these situations, hypoxia is prominent with its attendant hyperventilation and cyanosis, which are more marked clinical features than is dyspnea.

3. *Musculoskeletal or mechanical disorders* of the thoracic cage, as in *kyphoscoliosis,* thoracoplasty, poliomyelitis, and muscular dystrophy, may sometimes disturb pulmonary function to the extent of causing cor pulmonale. The common denominator of all these disorders is an uneven ventilation-perfusion relationship, with regional emphysema combined with fibrosis in other parts of the lungs. Regional alveolar hypoventilation with right-to-left shunting of unaerated blood develops, so that there results a combination of hypoxic pulmonary vasoconstriction and anatomic restriction of the capillary bed. Alveolar hypoventilation, owing to extreme obesity or, occasionally, to an apparent intrinsic hyposensitivity of the respiratory center to carbon dioxide, infrequently results in hypoxic pulmonary vasoconstriction and a functional form of cor pulmonale which is completely reversible when the underlying disorder has been promptly recognized and adequately treated.

(Continued on page 236)

EMPHYSEMA,
THE MOST COMMON
CAUSE OF COR PULMONALE

CHRONIC COR PULMONALE

(Continued from page 235)

PULMONARY
FIBROSIS: MAY
BE SECONDARY
TO SILICOSIS,
ASBESTOSIS,
HEMOSIDEROSIS,
TUBERCULOSIS,
BLASTOMYCOSIS,
FIBROCYSTIC DISEASE OF THE
PANCREAS, SCHISTOSOMIASIS,
X-RAY THERAPY OF BREAST;
POSSIBLY PRIMARY

ORGANIZED
AND CANALIZED
THROMBUS IN A
SMALL PULMONARY
VESSEL

P-A VIEW

KYPHO-
SCOLIOSIS

LATERAL
VIEW

ORGANIZED THROMBUS IN
A LARGE PULMONARY ARTERY

4. *Primary disease of the pulmonary vessels themselves* comprises the fourth important group of causes. These are distinguished by the absence of intrinsic pulmonary disease or other apparent etiologic factors. In some instances, widespread organization of apparent pulmonary *emboli* and *thrombi* of various ages are discovered at autopsy, and no history of pulmonary embolism can be found in retrospect. The lesions at the arteriolar and capillary levels are often indistinguishable in cases of so-called primary pulmonary hypertension in which there is no suspicion of multiple emboli. In both instances there are variable degrees of intimal hyperplasia, vascular occlusion, and recanalization, with medial hypertrophy of the muscular arteries and *arteriosclerosis* of the larger vessels. These microscopic changes may be either the cause or the result of hypertension in the pulmonary circuit, and considerable controversy exists over the pathogenesis of this situation. At times, the disorder seems to be familial, and it occurs more often in women than in men. When there is a history of complicated pregnancy, the possibility of amniotic-fluid embolization occasionally is considered an initial factor.

The *clinical diagnosis* of cor pulmonale requires a high index of suspicion in regard to the patient with chronic lung disease of any type known to increase resistance in the pulmonary circulation. Usually, the initial symptoms are those of the underlying pulmonary disorder; therefore, cough and dyspnea are prominent even before there is detectable cardiac involvement. The latter can be suspected if prominence of the pulmonic component of S II is present, along with cyanosis, clubbing of the fingers, increased cervical venous pressure, or a left parasternal heave. This may be absent in many instances of obstructive lung disease when there is an increased anteroposterior diameter of the chest, in which

case there may be a prominent epigastric pulsation. Atrial- and ventricular-gallop sounds may appear along with the murmurs of tricuspid or pulmonic insufficiency, and these signs are accentuated on inspiration and decreased on expiration, in contradistinction to the similar physical signs in left ventricular failure.

With the advancing decompensation of cor pulmonale, the usual findings of dependent edema, ascites, cyanosis, and hepatomegaly may appear, but some care is necessary in evaluating the last, because of the low position of the right side of the diaphragm in many of these patients.

Roentgenographic examination is often disappointing, since it usually will show a normal cardiac silhouette or simply the changes caused by the underlying lung disease. Sometimes, *dilatation of the pulmonary artery* and its branches is evident, but enlargement of the right ventricle is difficult to demonstrate, espe-

cially when there is a low diaphragm or a barrel-shaped chest. Some prominence or increased convexity of the right ventricular-outflow tract may be seen in the right anterior-oblique projection. If congestive failure supervenes, the consequent right atrial enlargement can occasionally produce a prominence of the right lower cardiac silhouette and an increased transverse diameter in the *posteroanterior (P-A) projection*.

The *electrocardiogram* of chronic cor pulmonale may remain within normal limits until there is a fixed elevation of mean pulmonary pressure up to more than twice the normal value. Patients with chronic lung disease frequently have a vertical electrical position with clockwise rotation, which is responsible for some of the electrocardiographic changes attributed to *right ventricular hypertrophy*. One of the first

(Continued on page 237)

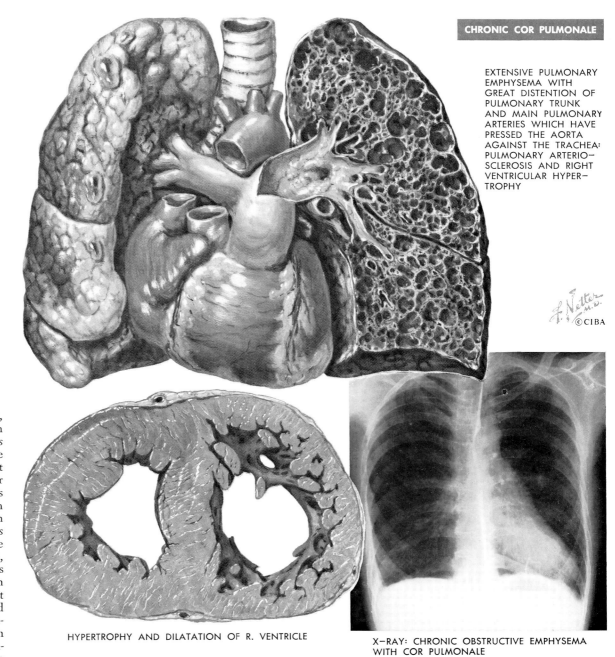

EXTENSIVE PULMONARY EMPHYSEMA WITH GREAT DISTENTION OF PULMONARY TRUNK AND MAIN PULMONARY ARTERIES WHICH HAVE PRESSED THE AORTA AGAINST THE TRACHEA: PULMONARY ARTERIO-SCLEROSIS AND RIGHT VENTRICULAR HYPER-TROPHY

HYPERTROPHY AND DILATATION OF R. VENTRICLE

X-RAY: CHRONIC OBSTRUCTIVE EMPHYSEMA WITH COR PULMONALE

R WAVES IN LEADS V₁ AND V₂ AS WELL AS S WAVES IN LEADS I, V₄, V₅, AND V₆ ARE INDICATIVE OF RIGHT VENTRICULAR HYPERTROPHY; PROMINENT P WAVES IN LEADS II, III, aV_F, V₁, AND V₂ SUGGEST RIGHT ATRIAL ENLARGEMENT

CHRONIC COR PULMONALE

(Continued from page 236)

reliable signs of cor pulmonale, however, is that of *right atrial enlargement,* with *prominence* and peaking of the P *waves* in leads II and III, and a relative increase in the initial component of P in the right precordial leads. When right ventricular hypertrophy develops, there is right axis deviation in the frontal plane, with increased amplitude of the R *waves* in the right precordium and deep S *waves* to the left, so that the R-S ratio may be greater than 1 over the right ventricle, and the electrical transition zone is shifted to the left. A delay appears in the intrinsicoid deflection over the right ventricular leads, up to 0.035 second or more, and the rSR pattern of incomplete or complete right bundle-branch block may appear. In advanced right ventricular hypertrophy, there may be an inversion of the T wave in leads II, III, and aV_F, as well as in the right precordial leads, but it should be remembered that, in early cor pulmonale, the absence of electrocardiographic abnormality does not exclude the possibility of pulmonary hypertension.

The technic of right-heart catheterization provides the most reliable method of studying pulmonary arterial and right ventricular pressures, which may occasionally reach systemic levels. When right ventricular failure is present, there is a characteristic elevation of the end-diastolic pressure in this chamber, together with a reduction in cardiac output as compared to normal values, but much less reduction than is the case with other forms of heart failure. Cardiac catheterization has also proved the reversibility of pulmonary hypertension. This depends, to some extent, on its underlying cause, but it justifies a vigorous therapeutic program for these patients, and modifies the dismal prognosis formerly assigned to them.

The *treatment* of chronic cor pulmonale depends primarily on the management of the underlying pulmonary disease. In the most common form of bronchopulmonary disorder associated with obstructive lung disease, the use of antibacterial agents to control infection, as well as bronchodilator agents, is of prime importance. Corticosteroids are occasionally justified, and the administration of these drugs by means of intermittent positive-pressure aerosol therapy has marked a major forward step in the available armamentarium. Intermittent positive-pressure breathing therapy also allows the administration of oxygen in a relatively safe manner, since increased ventilation is provided simultaneously, and the paradoxic respiratory depression, with consequent carbon dioxide retention in cases with emphysema, can be avoided.

Tracheostomy, sometimes on a permanent basis, can be most helpful in improving alveolar ventilation, particularly in patients with severe hypercapnia, and it occasionally is indicated as an emergency measure if the patient is comatose or extremely acidotic when first examined.

Cardiac measures, recommended in the treatment of decompensated cor pulmonale, include digitalization, which improves cardiac output, although there may be an initial rise in pulmonary-artery pressure resulting from the increased stroke volume. Sodium restriction and diuretic medications are indicated, as in other forms of congestive failure, and repeated small venesections are often advised, if the hematocrit reading is higher than 55, in order to reduce the augmented blood volume, as well as its viscosity, and the additional threat of thromboembolism. General supportive measures, with adequate rest and avoidance of excessive exertion, are advocated, as in other forms of cardiac failure, and the improvement in the functional state of many of these patients is most rewarding.

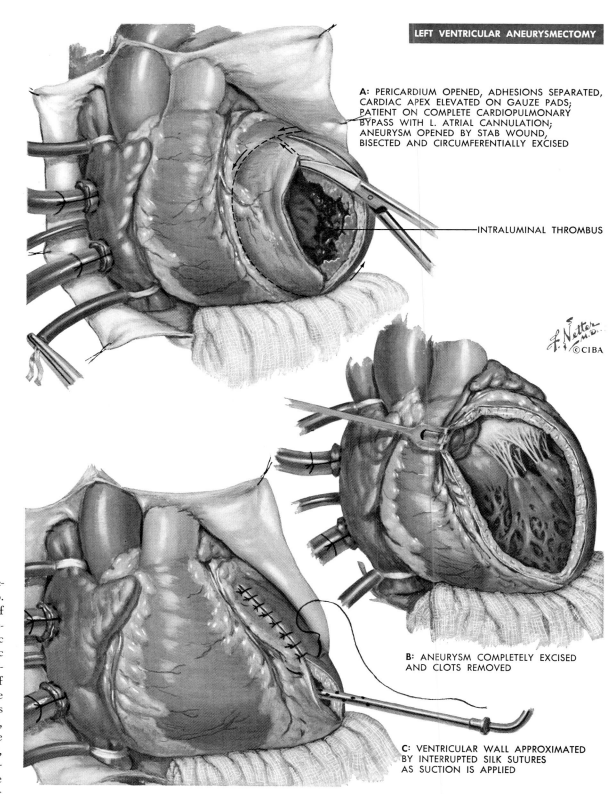

LEFT VENTRICULAR ANEURYSMECTOMY

A: PERICARDIUM OPENED, ADHESIONS SEPARATED, CARDIAC APEX ELEVATED ON GAUZE PADS; PATIENT ON COMPLETE CARDIOPULMONARY BYPASS WITH L. ATRIAL CANNULATION; ANEURYSM OPENED BY STAB WOUND, BISECTED AND CIRCUMFERENTIALLY EXCISED

INTRALUMINAL THROMBUS

B: ANEURYSM COMPLETELY EXCISED AND CLOTS REMOVED

C: VENTRICULAR WALL APPROXIMATED BY INTERRUPTED SILK SUTURES AS SUCTION IS APPLIED

Surgery for Coronary-Artery Disease

A new era of surgery for coronary arterial disease began nearly a decade ago. In 1958 Sones' revolutionary technic of selective coronary arteriography was presented to the medical world. This technic permitted, for the first time, a realistic appraisal of the patient suspected of having coronary disease. Proper utilization of coronary arteriography establishes the presence or absence of disease, localizes an existing myocardial-perfusion deficit, and assesses the functional status of the left ventricular muscle. Postoperatively, Sones' technic of selective coronary arteriography offers an assessment of the progress of the basic disease as well as of the success or failure of the surgical mission.

Since 1958 more than 10,000 patients have undergone selective coronary arteriography in the Cardiac Laboratory of the Cleveland Clinic, and approximately 1,500 of these patients have been surgically treated for the relief of myocardial ischemia. It is of interest that the basic surgical procedures utilized by the Cleveland Clinic team were in existence before coronary arteriography was available. Sones' contribution to the diagnosis and evaluation of coronary arterial disease has, more than any other procedure, given perspective to the surgical treatment.

Four basic categories of surgery are used in the Cleveland Clinic Hospital for treatment of coronary arterial disease. These are as follows: (1) reconstruction of the damaged left ventricle (*ventricular aneurysmectomy*), (2) direct relief of coronary arterial obstruction (*coronary arteriotomy*), (3) myocardial revascularization (*internal thoracic [mammary] artery-implant procedures*), and (4) *coronary-artery segmental replacement and bypass*. The operative approach is selected on the basis of the individual needs of the patient. The ramifications of coronary-artery disease are so great that no single operation is invariably applicable to patients who suffer from this disease. The need for individualizing the patient's status and his cardiac requirements cannot be overemphasized.

Ventricular Aneurysmectomy

Ventricular aneurysm occurs in a patient who has sustained a massive myocardial infarction. The rare exception is the aneurysm found in young persons who suffer a bizarre type of myopathy. Postinfarction aneurysm usually affects the anterior wall and the apex of the left ventricle that, in health, is perfused by the anterior interventricular (descending) branch of the left coronary artery. Aneurysm of the posterior left ventricle rarely occurs, even though massive infarction frequently develops in this area. The posterior wall of this ventricle supports its papillary muscle and chordae tendineae of the mitral valve; an infarction of sufficient magnitude to produce a ven-

(Continued on page 239)

CORONARY ARTERIOTOMY

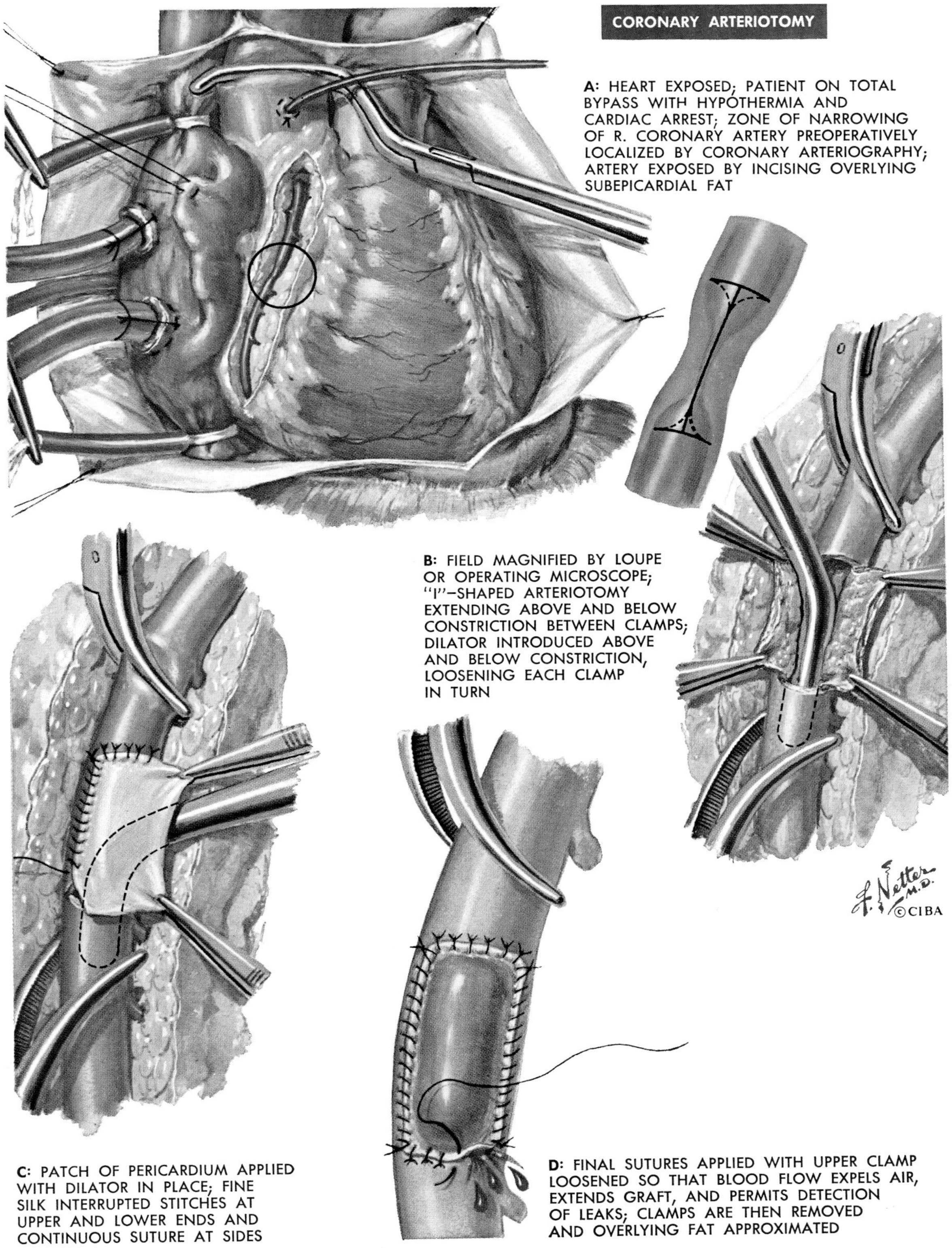

SURGERY FOR
CORONARY-ARTERY DISEASE

(*Continued from page 238*)

A: HEART EXPOSED; PATIENT ON TOTAL
BYPASS WITH HYPOTHERMIA AND
CARDIAC ARREST; ZONE OF NARROWING
OF R. CORONARY ARTERY PREOPERATIVELY
LOCALIZED BY CORONARY ARTERIOGRAPHY;
ARTERY EXPOSED BY INCISING OVERLYING
SUBEPICARDIAL FAT

B: FIELD MAGNIFIED BY LOUPE
OR OPERATING MICROSCOPE;
"I"-SHAPED ARTERIOTOMY
EXTENDING ABOVE AND BELOW
CONSTRICTION BETWEEN CLAMPS;
DILATOR INTRODUCED ABOVE
AND BELOW CONSTRICTION,
LOOSENING EACH CLAMP
IN TURN

C: PATCH OF PERICARDIUM APPLIED
WITH DILATOR IN PLACE; FINE
SILK INTERRUPTED STITCHES AT
UPPER AND LOWER ENDS AND
CONTINUOUS SUTURE AT SIDES

D: FINAL SUTURES APPLIED WITH UPPER CLAMP
LOOSENED SO THAT BLOOD FLOW EXPELS AIR,
EXTENDS GRAFT, AND PERMITS DETECTION
OF LEAKS; CLAMPS ARE THEN REMOVED
AND OVERLYING FAT APPROXIMATED

tricular aneurysm adds the unbearable burden of mitral incompetency to an acutely injured heart.

Ventricular aneurysm should be suspected in any patient who has sustained a major infarction, demonstrates a persistent increase in heart size, and is prone to ventricular arrhythmia or congestive failure. Angina pectoris, a feature of the disease preceding infarction, may no longer be present, because the pain receptors of the anterior wall are destroyed along with the myocardium itself. On occasion, the diagnosis may be established by roentgenographic study alone, although, in almost every instance, ventriculography (which accompanies coronary arteriography) will confirm the presence of ventricular aneurysm.

Ventricular aneurysmectomy is usually an elective procedure that is not undertaken until 4 to 6 months after the myocardial infarction occurred. Premature intervention adds to the risk of surgery; moreover, the line of demarcation between the destroyed tissue and the healthy residual myocardium is not apparent until fibrosis has become well advanced.

Technically, aneurysmectomy is a simple procedure. The heart is placed on *total bypass extracorporeal circulation*, but regional hypothermia and elective cardiac arrest are not required. Usually, the

pericardium is adherent to the aneurysm itself and must be *separated by sharp dissection*. The heart is then *elevated on gauze pads*, so that the left ventricle can be made more accessible, and — just as important — be the highest point in the surgical field, in order to *eliminate the risk of a systemic air embolus*. The *aneurysm is incised, through its midportion, by a stab wound* and is then opened to its upper and lower limits (see Plate 69: A). Usually, the aneurysm contains a laminated blood *clot*, and particular care is taken to recover any thrombotic material that may fall into the open left ventricle. The *aneurysm*, with its contained *thrombus*, is then *excised under direct vision*. The junction between the fibrous aneurysm and the residual myocardium is clearly demarcated (as suggested by the dotted line, Plate 69: A).

After the total removal of the aneurysm, the interior of the left ventricle can readily be inspected through the gaping defect created by the aneurysmectomy (see Plate 69: B). The intact aortic valve and the inferior aspect of the mitral valve also are easily seen. The *linear reconstruction of the left ventricle* is next accomplished by a *series of carefully placed, full-thickness, nonabsorbable sutures*. The interior of the left ventricle is *decompressed by a sterile aspirator* to remove excessive blood and retained air (see Plate 69: C).

Coronary Arteriotomy

Direct surgical relief of coronary obstruction is

(*Continued on page 240*)

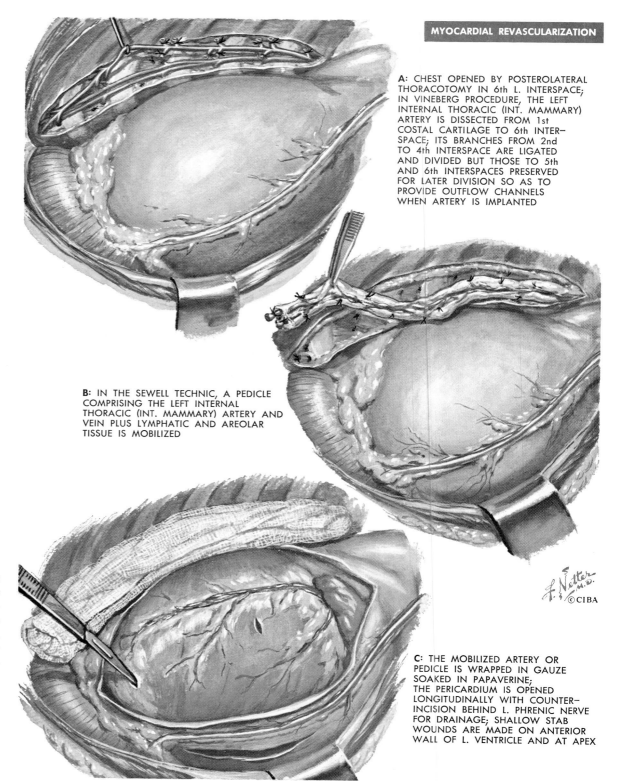

A: CHEST OPENED BY POSTEROLATERAL THORACOTOMY IN 6th L. INTERSPACE; IN VINEBERG PROCEDURE, THE LEFT INTERNAL THORACIC (INT. MAMMARY) ARTERY IS DISSECTED FROM 1st COSTAL CARTILAGE TO 6th INTERSPACE; ITS BRANCHES FROM 2nd TO 4th INTERSPACE ARE LIGATED AND DIVIDED BUT THOSE TO 5th AND 6th INTERSPACES PRESERVED FOR LATER DIVISION SO AS TO PROVIDE OUTFLOW CHANNELS WHEN ARTERY IS IMPLANTED

B: IN THE SEWELL TECHNIC, A PEDICLE COMPRISING THE LEFT INTERNAL THORACIC (INT. MAMMARY) ARTERY AND VEIN PLUS LYMPHATIC AND AREOLAR TISSUE IS MOBILIZED

C: THE MOBILIZED ARTERY OR PEDICLE IS WRAPPED IN GAUZE SOAKED IN PAPAVERINE; THE PERICARDIUM IS OPENED LONGITUDINALLY WITH COUNTER-INCISION BEHIND L. PHRENIC NERVE FOR DRAINAGE; SHALLOW STAB WOUNDS ARE MADE ON ANTERIOR WALL OF L. VENTRICLE AND AT APEX

SURGERY FOR CORONARY-ARTERY DISEASE

(Continued from page 239)

reserved for selected patients who present a segmental occlusion in a major coronary artery. The *localized obstruction*, amenable to direct surgery, develops in the dominant *right coronary artery*, which perfuses the posterior aspect of the left ventricle and the septum. Needless to say, *preoperative identification* of the segmental occlusion requires *precise coronary arteriography*.

The technic of *coronary arteriotomy* with patch-graft reconstruction uses *extracorporeal circulation*, and elective cardiac arrest may be of great help. The predetermined site of occlusion requires a generous exposure of the artery, well above and distal to the lesion in question. The surgeon and his first assistant may find it advantageous to use *low-power binocular loupes*. The *circle* (see Plate 70: A) denotes the bounds of the specific operative field. After the dissection of the vessel has been completed and the area of obstruction identified, a linear incision is made directly through the vessel wall and into the lumen. The *"I"-shaped arteriotomy incision* is shown schematically (see Plate 70: B). A longitudinal incision parallels the axis of the vessel and is terminated at each end, at right angles, with a tiny transverse incision, in order to obtain maximal luminal caliber. True endarterectomy is rarely attempted,

because distal dissection is likely to occur. *Gentle dilation* of the coronary artery with *metal sounds* is performed as an initial step and again as the final step of the *patch-graft reconstruction* (see Plate 70: B and C).

Comment. An analysis of the first 150 operations, at the Cleveland Clinic Hospital, in which arteriotomy and patch-graft reconstruction were performed shows that the procedure was used most frequently in a dominant right coronary artery. Direct operations upon the left coronary artery carry a far greater risk, because this vessel bifurcates to form the anterior interventricular (descending) and the circumflex branches. The technical problems of exposure and application of bifurcation grafts have not yet been resolved.

Internal Thoracic (Mammary) Artery-Implant Procedures

Myocardial revascularization may be accomplished by the implantation of a systemic artery within the ventricular myocardium, when a localized perfusion deficit exists. Vineberg's hypothesis, first suggested in 1945, was confirmed objectively, in 1961, when Sones catheterized 2 postoperative survivors and demonstrated a patent functioning implant in each patient. Since that time, more than 1,200 patients have undergone operation by the Cleveland Clinic surgical team for some form of internal thoracic (mammary) artery-implant procedure.

Vineberg's Implant. Vineberg's original implant opera-
(Continued on page 241)

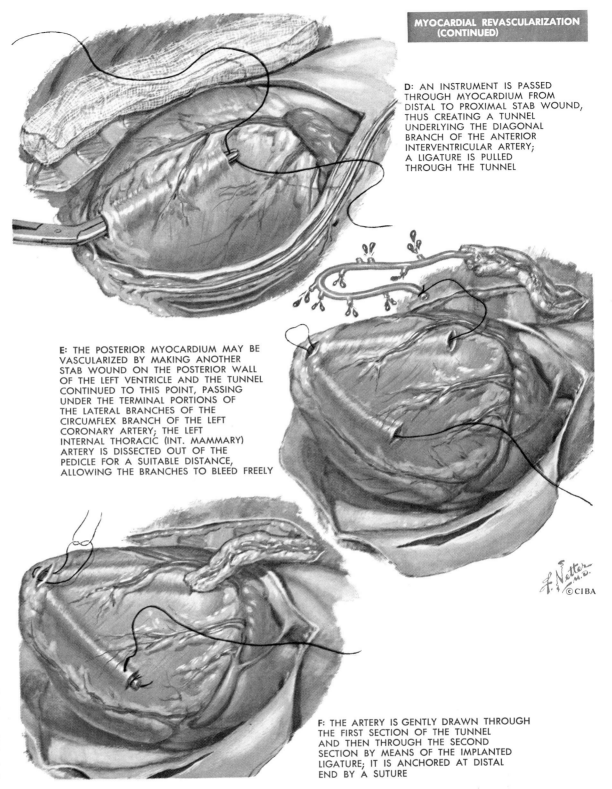

D: AN INSTRUMENT IS PASSED THROUGH MYOCARDIUM FROM DISTAL TO PROXIMAL STAB WOUND, THUS CREATING A TUNNEL UNDERLYING THE DIAGONAL BRANCH OF THE ANTERIOR INTERVENTRICULAR ARTERY; A LIGATURE IS PULLED THROUGH THE TUNNEL

E: THE POSTERIOR MYOCARDIUM MAY BE VASCULARIZED BY MAKING ANOTHER STAB WOUND ON THE POSTERIOR WALL OF THE LEFT VENTRICLE AND THE TUNNEL CONTINUED TO THIS POINT, PASSING UNDER THE TERMINAL PORTIONS OF THE LATERAL BRANCHES OF THE CIRCUMFLEX BRANCH OF THE LEFT CORONARY ARTERY; THE LEFT INTERNAL THORACIC (INT. MAMMARY) ARTERY IS DISSECTED OUT OF THE PEDICLE FOR A SUITABLE DISTANCE, ALLOWING THE BRANCHES TO BLEED FREELY

F: THE ARTERY IS GENTLY DRAWN THROUGH THE FIRST SECTION OF THE TUNNEL AND THEN THROUGH THE SECOND SECTION BY MEANS OF THE IMPLANTED LIGATURE; IT IS ANCHORED AT DISTAL END BY A SUTURE

SURGERY FOR CORONARY-ARTERY DISEASE

(Continued from page 240)

tion was performed through the *left pleural space* and utilized a naked *internal thoracic (mammary) artery*. The revascularization provided by this form of implant was limited to the anterior wall of the left ventricle and its interventricular septum. The experience at the Cleveland Clinic suggested that surgical failures, with this method, could be attributed to technical errors that resulted in damage to this delicate vessel.

Sewell's Pedicle Implant. This implant, which includes *artery, vein, muscle, and fibrous tissue,* resulted in a greater yield of functioning implants. The *Sewell procedure,* though, was accompanied by a significant increase in operative mortality, probably because of the need for a rather large tunnel to accommodate the bulky pedicle. Illustrated are the Vineberg procedure with the naked internal thoracic (mammary) artery (see Plate 71: A) and the dry, Sewell pedicle technic (Plate 71: B). The tunnel limits are created by separate *stab wounds* (Plate 71: C) that extend several millimeters into the *anterior wall of the left ventricle.* The selection of the *tunnel site* is based upon preoperative arteriographic findings and the localization of the functional demand for an improved blood supply.

Vineberg-Sewell Implant. In an effort to combine the low operative risk of Vineberg's implant with the better yield of the Sewell pedicle, a compromise procedure has been evolved. The Vineberg-Sewell pedicle implant (Plate 72: E) is currently used at the Cleveland Clinic Hospital.

The vessel is mobilized from the chest wall as a Sewell pedicle; then that portion of the vessel to be implanted is trimmed away from the redundant pedicle tissue. In this way, the best features of both Vineberg's and Sewell's operations are incorporated into a now-standardized procedure.

The Sewell pedicle offers a longer vessel for implantation, whereas Vineberg's naked artery retracts when taken away from the anterior chest wall. Since the ordinary pedicle is longer than is needed for an anterior implant, it has become common practice to make a second *tunnel* on the diaphragmatic aspect of the left ventricle. In this way, the implanted artery is brought into *intimate contact with the lateral and posterior interventricular (descending) branches of the left and right coronary arteries.*

Postoperative (mammary) arteriography has shown that a Vineberg-Sewell anteroposterior implant may form collateral connections to the anterior interventricular (descending) and the *lateral circumflex branches of the left coronary artery,* as well as to the posterior interventricular (descending) branches from a dominant right coronary artery. This collateral result, after the implantation of an internal thoracic (mammary) artery, has never been observed to occur in a simple anterior-wall implant of the Vineberg type.

Illustrated (Plate 72: E and F) are the principles

(Continued on page 242)

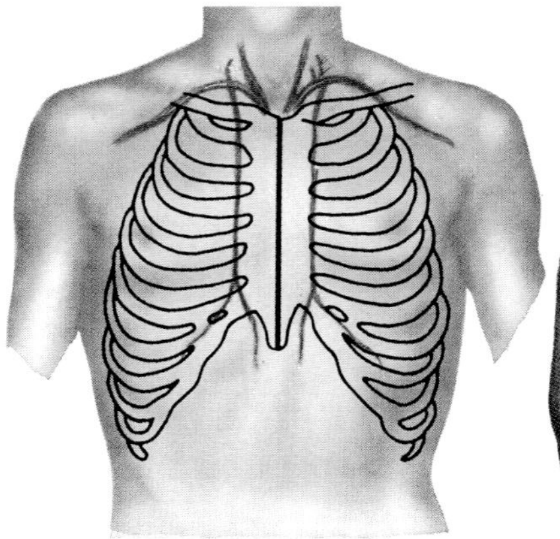

A: MIDLINE STERNUM—SPLITTING INCISION

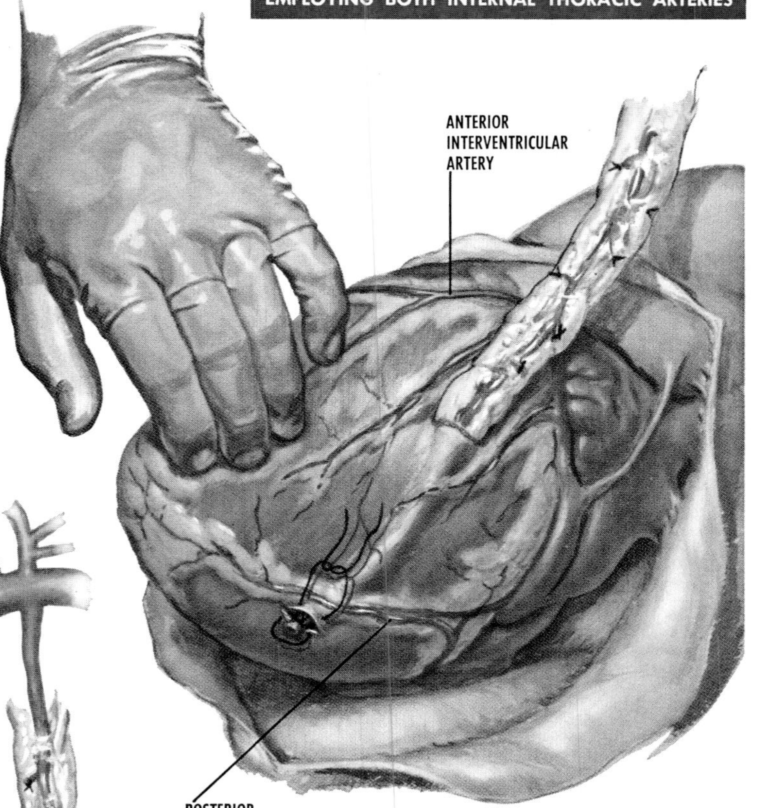

ANTERIOR
INTERVENTRICULAR
ARTERY

POSTERIOR
INTERVENTRICULAR
ARTERY

B: LEFT INTERNAL THORACIC (INTERNAL MAMMARY) ARTERY IMPLANTED INTO POSTERIOR WALL OF LEFT VENTRICLE, PASSING DEEP TO POSTERIOR INTER-VENTRICULAR ARTERY

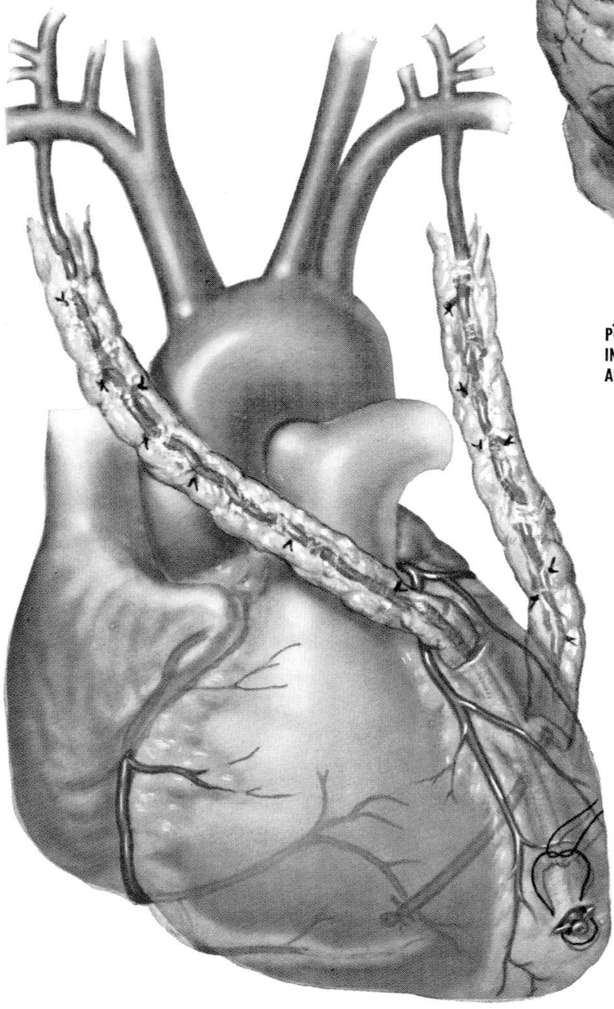

C: RIGHT INTERNAL THORACIC (INTERNAL MAMMARY) ARTERY IMPLANTED IN ANTERIOR WALL OF LEFT VENTRICLE, UNDERLYING OBLIQUE BRANCH OF ANTERIOR INTERVENTRICULAR ARTERY; IMPLANTED LEFT INTERNAL THORACIC ARTERY SHOWN IN PHANTOM

SURGERY FOR CORONARY-ARTERY DISEASE

(Continued from page 241)

of the anteroposterior tunnels. These are made separately, but the resultant implantation is an approximation of a healthy, systemic artery to all branches of the coronary blood supply of the left ventricle.

Bilateral Internal Thoracic (Mammary) Artery Implants. Greater appreciation of the revascularization potential by *internal thoracic (mammary) artery* implantation has led to a technic for bilateral internal thoracic artery implants. A *median-sternotomy incision* permits dissection of the pedicles of both the right and the left internal thoracic arteries. The pedicle dissection is identical to that undertaken for a single implant through a left-thoracotomy incision. The creation of a long *tunnel* on the lateral and diaphragmatic aspects of the *left ventricle* is not difficult. The beating heart may be elevated and rotated to expose the area of posterior perfusion deficit. It is now apparent that any portion of the left ventricular myocardium is amenable to implantation of an internal thoracic artery. The pedicle of the left internal thoracic artery is implanted along the lateral and diaphragmatic aspects of the left ventricle, where it may form collateral connections with all the *interventricular (descending) branches* of the left coronary artery and the dominant right coronary artery. The

anterior wall of the left ventricle will be served by the *right internal thoracic (mammary) artery* which may pass directly over or *under* the *anterior interventricular (descending) branch* of the left coronary artery.

The *bilateral* internal thoracic artery-implant procedure is intended for patients whose diffuse disease produces a perfusion deficit on both the anterior and the diaphragmatic aspects of the left ventricle. Postoperative arteriographic studies prove that revascularization, either by one or by both internal thoracic arteries, is feasible. It is now apparent that any area of perfusion deficit in the left ventricle can be improved by implantation of an internal thoracic artery if the affected myocardium is salvageable.

Interposed Saphenous-Vein Graft for Direct Coronary-Artery Surgery

After 6 years of experience with the pericardial patch graft, it is evident that this operation has value in selected patients with coronary-artery disease. The limitations of endarteriotomy with patch-graft reconstruction are determined by the extent and, to some degree, the nature of the underlying disease process. Frequently, the localized segmental obstruction, visualized at operation, is more extensive than had been suggested by the preoperative coronary arteriograms. In some patients the basic disease process has an inflammatory component, and surgical manipulation may accelerate degenerative occlusion at, or adjacent

(Continued on page 243)

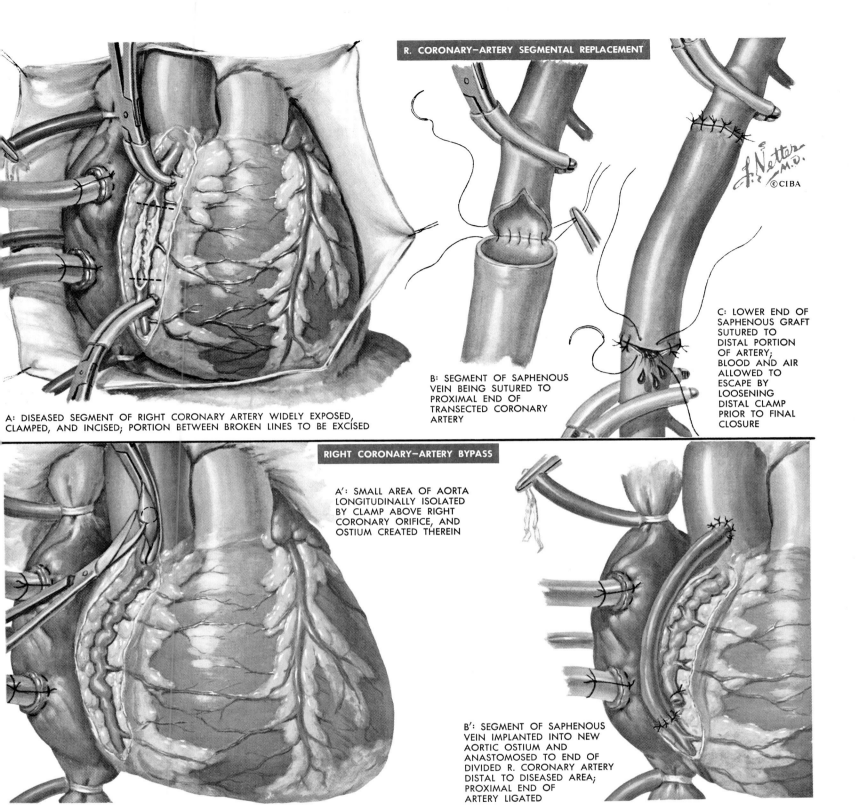

R. CORONARY–ARTERY SEGMENTAL REPLACEMENT

A: DISEASED SEGMENT OF RIGHT CORONARY ARTERY WIDELY EXPOSED, CLAMPED, AND INCISED; PORTION BETWEEN BROKEN LINES TO BE EXCISED

B: SEGMENT OF SAPHENOUS VEIN BEING SUTURED TO PROXIMAL END OF TRANSECTED CORONARY ARTERY

C: LOWER END OF SAPHENOUS GRAFT SUTURED TO DISTAL PORTION OF ARTERY; BLOOD AND AIR ALLOWED TO ESCAPE BY LOOSENING DISTAL CLAMP PRIOR TO FINAL CLOSURE

RIGHT CORONARY–ARTERY BYPASS

A': SMALL AREA OF AORTA LONGITUDINALLY ISOLATED BY CLAMP ABOVE RIGHT CORONARY ORIFICE, AND OSTIUM CREATED THEREIN

B': SEGMENT OF SAPHENOUS VEIN IMPLANTED INTO NEW AORTIC OSTIUM AND ANASTOMOSED TO END OF DIVIDED R. CORONARY ARTERY DISTAL TO DISEASED AREA; PROXIMAL END OF ARTERY LIGATED

SECTION V — PLATE 74

SURGERY FOR CORONARY-ARTERY DISEASE

(Continued from page 242)

to, the patch itself. A number of disappointments have, later, followed successful patch-graft reconstructions, thus prompting the search for a different form of direct surgical attack.

Right Coronary-Artery Segmental Replacement. The interposed *saphenous-vein graft* was first conceived and used in the Cleveland Clinic Hospital in September, 1967, by Rene G. Favaloro, M.D., a member of the Department of Thoracic and Cardiovascular Surgery of the Cleveland Clinic Foundation. During the next 5 months, over 50 operations of this type were performed, with 2 hospital deaths.

The procedure differs essentially from patch-graft reconstruction. A generous *segment of the diseased artery is excised,* and the continuity is reestablished by the patient's own venous tissue. When applied to the dominant *right coronary artery,* this procedure greatly extends the potential of direct coronary-artery surgery. Longer segments of diseased artery may be corrected, and, when necessary, a new *aortic ostium* may be made. Continuity is reestablished through a smooth endothelialized tube, in contrast to the irregular surface provided by a patched arterial segment. Experience with interposed vein-graft procedures indicates that they are less difficult, technically, than most of the patch-graft reconstructions.

Total bypass is made possible by extracorporeal circulation. (Elective cardiac arrest with regional hypothermia, which was utilized in most of the earlier patch-graft procedures, is not necessary.) As needed, over two thirds of the dominant right coronary artery may be *exposed* from the aortic ostium to the beginning of the posterior descending artery that perfuses the diaphragmatic aspect of the left ventricle. The predetermined occlusion is opened widely by a *linear*

(Continued on page 244)

243

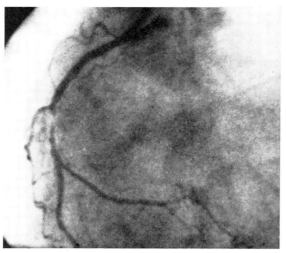

1: R. CORONARY ARTERIOGRAM; L. ANT. OBLIQUE PROJECTION; SEVERE OBSTRUCTION AT MIDDLE THIRD OF R. MAIN CORONARY ARTERY

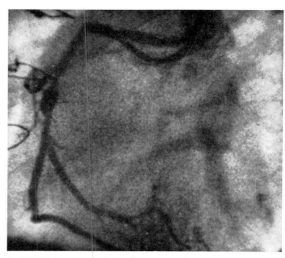

2: SAME PATIENT AS IN "1," NINE MONTHS AFTER ENDARTERIOTOMY AND PERICARDIAL PATCH GRAFT; OBSTRUCTION RELIEVED

SURGERY FOR CORONARY-ARTERY DISEASE

(Continued from page 243)

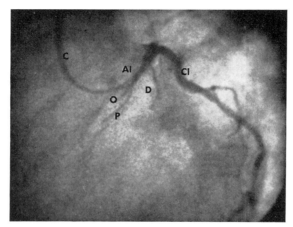

3: L. CORONARY ARTERIOGRAM; L. ANT. OBLIQUE PROJECTION; TOTAL OCCLUSION (O) OF ANT. INTER-VENTRICULAR BRANCH (AI) OF L. CORONARY ARTERY; D=A HIGH DIAGONAL BRANCH; P=A PERFORATING BRANCH; C=CATHETER; CI=CIRCUMFLEX BRANCH

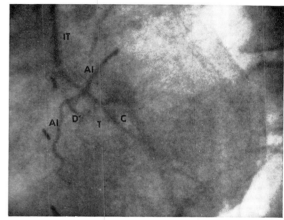

4: L. INT. THORACIC ARTERIOGRAM; SAME PT. AS IN "3," TEN MONTHS AFTER IMPLANTATION OF INT. THO-RACIC ARTERY (IT). THE LATTER HAS MADE CONNECTION AT "C" WITH A TERTIARY BRANCH (T) OF THE ANT. INTERVENTRICULAR (AI), AND, VIA THIS, A DISTAL DIAGONAL BRANCH (D') AND THE ANT. INTERVENTRIC-ULAR BEYOND THE OBSTRUCTION HAVE BEEN FILLED

arteriotomy, until good lumen is obtained above and below the segmental obstruction (Plate 74: A). The artery is then transected above and below, and the *diseased segment is removed*. The *saphenous vein*, obtained at the time of femoral-artery cannulation, is anastomosed *proximally* with interrupted fine arterial sutures (Plate 74: B). (The *cephalad* portion of the graft is used for the *proximal anastomosis*; obstruction produced by the vein valves may result *if the graft is inadvertently reversed!*) The *distal* anastomosis (Plate 74: C) is performed in a similar fashion; particular care being taken to avoid a long vein graft, which might kink or buckle and predispose to subsequent occlusion.

Right Coronary-Artery Bypass. A new concept of *direct coronary-artery* surgery utilizes the saphenous-vein graft to *bypass* the proximal third of the diseased coronary artery. This technic is helpful when the underlying sclerotic process involves the ostium of the *right coronary artery*. It may be used when the diseased vessel, partially open, gives collateral support to an obstructed anterior descending branch in the left coronary artery.

The *new ostium* (Plate 74: A') is made 2 cm or more *above the origin of the right coronary artery*. The circular aortic incision is comparable in size to the

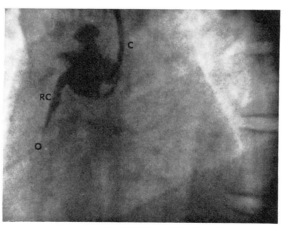

5: R. CORONARY ARTERIOGRAM; L. ANT. OBLIQUE PRO-JECTION; TOTAL OCCLUSION (O) OF R. CORONARY ARTERY (RC) ABOUT 2 CM FROM ITS ORIGIN; C=CATHETER

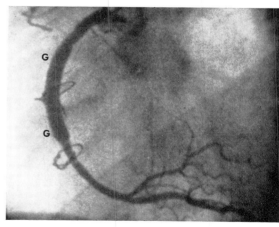

©CIBA

6: SAME PT. AS IN "5" AFTER OBLITERATED SEGMENT OF R. CORONARY ARTERY WAS REPLACED BY A SAPHENOUS—VEIN GRAFT (G), REESTABLISHING NORMAL BLOOD FLOW

lumen of the proximal *saphenous vein*. As shown (Plate 74: B'), the proximal segment of the diseased right coronary artery is left *in situ* to preserve whatever residual collateral support it can provide. Distally, this artery is ligated and divided, and the *lower end* of the *saphenous graft* is *connected* to the *distal segment* of the *right coronary artery*.

Follow-up Studies. Angiograms, made weeks or months after interposed vein-graft procedures have been car-

ried out, suggest that this newer approach may have greater application, in the direct surgical treatment of a coronary occlusive disease, than did the original patch-graft reconstruction. Certainly, this technic offers greater latitude, since longer segments of diseased artery may be removed or bypassed.

Application of the saphenous-vein-graft technic to the left coronary artery has not, as yet, been undertaken.

HEART IN HYPERTHYROIDISM

The striking relationship between thyotoxicosis and the circulation was recognized as early as 1786 by Parry, who described "enlargement of the thyroid gland in connection with enlargement or palpitation of the heart." In response to an *increase in metabolism,* the circulation becomes *hyperdynamic. Vasodilation* makes the skin flushed, warm, and moist. There is often a *rise in systolic blood pressure,* with a *drop in the diastolic,* and an *increase in the pulse pressure.* The pulse is vigorous, *rapid,* and (sometimes) irregular. The cardiac impulse is dynamic and may be displaced to the left. The heart sounds are forceful. The *velocity of blood flow is increased. Systolic ejection murmurs* are frequent. Edema of the lower extremities is common. The combination of dyspnea, tachycardia, arrhythmia, murmurs, and edema may suggest cardiac decompensation, but these are the regular accompaniments of the circulation in thyrotoxicosis. A variety of *electrocardiographic changes* have been described, including sinus tachycardia, *atrial fibrillation,* prolongation of the P-R interval, generalized St-T changes, and shortening of the Q-Tc interval. *Atrial fibrillation,* often *paroxysmal,* is particularly common in patients above the age of 40. Chest *roentgenograms* may show *moderate cardiac enlargement* and a *prominent pulmonary artery.*

The hemodynamic changes in thyrotoxic patients have been ascribed to the general increase in metabolic rate, to a greater sensitivity to catecholamines, and to a direct effect of thyroid hormones on the heart. The velocity of muscle shortening and the rate of tension development are augmented, and the duration of the active or the contractile state of cardiac muscle is decreased.

Early in the disease, while compensation persists, the *cardiac output is augmented* to a degree often relatively greater than the increase in body oxygen consumption; the arteriovenous oxygen difference may be decreased. The enhanced cardiac index is the result of the accelerated heart rate and, to a lesser extent, of the increase in stroke volume. In response to exercise, there is a further increase in rate and in cardiac output. The hemodynamic changes occur without a significant variation in pressure in the right atrium or the pulmonary artery. Of particular importance is the *distribution* of the greater output. Flow to the skin and muscles is improved, but there is no increase in cerebral or splanchnic

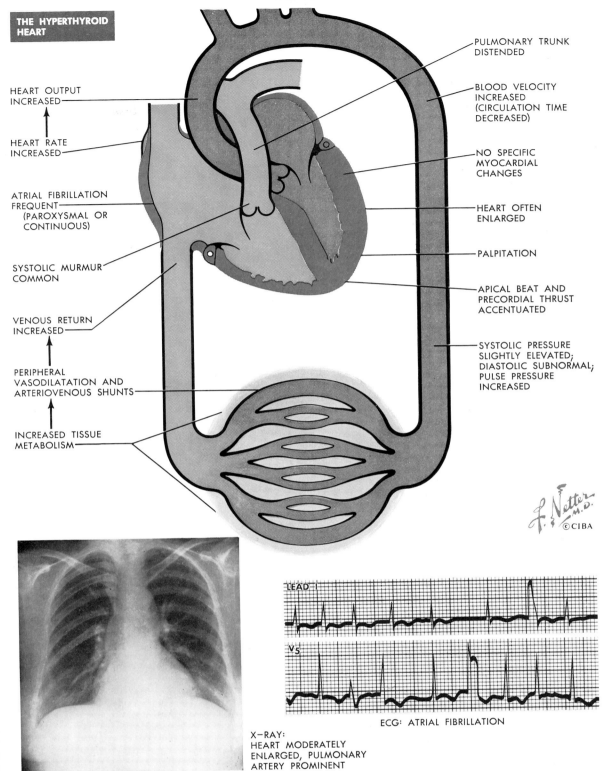

THE HYPERTHYROID HEART

HEART OUTPUT INCREASED

HEART RATE INCREASED

ATRIAL FIBRILLATION FREQUENT (PAROXYSMAL OR CONTINUOUS)

SYSTOLIC MURMUR COMMON

VENOUS RETURN INCREASED

PERIPHERAL VASODILATATION AND ARTERIOVENOUS SHUNTS

INCREASED TISSUE METABOLISM

PULMONARY TRUNK DISTENDED

BLOOD VELOCITY INCREASED (CIRCULATION TIME DECREASED)

NO SPECIFIC MYOCARDIAL CHANGES

HEART OFTEN ENLARGED

PALPITATION

APICAL BEAT AND PRECORDIAL THRUST ACCENTUATED

SYSTOLIC PRESSURE SLIGHTLY ELEVATED; DIASTOLIC SUBNORMAL; PULSE PRESSURE INCREASED

X-RAY: HEART MODERATELY ENLARGED, PULMONARY ARTERY PROMINENT

LEAD I

V5

ECG: ATRIAL FIBRILLATION

flow. The additional renal blood flow parallels the general increase in oxygen consumption; coronary blood flow is augmented, but it constitutes a normal fraction of the increased cardiac output.

The patient previously afflicted with coronary-artery disease may, under the burden of this load, develop angina pectoris. Similarly, in the presence of rheumatic valvular deformity, congestive heart failure may supervene. Of great interest is the question whether the normal heart may eventually fail as the result of increased cardiac work of long duration. Pathologic examination reveals no characteristic lesion, but, in animals and in man, prolonged hyperthyroidism results in cardiac hypertrophy. When the heart fails in thyrotoxicosis, the cardiac output falls, though not to absolute low levels. The output is low, however, in relation to body oxygen consumption. The stroke index falls, the response to exercise is poor,

and the pressures in the right atrium and pulmonary artery are elevated.

The response to *therapy* is dramatic. The velocity of blood flow decreases, and the peripheral resistance rises. As the heart rate falls, the cardiac output and the right and left ventricular work decrease, and the myocardial oxygen consumption returns to normal. Where angina pectoris and congestive failure have developed, striking improvement may be experienced. Even in the absence of recognizable heart disease, evidences of congestive heart failure may persist or recur, despite the euthyroid state. The same is true of atrial fibrillation; after the return to normal thyroid function, sinus rhythm may recur spontaneously or in response to antiarrhythmic therapy, although, in a substantial group of patients, and particularly those with congestive heart failure, atrial fibrillation may persist.

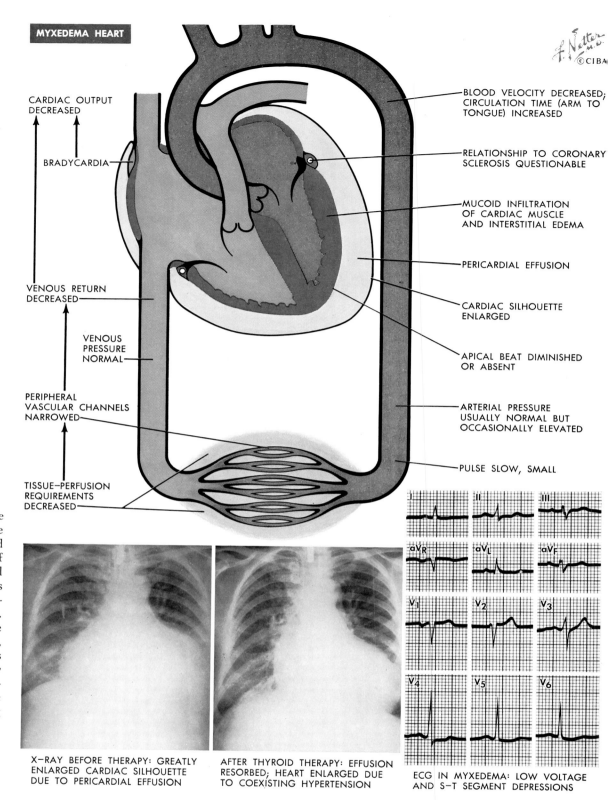

MYXEDEMA HEART

CARDIAC OUTPUT DECREASED

BRADYCARDIA

VENOUS RETURN DECREASED

VENOUS PRESSURE NORMAL

PERIPHERAL VASCULAR CHANNELS NARROWED

TISSUE–PERFUSION REQUIREMENTS DECREASED

BLOOD VELOCITY DECREASED; CIRCULATION TIME (ARM TO TONGUE) INCREASED

RELATIONSHIP TO CORONARY SCLEROSIS QUESTIONABLE

MUCOID INFILTRATION OF CARDIAC MUSCLE AND INTERSTITIAL EDEMA

PERICARDIAL EFFUSION

CARDIAC SILHOUETTE ENLARGED

APICAL BEAT DIMINISHED OR ABSENT

ARTERIAL PRESSURE USUALLY NORMAL BUT OCCASIONALLY ELEVATED

PULSE SLOW, SMALL

X-RAY BEFORE THERAPY: GREATLY ENLARGED CARDIAC SILHOUETTE DUE TO PERICARDIAL EFFUSION

AFTER THYROID THERAPY: EFFUSION RESORBED; HEART ENLARGED DUE TO COEXISTING HYPERTENSION

ECG IN MYXEDEMA: LOW VOLTAGE AND S–T SEGMENT DEPRESSIONS

HEART IN MYXEDEMA

In *myxedema* the circulation can be considered *hypodynamic* but adequate for the diminished flow requirements and decreased body oxygen consumption of this condition. The patient's skin is cool and thickened — an evidence of changes in the skin but also of *peripheral* vaso-constriction and *retarded velocity of flow.* The neck veins are not distended. The *cardiac impulse is sluggish* and feeble, the *pulse is slow,* and the heart sounds are muffled. The *blood pressure is usually normal* but may be elevated. The *electro-cardiogram* often contains characteristic (but not diagnostic) changes, including *low voltage,* flattening or *inversion of the T waves,* and an increased P-R interval. On the *X-ray plate* the *cardiac silhouette is increased in size.* In large part, this image is due to *pericardial effusion,* the withdrawal of which may reveal that the actual heart size is normal.

The level of thyroid function profoundly affects the contractile state of cardiac muscle. Muscles from hypothyroid animals develop tension at a slower rate, but this is compensated for by a prolonged period of contraction.

The *cardiac output is decreased,* as a result not only of the slow rate but also of a small stroke volume. On the other hand, the ratio of cardiac output to total oxygen consumption is normal. The pressures in the right atrium and pulmonary artery generally are normal. In response to exercise, the cardiac output, rate, and stroke volume are capable of rising.

The low output of the myxedematous heart is in contrast with that of cardiac decompensation. In the latter condition the output is low and not proportional to the body oxygen consumption, pressures are high in the right atrium, and, in response to exercise, there is an inadequate increase in cardiac output, with a marked elevation of atrial pressure.

Definitive pathologic data on the state of the heart in untreated hypothyroidism are meager. The heart has been described as flabby, pale, and dilated. Fibrous-tissue replacement and infiltration have been described. *Microscopic* changes include swelling of muscle cells, degeneration of muscle fibers, *fatty infiltration,* and *interstitial edema* with accumulation of interstitial fluid which is *mucinous* and has a high protein and nitrogen content. It is clear that the conditions are difficult to evaluate, because they occur also in the changes caused by aging. It is commonly stated that the hypercholesterolemia of myxedema leads to an increased incidence of *atherosclerosis,* but critical evaluation of the data leaves many questions unanswered, and the relationship between serum cholesterol, hypothyroidism, and atherosclerosis remains to be clarified.

The *changes in the circulation* in myxedema are *reversed by thyroid substitution therapy.* The heart size shrinks, cardiac output rises, ECGs normalize, the velocity of blood flow increases, peripheral flow becomes greater, and the blood pressure, if elevated, may fall. Since primary myxedema is a disease of later life, when coronary-artery disease may also be present, therapy should be undertaken cautiously, lest angina pectoris or even myocardial infarction be precipitated.

TRICHINOSIS

♀ (3 X 0.065 mm)

♂ (1.5 X 0.037 mm)

F. Netter
©CIBA

CYST WALLS DIGESTED, LIBERATING LARVAE

LARVAE DEVELOP INTO MATURE MALES AND FEMALES IN INTESTINE OF HOST AND COPULATE

INFECTED PORK EATEN BY HOGS AS SCRAPS IN GARBAGE

INFECTED, INCOMPLETELY COOKED PORK EATEN BY MAN

GRAVID FEMALES DEPOSIT YOUNG IN MUCOSA OF INTESTINE

YOUNG TRICHINAE (100 X 6μ) MIGRATE VIA LACTEALS, THORACIC DUCT, AND BLOOD–STREAM TO MUSCLES

TRICHINA LARVAE GROW AND ENCYST IN SKELETAL MUSCLES OF HOSTS: HOGS AND MAN (MUSCLE PAINS)

TRICHINA LARVAE, WHICH INVADE BUT DO <u>NOT</u> ENCYST IN THE HEART, MAY CAUSE SEVERE MYOCARDITIS

POSITIVE REACTION WITHIN 20 MINUTES AFTER INTRADERMAL INJECTION OF ANTIGEN

CHARACTERISTIC EDEMA OF EYELIDS AND FACE IN ACUTE TRICHINOSIS: PULMONARY, CNS, AND CUTANEOUS SYMPTOMS AS WELL AS FEVER MAY APPEAR; EOSINOPHILIA IS PRESENT

TRICHINOSIS

Trichinosis is caused by the round worm *Trichinella spiralis.* Its *life cycle* runs as follows: When *raw* or *incompletely cooked pork* or a *pork product* containing living trichina larvae is eaten, the *walls* of the *cysts are digested,* liberating the *microscopic larvae.* Within the *small intestine of the host,* the freed *larvae maturate,* during the next 2 days, to adult *male* (1 to 3 mm long) or *female* (2 to 4 mm long) worms, and *copulate.* Beginning 5 days after ingestion of the infected meat and, in man, continuing for as long as 12 weeks, the *gravid adult female* worms, which are partially embedded in the *mucosal wall* of the small bowel, give birth to *larvae* (the second generation). The latter (80 to 120 microns by 6 microns) successively enter the *lacteals* of the *intestinal villi,* the cavity of the right ventricle, the pulmonary capillaries, and the *systemic circulation.* Although they may also enter various organs of the body, by predilection they penetrate *skeletal muscle fibers.* Here they enlarge progressively, simultaneously causing degeneration of the fibers and provoking a local reaction characterized by *edema,* hyperemia, and granulomatous and *eosinophilic* inflammation. Approximately 30 days after invasion of the muscle fibers, the larvae, which now have assumed a characteristic coiled appearance, attain their maximal size and become *encapsulated.* Gravid adult female worms continue to give birth to additional larvae, which invade additional muscle fibers. In nature, the life cycle of the parasite is completed when a carnivorous mammal becomes infected with the parasite, as the result of ingesting the flesh of another animal containing living larvae.

The *incubation period* usually ranges between 7 and 10 days, but it may be as short as 1 day or as long as 28 days. As a rule, the first *symptoms* are *intestinal,* the mucosa of the small bowel being irritated by partial penetration of the larvae, *excysted from* the digested *infected meat,* and the adult worms developing from them. Symptoms include nausea, vomiting, abdominal cramps, and diarrhea or constipation. They usually last approximately 1 week. Symptoms of the *muscular phase* generally begin about 1 week after infection. As a rule, the first one noted by the patient is *edema of the eyelids.* It is followed by pain, tenderness, and *swelling of the face,* and by *pain* on movement of any of the *voluntary muscles.* The severity of this phase depends on the number of second-generation larvae invading the tissues of the host. In a severe or moderately severe infection, this phase lasts from 4 to 8 weeks and is accompanied by *fever* (up to 104 degrees) and weakness. Incidental involvement of other organs may cause *bronchitis or bronchopneumonia, encephalitis or meningismus,* a *cutaneous*

rash, the sensation of insects or worms crawling beneath the skin, *myocarditis,* or *arterial thrombosis.* Among patients hospitalized because of trichinosis, the mortality rate is approximately 5 percent. The stage of convalescence usually is rapid.

The most frequent serious complication is granulomatous *myocarditis,* attended by congestive heart failure or terminated by sudden unexpected death during the sixth to the eighth week of the infection. The heart is regularly involved, the young larvae invading the myocardium. They *never,* however, *encyst* there. As a rule, *electrocardiographic* changes appear during the second month of the infection. Occasionally, large arteries of the brain or of an extremity become thrombosed, owing, apparently, to hypercoagulability of the blood. Recovery from myocarditis is usually complete.

Eosinophilia begins about 10 days after infection, reaches its peak during the third week, and usually disappears after 6 months. Although moderately severe infections are often attended by eosinophilia of 35 percent or

(not rarely) as much as 70 percent or more, the degree of eosinophilia does not parallel the severity of infection. An abrupt fall from a high level to 1 percent or zero is ominous. In the *diagnosis,* a *skin test* is performed by *intradermal injection of an antigen,* prepared from an extract of powdered larvae. A *positive immediate reaction* (evoked beginning 17 days postinfection), consists of a soft wheal, 7 to 10 mm in diameter, appearing *within 15 to 20 minutes;* it is surrounded by an area of bright erythema and disappears within 1 hour. Other diagnostic technics include precipitin, flocculation, hemagglutination, complement-fixation, and fluorescent-antibody tests, most of which yield positive reactions beginning 17 to 30 days after infection. Biopsy is diagnostic if encysting larvae, accompanied by a characteristic myositis, are found.

In the *management* of the patient, bed rest, symptomatic *treatment,* and the use of steroids are indicated.

The microscopic slide is reproduced through the courtesy of John G. Batsakis, M.D.

CHAGAS' DISEASE

Chagas' disease is a menace to millions of people in South-Central America. The *parasite* Trypanosoma cruzi enters the body, usually through the *bite* of a reduviid bug, or by the transfusion or inoculation of contaminated blood. The parasite *circulates* only in its *trypanosomal form*. It *enters a body cell, transforms* to a *leishmania form,* and *multiplies* to form a leishmanial cyst which *ruptures* the invaded cell. In this stage the parasites are released and then transformed into trypanosomes, which circulate in the blood and invade other cells, thus continuing the cycle. The *cardiac muscle cells* are favored in the majority of cases, but, with some strains in particular areas, there is an equal or greater proclivity for the peripheral *ganglion cells* to be invaded or destroyed. In the rarer acute cases, all cells and tissues may be invaded, but in chronic cases the major damage falls on the cardiac muscle cells and the peripheral ganglion cells.

In the *myocardium* there is a parasitic myocarditis, though to demonstrate the actual parasite may require a prolonged search. Foci of cell necrosis with an *inflammatory-cell infiltrate,* which, in the early cases, includes many eosinophils, are found. Probably some ruptured fibers can recover, but others die and are replaced by fibrous tissue.

The invasion is probably reduced as immunity develops, one manifestation of this being the complement-fixation reaction which is so important in *diagnosis*. A positive reaction is generally held to indicate the presence in the body of living parasites, and, since lifelong serum positivity is usual, it would suggest that persisting damage is being done to the body cells. The heart becomes grossly enlarged and very heavy but rather feeble in action. In those patients who develop congestive failure, death may result at any time. The disease is much dreaded because sudden death can occur in affected individuals who are in apparent good health and are unaware of their infection. This is particularly common in young adult males and is often — but not necessarily — brought on by exertion. The precise cause is obscure.

While the disease in some geographic areas seems mainly to be a parasitic myocarditis with a variable progression, in other areas it is accompanied by a variety of lesions in other organs which appear to be the consequences of peripheral ganglion-cell destruction. In hollow organs these are manifested by tubular dilatations; thus megaesophagus, megacolon, or a comparable lesion of any part of the *gastrointestinal tract,* including the

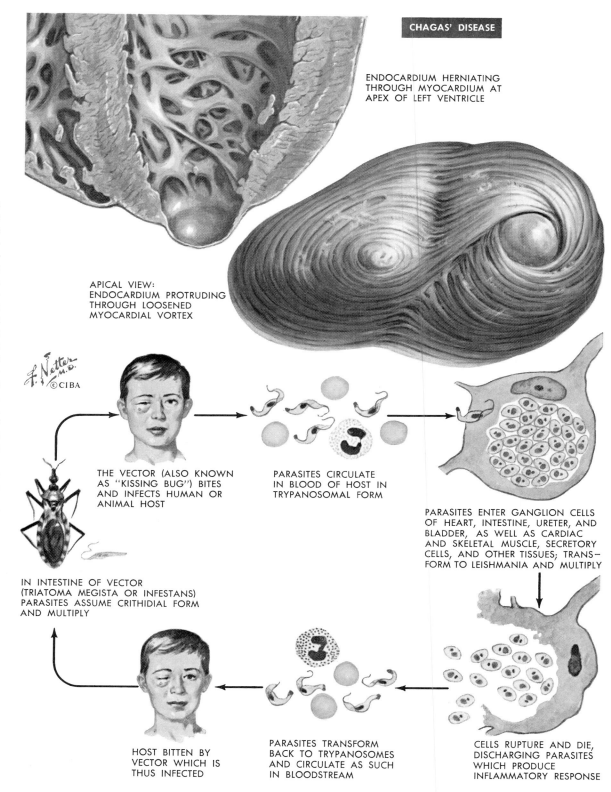

CHAGAS' DISEASE

ENDOCARDIUM HERNIATING THROUGH MYOCARDIUM AT APEX OF LEFT VENTRICLE

APICAL VIEW: ENDOCARDIUM PROTRUDING THROUGH LOOSENED MYOCARDIAL VORTEX

THE VECTOR (ALSO KNOWN AS "KISSING BUG") BITES AND INFECTS HUMAN OR ANIMAL HOST

PARASITES CIRCULATE IN BLOOD OF HOST IN TRYPANOSOMAL FORM

PARASITES ENTER GANGLION CELLS OF HEART, INTESTINE, URETER, AND BLADDER, AS WELL AS CARDIAC AND SKELETAL MUSCLE, SECRETORY CELLS, AND OTHER TISSUES; TRANSFORM TO LEISHMANIA AND MULTIPLY

IN INTESTINE OF VECTOR (TRIATOMA MEGISTA OR INFESTANS) PARASITES ASSUME CRITHIDIAL FORM AND MULTIPLY

HOST BITTEN BY VECTOR WHICH IS THUS INFECTED

PARASITES TRANSFORM BACK TO TRYPANOSOMES AND CIRCULATE AS SUCH IN BLOODSTREAM

CELLS RUPTURE AND DIE, DISCHARGING PARASITES WHICH PRODUCE INFLAMMATORY RESPONSE

gallbladder or bile duct, may be found. There also may be comparable dilatations of the *urinary bladder* and *ureters*. Much of the ganglion-cell destruction takes place in the early stages of infestation, with the dilatations occurring at variable intervals thereafter.

Studies of the cardiac ganglion cells show that these may also be affected, and this loss, as in other organs, results in a parasympathetic deprivation, the effects of which have not been fully explored. One cardiac lesion which develops is a loosening and slackening of the myocardial muscle bundles, producing dilatation of the pulmonary conus and thinning of the ventricular vessels at the apex, so that the *endocardium herniates* and becomes attached to the epicardium. The *apical lesions* in either or both ventricles may range from a deep, narrow cleft to a smooth-domed *protrusion* 2 to 3 cm in diameter and often filled with a thrombus. Oddly enough, these aneu-

rysms rarely rupture, perhaps because the muscle tautens during systole, and this protects them from the force — feeble though it may be — of ventricular ejection.

Much that is concerned with Chagas' disease is controversial and much remains to be discovered, but it is the commonest recognized parasitic myocarditis in the world. A history of exposure to infection, residence in an affected area, cardiomegaly, and the presence of a positive complement-fixation reaction are important points in the *clinical diagnosis*. The presence of a myocarditis, chronic in type, with variable degrees of fibrosis, in a large, heavy heart should lead to a search for the parasite. The presence of apical aneurysms appears unique to this disease. The existence of a mega syndrome, in an individual who has had a possible exposure to infection, should alert the clinician to the possibility of coexistent cardiac damage.

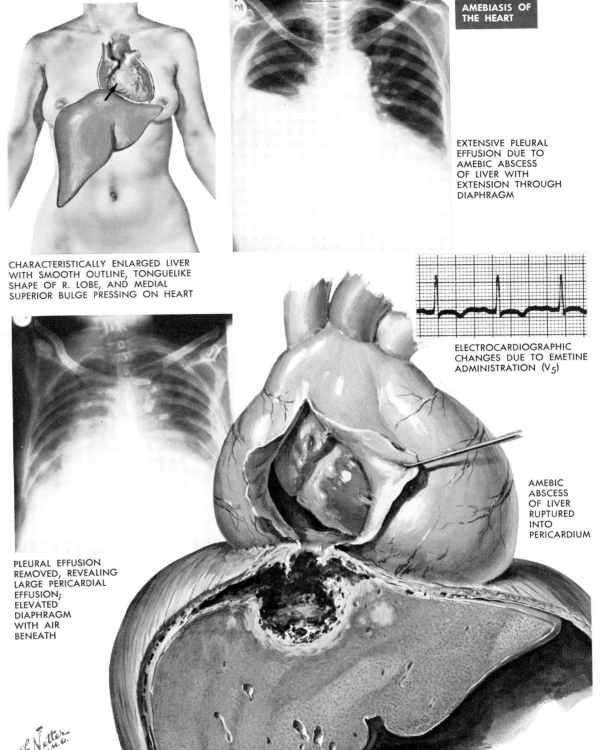

CHARACTERISTICALLY ENLARGED LIVER WITH SMOOTH OUTLINE, TONGUELIKE SHAPE OF R. LOBE, AND MEDIAL SUPERIOR BULGE PRESSING ON HEART

AMEBIASIS OF THE HEART

EXTENSIVE PLEURAL EFFUSION DUE TO AMEBIC ABSCESS OF LIVER WITH EXTENSION THROUGH DIAPHRAGM

ELECTROCARDIOGRAPHIC CHANGES DUE TO EMETINE ADMINISTRATION (V₅)

PLEURAL EFFUSION REMOVED, REVEALING LARGE PERICARDIAL EFFUSION; ELEVATED DIAPHRAGM WITH AIR BENEATH

AMEBIC ABSCESS OF LIVER RUPTURED INTO PERICARDIUM

AMEBIC PERICARDITIS

Amebiasis, transmitted by the protozoan *Entamoeba histolytica*, is considered to be initially and predominantly an intestinal disease, but it involves the liver in a substantial proportion of the cases.

The infective encysted form of the parasite, communicated from man to man (without an intermediate host) by water, food, etc., which has been contaminated by human fecal material, enters the intestinal tract by the mouth, passes through the stomach, and loses its cystic wall in the small intestine (see CIBA COLLECTION, Vol. 3/II, page 155, and Vol. 3/III, page 102). There, the *cyst* (5 to 20 microns in diameter), having matured during its passage, releases from 1 to 4 *trophozoites* (vegetative form) which, in contrast to the cyst, are mobile but do not survive outside the host's body. The amebas, which have attached themselves to the colonic wall, migrate into the crypts and penetrate the epithelium and muscularis. From the submucosa, the amebas move along to other organs, particularly the liver, creating there the chronic, nonsuppurative form of amebic hepatitis or producing abscesses. Other trophozoites are excreted in the encysted form, thus maintaining the life cycle.

The above-described events may proceed with only mild *symptoms* (not necessarily associated with the bowels) and thus may account for the "carrier stage." Upon careful examination of the feces, however, this stage may be detected in as much as 10 percent of the population in endemic United States areas. Some disturbances of the host-parasite relationship result in the activation of the dormant form of the ameba, causing the *clinical picture* of colitis, dysentery, or liver abscess.

Another manifestation of amebiasis, which is very rare, is *amebic pericarditis*. Until 1964 only 65 cases of this condition had been recorded in the world's medical literature. More recently, another 25 cases have been reported in South Africa. Pericardial involvement in amebiasis almost invariably occurs by direct extension from an *amebic abscess* of the left lobe of the *liver*. Only occasionally does amebic pericarditis result from a lung abscess or an abscess in the right lobe of the liver.

The salient *features* are epigastric pain, a palpable mass in the epigastrium or left hypochondrium, tenderness over the liver area, dyspnea, a pericardial friction rub, and high temperature. X-ray studies usually show an *elevated* left *diaphragm* and enlargement of the heart shadow. As a rule, there are mild anemia and polymorphonuclear leukocytosis. The ECG provides positive *diagnostic help* by showing the usual signs of pericarditis, *e.g.*, generalized S-T segment elevation, inverted T waves, or low voltage.

Emetine and chloroquine administration is the *treatment* of choice; however, pericardial aspiration, often repeated, is usually necessary. Amebic pericarditis is a fatal disease in more than 50 percent of the cases, and, even if the patient survives, he runs a high risk of developing constrictive pericarditis, necessitating pericardiectomy.

Another *diagnostic link* between amebiasis and the heart is a penetrating precordial pain or discomfort which often occurs in chronic amebiasis and frequently is thought to be due to heart disease. Radi-

ologically, one can observe a *characteristic configuration of the liver*. It consists of a *tonguelike* descending *enlargement of the right lobe*, with or without an elevation of the right dome and/or a *bulging* near the cardiac shadow. This bulging is probably responsible for the complaints *thought* to derive from the heart. In fact, these *symptoms* are caused by the elevation of the diaphragm owing to hepatomegaly, which is extremely common in amebiasis.

A final association between the heart and amebic infection is that provided by the toxic effect of *emetine* on the heart. *Treatment* with emetine causes, in a large proportion of cases, various *ECG* abnormalities — mainly flattening and inversion of the P and T waves — which are practically always reversible and should cause no anxiety to the physician. Emetine is contraindicated only in the presence of serious cardiac disease.

ECHINOCOCCUS CYST (HYDATID DISEASE)

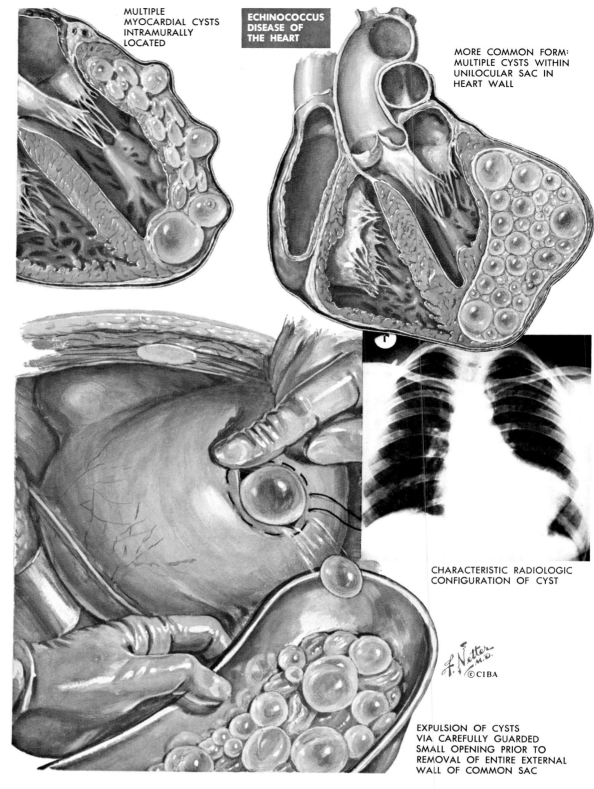

MULTIPLE MYOCARDIAL CYSTS INTRAMURALLY LOCATED

ECHINOCOCCUS DISEASE OF THE HEART

MORE COMMON FORM: MULTIPLE CYSTS WITHIN UNILOCULAR SAC IN HEART WALL

CHARACTERISTIC RADIOLOGIC CONFIGURATION OF CYST

EXPULSION OF CYSTS VIA CAREFULLY GUARDED SMALL OPENING PRIOR TO REMOVAL OF ENTIRE EXTERNAL WALL OF COMMON SAC

The pathogenesis of *echinococcus disease,* the life cycle of its causative parasite (Echinococcus granulosus, a species of Taenia echinococcus), which is a tapeworm, the contamination of man by infected dogs, and the distribution of the endemic areas in the world have been described in the CIBA COLLECTION, Vol. 3/III, page 104.

Even in endemic regions, the *heart* is rarely affected by echinococcus disease, the incidence of primary myocardial involvement being less than 2 percent in human echinococciasis. The parasitic six-hooked embryo reaches the myocardium through the coronary circulation, having passed through the gastric or intestinal mucosa into the portal circulation, and through both the hepatic and the pulmonary capillary beds. It can establish itself and develop into an echinococcus *cyst* in almost any part of the *myocardium,* but cysts are mostly located in the *walls of the ventricles.* There is a higher incidence of cysts in the myocardium of the left ventricle, because its vascular bed is more abundant. The developing parasitic membranous cyst is surrounded by a fibrous *sac* or capsule, the adventitia. When it grows larger, the cyst may protrude into a cardiac cavity, the pericardial sac, or both, its greater and more prominent part usually projecting toward the pericardium.

Primary echinococcus cyst of the heart is mostly single and slow-growing. Less often, more than one cyst and, rarely, *multiple cysts* may develop. A single cyst infrequently remains univesicular and intact. The adventitial capsule usually contains degenerated fragments of the ruptured original membranous cyst (the mother cyst), multiple — sometimes even hundreds — of both unruptured and ruptured daughter cysts varying in size, and free hydatid fluid. Rupture of the membranous cyst is favored greatly because of the repeated trauma inflicted by the continuous heart movement. When the membranous cysts rupture, they may die, and the content of the adventitia becomes caseous and inspissated. Calcification of the adventitial capsule may develop.

During the progressive enlargement of the cyst, disastrous complications can occur. The cyst may rupture into a cardiac cavity or into the pericardial sac. Such ruptures may cause sudden death, owing to anaphylactic shock and to hydatid embolism which is usually cerebral (less frequently, pulmonary). If the person survives, hematogenous dissemination occurs (more commonly, in the central nervous system), with the eventual development of multiple metastatic or secondary cysts in the brain, usually with a fatal outcome. Rupture into the pericardial sac produces acute hydatid pericarditis. Implantation of brood capsules and scolices in the pericardium leads to chronic hydatid pericarditis (hydatidopericardium) with fibrous-tissue reaction and secondary cyst formation.

Clinically, the uncomplicated single cyst, when small, and particularly if dead, may be asymptomatic. As it grows larger, atypical or even undetermined *symptoms* may appear but these do not lead to the *diagnosis. Radiographically,* an eccentric deformity, protruding from the contour of the cardiac shadow, is shown, generally as a circular or ovoid, homogeneous, well-defined opacity continuous with the outline of the heart silhouette. Calcification may appear also; this is more distinct on *tomography.* Transmitted cardiac pulsation in the opacity is demonstrated on *fluor-*oscopy. The *electrocardiogram* may be very useful in the diagnosis and in the more accurate localization of the cyst. Myocardial ischemia and conduction changes are shown more commonly in the ECG. *Angiocardiography* is a valuable adjunct to the radiological investigation, whereas *heart catheterization* is of no diagnostic value. The Casoni intradermal test and the Weinberg test add greatly to the establishment of the diagnosis. The correlation of radiographic and angiocardiographic findings with ECG changes, supplemented by positive biological tests and eosinophilia, in a person living in an endemic region, should lead to the diagnosis of cardiac echinococcus disease.

The *treatment* should aim at the *removal of the cyst.* In certain instances, surgery should be performed under extracorporeal circulation. If the cyst has not ruptured into a heart chamber, surgery probably will result in a cure of the disease.

MYXOMA: CHARACTERISTICALLY
ORIGINATING FROM INTERATRIAL
SEPTUM AND ALMOST FILLING
L. ATRIUM; R. VENTRICULAR
HYPERTROPHY

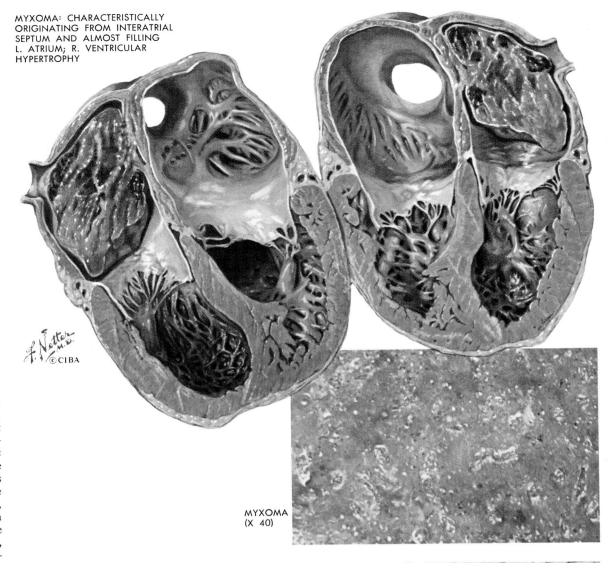

MYXOMA
(X 40)

HEART TUMORS

Myxomas

Primary tumors of the heart are rare. There are fibromas, lipomas, angiomas, and sarcomas, but more than 50 percent of the observed cases are *myxomas,* arising from the endocardium of the *left* (rarely, of the right) *atrium.* They are most common in persons between the ages of 30 and 60 years, and they occur more frequently in women than in men. Often, they develop in the region of the fossa ovalis and have a thin pedicle. The tumors are sometimes small, like a bean, but they may grow to large, smooth, ball-like or villous structures, *filling the atria* almost entirely, but leaving the rest of the endocardium and myocardium unchanged. On a cut surface the myxomas are gelatinous and often show patchy hemorrhagic areas.

Microscopically, myxomas of the atria demonstrate large stellate cells embedded in a myxomatous ground substance, resembling Wharton's jelly. In other areas, collagen and elastic fibers and numerous small blood vessels may be present. Therefore, some tumors may be called myxofibromas, elastomyxomas, or fibroangiomyxomas. Because of the delicate vessels, hemorrhages occur quite easily, and these can be demonstrated as iron deposits. Secondary parietal thromboses may develop, and these can be organized and fuse with the surrounding endocardium. In such thrombosed and organized structures, the original primary tumor may be difficult to assess.

Clinically, in patients with myxoma of the left atrium, there may be fainting after a sudden change to the upright position. These episodes can occur when the tumor is obstructing the mitral valve. In some patients, peripheral vascular disorders may be noted, and these are associated with trophic changes in the nails and skin. The tumor, located in the *left* atrium, may produce chronic passive congestion of the lungs, as in mitral stenosis. Tumors of the *right* atrium lead to early congestion of the abdominal organs. Death may be either sudden or a delayed

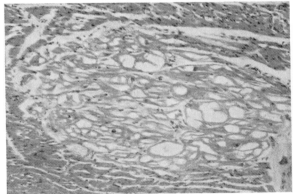

RHABDOMYOMA (X 40)

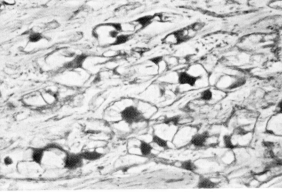

RHABDOMYOSARCOMA (X 40)

consequence of chronic congestive heart failure.

Angiocardiography can help to differentiate between mitral stenosis and a tumor of the left atrium. Surgical removal of such myxomas is possible and, almost invariably, is indicated. Open-heart surgery, with complete pulmonary bypass, is employed.

Rhabdomyomas

Rhabdomyoma, a congenital nodular glycogenic degeneration of myocardial fibers, may be found as single or multiple nodules, especially in the hearts of infants or children. Rhabdomyomas are often observed in cases with tuberous sclerosis or other malformations of the heart, blood vessels, and kidneys. Some of the nodules are so small that they can be discovered only by *microscopic* examination; others may be as large as chestnuts. Rhabdomyomas are localized and are

separated from uninvolved myocardium. Sometimes a fibrous capsule may exist. The cells of rhabdomyomas are arranged irregularly. The size of their nuclei varies only slightly, but the cytoplasm is engorged with *glycogen.*

Rhabdomyosarcoma, a malignant variant of the rhabdomyoma, grows invasively. It may perforate into the lumen of the cardiac chambers and metastasize. In rhabdomyosarcomas the size of the nuclei varies considerably, in contrast to rhabdomyoma. There are giant nuclei with large nucleoli and so-called spider cells with reduced, stringlike cytoplasm. All the remaining spaces of the cells are filled with glycogen.

Rhabdomyoma is considered to be a tissue malformation, resulting from a localized disorder of glycogen metabolism caused by an enzyme defect. *Clinical manifestations* depend on the size and localization of the tumorlike nodules.

METASTATIC HEART TUMORS

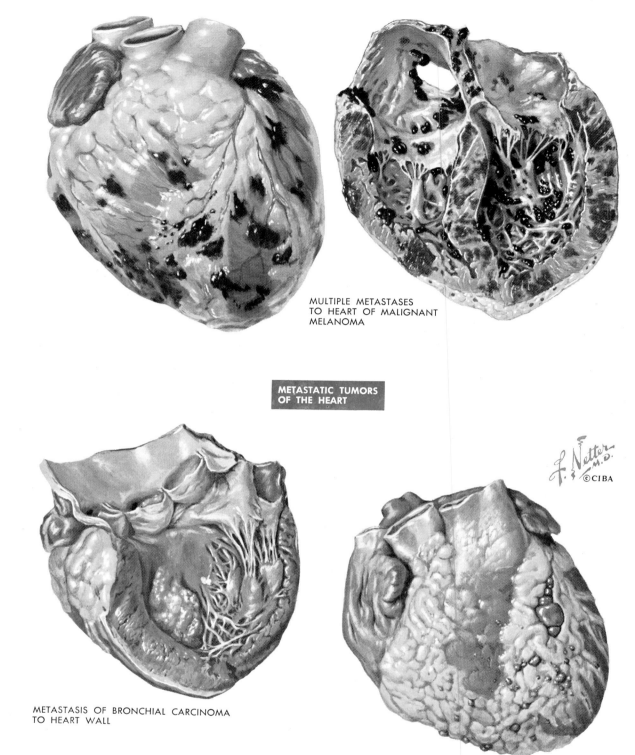

MULTIPLE METASTASES TO HEART OF MALIGNANT MELANOMA

METASTATIC TUMORS OF THE HEART

METASTASIS OF BRONCHIAL CARCINOMA TO HEART WALL

LYMPHANGIAL SPREAD OF METASTATIC BRONCHIAL CARCINOMA

Metastatic tumors of the heart may be present in 6 percent of all the autopsies which reveal malignant neoplasms. Among carcinomas, *bronchiogenic carcinoma* is the most frequent primary tumor metastasizing to the heart.

Some metastases may be discovered only by *microscopic* examination, but others may be so large that the *entire wall* of one chamber or the septum is involved. The spread of carcinoma from the lung may be hematogenous, lymphangial, or by direct extension. The metastases involve the pericardium and myocardium and, rarely, the endocardium may also be involved.

Besides bronchiogenic carcinoma, metastases to the heart are found in cases of carcinoma of the breast and carcinoma of the thyroid gland. In addition, almost every other carcinoma may metastasize to the heart. Sarcomas may also metastasize to the heart. In 44 percent of the *malignant melanomas*, metastases to the heart and the pericardium can be found. The epicardium, myocardium, and endocardium may be dotted by pigmented metastases.

Even if large areas of the myocardium are affected by metastases, no *clinical symptoms* may be observed. Also, retrospective analyses of the clinical data and autopsy findings can correlate only about 10 per-

cent of the clinical signs and anatomical changes.

Heart failure due to metastases rarely develops. Secondary tumor nodules involving the conduction system can cause abnormalities in the atrioventricular conduction, and these can be demonstrated by the *electrocardiogram*. Involvement of the pericardium by metastatic carcinoma may lead to inflow stasis, either through pericardial effusion (at times, hemorrhagic) or, less commonly, through constriction of the heart by an encasing layer of tumor. If metastases reach the endocardium of the ventricles or the atria, they can initiate parietal thromboses. Within the embolic material of such thrombi, tumor cells occasionally may be found.

F. Netter
©CIBA

CARDIAC TAMPONADE

PATIENT IN VARIABLE DEGREES OF SHOCK OR IN EXTREMIS

NECK VEINS DISTENDED

HEART SOUNDS DISTANT

DECREASED ARTERIAL AND PULSE PRESSURES OFTEN EXIST BUT NOT PATHOGNOMONIC

VENOUS PRESSURE ELEVATED (PATHOGNOMONIC)

PERICARDIAL TAP AT LARREY'S POINT (DIAGNOSTIC AND DECOMPRESSIVE)

IN CARDIAC TAMPONADE VENOUS PRESSURE RISES PROGRESSIVELY AND LINEARLY; ARTERIAL PRESSURE MAY BE NORMAL OR ELEVATED AND IS DIAGNOSTICALLY UNRELIABLE

PENETRATING HEART WOUNDS

Classification and Evaluation

Patients with penetrating wounds of the heart can be classified in three general groups:

1. People who have received extensive lacerations or large-caliber gunshot wounds comprise this group. These patients die almost immediately, as a result of rapid and voluminous blood loss.

2. The second group includes those with small wounds of the heart, caused by ice picks, knives, or other small agents (measuring from several millimeters to 2.5 cm in length), who, because of the development of *cardiac tamponade*, reach the hospital alive.

The potentially lethal complication of cardiac tamponade results from the existence of a tough, fibrous, nonextensible sac encasing the heart and the roots of the great vessels. Were it not for this sac, practically all heart wounds would present a hopeless situation because of voluminous blood loss, such as that which occurs with wounds of the great vessels outside the pericardium. Cardiac tamponade, by bringing pressure to bear on the bleeding heart wall, also plays an important role in controlling the hemorrhage.

3. In the third group are those with associated serious injuries in the chest and/or elsewhere in the body, which, in themselves, may contribute to death.

That the penetrating heart wound is a truly serious injury is shown by studies made both at the Harlem Hospital Center and in the Office of the Medical Examiner of the City of New York. These studies indicate that less than 40 percent of the patients with penetrating wounds of the heart reach a hospital alive. However, once they get there and receive prompt definitive therapy, the chance for recovery is high, ranging from 80 to 95 percent or more.

It should be emphasized that the condition of the patient, on admission to the hospital, must not be used as an index of the severity of the injury. There are moribund patients, with no *blood pressure* and a *nonperceptible pulse*, who survive operation and recover; on the other hand, there are patients in fair condition, with a systolic blood pressure ranging from 80 mm Hg to normal and a fair-to-good pulse, who die before surgery can be instituted. Therefore, an extremely grave status of the patient should never suggest that the case is hopeless; neither should the presence of a seemingly stabilized clinical picture lead to a false sense of security.

The vast majority of cardiac injuries are caused by knives, bullets, or other penetrating agents. The knives are frequently of the switchblade variety, usually having a blade about 6 in. long.

The thoracic "danger area" and the *approximate relative distribution of penetrating heart wounds* are revealing (see page 254). The types of wounds vary. There may be a simple laceration (nick) in the wall of the heart, penetration into the wall without entering the cardiac chamber (intramural), penetration into the cardiac chamber (intraluminal), or actual perforation through one or more chambers. The vast majority are of the intraluminal variety. In a small percentage of patients, a solitary laceration of the pericardium exists without cardiac involvement.

Causes of Death

The immediate cause of death is either exsanguination, cardiac tamponade, or interference with the conduction mechanism.

The delayed causes include sepsis, massive cerebral embolism with infarction from a mural thrombus of the left ventricle, cardiac failure due to valvular or interventricular septal injury, and constrictive pericarditis.

Cardiac Tamponade. Acute hemopericardium, of sufficient quantity to cause cardiac tamponade, constitutes the basic pathologic sequel to heart wounds, whether they are due to either penetrating or nonpenetrating trauma. Tamponade is a double-edged sword, for it is both lethal and lifesaving. There is little doubt that, up to a point, it contributes to the reduction or cessation of hemorrhage from the cardiac wound, but, beyond that point, a continuance of its action produces *profound shock which proves fatal*, unless promptly relieved.

Acute cardiac tamponade results in three major physiologic alterations:

1. *On the venous side* the increased intrapericardial pressure restricts venous return to the right ventricle during diastole. This produces an elevation of right ventricular end-diastolic pressure which is reflected back to the right atrium as an *elevated central venous pressure*.

2. *On the arterial side* the resultant cardiac compression reduces cardiac output. This leads to a *fall in blood*

(Continued on page 254)

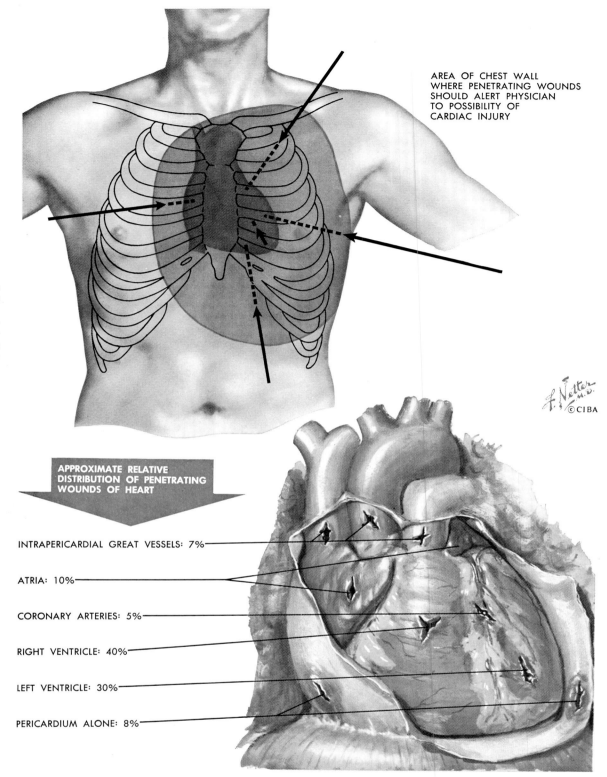

AREA OF CHEST WALL WHERE PENETRATING WOUNDS SHOULD ALERT PHYSICIAN TO POSSIBILITY OF CARDIAC INJURY

APPROXIMATE RELATIVE DISTRIBUTION OF PENETRATING WOUNDS OF HEART

INTRAPERICARDIAL GREAT VESSELS: 7%

ATRIA: 10%

CORONARY ARTERIES: 5%

RIGHT VENTRICLE: 40%

LEFT VENTRICLE: 30%

PERICARDIUM ALONE: 8%

Penetrating Heart Wounds

(Continued from page 253)

pressure (see page 253) and a reduction in coronary filling factors which predispose to myocardial hypoxia and failure.

3. *On the systemic side* the reduced cardiac output leads to generalized vasoconstriction which, in turn, causes an increase in peripheral vascular resistance. This factor may be responsible for the maintenance of near-*normal or even higher-than-normal blood pressure,* during the early stage, despite a progressively falling cardiac output and a *progressively rising venous pressure* (see page 253).

CLINICAL EFFECTS OF CARDIAC TAMPONADE. The effects of small quantities of blood in the pericardial sac are negligible, but, when the volume reaches 150 to 200 ml, severe shock may develop, often abruptly, because the *pericardium* cannot be stretched. At this critical point the addition or removal of as little as 10 to 20 ml of blood may spell the difference between life and death. In some patients the amount of blood in the pericardial sac is insufficient to produce detectable tamponade, and both cardiac and pericardial wounds heal spontaneously.

The final outcome depends on the interplay of three important variables — the cardiac wound, the pericardial wound, and the hemopericardium.

Diagnosis of Cardiac Injury

Diagnosis generally is easy if the physician maintains a high degree of suspicion of cardiac injury in every chest wound he encounters. Wounds of the upper abdomen, axillary region, posterior chest wall, and base of the neck also may be associated with heart injury. Wounds caused by ice picks or other small instruments are readily missed.

Occasionally, one observes a progressive rise in blood pressure, to 160 mm Hg or more over a period of hours. The author has seen this in three patients in whom not only bleeding cardiac wounds but also significant degrees of hemopericardium and intrapericardial clot formation were found at operation.

Shock weighs heavily in favor of a diagnosis of cardiac injury when the degree of shock seems out of proportion to the severity of the wound or the loss of blood. After cardiac injury there may be a symptom-free interval, of several minutes to several hours, followed suddenly by deep shock, and it may be difficult to tell whether the shock is due to tamponade or to blood loss.

Tamponade can be recognized easily by history or by physical examination alone. The classic *clinical* features are muffled and *distant heart tones,* falling or absent arterial pressure, and elevated venous pressure. The circulatory collapse is out of proportion to the blood loss. When tamponade persists, the *cervical veins,* especially the external jugulars, become *full and tense.* The *aspiration of blood* from the pericardial sac confirms the *diagnosis* of hemopericardium (see page 253).

Frequently, the respiration is rapid and sighing, and the excursions usually are irregular. Dyspnea, air hunger, and extreme thirst are common.

X-ray plates, including fluoroscopy, and venous-pressure readings may be helpful but are not absolutely necessary to establish a diagnosis. The X-ray film may demonstrate a widening of the cardiac silhouette, and *fluoroscopy* may reveal a diminution of cardiac pulsations. On the other hand, these commonly used studies may be of no value, since death can occur from a hemopericardium which is too small to cause any noticeable changes in the pulsations or in the size and contour of the cardiac shadow. Restlessness of the patient makes such studies difficult, but they are important in ruling out hemothorax and pneumothorax.

Venous-pressure readings are *pathognomonic* (see page 253) when increased, but they may be normal or even below normal when moderate to severe intrathoracic bleeding is present. Venous pressure constitutes an excellent means of differentiating shock due to cardiac tamponade from that due to hemorrhage. A systemic pressure of 12 cm H_2O or higher suggests cardiac tamponade; one of 5 cm or lower indicates a significant blood loss.

Electrocardiography is not particularly helpful. For several hours after the injury, the tracings may show little deviation from normal; hence they are of little value when needed most.

Immediate Treatment

Prompt, definitive therapy is imperative. This includes (1) antishock therapy, (2) pericardiocentesis, and (3) thoracotomy with pericardiotomy and suture of the wound.

Antishock Therapy. The patient is placed immediately in a moderate Trendelenburg position, oxygen is adminis-
(Continued on page 255)

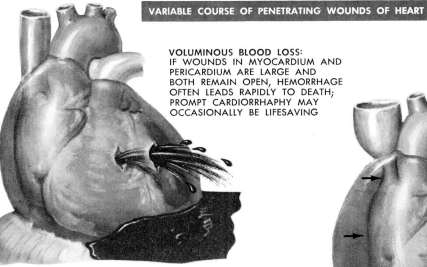

VARIABLE COURSE OF PENETRATING WOUNDS OF HEART

VOLUMINOUS BLOOD LOSS:
IF WOUNDS IN MYOCARDIUM AND PERICARDIUM ARE LARGE AND BOTH REMAIN OPEN, HEMORRHAGE OFTEN LEADS RAPIDLY TO DEATH; PROMPT CARDIORRHAPHY MAY OCCASIONALLY BE LIFESAVING

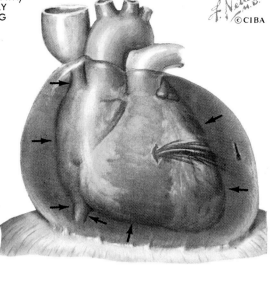

EARLY TAMPONADE:
IF MYOCARDIAL WOUND REMAINS OPEN AND PERICARDIAL WOUND SEALS OFF, CARDIAC TAMPONADE RESULTS AND MAY RAPIDLY CAUSE DEATH UNLESS RELIEVED BY PERICARDIOCENTESIS. THIS MAY ALSO BE EFFECTIVE DEFINITIVE THERAPY BUT CARDIORRHAPHY IS PREFERRED

PENETRATING HEART WOUNDS

(*Continued from page 254*)

tered, and a rapid intravenous infusion, of physiologic saline solution, plasma, or both, is started. As soon as blood is available, it is substituted for these solutions.

If there should be a delay in typing and crossmatching, O-negative blood should be used. On occasion, autotransfusion is lifesaving. It should be resorted to when indicated, while bank blood is being crossmatched.

Narcotics, if necessary, should be used judiciously, since restlessness is usually a reflection of cerebral hypoxia, and further depression of the cardiorespiratory centers may prove fatal.

Pericardiocentesis. With tamponade, immediate aspiration is mandatory and often lifesaving. Many authorities advocate pericardial aspiration as the sole means of treatment. They operate only when (1) several aspirations fail to relieve tamponade, (2) tamponade rapidly occurs after aspiration, or (3) hemorrhage persists.

Thoracotomy with Pericardiotomy and Suture of the Wound. All surgeons agree that when the cardiac wound is complicated by persistent and profuse hemorrhage, an immediate thoracotomy, with pericardiotomy and direct repair of the wound, is mandatory.

Associated injuries to the lung and to the internal mammary, intercostal, and great vessels, which result in pneumothorax, hemothorax, or hemopneumothorax, and life-threatening injuries of structures other than those involving the heart also must receive appropriate emergency care.

The anesthetic agent and the technic to be used will vary with the condition of the patient. In the comatose patient, no anesthesia is required initially. In the patient with profound hypotension, regional anesthesia (using 0.5 to 1 percent procaine hydrochloride) with oxygen therapy is preferred. In the patient with a relatively stable cardiovascular system, general anesthesia is employed. The agent most commonly used is cyclopropane, although halothane (Fluothane®) has been used frequently.

Endotracheal intubation, with assisted respiration, is preferred. Very often, however, this is not performed until the pericardium has been opened or the heart wound repaired. This is a detail of extreme importance. Positive airway pressure, by further increasing intrathoracic pressure, augments the severity of tamponade of the heart and venae cavae, and it may rapidly convert a markedly reduced cardiac output to none at all.

Operative Methods

Thoracotomy. Cardiac wounds, regardless of their location, are best dealt with through

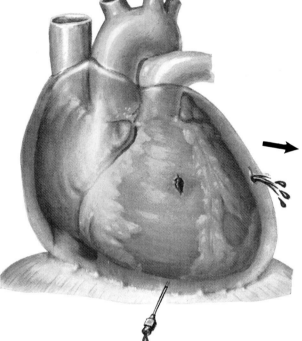

EARLY STABILIZATION:
IF MYOCARDIAL WOUND IS SEALED BY CLOT, VARIABLE DEGREES OF HEMOPERICARDIUM RESULT, AND IF RELIEVED BY SEEPAGE OR TAP, EFFECTIVE HEART ACTION MAY CONTINUE AND PATIENT SURVIVE

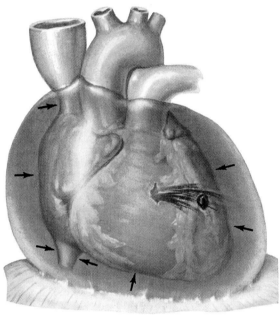

DELAYED TAMPONADE:
AFTER HOURS, DAYS, OR WEEKS THE CLOT MAY DISLODGE AND FATAL TAMPONADE RESULT; THIS EMPHASIZES DESIRABILITY OF PROMPT OPERATIVE THERAPY

a left transpleural thoracotomy, planned to afford maximum exposure. The right-side approach may be necessary, however, when the wound of entrance indicates an injury through the right chest.

In spite of the urgency of exploration, a deliberate, systematized routine, operating speedily but not hastily and observing meticulously the principles of surgical technic, must be followed.

Unless the *incisions* in the *skin*, underlying *muscles, intercostal spaces, and cartilages* are made some distance away from each other, in association with a careful chest-wall closure, the complications of wound breakdown, infection, and a chest-wall sinus tract are prone to occur.

The most crucial point of the operation is that moment when cardiac compression is released. Just as the pericardial sac is opened, uncontrollable brisk bleeding and clot formation are frequently encountered, with blood welling up in the wound, gushing forth in all directions, and often spurting several feet or more into the air. Therefore, before the pericardium is incised, it is essen-

tial to be very mindful of the following considerations:

1. Providing adequate exposure, through a *limited* thoracic incision, of the structures contained in the pericardial sac is virtually impossible, and the cutting of ribs to improve exposure, at a time when seconds count, may prove disastrous.

2. There must be a preconceived plan of action. The surgeon must pause to see that all necessary instruments (particularly, rakes, *Kocher clamps*, Asepto® *syringes filled with saline solution*, and proper suture material, already threaded on needles) are in readiness. Also, instructing the members of the team as to the steps which are to be followed and the rapidity with which they are to be performed often proves fruitful.

3. There must be sufficient amounts of blood and blood substitutes. This is lifesaving in exsanguination.

Attention to these three factors often makes the management of a most complex and potentially lethal situation appear simple and logical.

(*Continued on page 256*)

A: CURVED "Y"–SHAPED INCISION IN SKIN AND PECTORALIS MAJOR MUSCLE (BLUE); INCISION OF INTERCOSTAL AND PECTORALIS MINOR MUSCLES AND SECTION OF COSTAL CARTILAGES (RED)

PENETRATING HEART WOUNDS

(Continued from page 255)

Three crucial maneuvers spell the difference between life and death. These are as follows:

1. Soon after entry into the thoracic cavity, the first assistant elevates the *sternum* with two rakes. This maneuver is of value, since it places the assistant in a ready position to permit instantaneous *retraction* and fixation of the pericardium when it is presented to him at the time of pericardiotomy.

2. The surgeon *grasps the pericardium* with a *Kocher clamp* and *opens it* in its entire length (anterior to the phrenic nerve) from its base on the diaphragm to the upper narrower part surrounding the great vessels. The edges of the pericardium are grasped with two additional Kocher clamps. (Kochers, unlike Allis clamps, eliminate the chances of slipping or of obtaining a poor hold on the pericardium.) As the surgeon retracts the pericardium with the Kocher clamps — to the left and then up and over the sternum — the first assistant releases the rakes from under the sternum, and then reapplies them to retract the pericardium to the desired degree. This causes practically the entire heart to lie in the left hemithorax, resulting in excellent exposure. If necessary, the exposure can be enhanced further by forceful elevation of the sternum.

3. Just as the pericardium is incised, the second assistant forcefully flushes out the area with copious amounts of warm saline solution. This maneuver rapidly clears the field of blood and quickly brings the bleeding point into view. (Suction and mopping, to clear the field of blood and clots, are most ineffective. Also, blind digital palpation to locate the wound is dangerous, because it often results in cardiac irregularities and standstill.) With the bleeding point in view, *digital compression* over the wound will *adequately control the hemorrhage*.

These steps are performed in rapid succession and require no more than several seconds. At this point, the heart promptly resumes its normal activity, and the surgeon can pause, take inventory, and then proceed, without undue haste, to place the sutures in the myocardium.

The myocardial wound is closed with interrupted oo or ooo silk sutures, swaged on fine, curved, atraumatic needles. The suture is placed under the occluding finger and then tied; this is repeated with each suture until the wound has been completely closed. This is done best without any crisscrossing of sutures for hemostatic purposes, and without help from assistants. Two or three sutures usually prove sufficient. Each suture is passed down to — but not through — the endocardium (for fear of a mural thrombus).

The heart muscle, which is soft and

B: SKIN AND PECTORALIS MAJOR MUSCLE HAVE BEEN DIVIDED AND REFLECTED; INTERCOSTAL AND PECTORALIS MINOR MUSCLES ARE DIVIDED IN 4th INTERSPACE

C: 3rd, 4th, and 5th COSTAL CARTILAGES DIVIDED OVER A FLAT RIBBON RETRACTOR WHICH PROTECTS UNDERLYING STRUCTURES

friable because of myocardial hypoxia, may require mattress sutures reinforced with small pledgets of Teflon® felt. This measure adds safety to the placement of these sutures.

A wound near a *coronary vessel* should be closed by passing a mattress-type suture beneath the vessel so as to avoid it. If feasible, a coronary vessel that is cut must be ligated just proximal to the injury, using 6-o or 7-o silk sutures.

For an *auricular wound* a noncrushing clamp is very effective. However, simply grasping the wound edges with Allis clamps is equally effective. Auricular wounds are closed with interrupted or continuous 4-o or 5-o arterial-silk sutures.

Lacerations of the aorta and other *great vessels* are clamped tangentially with a noncrushing clamp, and closure is accomplished with simple interrupted or continuous sutures of 5-o arterial silk. The apical traction suture of Beck, for exposure of the posterior aspect of the heart, is valuable, but it is also dangerous. This suture

may cut through, inflicting troublesome wounds that often require repair.

The back part of the heart can be exposed by simple manual luxation, with the fingers spread apart. For torrential bleeding, some authorities advocate temporary occlusion of the venae cavae. The author has not had the occasion to resort to this measure.

On the left side, the pericardial sac is left wide open to allow free drainage into the pleural cavity. On the right side, the sac is closed loosely, lest there be dislocation and strangulation of the heart. A catheter is placed in the pleural cavity and is attached to an underwater negative-pressure drainage system; it is allowed to remain in place from 24 to 48 hours.

Closure of the *thoracotomy* wound is done with great care. The sectioned cartilages are approximated and sutured together with chromic catgut #1, swaged on a cutting needle. Postoperative management is similar to that of any procedure for open thoracotomy.

(Continued on page 257)

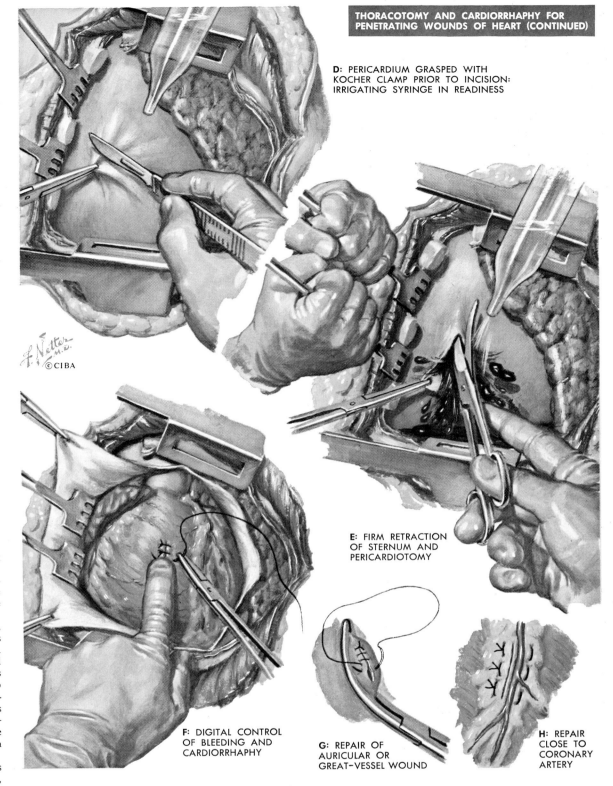

D: PERICARDIUM GRASPED WITH KOCHER CLAMP PRIOR TO INCISION: IRRIGATING SYRINGE IN READINESS

E: FIRM RETRACTION OF STERNUM AND PERICARDIOTOMY

F: DIGITAL CONTROL OF BLEEDING AND CARDIORRHAPHY

G: REPAIR OF AURICULAR OR GREAT-VESSEL WOUND

H: REPAIR CLOSE TO CORONARY ARTERY

PENETRATING HEART WOUNDS

(Continued from page 256)

Pericardiocentesis Versus Open Operation

The results with pericardiocentesis as the primary method of treatment are best shown by Beall and his associates in an excellent review of a large series of patients with penetrating wounds of the heart. They reported 78 patients thus treated, with a mortality of 5.5 percent of those requiring only aspiration. Among 23 patients who did not respond to pericardiocentesis, the mortality was only 26.7 percent if *cardiorrhaphy* was carried out immediately, but it rose to 62.5 percent if cardiac action was allowed to stop before thoracotomy was employed. Of the more desperate cases, 12 were treated primarily by cardiorrhaphy, with 33 percent mortality.

As can be seen from these figures, a direct comparison of results would be entirely misleading, since the results following pericardiocentesis are highly selective, omitting patients with large wounds and massive hemorrhage. In addition, this study shows that the mortality figures increase with the degree of conservatism exercised during the initial phase of treatment.

A review of the literature is confusing, since proponents of both pericardiocentesis and surgery report excellent results. Ravitch reported no mortality in 31 patients treated by aspiration alone, but the same results have also been reported (elsewhere) in 10 consecutive patients, all treated by thoracotomy. An additional 11 consecutive patients were treated surgically, also without mortality. Clearly, survival rates depend more on the nature and severity of the injury than on the form of treatment.

Maynard *et al.* reviewed 113 patients treated from June, 1955, through June, 1963. Of these, 58 operations showed a mortality of only 8.6 percent — a considerable reduction over their earlier series. This reduction is attributable, primarily, to accumulated experience, improved surgical and anesthesiologic technics, and the use of blood, plasma, and other intravenous fluids.

Reasons for Favoring Thoracotomy. There is no question of the value of pericardial aspiration as definitive therapy for a solitary heart wound complicated solely by hemopericardium and tamponade.

Practically, however, the author is convinced that pericardiocentesis, as initial therapy for hemopericardium, followed by prompt, definitive surgical intervention, is preferable to conservative management by aspiration. Pericardiocentesis, employed preoperatively for acute hemopericardium or tamponade, helps tide the patient over

that hazardous period of shock until surgery can be done.

For excellent results, the surgical team must be skilled in thoracotomy. For the occasional operator, confronted by a solitary heart wound complicated solely by a tamponade, nonoperative intervention with pericardiocentesis may be safer, since some of these patients do survive with aspiration alone and sometimes even without aspiration. Nevertheless, when the problem is continuous exsanguination, thoracotomy, with pericardiotomy and suture, offers the only chance for survival.

The reasons for preferring surgery to conservative treatment with aspiration as definitive therapy are these:

1. The site of injury can be determined with precision.
2. The type of injury can be adequately ascertained.
3. In about 50 percent of the patients, large intrapericardial hemorrhagic clots are found. These prevent effective withdrawal of blood from the sac, and a negative tapping may lull one into a false sense of security.
4. Secondary hemorrhage (delayed hemopericardium) has occurred variously after hours, days, or even weeks

following the injury in a significant number of patients.

5. The technic of aspiration, as usually done with the patient supine, is simple, but it risks laceration of the myocardium or the left coronary artery.
6. The incomplete evacuation of hemopericardium may result in the development of chronic pericardial effusions, adhesive pericarditis, or the constrictive syndrome.
7. A traumatic ventricular aneurysm may result near the epicardial opening, and a traumatic aneurysm of a coronary vessel may rupture.
8. The patients who do well with aspiration may continue on to survival, but the patients who do badly or are not helped by aspiration either die or are subjected to surgery as the only recourse. Thus, pericardiocentesis is fundamentally a trial-and-error procedure.

Thoracotomy, with pericardiotomy and direct repair of the wound, is the most effective definitive treatment. Pericardiocentesis is to be employed as definitive treatment only in special situations; it is not to be regarded as a recommended procedure.

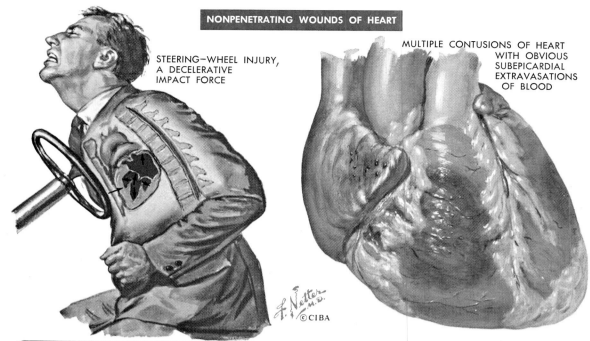

NONPENETRATING WOUNDS OF HEART

STEERING-WHEEL INJURY,
A DECELERATIVE
IMPACT FORCE

MULTIPLE CONTUSIONS OF HEART
WITH OBVIOUS
SUBEPICARDIAL
EXTRAVASATIONS
OF BLOOD

NONPENETRATING HEART WOUNDS

Cardiac Contusion

On the basis of autopsy studies, experimental data, and the notable incidence of clinical diagnosis in recent years, *contusion* is identified as the most common and also the basic injury of *blunt heart trauma*. It has been recorded in falls from heights (accelerative force); as a casualty of indirect force, *i.e.,* force applied to the abdomen and extremities and transmitted to the heart via the intravascular hemodynamic route; and as incident to the passage of high-velocity bullets and missile fragments through the abdomen or chest or from blast explosions in the air or water. The latter generate pressure waves whose energy is damaging to the tissues.

The major cause of contusion, however, is direct impact force applied violently to the precordium by a solid blunt object. Currently, the agent frequently involved is the auto accident, in which the chest wall is hurled against the *steering wheel* when the forward momentum of the vehicle is suddenly stopped (*decelerative force*). Uniquely, and more often than not, impact contusion occurs without fracture of the bony thorax and with an intact pericardium.

Pathology. The contused heart may reveal either a discrete area or disseminated foci of *hemorrhage* in the heart wall. In most instances, hemorrhage apparently originates at the endocardium, ranging from *subendocardial, mural,* and *valvular* petechiae to frank hemorrhage which may remain subendocardial or may spread interstitially through and across the myocardium to the *epicardium*. It may be confined within the myocardium or be complicated by lacerations of the endo- or epicardial surfaces—lesions which are conducive to the formation of endocardial and mural thrombi and to acute *hemopericardium*. Contusion also includes *myocardial* damage — from an innocuous bruise, to the *disruption and separation of muscle fibers,* to their total devitalization. Vascular damage ordinarily is restricted to the capillaries, the arterioles and coronary branches rarely being involved.

Although it has been suggested that contusive injury could initiate coronary thrombosis, it is generally agreed that this happens almost exclusively to the diseased atheromatous vessel. Pericardial effusions occur (usually during the second week) in over 50 percent of lesions uncomplicated by a pericardial tear. A fibrinous reaction at the contusion site may cause pain, a friction rub, and adhesion to the

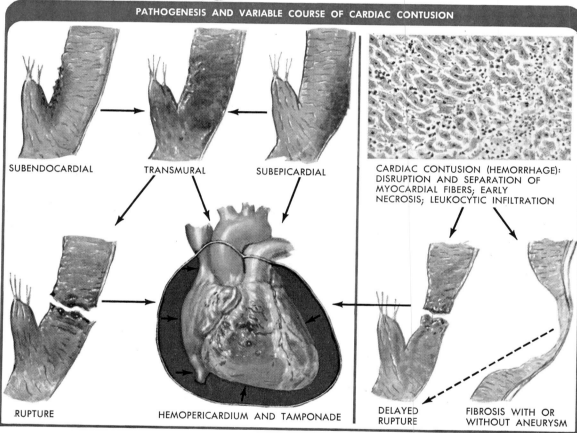

PATHOGENESIS AND VARIABLE COURSE OF CARDIAC CONTUSION

SUBENDOCARDIAL TRANSMURAL SUBEPICARDIAL

CARDIAC CONTUSION (HEMORRHAGE): DISRUPTION AND SEPARATION OF MYOCARDIAL FIBERS; EARLY NECROSIS; LEUKOCYTIC INFILTRATION

RUPTURE HEMOPERICARDIUM AND TAMPONADE DELAYED RUPTURE FIBROSIS WITH OR WITHOUT ANEURYSM

pericardium. A severe contusion projects a continuing degeneration and *necrosis* of damaged tissue, which may terminate in (1) *delayed rupture* or (2) a scarred (*fibrotic*) and weakened area that, under the intermittent intracardiac pressure, may give way to *aneurysm* formation.

Clinical Comment. The *diagnosis* of contusion has now achieved full acceptance as a clinical and legal entity, based on (1) an appropriate history, (2) clinical evidence, and (3) ECG findings and laboratory data.

Pain may be immediate or may occur up to 24 hours, or even days, later. It is retrosternal or anginal, often simulating that of coronary thrombosis. It is refractory to nitroglycerin and responsive to oxygen.

Functional disturbances include tachycardia (usually paroxysmal) and, rarely, bradycardia. Supraventricular disturbances are evidenced by ectopic beats, auricular flutter, and fibrillation. "Ticktack" heart

sounds, suggesting cardiac dilatation, are detectable by a rising venous pressure and a falling arterial pressure, parameters also suggestive of *pericardial tamponade*.

All types of *ECG alteration*, including conduction disturbances, have been noted. Chiefly affected are the ventricular complex, the S-T segment, and the T wave (exaggerated amplitude). The location of the lesion undoubtedly influences the type of arrhythmia and ECG alteration.

Laboratory data are of little value. Elevation of SGOT, LDH, and other enzymes is meaningful only if cardiac contusion is the sole injury.

Cardiac Rupture

With rare exceptions, cardiac *rupture*, involving
(Continued on page 259)

NONPENETRATING HEART WOUNDS

(Continued from page 258)

any or all chambers, causes immediate or early fatality. It is of interest that, in the resilient juvenile chest, cardiac rupture has been (not infrequently) a result of impact or compressive trauma without damage to the bony thorax and its soft tissues. In a study of 138 cases of rupture, Bright and Beck concluded that about 30 patients, who had lived longer than 1 hour, might have been helped by surgery, since their injuries were not so extensive as to preclude repair. The American literature now records 2 successful interventions for rupture, the first by Desforges and the other, recently, by Bogedain *et al.*

Interventricular Septal Rupture

An isolated interventricular septal defect is a rare lesion. When it stems from *septal rupture,* it may be manifest immediately or early. It is more common, however, as a sequel to septal *myocardial* contusion, appearing from the second week to months after the trauma. Currently, steering-wheel impact is the chief etiological agent. Bright and Beck considered the end of diastole, with the *ventricles* full and the tricuspid and mitral *valves* closed, as the moment in the cardiac cycle most propitious for septal rupture or contusion.

Time is required for a contusion fistula to become clearly delineated, its size and anatomic pattern established, and its borders defined by scar tissue and viable myocardium. If trauma has seriously or extensively involved the muscle surrounding the defect, progressive necrosis ultimately may produce a defect of a size incompatible with life. The defects observed at surgery have been irregular, sinuous, and even possessed of multiple orifices.

Diagnosis. This is made on (1) the history, (2) a holosystolic murmur and thrill along the lateral sternal border at the fourth or fifth interspace, and (3) a contusion defect (not always present) just above the apex: Right-heart catheterization for the collection of hemodynamic data on pressures and on oxygen saturation in the right ventricle, the pulmonary artery, and the superior vena cava, is essential. Left ventricular retrograde angiography may be valuable for detecting possible combined valvular lesions. The symptoms and course depend primarily on the volume of blood shunted into the right ventricle and the pulmonary circuit.

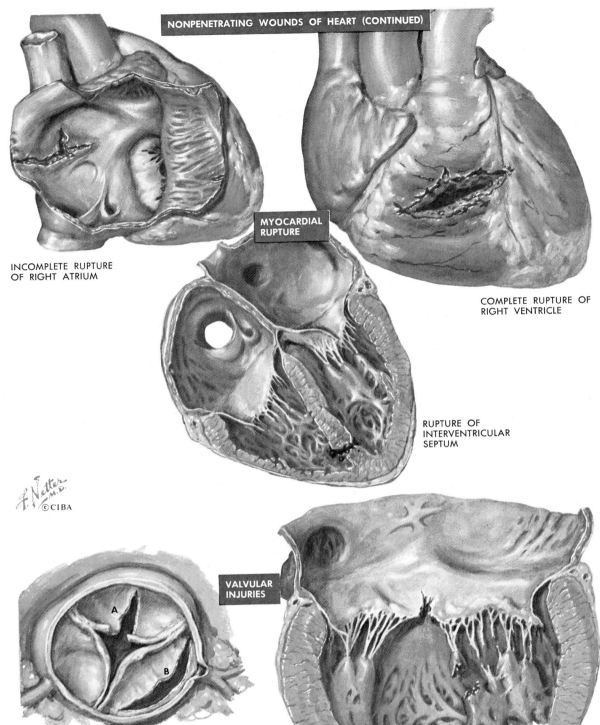

NONPENETRATING WOUNDS OF HEART (CONTINUED)

INCOMPLETE RUPTURE OF RIGHT ATRIUM

MYOCARDIAL RUPTURE

COMPLETE RUPTURE OF RIGHT VENTRICLE

RUPTURE OF INTERVENTRICULAR SEPTUM

VALVULAR INJURIES

RUPTURE OF AORTIC VALVE
A: CUSP ITSELF
B: ATTACHMENT TO RIM OF ORIFICE

RUPTURE OF CHORDAE TENDINEAE AND/OR PAPILLARY MUSCLE AND, RARELY, THE VALVE CUSPS

The pulmonary vascular resistance that develops is the key factor.

Treatment. Surgical repair is made under extracorporeal circulation (ECC). To date, about 10 cases of blunt traumatic defect have been repaired by suture.

Valvular Injuries

Endothelial tears, hemorrhage into the valve cusps, and rupture are the valvular injuries encountered at postmortem. Rupture, the most frequent, comes from impact force to the precordium, from indirect force, and from cardiac strain — a specific indirect force associated with an intense or excessive physical effort, mediated through the vascular route, and affecting almost exclusively the aortic valve (particularly in hypertensive, atherosclerotic patients). Ruptures occur when the valves are subjected to the greatest

internal pressure: for the aortic valves, at the end of systole; for the mitral and tricuspid valves, at the beginning of ventricular systole.

Rupture of the aortic valve may involve the *cusps* themselves or the *site of their attachment to the rim of the orifice.* Rupture of the mitral or tricuspid valves usually implicates the *chordae tendineae,* the *papillary muscles,* and (rarely) the cusps. The majority of ruptured valves have been diseased, with acute inflammation, the residual stigmas of bacterial endocarditis, valvulitis, or atherosclerotic changes. The valvular incompetence precipitated by rupture may not be sufficiently severe to induce an immediate or early fatality. When stabilization occurs, the physical signs specific for the valvular lesion may be detected, and further investigation may be carried out by cardiac catheterization and angiocardiography. Valve repair under ECC or valve substitution is now possible.

DISEASES OF PERICARDIUM

The pericardium may be involved in many varieties of disease processes, as can be seen from the classification of diseases of the pericardium by Wolff and Wolff (reproduced by permission from Annual Review of Medicine, Volume 16:22, 1965, and the authors).

I. Fibrinous or "dry" pericarditis (including hemopericardium with recognizable effusion)
   A. Infections
      1. Bacterial: wide variety of organisms including pneumococcus, streptococcus, staphylococcus, meningococcus, and in typhoid fever, tuberculosis, brucellosis, bacillary dysentery, melioidosis, salmonellosis, plague, tularemia, and subacute bacterial endocarditis
      2. Viral: Coxsackie, influenza, ECHO, chickenpox, mumps, lymphogranuloma venereum
      3. Rickettsial: Q fever, typhus, boutonneuse fever
      4. Protozoan: amebiasis, Chagas' disease, toxoplasmosis
      5. Mycotic: actinomycosis, histoplasmosis, blastomycosis, coccidioidomycosis
      6. Helminthic: echinococcus, dracunculosis
      7. Miscellaneous: yaws, infectious mononucleosis, primary atypical pneumonia
   B. Trauma
      1. Direct
         a. Penetrating injury
            1. Stab wounds, foreign bodies, sternal marrow aspiration
            2. Percutaneous puncture for left-heart catheterization
         b. Perforation of heart wall during right-heart catheterization
         c. Surgical pericardiotomy (postpericardiotomy syndrome)
         d. Radiation
         e. Electrical
      2. Indirect
         Nonpenetrating chest trauma
   C. Neoplastic diseases: including mesothelioma, reticulum-cell sarcoma, angiomatosis, hemangiopericytoma, thymoma, leukemia, Hodgkin's disease, lymphoblastoma, metastatic carcinoma, teratocarcinoma
   D. Drug-induced: hydralazine, psicofuranine, phenylbutazone, tetracycline, streptomycin, methylthiouracil, quinidine, anticoagulants
   E. Connective-tissue disorders
      1. Acute rheumatic fever
      2. Lupus erythematosus disseminata
      3. Rheumatoid arthritis, Reiter's syndrome
   F. Sensitivity states and autoimmunization
      1. Serum sickness
      2. ? Postmyocardial-infarction syndrome
      3. ? Recurrences of pericarditis regardless of etiology of first attack
      4. ? Following thoracic and extrathoracic surgery

5. Immunization for smallpox, tetanus, diphtheria
   G. Myocardial infarction
   H. Aortic dissection and ruptured luetic or mycotic aneurysm
   I. Metabolic
      1. Azotemia
      2. Hemochromatosis
      3. Gout
   J. Miscellaneous
      1. Acute pericardial fat necrosis
      2. Sarcoid
      3. Giant-cell arteritis
      4. Polyserositis
      5. Blood dyscrasias
      6. Pulmonary infiltration and eosinophilia syndrome
      7. Necrotizing angiitis
II. Pericardial effusion
   A. May occur in most of above
   B. Congestive heart failure

C. Myxedema
D. Cholesterol pericarditis
E. Chylopericardium
F. Anemia
G. Scleroderma
H. Thoracic-duct communication with pericardium
I. "Chronic effusive pericarditis"
J. Endomyocardial fibrosis
III. Constrictive pericarditis of multiple etiologies, most often tuberculosis
IV. Congenital affections of pericardium
   A. Partial or complete absence
   B. Chronic effusion in association with congenital heart disease
   C. In association with hypoplastic anemia and Cooley's anemia
   D. In association with Friedreich's ataxia
   E. Bronchogenic cyst
   F. Hygroma

(Continued on page 261)

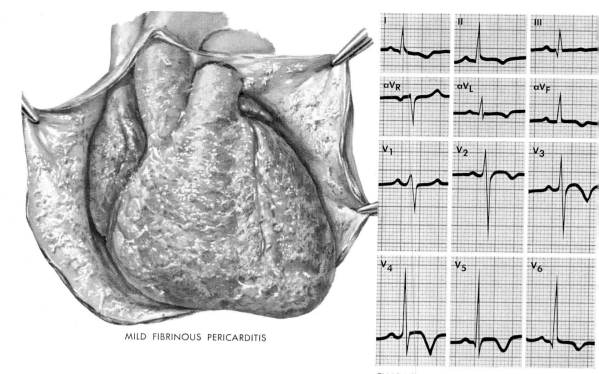

MILD FIBRINOUS PERICARDITIS

CHARACTERISTIC ECG CHANGES: T WAVE INVERSION IN ALL LEADS EXCEPT aV_R AND V_1; ISOELECTRIC IN LEAD III

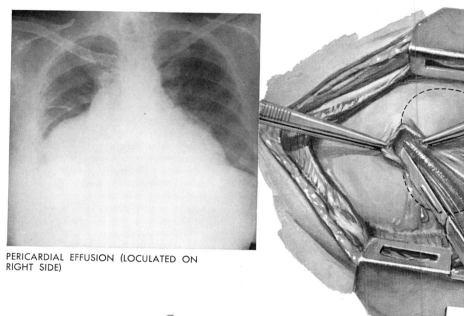

PERICARDIAL EFFUSION (LOCULATED ON RIGHT SIDE)

PERICARDIAL EFFUSION; PLEUROPERICARDIAL WINDOW BEING CREATED AND BIOPSY TAKEN VIA INCISION IN 5th LEFT INTERCOSTAL SPACE

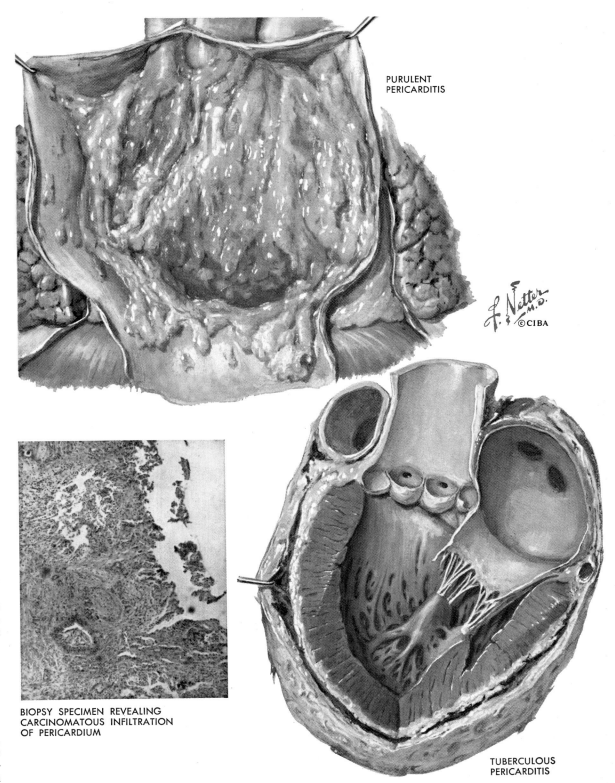

PURULENT
PERICARDITIS

BIOPSY SPECIMEN REVEALING
CARCINOMATOUS INFILTRATION
OF PERICARDIUM

TUBERCULOUS
PERICARDITIS

Diseases of Pericardium

(Continued from page 260)

Acute pericarditis may occur as acute fibrinous, serofibrinous, purulent, or hemorrhagic forms. *Fibrinous pericarditis* (see also page 168) is the type usually seen in rheumatic fever, benign nonspecific (see page 180), or viral pericarditis. *Purulent pericarditis* usually results from bacterial infection with such organisms as pneumococcus, staphylococcus, or streptococcus. *Hemorrhagic pericarditis,* which must be distinguished from hemorrhage into the pericardium, is most often noted when the etiology is *malignancy* or injury involving the pericardium. Following the acute condition, *adhesive pericarditis* (see also pages 170 and 262) may develop. This rarely occurs after the acute fibrinous or the serofibrinous forms; it is more likely to result from purulent or hemorrhagic pericarditis. The chronic adhesive form is also seen in *tuberculous pericarditis,* where the pericardium often becomes thickened. Constriction of either or both of the heart's inflow and outflow tracts can result from chronic adhesive pericarditis and may require surgical treatment.

The incidence of the common forms of acute pericarditis is given by Reeves (Amer. J. med. Sci., 34:225, 1953) as follows:

Rheumatic fever	40.6%
Bacterial infection	19.8%
Tuberculosis	7.3%
Benign nonspecific	10.4%
Uremia	11.5%
Neoplasm	3.1%
"Collagen" disease	2.1%

Pericarditis has a tendency to recur, and this is true particularly of the type classified as nonspecific. Careful bacteriological studies have shown a viral origin in some cases; however, many are not due to a virus infection but probably result from an autoimmune reaction, since the recurrences can be suppressed by steroid therapy in these cases.

Acute Pericarditis

Symptoms. The onset of pericarditis usually is accompanied by severe chest pains. However, there are cases in which pain is not a prominent symptom and may even be absent, especially when *pericardial effusion* appears early. The pain usually is substernal and may radiate to the left shoulder and arm or to the neck. The character of the pain may closely simulate that of the onset of acute myocardial infarction, thus presenting a difficult diagnostic problem. If there is pleural involve-

ment, the pain may be increased by deep inspiration.

With the development of effusion, dyspnea becomes the more prominent symptom. This is probably due to mechanical pressure on the lungs, compressing not only the alveolar structure but also the smaller bronchial branches.

Associated symptoms depend on the etiology of pericarditis. In acute inflammatory conditions, chills, fever, and sweating often are present.

Signs. The most important physical sign is a pericardial friction rub. Usually, it is heard best just to the left of the sternum and is fairly well localized. It is a to-and-fro scraping sound, and it seems to be closer to the ear than other cardiac sounds or murmurs. In pericarditis due to inflammatory conditions or to myocardial infarction, the rub may be heard for only a short time, but it is usually persistent when pericarditis is due to neoplasm. The friction rub may be

heard in the presence of considerable pericardial effusion, even as much as 1 liter. This is due to the accumulation of fluid at the sides and lower portions of the pericardium rather than at the base.

In the presence of a significant amount of effusion, the heart sounds will diminish in intensity, and, on percussion, the area of cardiac dullness will be increased. An area of dullness, with bronchial breathing, may be noted below the angle of the left scapula (Ewart's sign). Occasionally, there may be so much pericardial fluid that it interferes with cardiac function (cardiac tamponade) (see page 253). Venous pressure rises, the heart rate increases, the pulse becomes small, and there may then be a diminution in the amplitude of the pulse during inspiration (paradoxical pulse). Blood pressure may fall as much as 20 mm Hg at the end of inspiration. The rapidity of

(Continued on page 262)

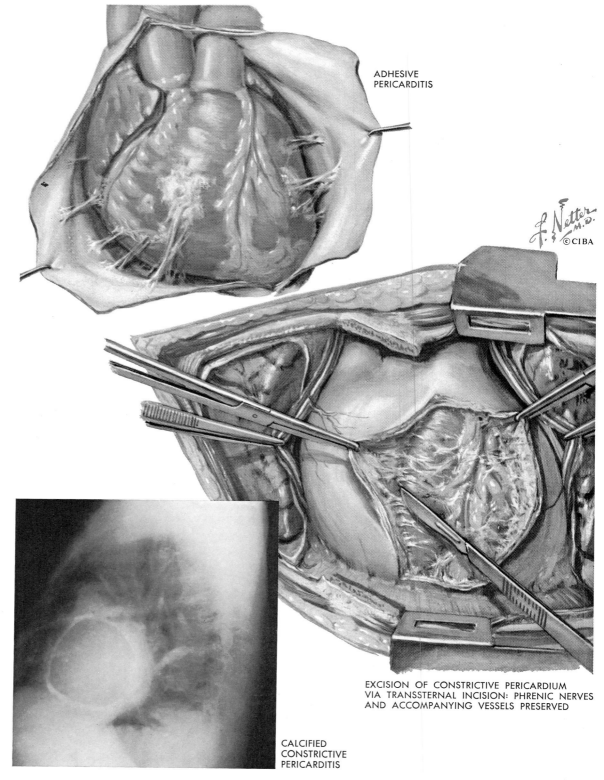

ADHESIVE
PERICARDITIS

EXCISION OF CONSTRICTIVE PERICARDIUM
VIA TRANSSTERNAL INCISION: PHRENIC NERVES
AND ACCOMPANYING VESSELS PRESERVED

CALCIFIED
CONSTRICTIVE
PERICARDITIS

Diseases of Pericardium

(*Continued from page 261*)

formation of pericardial effusion is an important factor in determining whether tamponade will occur. A small, rapidly developing effusion may cause tampònade, whereas a large one which has developed slowly over several weeks, as in tuberculous pericardial effusion, will not cause tamponade.

X-rays of the chest, particularly if serial films are taken, will demonstrate the presence of pericardial effusion. However, the fluid volume must be at least 250 cc before a significant change in the cardiac shadow makes possible a definite diagnosis. The cardiac silhouette, depending on the amount of fluid present, will assume a pear-shaped or water-bottle form. On fluoroscopy, the cardiac pulsations may be diminished or even absent in the case of a large effusion.

The *electrocardiogram* (see page 260) will aid in the diagnosis of pericarditis. It is particularly helpful in ruling out acute myocardial infarction. An elevation of the RS-T segment usually occurs in all three standard leads, whereas in myocardial infarction, depending upon the location of the infarct, only lead I or leads II and III are involved. Reciprocal elevation of the RS-T segment in lead I and depression in lead III, as is seen in myocardial infarction, is not observed in pericarditis. The shape of the RS-T segment also differs from that seen in myocardial infarction. There is an upward concavity, whereas in myocardial infarction there is an upward convexity. After a few days, the *T waves* at first become flattened and later *inverted*. If pericardial effusion is present, there may be a decrease in voltage of the QRS group.

Purulent Pericarditis

This condition may not be recognized because of the general disease of which it is a part. However, changes in the electrocardiogram suggesting pericarditis, X-ray evidence of pericardial effusion, or fluoroscopic evidence of diminished cardiac pulsations may call attention to the condition. The *clinical sign* of a pericardial rub is also helpful.

Antibiotics and early *surgical drainage* are indicated, and, when used early, they substantially reduce the mortality rate, which would otherwise be close to 100 percent.

Tuberculous Pericarditis

This complication usually results from an extension of a contiguous tuberculous process either in the lungs or in the lymph nodes. It starts as a fibrinous reaction, with or without effusion; then, thickening of the pericardium develops, owing to the formation of tubercles, caseation, and fibrosis. The thickened *adherent pericardium* assumes a shaggy appearance. *Constrictive pericarditis* may occur at this period, or later, when *calcification* results. The treatment, in the early stages before constriction, is by the conventional method of dealing with tuberculosis, namely, by administering isoniazid and paraaminosalicylic acid for a long period of time, usually 18 months to 2 years. When constriction is present, surgical treatment is required also.

Nonspecific Pericarditis

This *recurrent* type, such as that associated with autoimmune reactions, postcommissurotomy pericarditis, and postmyocardial-infarct pericarditis, is often benefited by steroid therapy. Such treatment simply suppresses the signs and symptoms and, therefore, usually must be continued for a long period of time.

In the case of pericardial effusion, a pericardial tap is required only when tamponade threatens or for diagnostic purposes, as in suspected malignancy. A method frequently employed, at present, is a *surgical* approach (see page 260) by the removal of fluid through a *window*, at which time a *biopsy* can be obtained and, if necessary, cannulization from the pericardium to the left pleural cavity can be performed. Fluid formed in the pericardial sac then passes into the left pleural cavity, from which it is absorbed.

The ECG and X-ray are reproduced through the courtesy of Dr. Lawrence Gould.

HEART TRANSPLANTATION

Transplantation of the heart has been surgically feasible since 1960 when the essence of the surgical method was propounded. The important restrictions of the immune reaction and recipient selection remain, even though clinical experience was begun with the work of Barnard in South Africa and Kantrowitz in New York. These illustrations show, in general, the surgical methods for *heart transplantation* which were developed at the Stanford University School of Medicine during the past 8 years.

At the outset of the experimental work, one of the most important constituents of the entire project was the technic of *extracorporeal circulation*. It may well be that lack of detailed attention to the modality of extracorporeal circulation has been more responsible for the high incidence of laboratory failure, in heart transplantation, than any other single factor. For example, the bubble oxygenator with hemodilution has been the extremely popular form of cardiopulmonary bypass in man, but, with laboratory animals, a better form of pump oxygenator is mandatory to the achievement of routine survival after orthotopic cardiac homotransplantation.

In the beginning there were several problems that required solution before any animal could be expected to survive after orthotopic homotransplantation of the heart. The most immediate of these obstacles lay in the realm of the surgical method and its development. Another very important problem was the protection of the donor heart against irreversible damage from the time it was removed to that moment when coronary circulation could be reestablished. Also, an extremely important element in the heart-transplantation physiological process was an assessment of the effect of total cardiac denervation. For decades, Russian physiologists have insisted that no organ completely separated from the central nervous system could approach physiological levels of performance. These opinions, of course, were precipitated from the early work of Pavlov and his colleagues. Finally, maintenance of "life" of the recipient had to be assured for that period when his own cardiopulmonary function was interrupted. For this lesser problem the rotating-disc *oxygenator* and roller *pump* were successfully applied.

We found, early, that peripheral venous *cannulation* was extremely helpful because of the complete absence, in the operative field, of tubing and catheters. Only one clamp is necessary to separate the inflow elements of the heart from the outflow tract. In the dog, a Satinsky noncrushing clamp is placed across the transverse sinus as far cephalad as possible. In man, dissection, individually, of the *pulmonary trunk* and *aorta* permits a single

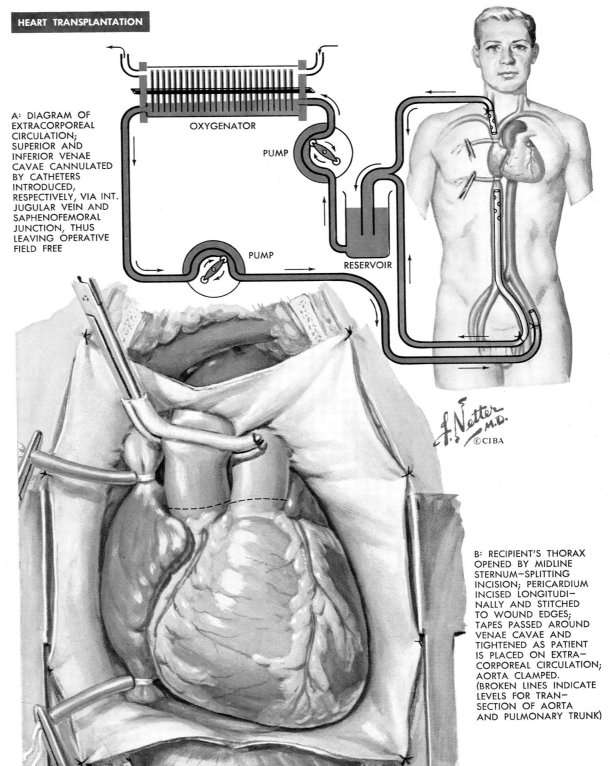

A: DIAGRAM OF EXTRACORPOREAL CIRCULATION; SUPERIOR AND INFERIOR VENAE CAVAE CANNULATED BY CATHETERS INTRODUCED, RESPECTIVELY, VIA INT. JUGULAR VEIN AND SAPHENOFEMORAL JUNCTION, THUS LEAVING OPERATIVE FIELD FREE

OXYGENATOR

PUMP

PUMP

RESERVOIR

B: RECIPIENT'S THORAX OPENED BY MIDLINE STERNUM—SPLITTING INCISION; PERICARDIUM INCISED LONGITUDI-NALLY AND STITCHED TO WOUND EDGES; TAPES PASSED AROUND VENAE CAVAE AND TIGHTENED AS PATIENT IS PLACED ON EXTRA-CORPOREAL CIRCULATION; AORTA CLAMPED. (BROKEN LINES INDICATE LEVELS FOR TRAN-SECTION OF AORTA AND PULMONARY TRUNK)

occlusive clamp across the ascending aorta, midway between the valve and the innominate artery. Left thoracotomy is the approach of choice in animals, but, in man, the *midline sternotomy* provides optimal exposure. Protection of the heart transplant is achieved by local cooling through the use of physiological saline solution at 2 to 4° C. The pericardium is sutured to the edges of the incision in such a way as to provide a well which can be filled with cold saline. Slush or particulate cold solution not only is injurious to thin atrial walls but has been implicated in damage to the phrenic nerves. Accordingly, liquid saline, seeking its own level, provides an excellent bath for local cardiac refrigeration. Peripheral *cannulation* of the *venae cavae* is achieved by means of the *right internal jugular* and *left saphenous veins*. The decannulated internal jugular vein can be either sutured or ligated. The saphenous vein is simply ligated at its femoral

junction. Number 28 French *catheters* are utilized for adult venae cavae. Venous pressure is monitored by means of a common iliac catheter inserted through the right saphenous vein. This catheter remains in place throughout the early postoperative period. The intrapericardial venae cavae of the recipient are looped by means of umbilical *tapes*, and occlusion is effected with rubber chokers.

This illustration reveals the essence of the surgical method, which depends upon retention, in the host, of portions of both *atria* and the *interatrial septum* to which the transplant is sutured. Individual sections of the four *pulmonary veins* at both venae cavae would provide an unnecessary, time-consuming, technical challenge. Accordingly, after division of the *aorta* and *pulmonary trunk* immediately above their respective semilunar valves, the atria are incised in such a

(Continued on page 264)

HEART TRANSPLANTATION

(*Continued from page 263*)

way as to leave intact portions of the *right* and *left atrial walls* and the atrial septum of the *recipient*. In man, because of the disproportion between the normal donor heart and the larger recipient organ, the donor heart is removed by individual division of each of the six inflow veins. In dogs, where there is no such disproportion between donor and recipient hearts, the donor heart is removed in precisely the same way as the recipient organ. Conceivably, in infants and children, the donor heart may be of the same size as that of the recipient. In such an event, individual section of donor inflow vessels would not be necessary.

Resuscitation of the donor heart is mandatory before proceeding with thoracotomy in the recipient. The donor is placed in conduit with extracorporeal circulation, in precisely the same manner as the recipient, as soon after pronouncement of death as possible. Ventricular fibrillation of the donor heart routinely develops, and no attempt is made to convert this arrhythmia to an effective contraction. Care must be taken to prevent distention of the donor heart while in cardiac arrest.

One of the most interesting observations, in transposing the laboratory experience to human application, was the marked similarity between the procedure in dogs and its application to man. The homotransplant between dogs is infinitely more difficult, technically, than its human counterpart. It has been well stated that any surgical method which achieves some success in dogs is more easily applied to the human. The annals of cardiac surgery — beginning with the Blalock-Taussig operation and embracing such more recent technics as control cross-circulation, general hypothermia, and various methods of extracorporeal circulation — bear out this axiom, to and including homotransplantation of the heart.

To gain as much donor atrium as possible, incisions are made posteriorly on the donor heart, connecting the *pulmonary venous orifices* on the *left atrium* and the *vena caval orifices* on the *right atrium*. The extended *atrial septum* is then sutured to the remnants of the recipient atria in precisely the same way as in the laboratory. It is quite probable that no adult donor heart will be too small for any recipient bed if the donor atria are extended in this manner. The better the anatomic match between donor and recipient heart, the less need for preserving the entire donor atria.

The *donor heart* is removed *after* excision of the recipient heart. The donor heart is immediately placed in a bowl of cold saline solution and transported to the recipient table. The huge pericardial well of the recipient is flooded with cold saline,

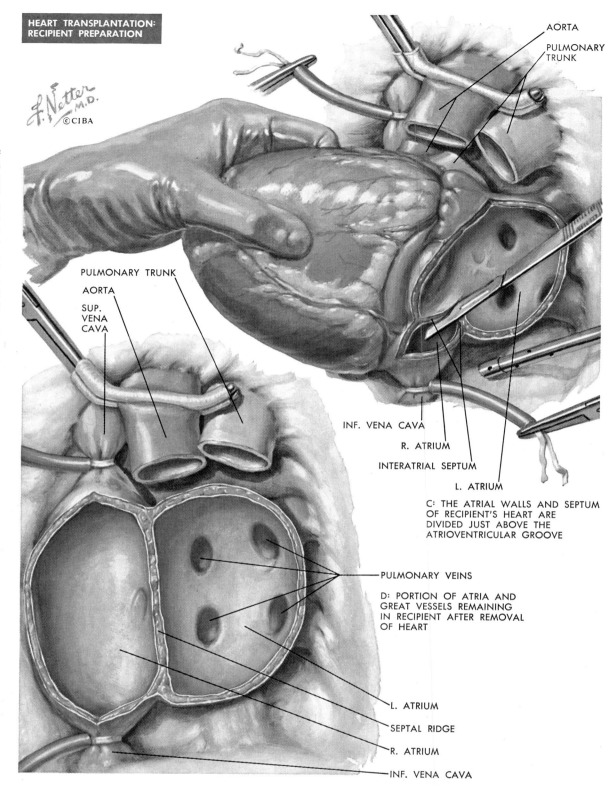

HEART TRANSPLANTATION: RECIPIENT PREPARATION

PULMONARY TRUNK
AORTA
SUP. VENA CAVA

AORTA
PULMONARY TRUNK

INF. VENA CAVA
R. ATRIUM
INTERATRIAL SEPTUM
L. ATRIUM

C: THE ATRIAL WALLS AND SEPTUM OF RECIPIENT'S HEART ARE DIVIDED JUST ABOVE THE ATRIOVENTRICULAR GROOVE

PULMONARY VEINS

D: PORTION OF ATRIA AND GREAT VESSELS REMAINING IN RECIPIENT AFTER REMOVAL OF HEART

L. ATRIUM
SEPTAL RIDGE
R. ATRIUM
INF. VENA CAVA

and the donor heart is removed from the vehicle transport and placed in the pericardial well. After guy sutures, at each end of the left atrial cavity of the recipient, have been united to the extent of the left atrium of the donor, a simple over-and-over suture is utilized for joining, first, the left atria and, second, the right atria. In the dog with a left thoracotomy, the more distal suture union, *i.e.*, the right atrial anastomosis, is accomplished first, but in the human with midline sternotomy, the distal inflow anastomosis is the left atrial union. After the inflow tracts have been united, a small catheter is placed in the left atrial appendage of the donor heart, and cold saline is used to fill the left side of the heart and expel all air which has been trapped in the pulmonary veins of the host, as well as that in the combined left atrium and the donor left ventricle. The last plate (see page 266) illustrates the left atrial *catheter* as well as *air* and

fluid emanating from the *aorta* before completion of the *aortic anastomosis*.

The aorta is easily sutured. The donor aorta may be incised transversely to make the necessary adjustment to a larger recipient aorta. The *aortic clamp* is removed after completion of the aortic anastomosis, and a small bulldog clamp is placed across the donor pulmonary artery. The caval tape is removed, and vigorous ventricular fibrillation of the donor heart commences. Local cooling of the heart is discontinued at this point, and, before suturing the pulmonary arteries, all atrial *suture lines* are very carefully *inspected* to identify any significant bleeding areas. The pulmonary arteries are then united leisurely, because the heart is now receiving its first coronary perfusion after a period of approximately 60 minutes of hypoxia, while cardiac viability was maintained entirely

(*Continued on page 265*)

HEART TRANSPLANTATION: DONOR HEART

HEART TRANSPLANTATION

(Continued from page 264)

through the expedient of local cooling.

Defibrillation of the ventricles is usually not spontaneous but is readily effected by means of a single d-c shock of 10 to 25 watt-seconds. The recipient is placed in the Trendelenburg position, and a needle hole is established at the apex of the ascending aorta, so that any residual air is expelled without reaching the cerebral circulation or the coronary arteries. The patient is then removed from his extracorporeal source of support, after some 15 to 20 minutes of partial bypass. Approximately 1 hour and 20 minutes of bypass are required. The total operating time does not exceed 4 hours.

A myocardial electrode is sutured into the right ventricle for the dual purpose of satisfying any need for artificial pacing of the transplant and to furnish specific information with respect to the electrocardiogram derived. When fluid collects in the pericardium, as almost always will be the case in patients having undergone transplantation of the heart, the R wave of the electrocardiogram is obscured unless the tracing is made from an implanted sensor. The best information and, in fact, the only consistently reliable herald of early homograft rejection of the heart is the changing amplitude of the R wave of the electrocardiogram.

It has been well demonstrated, in animals, that the daily administration of immune-suppression drugs almost always results in death, owing to drug toxicity. Accordingly, a program of intermittent immune suppression was developed, in the laboratory, which culminated in the long-term survival of dogs after orthotopic transplantation of the heart. The supposition was necessarily made that rejection of the heart is not a threat of constant intensity but may come in waves of varying strength. It could well be that the so-called wave of rejection is undetectable until sufficient myocardial damage has accrued to change the amplitude of the highest deflection of the ECG. However, the important fact is that the point of the natural history of homograft rejection, when the only detectable evidence of rejection lies in the R wave, is still a phase from which recovery is possible. At that time, rejection has not developed to an irreversible degree. Therefore, the demand utilization of immune-suppressing chemicals can reverse the effects of homograft rejection as delineated by the sensing mechanism of the ECG. Imuran® and methylprednisolone are the most commonly used immune suppressants. Many other physiological parameters have been measured in the laboratory to determine early signs of graft rejection, but, after careful study of cardiac output, left ventricular upstroke, venous and arterial pressures, and enzymatic values, the R wave of the ECG appears

to be the only reliable early indicator of graft rejection. It is probably very significant that, after heart transplantation, laboratory animals which have been treated with the same program of immune suppression as have renal transplants cannot survive for long-term observation. Wound infections, liver failure, severe loss of weight, and other manifestations of drug toxicity suggest that a schedule of intermittent or demand therapy is essential in securing long-term survival of the organism with cardiac homotransplantation.

Most patients who have progressed to the point where transplantation of the heart is justifiable will require tracheotomy. It is possible to perform a tracheotomy which does not contaminate the midline sternotomy. Careful application of plastic tape will readily separate the tracheotomy from the upper margin of the chest incision. The Engstrom respirator is extremely helpful in the early postoperative period,

and it may take many days or weeks of supportive ventilation before the patient can be weaned from the respirator. The tracheotomy should be changed at least twice a day, because of the tendency of patients taking immune suppressants to develop infections. The tracheotomy should be suctioned with a new and sterile catheter on each occasion, and the nurse should wear sterile gloves when tracheotomy care is being given. Only with these precautions can important pulmonary contamination and infection be prevented.

Moral, Ethical, and Social Implications of Human Heart Transplantation

The several years' delay between successful application of orthotopic homotransplantation of the heart

(Continued on page 266)

ORIFICES OF PULMONARY VEINS

LEFT ATRIUM

PULMONARY TRUNK

AORTA

ORIFICE OF SUPERIOR VENA CAVA

RIGHT ATRIUM

INTERATRIAL GROOVE

ORIFICE OF INFERIOR VENA CAVA

E: HEART REMOVED FROM DONOR BY SEVERING SUPERIOR AND INFERIOR VENAE CAVAE, PULMONARY VEINS, AORTA, AND PULMONARY TRUNK (VIEWED FROM REAR). (BROKEN LINES INDICATE INCISIONS TO CONNECT CAVAL ORIFICES AND VEIN ORIFICES, THUS OPENING THE ATRIA WITHOUT DIVIDING THE SEPTUM)

F: THE FLAPS CREATED BY THE INCISIONS INDICATED ABOVE HAVE BEEN TURNED OUT AND DRAWN LONGITUDINALLY BY SUTURES, THUS EXTENDING THE SEPTUM AND ATRIAL WALLS TO ACCOMMODATE TO LARGER HEART OF RECIPIENT

G: DIAGRAM TO INDICATE SUCCESSIVE CONTINUOUS SUTURES TO BE EMPLOYED IN UNITING DONOR HEART TO RECIPIENT AS ILLUSTRATED IN NEXT PLATE

LEFT ATRIUM   RIGHT ATRIUM

RIGHT ATRIUM   LEFT ATRIUM

DONOR HEART

RECIPIENT

Heart Transplantation

(Continued from page 265)

in animals and its use in man was the result of numerous factors. Experience with immune suppression in renal transplantation was clearly very important in the initiation of heart transplants. Long-term laboratory observations were likewise of value in determining if the absence of central-nervous-system reflexes had prohibitively deleterious effects on cardiac performance. Also experimentally, a demand form of immune suppression was formulated to cope specifically with the heart transplants. Merely transposing accepted immune chemotherapy from kidney transplants to heart transplants tends to oversimplify the problem.

One of the most challenging and difficult aspects of human heart homotransplantation is selection of the recipient. The heart is a strong organ, and it may well be that any patient whose heart has failed to the point where replacement is indicated has a certain amount of irreversible damage of other organ systems. Obviously, cardiac transplantation, at this point in history, has very little to offer the individual who expires suddenly from massive myocardial infarction. The coronary care unit, now a fixture at almost every hospital of any size, has markedly reduced early mortality from ventricular fibrillation and other arrhythmias secondary to acute coronary-artery occlusions. This unit has been so effective, in fact, that the acute coronary-disease patient seems an unlikely choice for heart transplantation at the present time.

Probably the most satisfactory type of adult who may be considered for heart transplantation is the one with severe myocarditis. Such individuals often present a relatively long history of marginal compensation, but with increasingly frequent episodes of decompensation. This kind of patient does not rally, as will the usual individual suffering from coronary-artery disease. In the last stages of myocarditis, only transplantation of the heart would seem to have any therapeutic application. The secondary effects of coronary-artery disease, such as ventricular aneurysm or mitral-valve insufficiency or ventricular septal defect, frequently are well treated by conventional open-heart surgery, but no such program is available for the patient in the terminal phases of myocarditis. The etiologic factors in unrelenting myocarditis are not well understood, but viral infections are thought to play a role. We have seen one patient with postirradiation myocarditis.

Another important application of heart transplantation, in its present state of development, refers to the infant with a cardiac anomaly for which there is no corrective operation and no palliative procedure. Great difficulty will be encountered in this group of candidates, not only because of a paucity of donors but

HEART TRANSPLANTATION: SUTURE METHOD

H: LEFT SIDE OF EXTENDED INTERATRIAL SEPTUM OF DONOR HEART SUTURED TO SEPTAL STUMP OF RECIPIENT; SUTURE WILL THEN BE CONTINUED TO UNITE THE LEFT ATRIAL WALLS AS INDICATED BY ARROWS

I: RIGHT SIDE OF EXTENDED INTERATRIAL SEPTUM OF DONOR HEART SUTURED TO SEPTAL STUMP OF RECIPIENT; SUTURE WILL THEN BE CONTINUED TO UNITE THE RIGHT ATRIAL WALLS AS INDICATED BY ARROWS

J: AORTAS ALMOST COMPLETELY ANASTOMOSED; LEFT HEART FLUSHED OUT WITH SALINE VIA CATHETER IN LEFT ATRIUM TO REMOVE ALL AIR BEFORE FINAL CLOSURE; HEART IS THEN LIFTED FROM ITS BED AND ALL SUTURE LINES INSPECTED PRIOR TO REMOVAL OF AORTIC CLAMP AND ANASTOMOSIS OF PULMONARY TRUNKS; HEART IS IMMERSED IN COLD SALINE FOR ENTIRE PERIOD OF HYPOXIA

also because of the technical problems that are certain to arise. On the plus side of the ledger, however, is the observation that puppies, after cardiac transplantation, show a very mild degree of cardiac rejection and require only sporadic immune-suppression therapy.

After the successful transplantation of the liver by Starzl and his associates, it was clear that transplantation of unpaired organs had been established. The general public appeared to be ready for the concept that death of the individual occurs in a stepwise fashion, with the brain dying first, and with the heart, liver, and kidneys suffering irreversible damage at some period after brain death had occurred. Irreversibly damaged organs clearly cannot be transplanted, and various methods are necessary to resuscitate the heart in a prospective donor who has suffered brain death. The same truth obtains for livers and kidneys

to be transplanted. Perhaps of a more controversial nature is recipient selection rather than donor selection. Only time and practice will permit the evolution of satisfactory criteria for transplant recipients.

Summary. The advent of clinical heart transplantation must not be construed to relegate the development of heart-assist devices to total obscurity. Although it is certainly a fact that, to date, the artificial apparatus has not competed well with laboratory heart transplants, it would be useful to have available some mechanical heart devices which would maintain the potential transplant recipient, much as hemodialysis units are utilized in preparing patients for kidney transplants. The future of heart replacement has by no means been settled with the initial application of homotransplantation. The way ahead is certainly as difficult as the modicum of success thus far achieved.

GLOSSARY OF ABBREVIATIONS

A — A band
ADP — adenosine diphosphate
AMP — adenosine monophosphate
ATP — adenosine triphosphate
C — creatine
CoA — coenzyme A
COMT — catechol-O-methyl transferase
CoQ — coenzyme Q
CP — creatine PO_4
CPK — creatine phosphokinase
CY.A — cytochrome A
CY.B — cytochrome B
CY.C — cytochrome C
d-c — direct current
DPN — diphosphopyridine nucleotide
DPNH — reduced diphosphopyridine nucleotide
Ⓔ — electron
ECC — extracorporeal circulation
ECHO — enteric cytopathogenic human orphan virus
E.S.R. — erythrocyte sedimentation rate
FAD — flavin adenine dinucleotide
$FADH_2$ — flavin adenine nucleotide
GOT — glutamic oxalacetic transaminase

H — H band
H — H disc
H — H zone
H. and E. stain — hematoxylin and eosin stain
I — I band
LDH — lactic dehydrogenase
M — M line
MAO — monamine oxidase
NEFA — nonesterified fatty acids
PP′ — pyrophosphate
SCPK — serum creatine phosphokinase
SGOT — serum glutamic oxalacetic transaminase
SHBD — serum alpha hydroxybutyric dehydrogenase
SLDH — serum lactic dehydrogenase
$SLDH_1$ — serum lactic dehydrogenase, isoenzyme$_1$
SLE — systemic lupus erythematosus
TPN — triphosphopyridine nucleotide
TPNH — reduced triphosphopyridine nucleotide
UDP — uridinediphosphate
UDPG — uridinediphosphoglucose
UTP — uridine triphosphate
VCG — vectorcardiogram
W — "wedge" pressure
Z — Z line

SELECTED REFERENCES

Section I

PLATE NUMBER

ARNULF, G.: *La résection du plexus préaortique dans l'angine de poitrine*, J. Chir. (Paris), 66:97, 1950.   17, 18

BIRKETT, D. A., APTHORP, CHAMBERLAIN, HAYWARD AND TUCKWELL: *Bilateral upper thoracic sympathectomy in angina pectoris, Results in 52 cases*, Brit. med. J., 2:187, 1965.   17, 18

BRAEUCKER, W.: *Der Brustteil des vegetativen Nervensystems und seine klinisch-chirurgische Bedeuting*, Beitr. Klin. Tuberk., 66:1, 1927.   17, 18

FAWCETT, D. W.: *The sarcoplasmic reticulum of skeletal and cardiac muscle*, Circulation, 24:336, 1961.   20

HANTZ, E.: *Contribution à l'Etude Anatomique et Expérimentale du Plexus Préaortique pour le Traitement de l'Angine de Poitrine*, L. Pidancet, Lyon, 1951.   17, 18

HOFFMAN, B. F., PAES DE CARVALHO, DE MELLO AND CRANEFIELD: *Electrical activity of single fibers of the atrioventricular node*, Circulat. Res., 7:11, 1959.   12–14

HUXLEY, A. F.: *Muscle structure and theories of contraction*, Progr. Biophys., 7:255, 1957.   19

HUXLEY, H. E.: *Muscle cells* in *The Cell*, Brachet, J., and Mirsky, Editors, Academic Press, London, 1960.   19

——: *The contractile structure of cardiac and skeletal muscle*, Circulation, 24:328, 1961.   19

JAMES, T. N.: *Anatomy of the sinus node of the dog*, Anat. Rec., 143:251, 1962.   13

——: *Morphology of the human atrioventricular node, with remarks pertinent to its electrophysiology*, Amer. Heart J., 62:756, 1961.   14

——: *The connecting pathways between the sinus node and A-V node and between the right and left atrium in the human heart*, Amer. Heart J., 66:498, 1963.   12

JONESCO, D., AND ENACHESCO: *Nerfs cardiaques naissant de la chaîne thoracique du sympathique, au-dessous du ganglion stellaire. Les nerfs cardiaques thoracique chez quelques mammifères*, C. R. Soc. Biol. (Paris), 97:977, 1927.   17, 18

KAWAMURA, K.: *Electron microscope studies on the cardiac conduction system of the dog. I. The Purkinje fibers*, Jap. Circulat. J., 25:594, 1961.   14

——: *Electron microscope studies on the cardiac conduction system of the dog. II. The sinoatrial and atrioventricular nodes*, Jap. Circulat. J., 25:973, 1961.   13, 14

KHABAROVA, A. Y.: *The Afferent Innervation of the Heart* (Translation by Haigh, B.), Pitman Medical Pub. Co., London, 1963.   17, 18

LEV, M.: *The conduction system* in *Pathology of the Heart*, Gould, S. E., Editor, 2nd ed., Chapter 4, Charles C Thomas, Springfield, Ill., 1960.   12

MILLER, M. R., AND KASAHARA: *Studies on the nerve endings in the heart*, Amer. J. Anat., 115:217, 1964.   17, 18

MITCHELL, G. A. G.: *Cardiac innervation*, Manch. Med. Gaz., 34:61, 1955.   17, 18

Section I (continued)

PLATE NUMBER

——: *Cardiovascular Innervation*, Williams & Wilkins Company, Baltimore, E. & S. Livingstone, Ltd., Edinburgh, 1956.   17, 18

——: *The discoverers of the thoracic cardiac nerves*, Edinb. med. J., 56:156, 1949.   17, 18

——, AND WARWICK: *The dorsal vagal nucleus*, Acta anat. (Basel), 25:371, 1955.   17, 18

MOLLARD, J.: *Les nerfs du coeur*, Rev. gén. Histol., 3:1, 1908.   17, 18

MORALES, M. F., AND WATANABE: *The ATPases of muscle proteins*, Circulation, 24:390, 1961.   19

MUIR, A. R.: *Further observations on the cellular structure of cardiac muscle*, J. Anat. (Lond.), 99:27, 1965.   20

——: *Observations on the fine structure of the Purkinje fibers in the ventricles of the sheep's heart*, J. Anat. (Lond.), 91:251, 1957.   14

NELSON, D. A., AND BENSON: *On the structural continuities of the transverse tubular system of rabbit and human myocardial cells*, J. Cell Biol., 16:297, 1963.   20

PAES DE CARVALHO, A.: *Cellular electrophysiology of the atrial specialized tissues*, in *The Specialized Tissues of the Heart*, Elsevier Pub. Co., Amsterdam, 1962.   12–14

——, AND DE ALMEIDA: *Spread of activity through the atrioventricular node*, Circulat. Res., 8:801, 1960.   12–14

——, DE MELLO AND HOFFMAN: *Electrophysiological evidence for specialized fiber types in rabbit atrium*, Amer. J. Physiol., 196:483, 1959.   12–14

PALADE, G. E.: *Blood capillaries of the heart and other organs*, Circulation, 24:368, 1961.   20

POLLOCK, L. J., AND DAVIS: *Visceral and referred pain*, Ass. Res. nerv. Dis. Proc., 15:210, 1935; also, Arch. Neurol. Psychiat. (Chicago), 34:1041, 1935.   17, 18

SONES, JR., F. M.: *Cine coronary arteriography*, Anesth. Analg. Curr. Res., 46:499, 1967.   20

SPALTEHOLZ, W.: *Handatlas der Anatomie des Menschen*, Band II: *Regionen, Muskeln, Faszien, Herz, Blutgefässe*, 13th ed., S. Hirzel, Leipzig, 1933.   1–11, 15, 16

SPIRO, D., AND SONNENBLICK: *Comparison of the ultrastructural basis of the contractile process in heart and skeletal muscle*, Circulat. Res., 15:II-14, 1964.   19

STENGER, R. J., AND SPIRO: *Structure of the cardiac muscle cell*, Amer. J. Med., 30:653, 1961.   20

——, AND ——: *The ultrastructure of mammalian cardiac muscle*, J. Biophys. Biochem. Cytol., 9:325, 1961.   20

TANDLER, J.: *Anatomie des Herzens* in Bardeleben's *Handbuch der Anatomie des Menschen*, Gustav Fisher, Jena, 1913.   1–11, 15, 16

THAEMERT, J. C.: *Ultrastructure of cardiac muscle and nerve contiguities*, J. Cell Biol., 29:156, 1966.   20

TRAUTWEIN, W., AND UCHIZONO: *Electron-microscopic and electrophysiologic study of the pacemaker in the sino-atrial node of

Section I (continued)

PLATE NUMBER

the rabbit heart*, Z. Zellforsch., 61:96, 1963.   13

TRUEX, R. C., BISHOF AND DOWNING: *Accessory atrioventricular muscle bundles. II. Cardiac conduction system in a human specimen with Wolff-Parkinson-White Syndrome*, Anat. Rec., 137:417, 1960.   12

——, AND SMYTHE: *Comparative morphology of the cardiac conduction tissue in animals* in *Comparative Cardiology*, ed. by Hecht, H. H., and Detweiler, Ann. N. Y. Acad. Sci., 127:19, 1965.   14

WAGNER, M. L., LAZZARA, WEISS AND HOFFMAN: *Specialized conducting fibers in the interatrial band*, Circulat. Res., 18:502, 1966.   12

WALMSLEY, T.: *The Heart* in *Elements of Anatomy*, Quain, J., Longmans, Green and Co., London, 1929.   1–11, 15, 16

WHITE, J. C., AND BLAND: *Surgical relief of severe angina pectoris. Methods employed and end results in 83 patients*, Medicine (Baltimore), 27:1, 1948.   17, 18

WILLIAMS, T. H.: *Mitral and tricuspid valve innervation*, Brit. Heart J., 26:105, 1964.   17, 18

Section II

AGRESS, C. M.: *Evaluation of the transaminase test*, Amer. J. Cardiol., 3:74, 1959.   53, 54

BACANER, M. B., LIOY AND VISSCHER: *Induced change in heart metabolism as a primary determinant of heart performance*, Amer. J. Physiol., 209:519, 1965.   1–4

BAYDAR, I. D., WALSH AND MASSIE: *A vectorcardiographic study of bundle branch block with the Frank lead system. Clinical correlation in ventricular hypertrophy and chronic pulmonary disease*, Amer. J. Cardiol., 15:185, 1965.   21

BECK, C. S., PRITCHARD AND FEIL: *Ventricular fibrillation of long duration abolished by electric shock*, J. Amer. med. Ass., 135:985, 1947.   56–58

BOCK, K. D., EDITOR: *Shock: Pathogenesis and Therapy*, An International Symposium, Chairman, U. S. von Euler, sponsored by CIBA-Stockholm, English and German ed., 1962.   55

BURCH, G. E., AND WINSOR: *A Primer of Electrocardiography*, Lea & Febiger, Philadelphia, 5th ed., 1966.   13, 18–20, 23, 25, 26

CALLAGHAN, J. C., AND BIGELOW: *Electrical artificial pacemaker for standstill of the heart*, Ann. Surg., 134:8, 1951.   33, 34

CARTER, W. A., AND ESTES: *Electrocardiographic manifestations of ventricular hypertrophy; a computer study of ECG-anatomic correlations in 319 cases*, Amer. Heart J., 68:173, 1964.   21

CENTER, S., AND NATHAN: *The synchronous pacer: Three years of clinical experience with 45 cases*, Ann. Surg., 164:862, 1966.   33, 34

CHARDACK, W. M., GAGE AND GREATBACH: *A transistorized, self-contained, implantable pacemaker for the long-term correction *of complete heart block,* Surgery, 48:643, 1960. 33, 34

—, —, FEDERICO, SCHIMERT AND GREATBACH: *The long-term treatment of heart block,* Progr. cardiovasc. Dis., 9:105, 1966. 33, 34

—, —, — AND —: *Five years' clinical experience with an implantable pacemaker: An appraisal,* Surgery, 58:915, 1965. 33, 34

CHÁVEZ RIVERA, I.: *"Coma, Síncope y Shock,"* Universidad Nacional Autónoma de México, Oficina Publicaciones, ed. 1966. 55

CHOU, TE-CHUAN, AND HELM: *Clinical Vectorcardiography,* Grune & Stratton, Inc., New York, 1967. 16, 18, 19

CONN, H. L., AND BRILLER, EDITORS: *The Myocardial Cell,* University of Pennsylvania Press, Philadelphia, 1966. 62–66

CORNE, R. A., PARKIN, BRANDENBURG AND BROWN: *Peri-infarction block: Postmyocardial-infarction intraventricular conduction disturbance,* Amer. Heart J., 69:150, 1965. 24

COURNAND, A.: *Pulmonary circulation. Its control in man, with some remarks on methodology* (Nobel Prize Lecture, 1956), Amer. Heart J., 54:172, 1957. 5

—, CHAIRMAN: *Symposium on cardiac output,* Fed. Proc., 4:183, 1945. 6

—, BALDWIN AND HIMMELSTEIN: *Cardiac catheterization,* in *Congenital Heart Disease: A Clinical and Physiological Study in Infants and Children,* Commonwealth Fund, New York, 1949. 7

—, BLOOMFIELD AND LAUSON: *Double lumen catheter for intravenous and intracardiac blood sampling and pressure recording,* Proc. Soc. exp. Biol., 60:73, 1945. 7

—, LAUSON, BLOOMFIELD, BREED AND BALDWIN: *Recording of right heart pressures in man,* Proc. Soc. exp. Biol., 55:34, 1944. 7

DE MELLO, W. C., AND HOFFMAN: *Potassium ions and electrical activity of specialized cardiac fibers,* Amer. J. Physiol., 199:1125, 1960. 10, 11

DIMOND, E. G.: *Electrocardiography and Vectorcardiography,* Little, Brown & Co., Boston, 1966. 16, 18, 19, 28, 30

DOUCET, P., WALSH AND MASSIE: *A vectorcardiographic and electrocardiographic study of left bundle branch block with myocardial infarction,* Amer. J. Cardiol., 17:171, 1966. 22

—, — AND —: *A vectorcardiographic study of right bundle branch block with the Frank lead system. Clinical correlation in myocardial infarction,* Amer. J. Cardiol., 16:342, 1965. 22

DOW, P.: *Estimations of cardiac output and central blood volume by dye dilution,* Physiol. Rev., 36:77, 1956. 6

EVANS, W.: *Faults in the diagnosis and management of cardiac pain,* Brit. med. J., 1:249, 1959. 32

FOWLER, N. O.: *Physical Diagnosis of Heart Disease,* The Macmillan Company, New York, 1963. 36, 40, 41, 43, 46–49, 51

FRIEDBERG, C. K.: *Diseases of the Heart,* 2nd ed., W. B. Saunders Company, Philadelphia, 1956. 40–43, 46–49, 51, 52

FRITTS, H. W., JR., AND COURNAND: *The application of the Fick principle to the measurement of cardiac output,* Proc. nat. Acad. Sci. (Wash.), 44:1079, 1958. 6

FURMAN, S., AND ROBINSON: *Stimulation of the ventricular endocardial surface in control of complete heart block,* Ann. Surg., 150:841, 1959. 33, 34

GADBOYS, H. L., WISOFF AND LITWAK: *Surgical treatment of complete heart block. An analysis of 36 cases,* J. Amer. med. Ass., 189:97, 1964. 33, 34

GALLETTI, P. M., AND BRECHER: *Heart-Lung Bypass: Principles and Techniques of Extracorporeal Circulation,* Grune & Stratton, Inc., New York, 1962. 59–61

GIBBON, J. H., JR.: *Application of a mechanical heart and lung application to cardiac surgery,* Minn. Med., 37:171, 1954. 59–61

—: *Extracorporeal maintenance of cardiorespiratory functions,* Harvey Lect., 53:186, 1959. 59–61

GOLDMAN, M. J.: *Principles of Clinical Electrocardiography,* 5th ed., Lange Medical Publications, Los Altos, 1964. 48–50

GOODMAN, L., AND GILMAN, EDITORS: *The Pharmacological Basis of Therapeutics,* 3rd ed., The Macmillan Company, New York, 1965. 62–66

GORLIN, G.: *Shunt flows and valve areas,* in *Intravascular Catheterization,* ed. by Zimmermann, 2nd ed. (pages 545-582), Charles C Thomas, Springfield, Ill., 1966. 9

GRANT, R. P.: *Clinical Electrocardiography,* McGraw-Hill Book Company, Inc., New York, 1957. 48–51

GREEN, H. D., AND KEPCHAR: *Control of peripheral resistance in major systemic vascular beds,* Physiol. Rev., 39:617, 1959. 1–4

HAMILTON, W. F.: *Measurement of cardiac output,* in *Handbook of Physiology,* Section 2 on Circulation, ed. by Hamilton, Vol. 1 (pages 551-584), Amer. Physiol. Soc., Bethesda, 1962. 6

HELLEMS, H. K., HAYNES, GOWDEY AND DEXTER: *Pulmonary capillary pressure in man,* J. clin. Invest., 27:540, 1948. 7

HERSHEY, S. G., EDITOR: *Shock,* Little, Brown & Co., Boston, 1964. 55

HILMER, W.: *About differential diagnosis of the negative T-waves. Myocardial infarction or anomaly of the excitation,* Cardiologia (Basel), 49:305, 1966. 32

HIMMELSTEIN, A., AND COURNAND: *Cardiac catheterization in the study of congenital cardiovascular anomalies,* Amer. J. Med., 12:349, 1952. 8

HIRSCH, E. Z.: *The effects of digoxin on the electrocardiogram after strenuous exercise in normal men,* Amer. Heart J., 70:196, 1965. 31

HOFFMAN, B. F., AND CRANEFIELD: *Electrophysiology of the Heart,* McGraw-Hill Book Company, Inc., New York, 1960. 10, 11

—, —, STUCKEY AND BAGDONAS: *Electrical activity during the P-R interval,* Circulat. Res., 8:1200, 1960. 10, 11

—, MOORE, STUCKEY AND CRANEFIELD: *Functional properties of the atrioventricular conduction system,* Circulat. Res., 13:308, 1963. 10, 11

—, PAES DE CARVALHO, DE MELLO AND CRANEFIELD: *Electrical activity of single fibers of the atrioventricular node,* Circulat. Res., 7:11, 1959. 10, 11

HOOKER, D. R., KOUWENHOVEN AND LANGWORTHY: *The Effect of Alternating Electric Currents on the Heart,* Amer. J. Physiol., 103:444, 1933. 56–58

INNES, I. R., AND NICKERSON: *Drugs acting on postganglionic adrenergic nerve endings and structures innervated by them (sympathomimetic drugs),* page 477 in *The Pharmacological Basis of Therapeutics,* ed. by Goodman and Gilman, The Macmillan Company, New York, 3rd ed., 1965. 63

JUDE, J. R., AND ELAM: *Fundamentals of Cardiopulmonary Resuscitation,* F. A. Davis Co., Philadelphia, 1965. 56–58

—, KOUWENHOVEN AND KNICKERBOCKER: *An experimental and clinical study of a portable external cardiac defibrillator,* Surg. Forum, 13:185, 1962. 56–58

—, — AND —: *External cardiac resuscitation,* Monogr. surg. Sci., 1:59, 1964. 56–58

KANTROWITZ, A., COHEN, RAILLARD, SCHMIDT AND FELDMAN: *The treatment of complete heart block with an implanted, controllable pacemaker,* Surg. Gynec. Obstet., 115:415, 1962. 33, 34

KOELLE, G. B.: *Neurohumoral transmission and the autonomic nervous system,* page 399 in *The Pharmacological Basis of Therapeutics,* ed. by Goodman and Gilman, The Macmillan Company, New York, 1965. 65

KOENIG, F.: *Lehrbuch die Allgemeinen Chirurgie,* pp. 60-61, Gottingen, 1883. 56–58

KORY, R. C., TSAZARIS AND BUSTAMONTE: *A Primer of Cardiac Catheterization* (pages 64-78), Charles C Thomas, Springfield, Ill., 1965. 9

KOUWENHOVEN, W. B., JUDE AND KNICKERBOCKER: *Closed-chest cardiac massage,* J. Amer. med. Ass., 173:1064, 1960. 56–58

—, MILNOR, KNICKERBOCKER AND CHESNUT: *Closed-chest defibrillation of the heart,* Surgery, 42:550, 1957. 56–58

LADUE, J. S., WRÓBLEWSKI AND KARMEN: *Serum glutamic oxaloacetic transaminase activity in human acute transmural myocardial infarction,* Science, 20:497, 1954. 53, 54

LAMB, L. E.: *Electrocardiography and Vectorcardiography. Instrumentation, Fundamentals and Clinical Application,* W. B. Saunders Co., Philadelphia, 1965. 16–19, 27

LARNER, J.: QUOTED BY ABDULLAH, M., TAYLOR AND WHELAN: *The enzymatic debranching of glycogen and the rôle of transferase,* in *Control of Glycogen Metabolism,* Ciba Foundation Symposium, J. and A. Churchill Ltd., London, and Little, Brown & Co., Boston, 1964. 1–4

LEVINE, S. A.: *Clinical Heart Disease,* 5th ed., W. B. Saunders Company, Philadelphia, 1958. 36, 42, 43, 46–51

—, AND HARVEY: *Clinical Auscultation of the Heart,* 2nd ed., W. B. Saunders Company, Philadelphia, 1959. 35, 36, 40–42, 48–50

LISTER, J. W., STEIN, KOSOWSKY, LAU AND DAMATO: *Atrioventricular conduction in man. Effect of rate, exercise, isoproterenol*

Section II (continued)

PLATE NUMBER

and atropine on the P-R interval, Amer. J. Cardiol., 16:516, 1965. — 29

LUISADA, A. A., EDITOR: *Cardiology: An Encyclopedia of the Cardiovascular System, Sponsored by the American College of Cardiology,* McGraw-Hill Book Company, Inc., New York, 1958-1963. — 42, 43, 46–52

—: *From Auscultation to Phonocardiography,* C. V. Mosby Co., St. Louis, 1965. — 35, 36, 38–42, 48–52

—: *Heart: A Physiologic and Clinical Study of Cardiovascular Diseases,* 2nd ed., Williams & Wilkins Company, Baltimore, 1954. — 40–43, 46–52

—: *The Heart Beat: Graphic Methods in the Study of the Cardiac Patient,* Paul B. Hoeber, Inc., New York, 1953. — 38–42, 48–51

—, AND SAINANI: *A Primer of Cardiac Diagnosis,* Warren H. Green, Inc., St. Louis, 1969. — 36, 40–43, 48–50

—, AND SLODKI: *The Differential Diagnosis of Cardiovascular Diseases,* Grune & Stratton, Inc., New York, 1965. — 36, 40–43, 48, 49, 52

MAASS, DR.: *Die Methode der Wiederbelebung bei Herztod nach Chloroformeinathmung,* Berl. klin. Wschr., 12:265, 1892. — 56–58

MAJOR, R. H., AND DELP: *Physical Diagnosis,* 6th ed., W. B. Saunders Company, Philadelphia, 1962. — 36, 46–50

MARRIOTT, H. J. L.: *Electrocardiographogenic suicide and lesser crimes,* J. Fla. med. Ass., 50:440, 1963. — 32

—: *Normal electrocardiographic variants simulating ischemic heart disease,* J. Amer. med. Ass., 199:325, 1967. — 32

—, AND NIZET: *Physiologic stimuli simulating ischemic heart disease,* J. Amer. med. Ass., 200:715, 1967. — 32

MARSHALL, H. W., HELMHOLZ AND WOOD: *Physiological consequences of congenital heart disease,* in *Handbook of Physiology,* Section 2 on Circulation, ed. by Hamilton, Vol. 1 (pages 417-487), Amer. Physiol. Soc., Bethesda, 1962. — 8

MARTINEZ, A.: *Aberrant ventricular conduction in the diagnosis of myocardial infarction,* Amer. J. Cardiol., 14:352, 1964. — 23

MAYER, S. E., WILLIAMS AND SMITH: *Adrenergic mechanisms in cardiac glycogen metabolism,* Ann. N. Y. Acad. Sci., 139:686, 1967. — 62

MELICHAR, F., JEDLICKA AND HAVLIK: *A study of undiagnosed myocardial infarctions,* Acta med. scand., 174:761, 1963. — 53, 54

MILLS, L. J., AND MOYER, EDITORS: *Shock and Hypotension: Pathogenesis and Treatment,* Grune & Stratton, Inc., New York, 1965. — 55

MOE, G. K., AND FARAH: *Digitalis and allied cardiac glycosides,* page 665 in *The Pharmacological Basis of Therapeutics,* ed. by Goodman and Gilman, The Macmillan Company, New York, 3rd ed., 1965. — 64, 66

NATHAN, D. A., CENTER, WU AND KELLER: *An implantable synchronous pacemaker for the long-term correction of complete heart block,* Amer. J. Cardiol., 11:362, 1963. — 33, 34

OLSON, E.: *Physiology of cardiac muscle,* Handbook of Physiology, Vol. I, Sec. 2, pages 199-235, American Physiological Society, Washington, D. C., 1962. — 1–4

Section II (continued)

PLATE NUMBER

PAES DE CARVALHO, A.: *Cellular electrophysiology of the atrial specialized tissues,* in *The Specialized Tissues of the Heart,* Elsevier Pub. Co., Amsterdam, 1962. — 10, 11

—, AND DE ALMEIDA: *Spread of activity through the atrioventricular node,* Circulat. Res., 8:801, 1960. — 10, 11

—, DE MELLO AND HOFFMAN: *Electrophysiological evidence for specialized fiber types in rabbit atrium,* Amer. J. Physiol., 196:483, 1959. — 10, 11

PREVOST, J. L., AND BATTELLI: *On some effects of electrical discharges on the heart of mammals,* C. R. Acad. Sci., 129:1267, 1899. — 56–58

PRUITT, R. D., WATT, JR., AND MURAO: *Left axis deviation: Its relationship to experimentally induced lesions of the anterior left bundle branch system in canine and primate hearts,* Ann. N. Y. Acad. Sci., 127:204, 1965. — 22

RICHARDS, D. W., JR.: *The contributions of right heart catheterization to physiology and medicine, with some observations on the physiopathology of pulmonary heart disease* (Nobel Prize Lecture, 1956), Amer. Heart J., 54:161, 1957. — 5

ROSALKI, S. B., AND WILKINSON: *Reduction of α-ketobutyrate by human serum,* Nature (Lond.), 188:1110, 1960. — 53, 54

ROSS, J., JR.: *Transseptal left heart catheterization: a new method of left atrial puncture,* Ann. Surg., 149:395, 1959. — 5

RUSHMER, R. F.: *Effects of nerve stimulation and hormones on the heart; the role of the heart in general circulatory regulation,* Handbook of Physiology, Vol. I, Sec. 2, pages 532-550, American Physiological Society, Washington, D. C., 1962. — 1–4

SARNA, R. N.: *Unusually tall and narrow U waves simulating hyperkalemic T waves. Report of 2 cases of hypochloremic alkalosis with hypokalemia,* Amer. Heart J., 70:397, 1965. — 31

SCHER, A. M.: *The sequence of ventricular excitation,* Amer. J. Cardiol., 14:287, 1964. — 14, 15

SCHIFF, M.: *Ueber direckte Reizung der Herzoberfiache,* Pflügers Arch. ges Physiol., 28:200, 1882. — 56–58

SEARS, G. A., AND MANNING: *Routine electrocardiography: Postprandial T-wave changes,* Amer. Heart J., 56:591, 1958. — 32

SETA, K., KLEIGER, HELLERSTEIN, LOWN AND VITALE: *Effect of potassium and magnesium deficiency on the electrocardiogram and plasma electrolytes of pure-bred beagles,* Amer. J. Cardiol., 17:516, 1966. — 31

SIMONSON, E.: *The concept and definition of normality,* Ann. N. Y. Acad. Sci., 134:541, 1966. — 12

—, TUNA, OKAMOTO AND TOSHIMA: *Diagnostic accuracy of the vectorcardiogram and electrocardiogram. A cooperative study,* Amer. J. Cardiol., 17:829, 1966. — 18, 19

SLEEPER, J. C., AND ORGAIN: *Differentiation of benign from pathologic T-waves in the electrocardiogram,* Amer. J. Cardiol., 11:338, 1963. — 32

SORENSEN, N. S.: *Creatine phosphokinase in the diagnosis of myocardial infarction,* Acta med. scand., 174:725, 1963. — 53, 54

Section II (continued)

PLATE NUMBER

TRAUTWEIN, W.: *Generation and conduction of impulses in the heart as affected by drugs,* Pharmacol. Rev., 15:277, 1963. — 62–66

VAN DAM, R. T., AND DURRER: *The T wave and ventricular repolarization,* Amer. J. Cardiol., 14:294, 1964. — 14, 15

WASSERBURGER, R. H., AND CORLISS: *Value of oral potassium salts in differentiation of functional and organic T-wave changes,* Amer. J. Cardiol., 10:673, 1962. — 32

—, AND LORENZ: *The effect of hyperventilation and Pro-Banthine on isolated RS-T segment and T-wave abnormalities,* Amer. Heart J., 51:666, 1956. — 32

WEBER, D. M., AND PHILLIPS, JR.: *A reevaluation of electrocardiographic changes accompanying acute pulmonary embolism,* Amer. J. med. Sci., 251:381, 1966. — 20

WEIDMANN, S.: *Elektrophysiologie der Herzmuskelfaser,* Huber, Bern, 1956. — 10, 11

WERKO, L.: *The dynamics and consequences of stenosis on insufficiency of the cardiac valves,* in *Handbook of Physiology,* Section 2, ed. by Hamilton, Vol. 1 (pages 645-680), Amer. Physiol. Soc., Bethesda, 1962. — 8

WHITE, P. D.: *Heart Disease,* 4th ed., The Macmillan Company, New York, 1959. — 42, 43, 46, 47, 49

WOOD, P. H.: *Diseases of the Heart and Circulation,* 2nd ed., J. B. Lippincott Company, Philadelphia, 1956. — 36, 43, 46–52

ZESAS, D. G.: *Ueber Massage des freigelegten Herzens beim Chloroformkollops,* Abl. Chir., 30:588, 1903. — 56–58

ZIMMERMAN, H. A.: *Intravascular Catheterization,* 2nd ed., Charles C Thomas, Springfield, Ill., 1966. — 48–52

—, SCOTT AND BECKER: *Catheterization of the left side of the heart in man,* Circulation, 1:357, 1950. — 5

ZOLL, P. M., FRANK, LARSKY, LINENTHAL AND BELGARD: *Long-term electric stimulation of the heart for Stokes-Adams disease,* Ann. Surg., 154:330, 1961. — 33, 34

—, LINENTHAL, GIBSON, PAUL AND NORMAN: *Termination of ventricular fibrillation in man by externally applied electric countershock,* New Engl. J. Med., 254:727, 1956. — 56–58

Section III

General References

BARRY, A.: *The aortic arch derivatives in the human adult,* Anat. Rec., 111:221, 1951.

BREMER, J. L.: *An interpretation of the development of the heart: the left aorta of reptiles,* Amer. J. Anat., 42:307, 1928.

CONGDON, E. D.: *Transformation of the aortic arch system during development of the human embryo,* Contr. Embryol. Carneg. Instn., 14:47, 1922.

DEVRIES, P. A., AND SAUNDERS: *Development of the ventricles and spiral outflow tract in the human heart,* Contr. Embryol. Carneg. Instn., 37:87, 1962.

GRÜNWALD, P.: *Die Entwicklung der Vena cava caudalis,* Z. mikr.-anat. Forsch., 43:275, 1938.

HAMILTON, W. J., BOYD AND MOSSMAN: *Human Embryology,* 3rd ed., Williams & Wilkins Company, Baltimore, 1963.

Section III (continued)

MALL, F. P.: *On the development of the human heart,* Amer. J. Anat., 13:249, 1912.

McCLURE, C. F. W., AND BUTLER: *The development of the vena cava inferior in man,* Amer. J. Anat., 35:331, 1925.

ODGERS, P. N. B.: *The development of the pars membranacea septi in the human heart,* J. Anat. (Lond.), 72:247, 1938.

——: *The formation of the venous valves, the foramen secundum and the septum secundum in the human heart,* J. Anat. (Lond.), 69:412, 1935.

PATTEN, B. M.: *Human Embryology,* 2nd ed., Blakiston Company, New York, 1953.

STREETER, G. L.: *Developmental horizons in human embryos. Description of age group XI, 13 to 20 somites, and age group XII, 21 to 29 somites,* Contr. Embryol. Carneg. Instn., 30:211, 1942.

——: *Developmental horizons in human embryos. Description of age group XIII, embryos about 4 or 5 millimeters long, and age group XIV, period of indentation of the lens vesicle,* Contr. Embryol. Carneg. Instn., 31:27, 1945.

——: *Developmental horizons in human embryos. Description of age groups XV, XVI, XVII, and XVIII, being the third issue of a survey of the Carnegie Collection,* Contr. Embryol. Carneg. Instn., 32:133, 1948.

TANDLER, J.: *Anatomie des Herzens,* in *Bardeleben's Handbuch der Anatomie des Menschen,* Gustav Fisher, Jena, 1913.

WATERSTON, D.: *The development of the heart in man,* Trans. roy. Soc. Edinb., 52 (II):257, 1908.

PLATE NUMBER

AÜER, J.: *The development of the human pulmonary vein and its major variations,* Anat. Rec., 101:581, 1948. — 12

BARRY, A.: *The functional significance of the cardiac jelly in the tubular heart of the chick embryo,* Anat. Rec., 102:289, 1948. — 4

CORNER, G. W.: *A well-preserved human embryo of 10 somites,* Contr. Embryol. Carneg. Instn., 20:81, 1929. — 5

DAVIS, C. L.: *Description of a human embryo having 20 paired somites,* Contr. Embryol. Carneg. Instn., 15:1, 1923. — 6

——: *Development of the human heart from its first appearance to the stage found in embryos of twenty paired somites,* Contr. Embryol. Carneg. Instn., 19:245, 1927. — 2, 4, 5

——: *The cardiac jelly of the chick embryo,* Anat. Rec., 27:201, 1924. — 4

GARDNER, E., GRAY AND O'RAHILLY: *Anatomy,* 2nd ed., page 403, W. B. Saunders Company, Philadelphia, 1963. — 15

GOSS, C. M.: *Development of the median coordinated ventricle from the lateral hearts in rat embryos with three to six somites,* Anat. Rec., 112:761, 1952. — 3

HERTIG, A. T., AND ROCK: *Two human ova of the pre-villous stage, having a developmental age of about seven and nine days, respectively,* Contr. Embryol. Carneg. Instn., 31:65, 1945. — 1

——, AND ——: *Two human ova of the pre-villous stage, having an ovulation age of about eleven and twelve days, respectively,* Contr. Embryol. Carneg. Instn., 29:127, 1941. — 1

HEUSER, C. H.: *A human embryo with 14*

Section III (continued)

PLATE NUMBER

pairs of somites, Contr. Embryol. Carneg. Instn., 22:135, 1930. — 5

KRAMER, T. C.: *The partitioning of the truncus and conus and the formation of the membranous portion of the interventricular septum in the human heart,* Amer. J. Anat., 71:343, 1942. — 9

LOS, J. A.: *The development of the human pulmonary veins and the coronary sinus in the human embryo,* Thesis, University of Leyden, 1958. — 12

PAYNE, F.: *General description of a 7 somite human embryo,* Contr. Embryol. Carneg. Instn., 16:117, 1924. — 4

VAN MIEROP, L. H. S., ALLEY, KAUSEL AND STRANAHAN: *Pathogenesis of transposition complexes. I. Embryology of the ventricles and great arteries,* Amer. J. Cardiol., 12:216, 1963. — 7–10, 13

——, ——, —— AND ——: *The anatomy and embryology of endocardial cushion defects,* J. Thorac. Cardiovasc. Surg., 43:71, 1962. — 7

Section IV

General References

EDWARDS, J. E., CAREY, NEUFELD AND LESTER: *Congenital Heart Disease,* Vols. I and II, W. B. Saunders Company, Philadelphia, 1965.

GASUL, B. M., ARCILLA AND LEV: *Heart Disease in Children,* J. B. Lippincott Co., Philadelphia, 1966.

KJELLBERG, S. R., MANNHEIMER, RUDHE AND JOHNSON: *Diagnosis of Congenital Heart Disease,* 2nd ed., Year Book Medical Publishers, Inc., Chicago, 1958.

NADAS, A. S.: *Pediatric Cardiology,* 2nd ed., page 453, W. B. Saunders Company, Philadelphia, 1963.

SHERMAN, F. E.: *An Atlas of Congenital Heart Disease,* Lea & Febiger, Philadelphia, 1963.

TAUSSIG, H. B.: *Congenital Malformations of the Heart,* page 354, The Commonwealth Fund, New York, 1947.

BEUREN, A. J.: *Differential diagnosis of the Taussig-Bing heart from complete transposition of the great vessels with a posteriorly overriding pulmonary artery,* Circulation, 21:1071, 1960. — 19

——, SCHULZE, EBERLE, HARMJANZ AND APITZ: *The syndrome of supravalvular aortic stenosis, peripheral pulmonary stenosis, mental retardation and similar facial appearance,* Amer. J. Cardiol., 13:471, 1964. — 22

BLALOCK, A., AND TAUSSIG: *The surgical treatment of malformations of the heart in which there is pulmonary stenosis or pulmonary atresia,* J. Amer. med. Ass., 128:189, 1945. — 18

BLAND, E. F., WHITE AND GARLAND: *Congenital anomalies of the coronary arteries: report of an unusual case associated with cardiac hypertrophy,* Amer. Heart J., 8:787, 1932-33. — 27

BRAUNWALD, E., GOLDBLATT, AYGEN, ROCKOFF AND MORROW: *Congenital aortic stenosis. I. Clinical and hemodynamic findings in 100 patients,* Circulation, 27:426, 1963. — 21, 22

Section IV (continued)

PLATE NUMBER

COLLETT, R. W., AND EDWARDS: *Persistent truncus arteriosus: a classification according to anatomic types,* Surg. Clin. N. Amer., 29:1245, 1949. — 26

DE LA CRUZ, M. V., ANSELMI, CISNEROS, REINHOLD, PORTILLO AND ESPINO-VELA: *An embryologic explanation for the corrected transposition of the great vessels: additional description of the main anatomic features of this malformation and its varieties,* Amer. Heart J., 57:104, 1959. — 25

DE VRIES, P. A., AND SAUNDERS: *Development of the ventricles and spiral outflow tract in the human heart. A contribution to the development of the human heart from age group IX to age group XV,* Contr. Embryol. Carneg. Instn., 37:87, 1962. — 25

EBSTEIN, W.: *Ueber einen sehr seltenen Fall von Insufficienz der Valvula tricuspidalis, bedingt durch eine tangeborene hochgradige Missbildung derselben,* Arch. Anat. Physiol. Wissensch. Med., 238, 1866. — 11

EDWARDS, J. E.: *The congenital bicuspid aortic valve* (Editorial), Circulation, 23:485, 1961. — 21

——: *The direction of blood flow in coronary arteries arising from the pulmonary trunk* (Editorial), Circulation, 29:163, 1964. — 3

EISENMENGER, V.: *Ursprung der Aorta aus Seichen Ventrikeln beim defecte des Septum Ventriculorum,* Wien. klin. Wschr., 11:25, 1898. — 19

FALLOT, A.: *Contribution a l'anatomie pathologique de la maladie bleue (cyanose cardiaque),* Marseille-méd., 25:77, 138, 207, 270, 341, 403, 1888. — 16

GARCIA, R. E., FRIEDMAN, KABACK AND ROWE: *Idiopathic hypercalcemia and supravalvular aortic stenosis. Documentation of a new syndrome,* New Engl. J. Med., 271:117, 1964. — 22

GARDNER, D. L., AND COLE: *Long survival with inferior vena cava draining into left atrium,* Brit. Heart J., 17:93, 1955. — 1

GLENN, W. W. L.: *Circulatory bypass of the right side of the heart. IV. Shunt between superior vena cava and distal right pulmonary artery — report of clinical application,* New Engl. J. Med., 259:117, 1958. — 10

GRANT, R. P.: *The embryology of the ventricular flow pathways in man,* Circulation, 25:756, 1962. — 23

——: *The morphogenesis of corrected transposition and other anomalies of cardiac polarity,* Circulation, 29:71, 1964. — 25

——: *The morphogenesis of transposition of the great vessels,* Circulation, 26:819, 1962. — 23

HANLON, C. R., AND BLALOCK: *Complete transposition of the aorta and the pulmonary artery. Experimental observations on venous shunts as corrective procedures,* Ann. Surg., 127:385, 1948. — 23

HARRIS, J. S., AND FARBER: *Transposition of the great cardiac vessels, with special reference to the phylogenetic theory of Spitzer,* Arch. Path., 28:427, 1939. — 23

IVEMARK, B. I.: *Implications of agenesis of the spleen on the pathogenesis of conotruncus anomalies in childhood. Analysis of heart malformations in splenic agenesis syndrome,* Acta paediat. (Uppsala), 44: (suppl. 104)1, 1955.   4

LEV, M., AND ROWLATT: *The pathologic anatomy of mixed levocardia. A review of thirteen cases of atrial or ventricular inversion with or without corrected transposition,* Amer. J. Cardiol., 8:216, 1961.   23, 25

NEUFELD, H. N., LUCAS, LESTER, ADAMS, ANDERSON AND EDWARDS: *Origin of both great vessels from the right ventricle without pulmonary stenosis,* Brit. Heart J., 24: 393, 1962.   19

PERNKOPF, E., AND WIRTINGER: *Das Wesen der Transposition im Gebiete des Herzens, ein Versuch der Erklärung auf entwicklungsgeschichtlicher Grundlage,* Virchows Arch. path. Anat., 295:143, 1935.   23

POMPE, J. D.: *Over idiopatische hypertrophie van het hart,* Ned. T. Geneesk., 76:304, 1932.   32

ROGER, H.: *Recherches cliniques sur la communication congénitale des deux coeurs, par inocclusion du septum interventriculaire,* Bull. Acad. Méd. (Paris), 8:1189, 1879.   13

SCHIEBLER, G. L., ADAMS, JR., ANDERSON, AMPLATZ AND LESTER: *Clinical study of twenty-three cases of Ebstein's anomaly of the tricuspid valve,* Circulation, 19:165, 1959.   11

——, EDWARDS, BURCHELL, DuSHANE, ONGLEY AND WOOD: *Congenital corrected transposition of the great vessels: a study of 33 cases,* Pediatrics, 27:(suppl.)851, 1961.   25

SHAHER, R. M.: *Complete and inverted transposition of the great vessels,* Brit. Heart J., 26:51, 1964.   23, 25

——, DUCKWORTH, KHOURY AND MOES: *The significance of the atrial situs in the diagnosis of positional anomalies of the heart,* Amer. Heart J., 73:32, 1967.   25

STEWART, J. R., KINCAID AND EDWARDS: *An Atlas of Vascular Rings and Related Malformations of the Aortic Arch System,* page 171, Charles C Thomas, Springfield, Ill., 1964.   29, 30

VAN MIEROP, L. H. S., ALLEY, KAUSEL AND STRANAHAN: *Ebstein's malformation of the left atrioventricular valve in corrected transposition, with subpulmonary stenosis and ventricular septal defect,* Amer. J. Cardiol., 8:270, 1961.   11, 25

——, ——, —— AND ——: *Pathogenesis of transposition complexes. I. Embryology of the ventricles and great arteries,* Amer. J. Cardiol., 12:216, 1963.   23, 25

——, PATTERSON AND REYNOLDS: *Two cases of congenital asplenia with isomerism of the cardiac atria and the sinoatrial nodes,* Amer. J. Cardiol., 13:407, 1964.   4

——, AND WIGLESWORTH: *Pathogenesis of transposition complexes. II. Anomalies due to faulty transfer of the posterior great artery,* Amer. J. Cardiol., 12:226, 1963.   16, 19

——, AND ——: *Pathogenesis of transposition complexes. III. True transposition of the great vessels,* Amer. J. Cardiol., 12:233, 1963.   23, 25

VAN PRAAGH, R., AND VAN PRAAGH: *Isolated ventricular inversion. A consideration of the morphogenesis, definition and diagno-*

---

sis of nontransposed and transposed great arteries, Amer. J. Cardiol., 17:395, 1966.   15, 25

——, AND ——: *The anatomy of common aorticopulmonary trunk (truncus arteriosus communis) and its embryological implications, A study of 51 necropsy cases,* Amer. J. Cardiol., 16:406, 1965.   26

——, ——, VLAD AND KEITH: *Diagnosis of the anatomic types of single or common ventricle,* Amer. J. Cardiol., 15:345, 1965.   15

Section V

AKBERIAN, M., YANKOPOULOS AND ABELMAN: *Hemodynamic studies in beriberi heart disease,* Amer. J. Med., 41:197, 1966.   45

ALEXANDER, C. S.: *Idiopathic heart disease. I. Analysis of 100 cases, with special reference to chronic alcoholism,* Amer. J. Med., 41:213, 1966.   46

ALLEN, A. C.: *Mechanism of localization of vegetations of bacterial endocarditis,* Arch. Path., 27:399, 1939.   17

——, AND SIROTA: *The morphogenesis and significance of degenerative verrucal endocardiosis (terminal endocarditis, endocarditis simplex, nonbacterial thrombotic endocarditis),* Amer. J. Path., 20:1025, 1944.   23

AMERICAN HEART ASSOCIATION, Proceedings of the Annual Meeting Council for High Blood Pressure Research, New York, 1952-1967.   58

ANGELL, W. W., AND SHUMWAY: *Resuscitative storage of the cadaver heart transplant,* Surg. Forum, 17:224, 1966.   94–97

——, DONG, JR., AND SHUMWAY: *A humoral substitute for nervous control in the dog heart transplant,* Surg. Forum, 18:223, 1967.   94–97

AVECILLA, M. J., AND NACLERIO: *Cardiac wounds treated by pericardiotomy and cardiorrhaphy. Report of seven recent cases with 100 per cent survival,* Harlem Hospital Bull., 9:1, 1956.   84–88

BAILEY, C. P., GLOVER AND O'NEILL: *The surgery of mitral stenosis,* J. thorac. Surg., 19:16, 1950.   26–31

BAIN, R. C., EDWARDS, SCHEIFLEY AND GERACI: *Right-sided bacterial endocarditis and endarteritis,* Amer. J. Med., 24:98, 1958.   16, 19

BALL, J. D., WILLIAMS AND DAVIES: *Endomyocardial fibrosis,* Lancet, 1:1049, 1954.   42

BARBER, H.: *Contusion of the myocardium,* Brit. med. J., 2:520, 1940.   89, 90

——, AND OSBORN: *A fatal case of myocardial contusion,* Brit. Heart J., 3:127, 1941.   89, 90

BARGMANN, W.: *Histologie und Mikroskopische Anatomie des Menschen,* 2nd ed., Georg Thieme Verlag, Stuttgart, 1956.   47, 48

BARRETT, N. R.: *The anatomy and the pathology of multiple hydatid cysts in the thorax,* Ann. roy. Coll. Surg. Eng., 26:362, 1960.   81

BEALL, A. C., JR., OCHSNER, MORRIS, COOLEY AND DeBAKEY: *Penetrating wounds of the heart,* J. Trauma, 1:195, 1961.   84–88

BECK, C. W.: *Contusions of the heart,* J. Amer. med. Ass., 104:109, 1935.   89, 90

BECKER, B. J. P.: *Idiopathic mural endocardial disease in South Africa,* Med. Proc. (Cape Town), 9:121-128; 147-158, 1963.   44

——, CHATGIDAKIS AND VAN LINGEN: *Cardiovascular collagenosis with parietal endocardial thrombosis. A clinicopathologic study of forty cases,* Circulation, 7:345, 1953.   44

BENEDETTI-VALENTINI, F., JR., EFFLER, GROVES AND SUAREZ: *La rivascolarizzazione del miocardio mediante impianto dell'arteria mammaria interna,* Estratto da Rassegna di Fisiopatologia Clinica E Terapeutica, 38:304, 1966.   69–75

BIERMAN, H. R., PERKINS AND ORTEGA: *Pericarditis in patients with leukemia,* Amer. Heart J., 43:413, 1952.   91–93

BLALOCK, A., AND RAVITCH: *A consideration of the non-operative treatment of cardiac tamponade resulting from wounds of the heart,* Surgery, 14:157, 1943.   84–88

BLAND, E. F., AND JONES: *Rheumatic fever and rheumatic heart disease. A twenty year report on 1000 patients followed since childhood,* Circulation, 4:836, 1951.   4–6, 11–14

BLEGEN, S. D.: *Post-partum congestive heart failure. Beri-beri heart disease,* Acta med. scand., 178:515, 1965.   45

BLUMENTHAL, H. T., EDITOR: *Cowdry's Arteriosclerosis,* 2nd ed., Charles C Thomas, Springfield, Ill., 1967.   51

BLUMGART, H. L., SCHLESINGER AND DAVIS: *Studies on the relation of the clinical manifestations of angina pectoris, coronary thrombosis, and myocardial infarction to the pathologic findings, with particular reference to the significance of the collateral circulation,* Amer. Heart J., 19:1, 1940.   52–56

——, —— AND ZOLL: *Angina pectoris, coronary failure and acute myocardial infarction. The role of coronary occlusions and collateral circulation,* J. Amer. med. Ass., 116:91, 1941.   52–56

BOAS, E. P.: *Angina pectoris and cardiac infarction from trauma or unusual effort, with consideration of certain medicolegal aspects,* J. Amer. med. Ass., 112:1887, 1939.   89, 90

BOCK, K. D., AND COTTIER: *Essential Hypertension,* Springer-Verlag, Berlin, 1960.   58

BOGEDAIN, W., CARPATHIOS, SUU AND MOOTS: *Traumatic rupture of myocardium. Successful surgical repair,* J. Amer. med. Ass., 197:1102, 1966.   89, 90

BOLANDE, R. P.: *The nature of the connective tissue abiotrophy in the Marfan syndrome,* Lab. Invest., 12:1087, 1963.   24

——, AND TUCKER: *Pulmonary emphysema and other cardiorespiratory lesions as part of the Marfan abiotrophy,* Pediatrics, 33: 356, 1964.   24

BONNABEAU, R. C., JR., STEVENSON AND EDWARDS: *Obliteration of the principal orifice of the stenotic mitral valve: A rare form of "restenosis,"* J. thorac. cardiovasc. Surg., 49:264, 1965.   6

BORDLEY, J., AND EICHNA: *A photographic study of the evolution of the retinal lesions in cases of arterial hypertension,* Trans. Ass. Amer. Phycns., 55:270, 1940.   60

Section V (continued)

BRIGDEN, W.: *Cardiac Amyloidosis*, Progr. cardiovasc. Dis., 7:142, 1964. — 37

——: *Uncommon myocardial diseases. The non-coronary cardiomyopathies*, Lancet, 2:1179, 1957. — 46

BRIGHT, E. F., AND BECK: *Nonpenetrating wounds of the heart. A clinical and experimental study*, Amer. Heart J., 10:293, 1935. — 89, 90

BRINK, A. J., AND WEBER: *Fibroplastic parietal endocarditis with eosinophilia. Löffler's Endocarditis*, Amer. J. Med., 34:52, 1963. — 43

BUCCINO, R. A., SPANN, POOL, SONNENBLICK AND BRAUNWALD: *Influence of the thyroid state on the intrinsic contractile properties and energy stores of the myocardium*, J. clin. Invest., 46:1669, 1967. — 76, 77

BUCK, R. C.: *Atherosclerosis and its Origin*, pages 1-37, Academic Press, Inc., New York, 1963. — 47

BURCH, G. E., AND PHILIPS: *Methods in the diagnostic differentiation of myocardial dilatation from pericardial effusion*, Amer. Heart J., 64:266, 1962. — 91-93

——, AND DE PASQUALE: *Viral myocarditis*, in *Cardiomyopathies*, J. & A. Churchill Ltd., London, 1964. — 39

BURCHELL, H. B., AND EDWARDS: *Rheumatic mitral insufficiency*, Circulation, 7:747, 1953. — 11

CAMPBELL, M., AND SHACKLE, J. W.: *A note on aortic valvular disease, with reference to etiology and prognosis*, Brit. med. J., 1:328, 1932. — 25

CANABAL, E. J., AND DIGHIERO: *Echinococcus disease of the heart; page 8 in Cardiology*, Vol. 3, ed. by Luisada, A. A., McGraw-Hill Book Company, New York, 1959. — 81

COBURN, A. F.: *The Factor of Infection in the Rheumatic State*, Williams & Wilkins Company, Baltimore, 1931. — 1

COCKSHOTT, W. P.: *Angiocardiography of endomyocardial fibrosis*, Brit. J. Radiol., 38:192, 1965. — 42

COOPER, F. W., JR., STEAD AND WARREN: *Beneficial effect of intravenous infusions in acute pericardial tamponade*, Ann. Surg., 120:822, 1944. — 84-88

CORT, J. H., FENCL, HEJL AND JIRKA, EDITORS: *Symposium on the Pathogenesis of Essential Hypertension*, State Medical Publishing House, Prague, 1961. — 58

COURNAND, A.: *Some aspects of the pulmonary circulation in normal man and in chronic cardiopulmonary diseases*, Circulation, 2:641, 1950. — 52-56

D'AUNOY, R., AND VON HAAM: *Aneurysm of the pulmonary artery with patent ductus arteriosus (Botallo's duct); report of two cases and review of the literature*, J. Path. Bact., 38:39, 1934. — 19

DAVIES, A. J., AND GERY: *The role of autoantibodies in heart disease*, Amer. Heart J., 60:669, 1960. — 91-93

DAVIES, J. N. P.: *Some considerations regarding obscure diseases affecting the mural endocardium*, Amer. Heart J., 59:600, 1960. — 43

Section V (continued)

——, AND BALL: *The pathology of endomyocardial fibrosis in Uganda*, Brit. Heart J., 17:337, 1955. — 42

——, AND HOLLMAN: *Becker type cardiomyopathy in a West Indian woman*, Amer. Heart J., 70:225, 1965. — 44

DAWBER, T. R., MOORE AND MANN: *Coronary heart disease in the Framingham study*, Amer. J. publ. Hlth., 47:4, 1957. — 52-56

DEMUTH, W. E., JR., BAUE AND ODOM: *Contusions of the heart*, J. Trauma, 7:443, 1967. — 89, 90

DESFORGES, G., RIDDER AND LENOCI: *Successful suture of ruptured myocardium after nonpenetrating injury*, New Engl. J. Med., 252:567, 1955. — 89, 90

DEW, H. R.: *Hydatid Disease*, The Australasian Medical Publishing Co., Sydney, 1928. — 81

DEXTER, L., DOCK, McGUIRE, HYLAND AND HAYNES: *Pulmonary embolism*, Med. Clin. N. Amer., 44:1251, 1960. — 52-56

DICKINSON, C. J.: *Neurogenic Hypertension*, Blackwell, Oxford, 1965. — 58

DIETRICH, A.: *Heart muscle damage by indirect trauma in warfare*, Virchows Arch. path. Anat., 237:393, 1922. — 89, 90

DOERR, W.: *Myokarditis*, verh. dtsch. Ges. Path., 51, 1967. — 39

DOGLIOTTI, G.: *Traumatismes du coeur et des gros vaisseaux*, Lyon chir., 60:74, 1960. — 89, 90

DONG, E., JR., FOWKES, HURLEY, HANCOCK AND PILLSBURY: *Hemodynamic effects of cardiac autotransplantation*, Circulation (Supp.), 29:77, 1964. — 94-97

——, HURLEY, LOWER AND SHUMWAY: *Performance of the heart two years after autotransplantation*, Surgery, 56:270, 1964. — 94-97

——, AND LOWER: *Transplantation of the heart*, in Norman, J. C., *Fundamentals of Cardiac Surgery*, Appleton-Century-Crofts, New York, 1967. — 94-97

——, ——, HURLEY AND SHUMWAY: *Transplantation of the heart*, Dis. Chest, 48:455, 1965. — 94-97

——, —— AND SHUMWAY: *Electrocardiographic observations after cardiac transplantation*, Clin. Res., 13:205, 1965 (abstr.). — 94-97

——, TSUJI, HANSEN AND SHUMWAY: *Rate control and the artificial heart*, Surg. Forum, 18:199, 1967. — 94-97

DOXIADES, T.: *Diagnostic procedures of chronic amoebiasis*, J. Amer. med. Ass., 187:719, 1964. — 80

DRESDALE, D. T.: *Primary pulmonary hypertension*, page 47 in *Cardiology*, Vol. 4, *Clinical Cardiology — Therapy*, ed. by Luisada, A. A., McGraw-Hill Book Company, New York, 1959. — 52-56

DRESSLER, W.: *The post-myocardial-infarction syndrome*, Arch. intern. Med., 103:28, 1959. — 91-93

DUBOST, C., SALVESTRINI, DUBERNET, LUCCHINI, SAAVEDRA, WILSON AND CACHERA: *Communication inter-ventriculaire traumatique. Fermeture chirurgicale sous circulation extra-corporelle*, Ann. Chir. Thorac. Cardiov., 4:448, 1965. — 89, 90

Section V (continued)

DULFANO, M. J., AND SEGAL: *Pulmonary heart disease. Clinical-physiologic variants*, Dis. Chest, 49:15, 1966. — 52-56

EDWARDS, J. E.: *Calcific aortic stenosis: Pathologic features*, Proc. Mayo Clin., 36:444, 1961. — 12

——: *Differential diagnosis of mitral stenosis. A clinicopathologic review of simulating conditions*, Lab. Invest., 3:89, 1954. — 6, 11

——: Editorial. *On the etiology of calcific aortic stenosis*, Circulation, 26:817, 1962. — 12

——: Editorial. *The congenital bicuspid aortic valve*, Circulation, 23:485, 1961. — 12

——: *Pathologic aspects of cardiac valvular insufficiencies*, Arch. Surg., 77:634, 1958. — 11, 13, 18, 20

EFFLER, D. B.: *Surgery for coronary artery disease*, Geriatrics, 22:129, 1967. — 69-75

——, GROVES AND FAVALORO: *Surgical repair of ventricular aneurysm*, Dis. Chest, 48:37, 1965. — 69-75

——, ——, SUAREZ AND FAVALORO: *Direct coronary artery surgery with endarterotomy and patch-graft reconstruction*, J. thorac. cardiovasc. Surg., 53:93, 1967. — 69-75

——, SONES, JR., FAVALORO AND GROVES: *Coronary endarterotomy with patch-graft reconstruction: Clinical experience with 34 cases*, Ann. Surg., 162:590, 1965. — 69-75

ELIOT, R. S., WOODBURN AND EDWARDS: *Conditions of the ascending aorta simulating aortic valvular incompetence*, Amer. J. Cardiol., 14:679, 1964. — 13

ELKIN, D. C.: *Discussion of Bigger, I. A.: Heart wounds. Report of 17 patients operated upon in Medical College of Virginia Hospitals and discussion of treatment and prognosis*, J. thorac. Surg., 8:239, 1939. — 84-88

ENGLE, M. A., AND ITO: *The postpericardiotomy syndrome*, Amer. J. Cardiol., 7:73, 1961. — 91-93

ERNSTENE, A. C.: *Complications and sequelae of acute myocardial infarction*, J. Amer. med. Ass., 150:1069, 1952. — 52-56

——: *Differential diagnosis of the pain of coronary heart disease*, Ann. intern. Med., 46:247, 1957. — 52-56

FAVALORO, R. G., EFFLER, GROVES, SONES, JR. AND FERGUSSON: *Myocardial revascularization by internal mammary artery implant procedures*, J. thorac. cardiovasc. Surg., 54:359, 1967. — 69-75

FAWCETT, D. W.: *The Peripheral Blood Vessels*, pages 17-44, Williams & Wilkins Company, Baltimore, 1963. — 47

FERRER, M. I., AND HARVEY: *Management of cor pulmonale*, N. Y. med. J., 57:2489, 1957. — 52-56

FISHBERG, A. M., AND OPPENHEIMER: *The differentiation and significance of certain ophthalmoscopic pictures in hypertensive diseases*, Arch. intern. Med., 46:901, 1930. — 60

FOLLIS, R. H., JR.: *Deficiency Disease*, Charles C Thomas, Springfield, Ill., 1958. — 45

FREEDBERG, A. S., BLUMGART, ZOLL AND SCHLESINGER: *Coronary failure: The clinical syndrome of cardiac pain intermediate between angina pectoris and acute myocardial infarction*, J. Amer. med. Ass., 138:107, 1948. — 52-56

273

Section V (continued)

	PLATE NUMBER

FRESEN, O.: *Die gestaltliche Betrachtung des Morbus*, Ergebn. ges. Tuberk.-u. Lung.-Forsch., 14:904, 1958. — 40

FRIEDBERG, C. K.: *Diseases of the Heart*, W. B. Saunders Company, Philadelphia, 1966. — 38, 40, 83

——: Editorial. *Cardiac pain, the electrocardiogram, serum transaminase and the diagnosis of myocardial infarction, subendocardial necrosis or myocardial ischemia*, Progr. cardiovas. Dis., 1:109, 1958. — 52–56

——, AND GROSS: *Pericardial lesions in rheumatic fever*, Amer. J. Path., 12:183, 1936. — 3, 5

FRENCH, J. E.: *Atherosclerosis in relation to the structure and function of the arterial intima with a special reference to the endothelium*, Int. Rev. exp. Path., 5:253, 1966. — 47

FRIEDENWALD, J. S.: *Disease processes versus disease pictures in interpretation of retinal vascular lesions*, Arch. Ophthal., 37:403, 1947. — 60

GEER, J. C.: *Fine structure of human aortic intimal thickening and fatty streaks*, Lab. Invest., 14:1764, 1965. — 48

——, McGILL AND STRONG: *The fine structure of human atherosclerotic lesions*, Amer. J. Path., 38:263, 1961. — 48

GELFMAN, R., AND LEVINE: *The incidence of acute and subacute bacterial endocarditis in congenital heart disease*, Amer. J. med. Sci., 204:324, 1942. — 16

GIFFORD, R. W., JR., McCORMACK AND POUTASSE: *The unilateral atrophic kidney and hypertension (Abstract)*, Amer. J. Cardiol., 15:131, 1965. — 49, 52–56, 61–63

GLYNN, A. A., GLYNN AND HOLBOROW: *Secretion of blood-group substances in rheumatic fever: A genetic requirement for susceptibility?*, Brit. med. J., 2:266, 1959. — 2

GOLDBLATT, H.: *The renal origin of hypertension*, Physiol. Rev., 27:120, 1947. — 52–56

GOULD, S. E.: *Pathology of trichinosis*, Amer. J. clin. Path., 13:627, 1943. — 78

——: *Trichinosis*, Charles C Thomas, Springfield, Ill., 1945. — 78

——, GOMBERG AND BETHELL: *Prevention of trichinosis by gamma irradiation of pork as a public health measure*, Amer. J. publ. Hlth., 43:1550, 1953. — 78

——, ——, ——, VILLELLA AND HERTZ: *Studies on Trichinella spiralis*, Amer. J. Path., 31:933, 1955. — 78

GRAETTINGER, J. S., MUENSTER, CHECCHIA, GRISSOM AND CAMPBELL: *A correlation of clinical and hemodynamic studies in patients with hypothyroidism*, J. clin. Invest., 37:502, 1958. — 76, 77

——, ——, SELVERSTONE AND CAMPBELL: *A correlation of clinical and hemodynamic studies in patients with hyperthyroidism with and without congestive heart failure*, J. clin. Invest., 38:1316, 1959. — 76, 77

GROSS, F., EDITOR: *Antihypertensive Therapy. Principles and Practice*, Springer-Verlag, 1966. — 58

GROSS, L.: *Cardiac lesions in Libman-Sacks disease, with consideration of its relationship to acute diffuse lupus erythematosus*, Amer. J. Path., 16:375, 1940. — 15

——, AND FRIEDBERG: *Lesions of the cardiac*

Section V (continued)

	PLATE NUMBER

valves in rheumatic fever, Amer. J. Path., 12:469; 855, 1936. — 3, 4

GUILFOIL, P. H., AND DOYLE: *Traumatic cardiac septal defect. Report of a case in which diagnosis is established by cardiac catheterization*, J. thorac. Surg., 25:510, 1953. — 89, 90

HALL, E. M.: *The heart*, in *Pathology*, 2nd ed., ed. by Anderson, W. A. D., Kimpton, London, 1953. — 38

HAMOLSKY, M. W., HURLAND AND FREEDBERG: *The heart in hypothyroidism*, in *Hypothyroidism: A Symposium*, ed. by Crispel, Pergamon Press, Ltd., New York, 1963. — 76, 77

HARKEN, D. E., ELLIS AND NORMAN: *The surgical treatment of mitral stenosis: Progress in developing controlled valvuloplastic technique*, J. thorac. Surg., 19:1, 1950. — 26–31

HARRIS, P. D., KOVALIK, MARKS AND MALM: *Factors modifying aortic homograft structure and function*, Surgery, 63:45, 1968. — 35, 36

HARVEY, R. M., FERRER, RICHARDS, JR. AND COURNAND: *Influence of chronic pulmonary disease on the heart and circulation*, Amer. J. Med., 10:719, 1951. — 52–56

HEGGTVEIT, H. A.: *Syphilitic aortitis. A clinicopathologic autopsy study of 100 cases, 1950 to 1960*, Circulation, 29:346, 1964. — 25

HERRICK, J. B.: *Clinical features of sudden obstruction of the coronary arteries*, J. Amer. med. Ass., 59:201, 1912. — 52–56

HOWARD, J. E., BERTHRONG, GOULD AND YENDT: *Hypertension resulting from unilateral renal vascular disease and its relief by nephrectomy*, Bull. Johns Hopk. Hosp., 94:51, 1954. — 49, 52–56, 61–63

HURLEY, E. J., DONG, JR., LOWER, HANCOCK, STOFER AND SHUMWAY: *An approach to extracorporeal surgery of the heart*, J. thor. cardiovasc. Surg., 44:776, 1962. — 94–97

——, ——, STOFER AND SHUMWAY: *Isotopic replacement of the totally excised canine heart*, J. surg. Res., 2:90, 1962. — 94–97

——, LOWER AND SHUMWAY: *Stokes-Adams attacks in transplanted hearts*, Surg. Forum, 16:218, 1965. — 94–97

HÜSSELMANN, H.: *Beitrag zum Amyloidproblem auf Grund von Untersuchungen an menschlichen Herzen*, Virchows Arch. path. Anat., 327:607, 1955. — 37

JAMES, T. N.: *Anatomy of the Coronary Arteries*, Hoeber Medical Books, Harper & Row, Publishers, New York, 1961. — 52–56

——: *Pathology of the cardiac conduction system in amyloidosis*, Ann. intern. Med., 65:28, 1966. — 37

JOACHIM, H., AND MAYS: *Case of cardiac aneurysm probably of traumatic origin*, Amer. Heart J., 2:682, 1927. — 89, 90

JORDAN, R. A., SCHEIFLEY AND EDWARDS: *Mural thrombosis and arterial embolism in mitral stenosis. A clinicopathologic study of fifty-one cases*, Circulation, 3:363, 1951. — 9, 10

KAPLAN, M. H., AND MEYESERIAN: *An immunological cross-reaction between group-A streptococcal cells and human heart tissue*, Lancet, 1:706, 1962. — 1

Section V (continued)

	PLATE NUMBER

KAUFMANN, E.: *Die Kreislauforgane*, in *Lehrbuch der Speziellen Pathologischen Anatomie*, 11th and 12th ed., ed. by Staemmler, Walter de Gruyter & Co., Berlin, 1954. — 38

KAY, J. H., AND EGERTON: *The repair of mitral insufficiency associated with ruptured chordae tendineae*, Ann. Surg., 157:351, 1963. — 89, 90

——, TOLENTINO, ANDERSON, BLOMMER, MEIHAUS AND LEWIS: *Surgical correction of traumatic partial separation of ventricular septum*, Calif. Med., 93:104, 1960. — 89, 90

KEAN, B. H., AND BRESLAU: *Parasites of the Human Heart*, Grune & Stratton, Inc., New York, 1964. — 81

KELLERT, E.: *Report of a case of cardiac injury with uninjured chest wall (indirect force to abdomen and extremities)*, J. Lab. clin. Med., 2:276, 1917. — 89, 90

KLEMPERER, P., POLLACK AND BAEHR: *Pathology of disseminated lupus erythematosus*, Arch. Path., 32:569, 1941. — 15

KÖBERLE, F.: *Enteromegaly and cardiomegaly in Chagas' disease*, Gut, 4:399, 1963. — 79

KULBS, F.: *Experimentelle Untersuchunger über Herz und Trauma*, Mitt. Grenzgeb. Med. Chir., 19:679, 1909. — 89, 90

KUMMEROW, F. A., EDITOR: *Metabolism of Lipids as Related to Atherosclerosis*, Charles C Thomas, Springfield, Ill., 1965. — 51

KUSCHNER, M., FERRER, HARVEY AND WYLIE: *Rheumatic carditis in surgically removed auricular appendages*, Amer. Heart J., 43:286, 1952. — 4

LEONARD, J. J., HARVEY AND HUFNAGEL: *Rupture of the aortic valve. A therapeutic approach*, New Engl. J. Med., 252:208, 1955. — 89, 90

LETTERER, E.: *Allgemeine Pathologie*, Georg Thieme Verlag, Stuttgart, 1959. — 37

LEVY, M. J., AND EDWARDS: *Anatomy of mitral insufficiency*, Progr. cardiovasc. Dis., 5:119, 1962. — 11

——, SIEGAL, WANG AND EDWARDS: *Rupture of aortic valve secondary to aneurysm of ascending aorta*, Circulation, 27:422, 1963. — 24

LIBMAN, E., AND SACKS: *A hitherto undescribed form of valvular and mural endocarditis*, Arch. intern. Med., 33:701, 1924. — 15

LILLEHEI, C. W., GOTT, DeWALL AND VARCO: *The surgical treatment of stenotic or regurgitant lesions of the mitral and aortic valves by direct vision utilizing a pump oxygenator*, J. thorac. Surg., 35:154, 1958. — 26–31

LÖFFLER, W.: *Endocarditis parietalis fibroplastica mit Bluteosinophilie. Ein eigenartiges Krankheitsbild*, Schweiz. med. Wschr., 66:817, 1936. — 43

LOGUE, B., AND TUTUNJI: *The use of steroids in pericarditis*, Amer. Heart J., 64:570, 1962. — 91–93

LOOGEN, F., AND BÖHM: *Isolierte Amyloidose des Herzens*, Z. Kreisl.-Forsch., 43:224, 1954. — 37

LOWER, R. R., DONG, JR., AND GLAZENER: *Electrocardiograms of dogs with heart homografts*, Circulation, 33:455, 1966. — 94–97

SUBJECT INDEX

(Numerals refer to pages, *not* plates. Boldface numerals indicate major emphasis. Meanings of abbreviations may be found in the glossary.)

INFORMATION ON CIBA COLLECTION VOLUMES

Since publication of its first volume, THE CIBA COLLECTION OF MEDICAL ILLUSTRATIONS has enjoyed an almost "unheard-of" reception from members of the medical community. The remarkable illustrations by Frank H. Netter, M.D. and text discussions by select specialists make these books unprecedented in their educational, clinical, and scientific value.

Volume 1   **NERVOUS SYSTEM**
". . . a beautiful bargain . . . and handsome reference work."
Psychological Record

Volume 2   **REPRODUCTIVE SYSTEM**
". . . a desirable addition to any nursing or medical library."
American Journal of Nursing

Volume 3/I   **DIGESTIVE SYSTEM** (**Upper Digestive Tract**)
". . . a fine example of the high quality of this series."
Pediatrics

Volume 3/II   **DIGESTIVE SYSTEM** (**Lower Digestive Tract**)
". . . a unique and beautiful work, worth much more than its cost."
Journal of the South Carolina Medical Association

Volume 3/III   **DIGESTIVE SYSTEM** (**Liver, Biliary Tract and Pancreas**)
". . . a versatile, multipurpose aid to clinicians, teachers, researchers,
and students . . ."   *Florida Medical Journal*

Volume 4   **ENDOCRINE SYSTEM and Selected Metabolic Diseases**
". . . another in the series of superb contributions made by CIBA . . ."
International Journal of Fertility

Volume 5   **HEART**
"The excellence of the volume . . . is clearly deserving of highest praise."
Circulation

Volume 6   **KIDNEYS, URETERS, AND URINARY BLADDER**
". . . a model of clarity of language and visual presentation . . ."
Circulation

In the United States, copies of all CIBA COLLECTION books may be purchased from the Medical Education Division, CIBA Pharmaceutical Company, Division of CIBA-GEIGY Corporation, Summit, New Jersey 07901. In other countries, please direct inquiries to the nearest CIBA-GEIGY office.